CRC Standard Probability and Statistics

Tables and Formulae

Editor

William H. Beyer
Associate Dean
Buchtel College of Arts and Sciences
The University of Akron
Akron, Ohio

CRC Press
Boca Raton Ann Arbor Boston

Library of Congress Cataloging-in-Publication Data

CRC standard probability and statistics tables and formulae / editor,
William H. Beyer.
p. cm.
Includes index.
ISBN 0-8493-0680-9
1. Mathematical statistics--Tables. 2. Probabilities--Tables.
I. Beyer, William H. II. Title: Standard Probability and statistics
tables and formulae.
QA276.25.C72 1990
519.5′0212--dc20 90-20779
CIP

Direct all inquiries to CRC Press, Inc., 2000 Corporate Blvd., N.W., Boca Raton, Florida, 33431.

International Standard Book Number 0-8493-0680-9

Library of Congress Number 90-20779
Printed in the United States

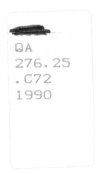

PREFACE

Statistics is a key technology of the present day

The pursuit of knowledge frequently involves data collection; and those responsible for the collection must appreciate the need for analyzing the data to recover and interpret the information contained therein. Today, statistics are being accepted as a universal language for the results of experimentation and research and the dissemination of information.

It has long been the established policy of CRC Press, Inc. to publish in handbook form the most up-to-date, authoritative, logically arranged, and readily usable reference material available. This *Handbook* is primarily a collection of expository material and tables that are useful in the statistical analysis of data and in statistics generally. Special attention has been given to include those tables which are most commonly employed in all phases of present-day academics and research, rather than highly specialized tables that are rarely used. The *Handbook* provides an important "aid" to the teaching profession, to the student, and to the many other users who require the table or fact for investigation or the creation of answers to today's challenging and complex problems.

The same successful format which characterized earlier editions of the *Handbook* and the companion *CRC Standard Mathematical Tables and Formulae* has been retained. Material is presented in a multi-sectional format, with each section containing a valuable collection of fundamental reference material — tabular and/or expository.

In the development of this *Handbook*, the first section is devoted entirely to the fundamental theories of probability and statistics. The primary objective here has been to bring together material widely scattered throughout existing literature. This *Handbook* is not intended to be a textbook; however, the material in this section is included only to serve the main objective of providing a sound and complete reference for statistical terminology and techniques.

Each section contains a valuable collection of statistical and/or mathematical tables. The introductory material devoted to each table was written to present a clear definition of the statistical functions involved and, wherever possible, the relationship between them. To facilitate the use of the tables, this introductory material is presented preceding each table. It was further decided to keep examples to a minimum, giving only the essentials needed for the understanding of the functions tabulated.

The Editor gratefully acknowledges the services rendered by Debbie Stone, Editorial Assistant, and by Paul Gottehrer, Editor, for the handling of the detail work which is so essential in the final production of this *Handbook*.

In line with the established editorial policies of CRC Press, Inc., this *Handbook* will be kept as up-to-date as possible. Revisions and anticipated uses of new material and tables will be introduced as the need arises. Suggestions for the inclusion of new material in subsequent editions and suggestions concerning accuracy of stated information are welcomed.

William H. Beyer

ACKNOWLEDGMENTS

Acknowledgment is made to the following authors, editors, and publishers whose material has been used in the *CRC Standard Probability and Statistics Tables and Formulae*, and for which permission has been received.

AMERICAN SOCIETY FOR TESTING MATERIALS STP-15C
ASTM Manual on Quality Control of Materials (1951)
XI.1—Factors for Computing Control Limits

AMERICAN STATISTICAL ASSOCIATION, JOURNAL OF
Vol. 32 (1937) 349—386, W. E. Ricker
III.4—Confidence Limits for the Expected Value of a Poisson Distribution
Vol. 41 (1946) 557—566, W. J. Dixon and A. M. Mood
X.1—Critical Values for the Sign Test
Vol. 46 (1951) 68—78, F. J. Massey, Jr.
Vol. 47 (1952) 425—441, Z. W. Birnbaum
X.7—Critical Values for the Kolmogorov-Smirnov One-Sample Statistic
Vol. 47 (1952) 583—621, W. H. Kruskal and W. A. Wallis
X.9—Kruskal-Wallis One-Way Analysis of Variance by Ranks

BARGMANN, ROLF E.
Department of Statistics
University of Georgia
Athens, Georgia
Part I. "General Linear Model"

BIOMETRIKA TRUSTEES; E. S. PEARSON AND H. O. HARTLEY
Cambridge University Press
Biometrika
Vol. 40 (1953) 74—86, R. Latscha
III.6—Tests of Significance in 2 × 2 Contingency Tables
Vol. 38 (1951) 112—130, E. S. Pearson and H. O. Hartley
VI.2—Power Functions of the Analysis-of-Variance Tests
Vol. 39 (1952) 422—424, H. A. David
VI.6—Percentage Points of the Maximum F-Ratio
Vol. 48 (1961) 151—165, H. L. Harter
VII.1—Expected Values of Order Statistics from a Standard Normal Population
Vol. 32 (1942) 301—310, E. S. Pearson and H. O. Hartley
VII.6—Simple Estimates in Small Samples
Vol. 34 (1947) 41—67, E. Lord
VIII.5—Substitute t-Ratios

Biometrika Tables for Statisticians

Vol. 1 (1962) 204—205	III.5 —Confidence Limits for Proportions
Vol. 1 (1962) 188—193	III.6 —Tests of Significance in 2 × 2 Contingency Tables
Vol. 1 (1962) 135	IV.3 —Power Function of the t-Test
Vol. 1 (1962) 130—131	V.1 —Percentage Points, Chi-Square Distribution
Vol. 1 (1962) 157—163	VI.1 —Percentage Points, F-Distribution
Vol. 1 (1962) 166—171	VIII.1 —Probability Integral of the Range
Vol. 1 (1962) 165	VIII.2 —Percentage Points, Distribution of the Range

Vol. 1 (1962) 176—177 VIII.3 —Percentage Points, Studentized Range
Vol. 1 (1962) 138 IX.1 —Percentage Points, Distribution of the Correlation Coefficient when $\rho = 0$
Vol. 1 (1962) 140—141 IX.2 —Confidence Limits for the Population Correlation Coefficient
Vol. 1 (1962) 139 IX.3 —The Transformation $z = \tanh^{-1} r$ for the Correlation Coefficient
Vol. 1 (1962) 211 X.11 —Critical Values of Kendall's Rank Correlation Coefficient
Vol. 1 (1962) 165 XI.2 —Percentage Points of the Distribution of the Mean Deviation

BIOMETRICS
Vol. 11 (1955) 1—42, D. B. Duncan
VIII.4 —Critical Values for Duncan's New Multiple Range Test

THE CHEMICAL RUBBER CO.
CRC Standard Mathematical Tables, 28th Edition, W. H. Beyer
II.1—The Normal Probability Function and Related Functions
II.3—Factors for Computing Probable Errors
II.4—Probability of Occurrence of Deviations
II.1—Cumulative Terms, Binomial Distribution (Revised)
III.2—Cumulative Terms, Poisson Distribution (Revised)
XII.3—Random Units
XIII.1—Exponential Functions
XIII.2—Sums of Powers of Integers
XIII.3—Factorials, Exact Values
XIII.4—Gamma Function, Beta Function
XIII.5—Coefficients for Orthogonal Polynomials
XIII.6—Derivatives
XIII.7—Integrals

DAVID, HERBERT A.
Department of Biostatistics
Iowa State University
Ames, Iowa
VIII.7—Analysis of Variance Based on Range

INSTITUTE OF EDUCATIONAL RESEARCH
Indiana University, Bloomington, Indiana
Vol. 1, No. 2 (1953), D. Auble
X.4—Critical Values of U in the Wilcoxon (Mann-Whitney) Two Sample Statistic

LEDERLE LABORATORIES
Some Rapid Approximate Statistical Procedures (1964) 20—28, F. Wilcoxon and R. A. Wilcox
X.2—Critical Values of T in the Wilcoxon Matched-Pairs Signed-Ranks Test
X.5—Critical Values for the Wilcoxon Rank Sum Test

MATHEMATICAL STATISTICS, ANNALS OF
Vol. 17 (1946) 178—197, C. D. Ferris, F. E. Grubbs, and C. L. Weaver
II.5—Operating Characteristic (OC) Curves for a Test on the Mean of a Normal Distribution with Known Standard Deviation
Vol. 31 (1960) 625—642, D. L. Heck
II.6—Charts of Upper 1%, 2.5% and 5% Points of the Distribution of the Largest Characteristic Root

Vol. 17 (1946) 178—197, C. D. Ferris, F. E. Grubbs, and C. L. Weaver
IV.6—Operating Characteristic (OC) Curves for a Test on the Mean of a Normal Distribution with Unknown Standard Deviation
V.4—Operating Characteristic (OC) Curves for a Test on the Standard Deviation of a Normal Distribution
VI.4—Operating Characteristic (OC) Curves for a Test on the Standard Deviations of Two Normal Distributions
Vol. 27 (1956) 427—451, A. E. Sarhan, B. G. Greenberg
VII.2—Variances and Covariances of Order Statistics
Vol. 22 (1951) 68—78, W. J. Dixon
VII.4—Critical Values for Testing Outliers
Vol. 17 (1946) 377—408, F. Mosteller
VII.5—Percentile Estimates in Large Samples
Vol. 31 (1960) 1122—1147, H. L. Harter
VIII.2—Percentage Points, Distribution of the Range
VIII.3—Percentage Points, Studentized Range
Vol. 20 (1949a) 257—267, J. E. Walsh
VIII.5—Substitute t-Ratios
Vol. 21 (1950) 112—116, R. F. Link
VIII.6—Substitute F-Ratio
Vol. 18 (1947) 50—60, H. B. Mann, D. R. Whitney
X.3—Probabilities for the Wilcoxon (Mann-Whitney) Two-Sample Statistic
Vol. 14 (1943) 66—87, C. Eisenhart and F. C. Swed
X.6—Distribution of the Total Number-of-Runs Test
Vol. 23 (1952) 435—441, F. J. Massey, Jr.
X.8—Critical Values for the Kolmogorov-Smirnov Two Sample Statistic
Vol. 9 (1938) 133—148, E. G. Olds and Vol. 20 (1949) 117—118, E.G. Olds
X.10—Critical Values of Spearman's Rank Correlation Coefficient

MCGRAW-HILL BOOK COMPANY
Selected Techniques of Statistical Analysis, C. Eisenhart, M. W. Hastay, W. A. Wallis
(1947) 102—107 II.2—Tolerance Factors for Normal Distributions
(1947) 284—309 V.3—Number of Observations for the Comparison of a Population Variance With a Standard Value Using the Chi-Square Test
VI.3—Number of Observations Required for the Comparison of Two Population Variances Using the F-Test
(1947) 390—391 VI.5—Cochran's Test for the Homogeneity of Variances
Introduction to Statistical Analysis, 2nd Edition, W. J. Dixon, F. J. Massey, Jr.
(1957) 405—407 VII.6—Simple Estimates in Small Samples

OLIVER AND BOYD, LTD., EDINBURGH, SCOTLAND
Design and Analysis of Industrial Experiments, O. L. Davies
Research Vol. 1 (1948) 520—525
(1956) 606—607 IV.4—Number of Observations for t-Test of Mean
(1956) 609—610 IV.5—Number of Observations for t-Test of Difference Between Two Means
(1956) 613—614 V.3—Number of Observations for the Comparison of a Population Variance With a Standard Value Using the Chi-Square Test
Statistical Tables for Biological, Agricultural, and Medical Research, R. A. Fisher, F. Yates
The Literary Executor of the Late Sir Ronald Fisher, F. R. S., Cambridge, Dr. Frank Yates, F. R. S., Rothamstead and Messrs. Oliver and Boyd, Ltd., Edinburgh, Scotland
(1938) 46 IV.1—Percentage Points, Student's t-Distribution
(1938) 98—103 XII.7—Orthogonal Polynomials

Quality Technology, Journal of
Vol. 7, No. 4 (1975) 200—201, L. S. Nelson
IV.2—Nomograph for Student's t-Distribution

THE ROYAL SOCIETY, LONDON, ENGLAND
Royal Society Mathematical Tables
Vol. 3 (1954) 2 XII.2—Number of Combinations

SPRINGER-VERLAG NEW YORK, INC.
Fünfstellige Funktionentafeln (1930), Hayashi, K.
XII.1—Number of Permutations

STANFORD UNIVERSITY PRESS
Tables of the Hypergeometric Probability Distribution, G. J. Lieberman and D. B. Owen
(1961) III.5—Hypergeometric Distribution

STATISTICAL PUBLISHING SOCIETY, CALCUTTA, INDIA
Sankhya
Vol. 4 (1940) 551—558 S. K. Banerjee, K. R. Nair
VII.3—Confidence Intervals for Medians

WRIGHT AIR DEVELOPMENT CENTER, WRIGHT-PATTERSON AFB
WADC Technical Report 58—484, H. L. Harter, D. S. Clemm, and G. H. Guthrie
Vol. II (1959) VIII.4—Critical Values for Duncan's New Multiple Range Test

JOHN WILEY & SONS, INC.
Experimental Designs, W. G. Cochran, G. M. Cox
(1957) Part I—Plans for Design of Experiments
Statistical Tables and Formulas, A. Hald
(1952) 66—69 III.3—Confidence Limits for Proportions
(1952) 44—45 V.2—Percentage Points, Chi-Square Over Degrees of Freedom Distribution
Statistics and Experimental Design, N. L. Johnson, F. C. Leone
Vol. 1 (1964) 412 X.10—Critical Values of Spearman's Rank Correlation Coefficient
Vol. 1 (1964) 320—341 XI.3—Cumulative Sum Control Charts

TABLE OF CONTENTS

I. PROBABILITY AND STATISTICS

DESCRIPTIVE STATISTICS

a) Ungrouped Data

The formulas of this section designated as *a*) apply to a random sample of size n, denoted by x_i, $i = 1, 2, \ldots, n$.

b) Grouped Data

The formulas of this section designated as *b*) apply to data grouped into a frequency distribution having class marks x_i, $i = 1, 2, \ldots, k$, and corresponding class frequencies f_i, $i = 1, 2, \ldots, k$. The total number of observations given by

$$n = \sum_{i=1}^{k} f_i$$

In the formulas that follow, c denotes the width of the class interval, x_o denotes one of the class marks taken to be the computing origin, and $u_i = \dfrac{x_i - x_o}{c}$. Then coded class marks are obtained by replacing the original class marks with the integers $\ldots, -3, -2, -1, 0, 1, 2, 3, \ldots$ where 0 corresponds to class mark x_o in the original scale.

Mean (Arithmetic Mean)

a) $$\bar{x} = \frac{1}{n}\sum_{i=1}^{n} x_i = \frac{x_1 + x_2 + \cdots + x_n}{n}$$

b.1) $$\bar{x} = \frac{1}{n}\sum_{i=1}^{k} f_i x_i = \frac{f_1x_1 + f_2x_2 + \cdots + f_kx_k}{n}$$

If data is coded

b.2) $$\bar{x} = x_o + c\,\frac{\sum_{i=1}^{k} f_i u_i}{n}$$

Weighted Mean (Weighted Arithmetic Mean)

If with each value x_i is associated a weighting factor $w_i \geq 0$, then $\sum_{i=1}^{n} w_i$ is the total weight, and

a) $$\bar{x} = \frac{\sum_{i=1}^{n} w_i x_i}{\sum_{i=1}^{n} w_i} = \frac{w_1x_1 + w_2x_2 + \cdots + w_nx_n}{w_1 + w_2 + \cdots + w_n}$$

Geometric Mean

a) $$\text{G.M.} = \sqrt[n]{x_1 \cdot x_2 \cdots x_n}$$

In logarithmic form

$$\log\,(\text{G.M.}) = \frac{1}{n}\sum_{i=1}^{n} \log x_i = \frac{\log x_1 + \log x_2 + \cdots + \log x_n}{n}$$

b) $\text{G.M.} = \sqrt[n]{x_1^{f_1} \cdot x_2^{f_2} \cdots x_k^{f_k}}$

In logarithmic form

$$\log\,(\text{G.M.}) = \frac{1}{n}\sum_{i=1}^{k} f_i \log x_i = \frac{f_1 \log x_1 + f_2 \log x_2 + \cdots + f_k \log x_k}{n}$$

Harmonic Mean

a) $\text{H.M.} = \dfrac{n}{\sum_{i=1}^{n} \dfrac{1}{x_i}} = \dfrac{n}{\dfrac{1}{x_1} + \dfrac{1}{x_2} + \cdots + \dfrac{1}{x_n}}$

b) $\text{H.M.} = \dfrac{n}{\sum_{i=1}^{k} \dfrac{f_i}{x_i}} = \dfrac{n}{\dfrac{f_1}{x_1} + \dfrac{f_2}{x_2} + \cdots + \dfrac{f_k}{x_k}}$

Relation Between Arithmetic, Geometric, and Harmonic Mean

$\text{H.M.} \le \text{G.M.} \le \bar{x}$, (Equality sign holds only if all sample values are identical.)

Mode

a) A mode M_o of a sample of size n is a value which occurs with greatest frequency, i.e., it is the most common value. A mode may not exist, and even if it does exist it may not be unique.

b) $M_o = L + c\dfrac{\Delta_1}{\Delta_1 + \Delta_2}$,

where L is the lower class boundary of the modal class (class containing the mode),
Δ_1 is the excess of modal frequency over frequency of next lower class,
Δ_2 is the excess of modal frequency over frequency of next higher class.

Median

a) If the sample is arranged in ascending order of magnitude, then the median M_d is given by the $\dfrac{n+1}{2}$ *nd* value. When n is odd, the median is the middle value of the set of ordered data; when n is even, the median is usually taken as the mean of the two middle values of the set of ordered data.

b) $M_d = L + c\dfrac{\dfrac{n}{2} - F_c}{f_m}$,

where L is lower class boundary of median class (class containing the median),
F_c is the sum of the frequencies of all classes lower than the median class,
f_m is the frequency of the median class.

Empirical Relation Between Mean, Median, and Mode

$$\text{Mean} - \text{Mode} = 3\,(\text{Mean} - \text{Median})$$

Quartiles

a) If the data is arranged in ascending order of magnitude, the *j*th quartile Q_j, $j = 1, 2$, or 3, is given by the $\frac{j(n+1)}{4}$th value. It may be necessary to interpolate between successive values.

b) The *j*th quartile Q_j, $j = 1, 2$, or 3, is obtained from formula *b*) for the median by counting $\frac{jn}{4}$ cases starting at the bottom of the distribution.

Deciles

a) If the sample is arranged in ascending order of magnitude, the *j*th decile D_j, $j = 1, 2, \ldots$, or 9, is given by the $\frac{j(n+1)}{10}$th value. It may be necessary to interpolate between successive values.

b) The *j*th decile D_j, $j = 1, 2, \ldots$, or 9, is obtained from formula *b*) for the median by counting $\frac{jn}{10}$ cases starting at the bottom of the distribution.

Percentiles

a) If the sample is arranged in ascending order of magnitude, the *j*th percentile P_j, $j = 1, 2, \ldots$, or 99 is given by the $\frac{j(n+1)}{100}$th value. It may be necessary to interpolate between successive values.

b) The *j*th percentile P_j, $j = 1, 2, \ldots$, or 99, is obtained from formulas *b*) for the median by counting $\frac{jn}{100}$ cases starting at the bottom of the distribution.

Mean Deviation

a) $$\text{M.D.} = \frac{1}{n}\sum_{i=1}^{n} |x_i - \bar{x}|$$

or

$$\text{M.D.} = \frac{1}{n}\sum_{i=1}^{n} |x_i - M_d|$$

where $\bar{x}$ is the mean and M_d is the median of the sample.

b) $$\text{M.D.} = \frac{1}{n}\sum_{i=1}^{k} f_i|x_i - \bar{x}|$$

or

$$\text{M.D.} = \frac{1}{n}\sum_{i=1}^{k} f_i|x_i - M_d|$$

where $\bar{x}$ is the mean and M_d the median of the sample.

Standard Deviation

a) $s = \sqrt{\dfrac{\sum_{i=1}^{n} (x_i - \bar{x})^2}{n-1}}$, where $\bar{x}$ is the mean of the sample.

For computational purposes,

$$s = \sqrt{\frac{\sum_{i=1}^{n} x_i^2 - n\bar{x}^2}{n-1}}$$

$$s = \sqrt{\frac{n \sum_{i=1}^{n} x_i^2 - \left(\sum_{i=1}^{n} x_i\right)^2}{n(n-1)}}$$

b) $s = \sqrt{\dfrac{\sum_{i=1}^{k} f_i(x_i - \bar{x})^2}{n-1}}$, where $\bar{x}$ is the mean of the sample.

For computational purposes

$$s = \sqrt{\frac{\sum_{i=1}^{k} f_i x_i^2 - n\bar{x}^2}{n-1}}$$

$$s = \sqrt{\frac{n \sum_{i=1}^{k} f_i x_i^2 - \left(\sum_{i=1}^{k} f_i x_i\right)^2}{n(n-1)}}$$

If data is coded,

$$s = c\sqrt{\frac{n \sum_{i=1}^{k} f_i u_i^2 - \left(\sum_{i=1}^{k} f_i u_i\right)^2}{n(n-1)}}$$

Variance

The variance is the square of the standard deviation.

Range

The range of a set of values is the difference between the largest and smallest values in the set.

Root Mean Square

a) $\text{R.M.S.} = \left[\frac{1}{n} \sum_{i=1}^{n} x_i^2\right]^{\frac{1}{2}}$

b) $\text{R.M.S.} = \left[\frac{1}{n} \sum_{i=1}^{k} f_i x_i^2\right]^{\frac{1}{2}}$

Interquartile Range

$$Q_3 - Q_1,$$

where Q_1 and Q_3 are the first and third quartiles.

Quartile Deviation (Semi-Interquartile Range)

$$\frac{Q_3 - Q_1}{2},$$

where Q_1 and Q_3 are the first and third quartiles.

Coefficient of Variation

$$V = \frac{100s}{\bar{x}},$$

where $\bar{x}$ is the mean and s the standard deviation of the sample.

Coefficient of Quartile Variation

$$V = 100\,\frac{Q_3 - Q_1}{Q_3 + Q_1},$$

where Q_1 and Q_3 are the first and third quartiles.

Standardized Variable (Standard Scores)

$$z = \frac{x_i - \bar{x}}{s},$$

where $\bar{x}$ is the mean and s the standard deviation of the sample.

Moments

a) The rth moment about the origin is given by

$$m'_r = \frac{1}{n}\sum_{i=1}^{n} x_i^{\,r}$$

The rth moment about the mean $\bar{x}$ is given by

$$m_r = \frac{1}{n}\sum_{i=1}^{n} (x_i - \bar{x})^r$$

If $\sum_{i=1}^{n} (x_i - \bar{x})^r$ is expanded by use of the binomial theorem, moments about the mean may be expressed in terms of moments about the origin.

b) The rth moment about the origin is given by

$$m'_r = \frac{1}{n}\sum_{i=1}^{k} f_i x_i^{\,r}$$

The rth moment about the mean $\bar{x}$ is given by

$$m_r = \frac{1}{n}\sum_{i=1}^{k} f_i (x_i - \bar{x})^r$$

If $\sum_{i=1}^{k} f_i(x_i - \bar{x})^r$ is expanded by use of the binomial theorem, moments about the mean may be expressed in terms of moments about the origin.

If data is coded

$$m_r' = c^r \frac{\sum_{i=1}^{k} f_i u_i^r}{n}$$

Coefficient of Skewness

$$\alpha_3 = \frac{m_3}{(m_2)^{3/2}},$$

where m_2 and m_3 are the second and third moments about the mean of the sample.

Coefficient of Momental Skewness

$$\frac{\alpha_3}{2} = \frac{m_3}{2(m_2)^{3/2}},$$

where m_2 and m_3 are the second and third moments about the mean of the sample.

Pearson's First Coefficient of Skewness

$$S_{k_1} = \frac{3(\bar{x} - M_o)}{s},$$

where $\bar{x}$ is the mean, M_o the mode, and s the standard deviation of the sample.

Pearson's Second Coefficient of Skewness

$$S_{k_2} = \frac{3(\bar{x} - M_d)}{s},$$

where $\bar{x}$ is the mean, M_d the median, and s the standard deviation of the sample.

Quartile Coefficient of Skewness

$$S_{k_Q} = \frac{Q_3 - 2Q_2 + Q_1}{Q_3 - Q_1},$$

where Q_1, Q_2, and Q_3 are the first, second, and third quartiles.

Coefficient of Kurtosis

$$\alpha_4 = \frac{m_4}{(m_2)^2},$$

where m_2 and m_4 are the second and fourth moments about the mean of the sample.

Coefficient of Excess (Kurtosis)

$$\alpha_4 - 3 = \frac{m_4}{(m_2)^2} - 3,$$

where m_2 and m_4 are the second and fourth moments about the mean of the sample.

Sheppards Corrections for Grouping

Let all class intervals be of equal length c. If the distribution of x has a high order of contact with the x-axis at both tails, (i.e., if the distribution of x has tails which are very nearly tangent to the x-axis), one may improve the grouped data approximation to the variance by adding Sheppard's correction $-\frac{c^2}{12}$. Thus

$$\text{corrected variance} = \text{grouped data variance} - \frac{c^2}{12}$$

Analogous corrections for grouped data sample moments

$$m'_r = \frac{1}{n}\sum_{i=1}^{k} f_i x_i^r \quad \text{and} \quad m_r = \frac{1}{n}\sum_{i=1}^{k} f_i(x_i - \bar{x})^r$$

yield improved estimates m'_{r_c} and m_{r_c} given by

$$m'_{1_c} = m'_1 \qquad m_{1_c} = m_1$$

$$m'_{2_c} = m'_2 - \frac{c^2}{12} \qquad m_{2_c} = m_2 - \frac{c^2}{12}$$

$$m'_{3_c} = m'_3 - \frac{c^2}{4}m'_1 \qquad m_{3_c} = m_3$$

$$m'_{4_c} = m'_4 - \frac{c^2}{2}m'_1 + \frac{7c^4}{240} \qquad m_{4_c} = m_4 - \frac{c^2}{2}m_2 + \frac{7c^4}{240}$$

Curve Fitting, Regression, and Correlation

The following formulas apply to a set of n ordered pairs $\{(x_i,y_i)\}$, $i = 1, 2, \ldots, n$. The assumptions of normal regression analysis are that the x's are fixed variables, and the y's are independent random variables having normal distributions with common variance σ^2. The assumptions of normal correlation analysis are that $\{(x_i,y_i)\}$ constitute a random sample from a bivariate normal population.

Curve Fitting

1. Polynomial Function

$$y = b_0 + b_1x + b_2x^2 + \cdots + b_mx^m$$

For a polynomial function fit by the method of least squares, the values of $b_o, b_1, \ldots, b_m$ are obtained by solving the system of $m + 1$ normal equations

$$\begin{aligned} nb_o + b_1\Sigma x_i + b_2\Sigma x_i^2 + \cdots + b_m\Sigma x_i^m &= \Sigma y_i \\ b_o\Sigma x_i + b_1\Sigma x_i^2 + b_2\Sigma x_i^3 + \cdots + b_m\Sigma x_i^{m+1} &= \Sigma x_iy_i \\ \cdots\cdots\cdots\cdots\cdots\cdots\cdots\cdots\cdots\cdots& \\ b_o\Sigma x_i^m + b_1\Sigma x_i^{m+1} + b_2\Sigma x_i^{m+2} + \cdots + b_m\Sigma x_i^{2m} &= \Sigma x_i^my_i \end{aligned}$$

2. Straight Line

$$y = b_0 + b_1x$$

For a straight line fit by the method of least squares, the values b_o and b_1 are obtained by solving the normal equations

$$\begin{aligned} nb_0 + b_1\Sigma x_i &= \Sigma y_i \\ b_0\Sigma x_i + b_1\Sigma x_i^2 &= \Sigma x_iy_i \end{aligned}$$

The solutions of these normal equations are

$$b_1 = \frac{n\Sigma x_iy_i - (\Sigma x_i)(\Sigma y_i)}{n\Sigma x_i^2 - (\Sigma x_i)^2}$$

$$b_0 = \frac{\Sigma y_i}{n} - b_1\frac{\Sigma x_i}{n} = \bar{y} - b_1\bar{x}$$

3. Exponential Curve

$$y = ab^x$$

or

$$\log y = \log a + (\log b)x$$

For an exponential curve fit by the method of least squares, the values $\log a$ and $\log b$ are obtained by fitting a straight line to the set of ordered pairs $\{(x_i, \log y_i)\}$.

4. Power Function

$$y = ax^b$$

or

$$\log y = \log a + b \log x$$

For a power function fit by the method of least squares, the values $\log a$ and b are obtained by fitting a straight line to the set of ordered pairs $\{(\log x_i, \log y_i)\}$.

Regression and Correlation

1. Simple Linear Regression.

For a regression of y on x

$$E(y/x) = b_0 + b_1 x,$$

where $E(y/x)$ is the mean of the distribution of y for a given x.

Standard Error of Estimate

$$s_e = \sqrt{\frac{\Sigma[y_i - (b_0 + b_1 x_i)]^2}{n - 2}},$$

where b_0 and b_1 are given by

$$b_1 = \frac{n\Sigma x_i y_i - (\Sigma x_i)(\Sigma y_i)}{n\Sigma x_i^2 - (\Sigma x_i)^2}$$

$$b_0 = \frac{\Sigma y_i}{n} - b_1 \frac{\Sigma x_i}{n} = \bar{y} - b_1 \bar{x}$$

2. Correlation.

An estimate of the population correlation coefficient ρ is given by

$$r = \frac{\Sigma(x_i - \bar{x})(y_i - \bar{y})}{\sqrt{[\Sigma(x_i - \bar{x})^2][\Sigma(y_i - \bar{y})^2]}}$$

or by the computing formula

$$r = \frac{n\Sigma x_i y_i - (\Sigma x_i)(\Sigma y_i)}{\sqrt{[n\Sigma x_i^2 - (\Sigma x_i)^2][n\Sigma y_i^2 - (\Sigma y_i)^2]}}$$

For grouped data

$$r = \frac{n\Sigma f x_i y_i - (\Sigma f_x x_i)(\Sigma f_y y_i)}{\sqrt{[n\Sigma f_x x_i^2 - (\Sigma f_x x_i)^2][n\Sigma f_y y_i^2 - (\Sigma f_y y_i)^2]}}$$

where f_x and f_y denote the frequencies corresponding to the class marks x and y, and f denotes the frequency of the corresponding cell of the correlation table.

If the data is coded

$$r = \frac{n\Sigma fuv - (\Sigma f_u u)(\Sigma f_v v)}{\sqrt{[n\Sigma f_u u^2 - (\Sigma f_u u)^2][n\Sigma f_v v^2 - (\Sigma f_v v)^2]}}$$

where the u's and v's are coded class marks. The frequencies f_u and f_v are defined analogous to f_x and f_y.

BASIC CONCEPTS FOR ALGEBRA OF SETS

I. *Algebra of Sets*

1. A set is a collection or an aggregate of objects, called "the elements of the set". If a is an element of set A, we write $a \in A$. If not then $a \notin A$.
   If a set contains only the element a, we denote it by $\{a\}$.
2. The *null set,* denoted by ϕ, is the set which has no elements.
3. Two sets A and B are called "equal",* written $A = B$
   if (1) every element of A is an element of B
   and (2) every element of B is an element of A.
4. If every element of set A is an element of set B, we call set A a "subset" of set B, written $A \subset B$ (or $B \supset A$).
   By convention $\phi \subset A$ for every set A.
5. If $A \subset B$ and if $B \subset A$, then A is called an *improper* subset of B—also $A = B$ by (3).
   If $A \subset B$ and if B includes at least one element which is not an element of A, then A is a *proper* subset of B.
   The symbol $\subset$ is sometimes used to mean *proper* inclusion, with $\subseteq$ meaning inclusion as defined above.
   $\neq \subset$ is sometimes also used for proper inclusion.
6. If all of the elements under consideration are elements of a universal set I, then for all sets A, $A \subset I$.
7. The set A', called the *complementary* set of A (relative to I), is the set which contains all the elements of I which are not elements of A.
8. Two binary operations on sets are $\cup$ and $\cap$.
   $A \cup B$, called the *union* (sometimes called the *join*) of sets A and B is the set of all elements which are elements of A or of B or of both.
   $A \cap B$, called the *intersection* (sometimes called the *meet*) of sets A and B is the set of all elements which are elements of *both A and B*.
9. Some properties of sets involving these relations:
   For all sets A, B, C in a universal set I. Only in those rules explicitly involving I, or those using complementation (which is defined in terms of I) is it necessary to assume that $A, B, C, \ldots,$ lie in a universal set.

A. (Closure)
   A_1: There is a unique set $A \cup B$
   A_2: There is a unique set $A \cap B$

B. (Commutative Laws)
   B_1: $A \cup B = B \cup A$
   B_2: $A \cap B = B \cap A$

C. (Associative Laws)
   C_1: $(A \cup B) \cup C = A \cup (B \cup C)$
   C_2: $(A \cap B) \cap C = A \cap (B \cap C)$

D. (Distributive Laws)
   D_1: $A \cup (B \cap C) = (A \cup B) \cap (A \cup C)$
   D_2: $A \cap (B \cup C) = (A \cap B) \cup (A \cap C)$

E. (Idempotent Laws)
   E_1: $A \cup A = A$
   E_2: $A \cap A = A$

F. Properties of I and ϕ
   F_1: $A \cap I = A$
   F_2: $A \cup \phi = A$
   F_3: $A \cap \phi = \phi$
   F_4: $A \cup I = I$

* This equality, as well as ordinary equality between numbers, is a special case of an *equivalence relation*. In general, an equivalence relation is any relation with the following three properties:
1. Reflexive Law: $A = A$.
2. Symmetric Law: If $A = B$, then $B = A$.
3. Transitive Law: If $A = B$ and $B = C$, then $A = C$.

G. Properties of $\subset$.

G_1: $A \subset (A \cup B)$
G_2: $(A \cap B) \subset A$
G_3: $A \subset I$
G_4: $\phi \subset A$
G_5: If $A \subset B$, then $A \cup B = B$
If $B \subset A$, then $A \cap B = B$

H. Properties of $'$.

H_1: For every set A, there is a unique set A'
H_2: $A \cup A' = I$
H_3: $A \cap A' = \phi$
H_4: $(A \cup B)' = A' \cap B'$
H_5: $(A \cap B)' = A' \cup B'$

I. *Duality*

If we interchange $\left\{\begin{matrix} \cup \text{ and } \cap \\ \phi \text{ and } I \\ \subset \text{ and } \supset \end{matrix}\right\}$ in any correct formula we obtain another correct formula.

J. The above Algebra of Sets is a representation of a *Boolean* Algebra, which may be defined:

Undefined concepts: Set H of elements $a, b, c, \ldots$
2 binary operations $\oplus$, $\otimes$

Postulates for all a, b, c, of H

P_1: $a \oplus b \in H$; P_1': $a \otimes b \in H$
P_2: $a \oplus b = b \oplus a$; P_2': $a \otimes b = b \otimes a$
P_3: $(a \oplus b) \oplus c = a \oplus (b \oplus c)$;
P_3': $(a \otimes b) \otimes c = a \otimes (b \otimes c)$
P_4: $a \oplus (b \otimes c) = (a \oplus b) \otimes (a \oplus c)$
P_4': $a \otimes (b \oplus c) = (a \otimes b) \oplus (a \otimes c)$
P_5: There exists an element Z in H, such that for every element a of H, $a \oplus Z = a$
P_5': There exists an element U in H, such that for every element a of H, $a \otimes U = a$
P_6: For every element a of H, there exists an element a' such that $a \oplus a' = U$ and $a \otimes a' = Z$

PROBABILITY

Definitions

A sample space S associated with an experiment is a set S of elements such that any outcome of the experiment corresponds to one and only one element of the set. An event E is a subset of a sample space S. An element in a sample space is called a sample point or a simple event (Unit subset of S).

Definition of Probability

If an experiment can occur in n mutually exclusive and equally likely ways, and if exactly m of these ways correspond to an event E, then the probability of E is given by

$$P(E) = \frac{m}{n}.$$

If E is a subset of S, and if to each unit subset of S, a non-negative number, called its probability, is assigned, and if E is the union of two or more different simple events, then the probability of E, denoted by $P(E)$, is the sum of the probabilities of those simple events whose union is E.

Marginal and Conditional Probability

Suppose a sample space S is partioned into rs disjoint subsets where the general subset is denoted by $E_i \cap F_j$. Then the marginal probability of E_i is defined as

$$P(E_i) = \sum_{j=1}^{s} P(E_i \cap F_j)$$

and the marginal probability of F_j is defined as

$$P(F_j) = \sum_{i=1}^{r} P(E_i \cap F_j)$$

The conditional probability of E_i, given that F_j has occurred, is defined as

$$P(E_i/F_j) = \frac{P(E_i \cap F_j)}{P(F_j)}, \qquad P(F_j) \neq 0$$

and that of F_j, given that E_i has occurred, is defined as

$$P(F_j/E_i) = \frac{P(E_i \cap F_j)}{P(E_i)}, \qquad P(E_i) \neq 0 .$$

Probability Theorems

1. If ϕ is the null set, $P(\phi) = 0$.
2. If S is the sample space, $P(S) = 1$.
3. If E and F are two events

$$P(E \cup F) = P(E) + P(F) - P(E \cap F).$$

4 If E and F are mutually exclusive events,

$$P(E \cup F) = P(E) + P(F).$$

5. If E and E' are complementary events,

$$P(E) = 1 - P(E').$$

6. The conditional probability of an event E, given an event F, is denoted by $P(E/F)$ and is defined as

$$P(E/F) = \frac{P(E \cap F)}{P(F)},$$

where $P(F) \neq 0$.

7. Two events E and F are said to be independent if and only if

$$P(E \cap F) = P(E) \cdot P(F).$$

E is said to be statistically independent of F if $P(E/F) = P(E)$ and $P(F/E) = P(F)$.

8. The events $E_1, E_2, \ldots, E_n$ are called mutually independent for all combinations if and only if every combination of these events taken any number at a time is independent.

9. *Bayes Theorem.*

   If $E_1, E_2, \ldots, E_n$ are n mutually exclusive events whose union is the sample space S, and E is any arbitrary event of S such that $P(E) \neq 0$, then

$$P(E_k/E) = \frac{P(E_k) \cdot P(E/E_k)}{\sum_{j=1}^{n} [P(E_j) \cdot P(E/E_j)]}$$

Random Variable

A function whose domain is a sample space S and whose range is some set of real numbers is called a random variable, denoted by $\mathbf{X}$. The function $\mathbf{X}$ transforms sample points of S into points on the x-axis. $\mathbf{X}$ will be called a discrete random variable if it is a random variable that assumes only a finite or denumerable number of values on the x-axis. $\mathbf{X}$ will be called a continuous random variable if it assumes a continuum of values on the x-axis.

Probability Function (Discrete Case)

The random variable $\mathbf{X}$ will be called a discrete random variable if there exists a function f such that $f(x_i) \geq 0$ and $\sum_i f(x_i) = 1$ for $i = 1, 2, 3, \ldots$ and such that for any event E,

$$P(E) = P[\mathbf{X} \text{ is in } E] = \sum_E f(x)$$

where $\sum_E$ means sum $f(x)$ over those values x_i that are in E and where $f(x) = P[\mathbf{X} = x]$. The probability that the value of $\mathbf{X}$ is some real number x, is given by $f(x) = P[\mathbf{X} = x]$, where f is called the probability function of the random variable $\mathbf{X}$.

Cumulative Distribution Function (Discrete Case)

The probability that the value of a random variable $\mathbf{X}$ is less than or equal to some real number x is defined as

$$F(x) = P(X \leq x)$$
$$= \Sigma f(x_i), \qquad -\infty < x < \infty,$$

where the summation extends over those values of i such that $x_i \leq x$.

Probability Density (Continuous Case)

The random variable **X** will be called a continuous random variable if there exists a function f such that $f(x) \geq 0$ and $\int_{-\infty}^{\infty} f(x)\,dx = 1$ for all x in interval $-\infty < x < \infty$ and such that for any event E

$$P(E) = P(\mathbf{X} \text{ is in } E) = \int_E f(x)\,dx.$$

$f(x)$ is called the probability density of the random variable **X**. The probability that **X** assumes any given value of x is equal to zero and the probability that it assumes a value on the interval from a to b, including or excluding either end point, is equal to

$$\int_a^b f(x)\,dx.$$

Cumulative Distribution Function (Continuous Case)

The probability that the value of a random variable **X** is less than or equal to some real number x is defined as

$$F(x) = P(\mathbf{X} \leq x), \qquad -\infty < x < \infty$$
$$= \int_{-\infty}^{x} f(x)\,dx.$$

From the cumulative distribution, the density, if it exists, can be found from

$$f(x) = \frac{dF(x)}{dx}.$$

From the cumulative distribution

$$P(a \leq \mathbf{X} \leq b) = P(\mathbf{X} \leq b) - P(\mathbf{X} \leq a)$$
$$= F(b) - F(a)$$

Mathematical Expectation

A. Expected Value

Let **X** be a random variable with density $f(x)$. Then the expected value of **X**, $E(\mathbf{X})$, is defined to be

$$E(\mathbf{X}) = \sum_x x f(x)$$

if **X** is discrete and

$$E(\mathbf{X}) = \int_{-\infty}^{\infty} x f(x)\,dx$$

if **X** is continuous. The expected value of a function g of a random variable **X** is defined as

$$E[g(\mathbf{X})] = \sum_x g(x) \cdot f(x)$$

if **X** is discrete and

$$E[g(\mathbf{X})] = \int_{-\infty}^{\infty} g(x) \cdot f(x)\,dx$$

if **X** is continuous.

Theorems

1. $E[a\mathbf{X} + b\mathbf{Y}] = aE(\mathbf{X}) + bE(\mathbf{Y})$
2. $E[\mathbf{X} \cdot \mathbf{Y}] = E(\mathbf{X}) \cdot E(\mathbf{Y})$ if **X** and **Y** are statistically independent.

B. MOMENTS

a. Moments About the Origin. The moments about the origin of a probability distribution are the expected values of the random variable which has the given distribution. The rth moment of **X**, usually denoted by μ'_r, is defined as

$$\mu'_r = E[\mathbf{X}^r] = \sum_x x^r f(x)$$

if **X** is discrete and

$$\mu'_r = E[\mathbf{X}^r] = \int_{-\infty}^{\infty} x^r f(x)\, dx$$

if **X** is continuous.

The first moment, μ'_1, is called the mean of the random variable **X** and is usually denoted by μ.

b. Moments About the Mean. The rth moment about the mean, usually denoted by μ_r, is defined as

$$\mu_r = E[(\mathbf{X} - \mu)^r] = \sum_x (x - \mu)^r f(x)$$

if **X** is discrete and

$$\mu_r = E[(\mathbf{X} - \mu)^r] = \int_{-\infty}^{\infty} (x - \mu)^r f(x)\, dx$$

if **X** is continuous.

The second moment about the mean, μ_2, is given by

$$\mu_2 = E[(\mathbf{X} - \mu)^2] = \mu'_2 - \mu^2$$

and is called the variance of the random variable **X**, and is denoted by σ^2. The square root of the variance, σ, is called the standard deviation.

Theorems

1. $\sigma^2_{c\mathbf{X}} = c^2\sigma^2_{\mathbf{X}}$
2. $\sigma^2_{c+\mathbf{X}} = \sigma^2_{\mathbf{X}}$
3. $\sigma^2_{a\mathbf{X}+b} = a^2\sigma^2_{\mathbf{X}}$

c. Factorial Moments. The rth factorial moment of a probability distribution is defined as

$$\mu'_{(r)} = E[\mathbf{X}^{[r]}] = \sum_x x^{[r]} f(x)$$

if **X** is discrete and

$$\mu'_{(r)} = E[\mathbf{X}^{[r]}] = \int_{-\infty}^{\infty} x^{[r]} f(x)\, dx$$

if **X** is continuous, where the symbol $x^{[r]}$ denotes the factorial expression

$$x^{[r]} = x(x - 1)(x - 2) \cdots (x - r + 1),\ r = 1, 2, 3, \ldots .$$

C. Generating Functions

a. Moment Generating Functions. The moment generating function (m.g.f.) of the random variable **X** is defined as

$$m_x(t) = E(e^{t\mathbf{X}}) = \sum_x e^{tx} f(x)$$

if **X** is discrete and

$$m_x(t) = E(e^{t\mathbf{X}}) = \int_{-\infty}^{\infty} e^{tx} f(x)\, dx$$

if **X** is continuous.
$E(e^{t\mathbf{X}})$ is the expected value of $e^{t\mathbf{X}}$. If $m_x(t)$ and its derivatives exist, $|t| < h^2$, the rth moment about the origin is

$$\mu'_r = m_x^{(r)}(0), \qquad r = 0, 1, 2, \ldots$$

where $m_x^{(r)}(0)$ is the rth derivative of $m_x(t)$ with respect to t, evaluated at $t = 0$. For

$$\begin{aligned} m_x(t) &= E(e^{t\mathbf{X}}) \\ &= E\left[1 + \mathbf{X}t + \frac{(\mathbf{X}t)^2}{2!} + \cdots\right] \\ &= 1 + \mu'_1 t + \mu'_2 \frac{t^2}{2} + \cdots \end{aligned}$$

Thus, the moments μ'_r appear as coefficients of $\frac{t^r}{r!}$, and $m_x(t)$ may be regarded as generating the moments ν_r. The moments μ_r may be generated by the generating function

$$M_x(t) = E[e^{t(\mathbf{X}-\mu)}] = e^{-\mu t} E(e^{t\mathbf{X}}) = e^{-\mu t} m_x(t) .$$

b. Factorial Moment Generating Function. The factorial moment generating function is defined as

$$E(t^{\mathbf{X}}) = \sum_x t^x f(x) \qquad \text{(probability generation function)}$$

if **X** is discrete and

$$E(t^{\mathbf{X}}) = \int_{-\infty}^{\infty} t^x f(x)\, dx$$

if **X** is continuous.

The rth factorial moment is obtained from the factorial moment generating function by differentiating it r times with respect to t and then evaluating the result when $t = 1$.

Theorems

1. If c is a constant, the m.g.f. of $c + \mathbf{X}$ is $e^{ct} m_x(t)$.
2. If c is a constant, the m.g.f. of $c\mathbf{X}$ is $m_x(ct)$.
3. If $\mathbf{Y} = \sum_{i=1}^{n} \mathbf{X}_i$, and $m_x(t)$ is the m.g.f. of $\mathbf{X}_i$, where $\mathbf{X}_1, \ldots, \mathbf{X}_n$ is a random sample from $f(x)$, then the m.g.f. of **Y** is $[m_x(t)]^n$.

D. Cumulant Generating Function

Let $m_x(t)$ be a m.g.f. If $\ln m_x(t)$ can be expanded in the form

$$c(t) = \ln m_x(t) = \kappa_1 t + \kappa_2 \frac{t^2}{2!} + \kappa_3 \frac{t^3}{3!} + \cdots + \kappa_r \frac{t^r}{r!} + \cdots ,$$

then $c(t)$ is called the cumulant generating function (semi-invariant generating function) and κ_r are called the cumulants (semi-invariants) of a distribution.

$$\kappa_r = c^{(r)}(0)$$

where $c^{(r)}(0)$ is the rth derivative of $c(t)$ with respect to t evaluated at $t = 0$.

E. Characteristic Functions

The characteristic function of a distribution is defined as

$$\phi(t) = E(e^{it\mathbf{X}}) = \sum_x e^{itx} \cdot f(x)$$

if **X** is discrete and

$$\phi(t) = E(e^{it\mathbf{X}}) = \int_{-\infty}^{\infty} e^{itx} \cdot f(x)\,dx$$

if **X** is continuous.
Here t is a real number, $i^2 = -1$, and $e^{it\mathbf{X}} = \cos(t\mathbf{X}) + i\sin(t\mathbf{X})$. The characteristic function also generates moments, if they exist for

$$i^r\mu'_r = \phi^{(r)}(0)$$

where $\phi^{(r)}(0)$ is the rth derivative of $\phi(t)$ with respect to t evaluated at $t = 0$.

Multivariate Distributions

A. Discrete Case

The k-dimensional random variable $(\mathbf{X}_1, \mathbf{X}_2, \ldots, \mathbf{X}_k)$ is a k-dimensional discrete random variable if it assumes values only at a finite or denumerable number of points $(x_1, x_2, \ldots, x_k)$. Define

$$P[\mathbf{X}_1 = x_1, \mathbf{X}_2 = x_2, \ldots, \mathbf{X}_k = x_k] = f(x_1, x_2, \ldots, x_k)$$

for every value that the random variable can assume. $f(x_1, x_2, \ldots, x_k)$ is called the joint density of the k-dimensional random variable. If E is any subset of the set of values that the random variable can assume, then

$$P(E) = P[(\mathbf{X}_1, \mathbf{X}_2, \ldots, \mathbf{X}_k) \text{ is in } E] = \sum_E f(x_1, x_2, \ldots, x_k)$$

where the sum is over all those points in E. The cumulative distribution is defined as

$$F(x_1, x_2, \ldots, x_k) = \sum_{x_1}\sum_{x_2} \cdots \sum_{x_k} f(x_1, x_2, \ldots, x_k).$$

B. Continuous Case

The k random variables $\mathbf{X}_1, \mathbf{X}_2, \ldots, \mathbf{X}_k$ are said to be jointly distributed if there exists a function f such that $f(x_1, x_2, \ldots, x_k) \geq 0$ for all $-\infty < x_i < \infty$, $i = 1, 2, \ldots, k$ and such that for any event E

$$\begin{aligned} P(E) &= P[(\mathbf{X}_1, \mathbf{X}_2, \ldots, \mathbf{X}_k) \text{ is in } E] \\ &= \int_E f(x_1, x_2, \ldots, x_k)\,dx_1\,dx_2 \cdots dx_k. \end{aligned}$$

$f(x_1, x_2, \ldots, x_k)$ is called the joint density of the random variables $\mathbf{X}_1, \mathbf{X}_2, \ldots, \mathbf{X}_k$.
The cumulative distribution is defined as

$$F(x_1, x_2, \ldots, x_k) = \int_{-\infty}^{x_1}\int_{-\infty}^{x_2} \cdots \int_{-\infty}^{x_k} f(x_1, x_2, \ldots, x_k)\,dx_k \cdots dx_2\,dx_1\,.$$

Given the cumulative distribution, the density may be found by

$$f(x_1, x_2, \ldots, x_k) = \frac{\partial}{\partial x_1} \cdot \frac{\partial}{\partial x_2} \cdots \frac{\partial}{\partial x_k} F(x_1, x_2, \ldots, x_k) .$$

Moments

The rth moment of $\mathbf{X}_i$, say, is defined as

$$E(\mathbf{X}_i^r) = \sum_{x_1} \sum_{x_2} \cdots \sum_{x_k} x_i^r f(x_1, x_2, \ldots, x_k)$$

if the $\mathbf{X}_i$ are discrete and

$$E(\mathbf{X}_i^r) = \int_{-\infty}^{\infty} \int_{-\infty}^{\infty} \cdots \int_{-\infty}^{\infty} x_i^r f(x_1, x_2, \ldots, x_k)\, dx_k \cdots dx_2\, dx_1$$

if the $\mathbf{X}_i$ are continuous.

Joint moments about the origin are defined as

$$E(\mathbf{X}_1^{r_1} \mathbf{X}_2^{r_2} \cdots \mathbf{X}_k^{r_k})$$

where $r_1 + r_2 + \cdots + r_k$ is the order of the moment.

Joint moments about the mean are defined as

$$E[(\mathbf{X}_1 - \mu_1)^{r_1} (\mathbf{X}_2 - \mu_2)^{r_2} \cdots (\mathbf{X}_k - \mu_k)^{r_k}].$$

Marginal and Conditional Distributions

If the random variables $\mathbf{X}_1, \mathbf{X}_2, \ldots, \mathbf{X}_k$ have the joint density function $f(x_1, x_2, \ldots, x_k)$, then the marginal distribution of the subset of the random variables, say, $\mathbf{X}_1, \mathbf{X}_2, \ldots, \mathbf{X}_p$ $(p < k)$, is given by

$$g(x_1, x_2, \ldots, x_p) = \sum_{x_{p+1}} \sum_{x_{p+2}} \cdots \sum_{x_k} f(x_1, x_2, \ldots, x_k)$$

if the $\mathbf{X}$'s are discrete, and

$$g(x_1, x_2, \ldots, x_p) = \int_{-\infty}^{\infty} \int_{-\infty}^{\infty} \cdots \int_{-\infty}^{\infty} f(x_1, x_2, \ldots, x_k)\, dx_{p+1} \cdots dx_{k-1}\, dx_k$$

if the $\mathbf{X}$'s are continuous.

The conditional distribution of a certain subset of the random variables is the joint distribution of this subset under the condition that the remaining variables are given certain values. The conditional distribution of $\mathbf{X}_1, \mathbf{X}_2, \ldots, \mathbf{X}_p$ given $\mathbf{X}_{p+1}, \mathbf{X}_{p+2}, \ldots, \mathbf{X}_k$ is

$$h(x_1, x_2, \ldots, x_p | x_{p+1}, x_{p+2}, \ldots, x_k) = \frac{f(x_1, x_2, \ldots, x_k)}{g(x_{p+1}, x_{p+2}, \ldots, x_k)}$$

if $g(x_{p+1}, x_{p+2}, \ldots, x_k) \neq 0$.

The variance σ_{ii} of $\mathbf{X}_i$ and the covariance σ_{ij} of $\mathbf{X}_i$ and $\mathbf{X}_j$ are given by

$$\sigma_{ii} = \sigma_i^2 = E[(\mathbf{X}_i - \mu_i)^2]$$

and

$$\sigma_{ij} = \rho_{ij}\sigma_i\sigma_j = E[(\mathbf{X}_i - \mu_i)(\mathbf{X}_j - \mu_j)]$$

where ρ_{ij} is the correlation coefficient and σ_i and σ_j are the standard deviations of $\mathbf{X}_i$ and $\mathbf{X}_j$.

A joint m.g.f. is defined as

$$m(t_1, t_2, \ldots, t_k) = E[e^{t_1 \mathbf{X}_1 + t_2 \mathbf{X}_2 + \cdots + t_k \mathbf{X}_k}]$$

if it exists for all values of t_i such that $|t_i| < h^2$.

The rth moment of $\mathbf{X}_i$ may be obtained by differentiating the m.g.f. r times with respect to t_i and then evaluating the result when all t's are set equal to zero. Similarly, a joint moment would be found by differentiatins the m.g.f. r_1 times with respect to t_1, . . . , r_k times with respect to t_k, and then evaluating the result when all t's are set equal to zero.

Probability Distributions

A. Discrete Case

1. *Discrete Uniform Distribution.* If the random variable $\mathbf{X}$ has a probability function given by

$$P(\mathbf{X} = x) = f(x) = \frac{1}{n}, \qquad x = x_1, x_2, \ldots, x_n,$$

then the variable $\mathbf{X}$ is said to possess a discrete uniform distribution.

Properties

When $x_i = i$ for $i = 1, 2, \ldots,$ and n

$$\text{Mean} = \mu = \frac{n+1}{2}$$

$$\text{Variance} = \sigma^2 = \frac{n^2 - 1}{12}$$

$$\text{Standard Deviation} = \sigma = \sqrt{\frac{n^2 - 1}{12}}$$

$$\text{Moment Generating Function} = m_x(t) = \frac{e^t(1 - e^{nt})}{n(1 - e^t)}$$

2. *Binomial Distribution.* If the random variable $\mathbf{X}$ has a probability function given by

$$P(\mathbf{X} = x) = f(x) = \binom{n}{x} \theta^x (1 - \theta)^{n-x}, \qquad x = 0, 1, 2, \ldots, n$$

where

$$\binom{n}{x} = \frac{n!}{x!(n - x)!},$$

then the variable $\mathbf{X}$ is said to possess a binomial distribution. $f(x)$ is the general term of the expansion of $[\theta + (1 - \theta)]^n$.

Properties

$$\text{Mean} = \mu = n\theta$$

$$\text{Variance} = \sigma^2 = n\theta(1 - \theta)$$

$$\text{Standard Deviation} = \sigma = \sqrt{n\theta(1 - \theta)}$$

$$\text{Moment Generating Function} = m_x(t) = [\theta e^t + (1 - \theta)]^n$$

3. *Geometric Distribution.* If the random variable $\mathbf{X}$ has a probability function given by

$$P(\mathbf{X} = x) = f(x) = \theta(1 - \theta)^{x-1}, \qquad x = 1, 2, 3, \ldots,$$

then the variable $\mathbf{X}$ is said to possess a geometric distribution.

Properties

$$\text{Mean} = \mu = \frac{1}{\theta}$$

$$\text{Variance} = \sigma^2 = \frac{1-\theta}{\theta^2}$$

$$\text{Standard Deviation} = \sigma = \sqrt{\frac{1-\theta}{\theta^2}}$$

$$\text{Moment Generating Function} = m_x(t) = \frac{\theta e^t}{1 - e^t(1-\theta)}$$

4. *Multinomial Distribution.* If a set of random variables $\mathbf{X}_1, \mathbf{X}_2, \ldots, \mathbf{X}_n$ has a probability function given by

$$P(\mathbf{X}_1 = x_1, \mathbf{X}_2 = x_2, \ldots, \mathbf{X}_n = x_n) = f(x_1, x_2, \ldots, x_n) = \frac{N!}{\prod_{i=1}^{n} x_i!} \prod_{i=1}^{n} \theta_i^{x_i}$$

where x_i are positive integers and each $\theta_i > 0$ for $i = 1, 2, \ldots, n$ and

$$\sum_{i=1}^{n} \theta_i = 1, \qquad \sum_{i=1}^{n} x_i = N,$$

then the joint distribution of $\mathbf{X}_1, \mathbf{X}_2, \ldots, \mathbf{X}_n$ is called the multinomial distribution. $f(x_1, x_2, \ldots, x_n)$ is the general term of the expansion of $(\theta_1 + \theta_2 + \cdots + \theta_n)^N$.

Properties

$$\text{Mean of } \mathbf{X}_i = \mu_i = N\theta_i$$

$$\text{Variance of } \mathbf{X}_i = \sigma_i^2 = N\theta_i(1 - \theta_i)$$

$$\text{Covariance of } \mathbf{X}_i \text{ and } \mathbf{X}_j = \sigma_{ij}^2 = -N\theta_i\theta_j$$

$$\text{Joint Moment Generating Function} = (\theta_1 e^{t_1} + \cdots + \theta_n e^{t_n})^N$$

5. *Poisson Distribution.* If the random variable $\mathbf{X}$ has a probability function given by

$$P(\mathbf{X} = x) = f(x) = \frac{e^{-\lambda}\lambda^x}{x!}, \qquad \lambda > 0,\ x = 0, 1, \ldots,$$

then the variable $\mathbf{X}$ is said to possess a Poisson distribution.

Properties

$$\text{Mean} = \mu = \lambda$$

$$\text{Variance} = \sigma^2 = \lambda$$

$$\text{Standard Deviation} = \sigma = \sqrt{\lambda}$$

$$\text{Moment Generating Function} = m_x(t) = e^{\lambda(e^t - 1)}$$

6. *Hypergeometric Distribution.* If the random variable $\mathbf{X}$ has a probability function given by

$$P(\mathbf{X} = x) = f(x) = \frac{\binom{k}{x}\binom{N-k}{n-x}}{\binom{N}{n}}, \qquad x = 0, 1, 2, \ldots, [n, k],$$

where $[n, k]$ means the smaller of the two numbers n, k, then the variable $\mathbf{X}$ is said to possess a hypergeometric distribution.

Properties

$$\text{Mean} = \mu = \frac{kn}{N}$$

$$\text{Variance} = \sigma^2 = \frac{k(N-k)n(N-n)}{N^2(N-1)}$$

$$\text{Standard Deviation} = \sigma = \sqrt{\frac{k(N-k)n(N-n)}{N^2(N-1)}}$$

7. *Negative Binomial Distribution*. If the random variable **X** has a probability function given by

$$P(\mathbf{X} = x) = f(x) = \binom{x+r-1}{r-1}\theta^r(1-\theta)^x, \qquad x = 0, 1, 2, \ldots;$$

then the variable **X** is said to possess a negative binomial distribution, known also as the Pascal or Pólya distribution.

Properties

$$\text{Mean} = \mu = \frac{r}{\theta}$$

$$\text{Variance} = \sigma^2 = \frac{r}{\theta}\left(\frac{1}{\theta} - 1\right) = \frac{r(1-\theta)}{\theta^2}$$

$$\text{Standard Deviation} = \sigma = \sqrt{\frac{r}{\theta}\left(\frac{1}{\theta} - 1\right)} = \sqrt{\frac{r(1-\theta)}{\theta^2}}$$

$$\text{Moment Generating Function} = m_x(t) = e^{tr}\theta^r[1 - (1-\theta)e^t]^{-r}$$

B. Continuous Case

1. *Uniform Distribution*. A random variable **X** is said to be distributed as the uniform distribution if the density function is given by

$$f(x) = \frac{1}{\beta - \alpha}, \qquad \alpha < x < \beta,$$

where α and β are parameters with $\alpha < \beta$.

Properties

$$\text{Mean} = \mu = \frac{\alpha + \beta}{2}$$

$$\text{Variance} = \sigma^2 = \frac{(\beta - \alpha)^2}{12}$$

$$\text{Standard Deviation} = \sigma = \sqrt{\frac{(\beta - \alpha)^2}{12}}$$

$$\text{Moment Generating Function} = m_x(t) = \frac{2}{(\beta - \alpha)t}\sinh\left[\frac{(\beta - \alpha)t}{2}\right]e^{\frac{\alpha+\beta}{2}t} = \frac{e^{\beta t} - e^{\alpha t}}{(\beta - \alpha)t}$$

2. *Normal Distribution*. A random variable **X** is said to be normally distributed if its density function is given by

$$f(x) = \frac{1}{\sqrt{2\pi}\,\sigma}e^{-(x-\mu)^2/2\sigma^2}, \qquad -\infty < x < \infty$$

where μ and σ are parameters, called the mean and the standard deviation or the random variable **X**, respectively.

Properties

$$\text{Mean} = \mu$$
$$\text{Variance} = \sigma^2$$
$$\text{Standard Deviation} = \sigma$$

$$\text{Moment Generating Function} = m_x(t) = e^{t\mu + \frac{\sigma^2 t^2}{2}}$$

Cumulative Distribution

$$F(x) = \int_{-\infty}^{x} \frac{1}{\sqrt{2\pi}\,\sigma} e^{-(x-\mu)^2/2\sigma^2}\,dx$$

Set $y = \dfrac{x-\mu}{\sigma}$ to obtain the cumulative standard normal.

3. *Gamma Distribution.* A random variable **X** is said to be distributed as the gamma distribution if the density function is given by

$$f(x) = \frac{1}{\Gamma(\alpha+1)\beta^{\alpha+1}} x^{\alpha} e^{-x/\beta}, \qquad 0 < x < \infty$$

where α and β are parameters with $\alpha > -1$ and $\beta > 0$.

Properties

$$\text{Mean} = \mu = \beta(\alpha+1)$$
$$\text{Variance} = \sigma^2 = \beta^2(\alpha+1)$$
$$\text{Standard Deviation} = \sigma = \beta\sqrt{\alpha+1}$$
$$\text{Moment Generating Function} = m_x(t) = (1-\beta t)^{-(\alpha+1)}, \qquad t < \frac{1}{\beta}.$$

4. *Exponential Distribution.* A random variable **X** is said to be distributed as the exponential distribution if the density function is given by

$$f(x) = \frac{1}{\theta} e^{-x/\theta}, \qquad x > 0$$

where θ is a parameter and $\theta > 0$.

Properties

$$\text{Mean} = \mu = \theta$$
$$\text{Variance} = \sigma^2 = \theta^2$$
$$\text{Standard Deviation} = \sigma = \sqrt{\theta^2}$$
$$\text{Moment Generating Function} = m_x(t) = (1-\theta t)^{-1}$$

5. *Beta Distribution.* A random variable **X** is said to be distributed as the beta distribution if the density function is given by

$$f(x) = \frac{\Gamma(\alpha+\beta+2)}{\Gamma(\alpha+1)\Gamma(\beta+1)} x^{\alpha}(1-x)^{\beta}, \qquad 0 < x < 1$$

where α and β are parameters with $\alpha > -1$ and $\beta > -1$.

Properties

$$\text{Mean} = \mu = \frac{\alpha+1}{\alpha+\beta+2}$$

$$\text{Variance} = \sigma^2 = \frac{(\alpha+1)(\beta+1)}{(\alpha+\beta+2)^2(\alpha+\beta+3)}$$

$$r\text{th moment about the origin} = \nu_r = \frac{\Gamma(\alpha+\beta+2)\Gamma(\alpha+r+1)}{\Gamma(\alpha+\beta+r+2)\Gamma(\alpha+1)}.$$

Sampling Distributions

Population—A finite or infinite set of elements of a random variable **X**.

Random Sample—If the random variables $X_1, X_2, \ldots, X_n$ have a joint density,

$$g(x_1, x_2, \ldots, x_n) = f(x_1)f(x_2) \cdots f(x_n)$$

where the density of each X_i is $f(x)$, then $X_1, X_2, \ldots, X_n$ is said to be a random sample of size n from the population with density $f(x)$.

Sampling Distributions

A random sample is selected from a population in which the form of the probability function is known, and from the joint density of the random variables a distribution, called the sampling distribution, of a function of the random variables is derived.

1. *Chi-Square Distribution.* If $Y_1, Y_2, \ldots, Y_n$ are normally and independently distributed with mean 0 and variance 1, then

$$\chi^2 = \sum_{i=1}^{n} Y_i^2$$

is distributed as Chi-Square (χ^2) with n degrees of freedom. The density function is given by

$$f(\chi^2) = \frac{(\chi^2)^{\frac{1}{2}(n-2)}}{2^{\frac{n}{2}}\Gamma\left(\frac{n}{2}\right)} e^{-\chi^2/2}, \qquad 0 < \chi^2 < \infty .$$

Properties

$$\text{Mean} = \mu = n$$
$$\text{Variance} = \sigma^2 = 2n$$

Reproductive Property of χ^2 - Distribution

If $\chi_1^2, \chi_2^2, \ldots, \chi_k^2$ are independently distributed according to χ^2 - distributions with $n_1, n_2, \ldots, n_k$ degrees of freedom, respectively, then $\sum_{j=1}^{k} \chi_j^2$ is distributed according to a χ^2 - distribution with $n = \sum_{j=1}^{k} n_j$ degrees of freedom.

2. *Snedecor's F-Distribution.* If a random variable **X** is distributed as χ^2 with m degrees of freedom (χ^2_m) and a random variable **Y** is distributed as χ^2 with n degrees of freedom (χ^2_n) and if **X** and **Y** are independent, then $F = \dfrac{\mathbf{X}/m}{\mathbf{Y}/n}$ is distributed as Snedecor's F with m and n degrees of freedom, denoted by $F(m, n)$. The density function of the F-distribution is given by

$$f(F) = \frac{\Gamma\left(\frac{m+n}{2}\right)\left(\frac{m}{n}\right)^{m/2} F^{(m-2)/2}}{\Gamma\left(\frac{m}{2}\right)\Gamma\left(\frac{n}{2}\right)\left(1 + \frac{m}{n}F\right)^{(m+n)/2}}, \qquad 0 < F < \infty.$$

Properties

$$\text{Mean} = \mu = \frac{n}{n-2}, \qquad n > 2$$

$$\text{Variance} = \sigma^2 = \frac{2n^2(m+n-2)}{m(n-2)^2(n-4)}, \qquad n > 4 .$$

The transformation $w = \dfrac{mF/n}{1 + \frac{mF}{n}}$ transforms the F-density into a Beta density.

3. *Student's t-Distribution.* If a random variable **X** is normally distributed with mean 0 and variance σ^2, and if $\mathbf{Y}^2/\sigma^2$ is distributed as χ^2 with n degrees of freedom and if **X** and **Y** are independent, then

$$t = \frac{\mathbf{X}\sqrt{n}}{\mathbf{Y}}$$

is distributed as Student's t with n degrees of freedom. The density function is given by

$$f(t) = \frac{\Gamma\left(\frac{n+1}{2}\right)}{\sqrt{n\pi}\,\Gamma\left(\frac{n}{2}\right)\left(1 + \frac{t^2}{n}\right)^{\frac{1}{2}(n+1)}}, \qquad -\infty < t < \infty .$$

Properties

$$\text{Mean} = \mu = 0$$

$$\text{Variance} = \sigma^2 = \frac{n}{n-2}, \qquad n > 2 .$$

SUMMARY OF SIGNIFICANCE TESTS: TESTING FOR THE VALUE OF A SPECIFIED PARAMETER

Hypothesis	Conditions	Test Statistic	Distribution of Test Statistic	Critical Region
1. $\mu = \mu_0$	Known σ	$z = \dfrac{(\bar{x} - \mu_0)\sqrt{n}}{\sigma}$	Normal	$z > z_\alpha$ if we wish to reject when $\mu > \mu_0$ $z < -z_\alpha$ if we wish to reject when $\mu < \mu_0$ $\|z\| > z_{\alpha/2}$ if we wish to reject when $\mu \neq \mu_0$
2. $\mu = \mu_0$	Unknown σ	$t = \dfrac{(\bar{x} - \mu_0)\sqrt{n}}{s}$	Student's t – with $(n - 1)$ d.f.	$t > t_{\alpha;n-1}$ if we wish to reject when $\mu > \mu_0$ $t < -t_{\alpha;n-1}$ if we wish to reject when $\mu < \mu_0$ $\|t\| > t_{\alpha/2;n-1}$ if we wish to reject when $\mu \neq \mu_0$
3. $\sigma = \sigma_0$		$\chi^2 = \dfrac{(n - 1)s^2}{\sigma_0^2}$	χ^2 with $n - 1$ d.f.	$\chi^2 > \chi^2_{\alpha;n-1}$ if we wish to reject when $\sigma > \sigma_0$ $\chi^2 < \chi^2_{1-\alpha;n-1}$ if we wish to reject when $\sigma < \sigma_0$ $\chi^2 < \chi^2_{1-\alpha/2;n-1}$ or $\chi^2 > \chi^2_{\alpha/2;n-1}$ if we wish to reject when $\sigma \neq \sigma_0$
4. $\theta = \theta_0$	Large sample. (For small samples, exact tests are based on tables of binomial probabilities)	$z = \dfrac{\frac{x}{n} - \theta_0}{\sqrt{\dfrac{\theta_0(1 - \theta_0)}{n}}}$ Continuity correction: Replace x in numerator of formula with $x - \frac{1}{2}$ or $x + \frac{1}{2}$, whichever makes z numerically smallest.	Normal	$z > z_\alpha$ if we wish to reject when $\theta > \theta_0$ $z < -z_\alpha$ if we wish to reject when $\theta < \theta_0$ $\|z\| > -z_{\alpha/2}$ if we wish to reject when $\theta \neq \theta_0$

SUMMARY OF SIGNIFICANCE TESTS: COMPARISON OF TWO POPULATIONS

Hypothesis	Conditions	Test Statistic	Distribution of Test Statistic	Critical Region
1. $\mu_x = \mu_y$	Known σ_x and σ_y	$z = \dfrac{\bar{x} - \bar{y}}{\sqrt{\dfrac{\sigma_x^2}{n_x} + \dfrac{\sigma_y^2}{n_y}}}$	Normal	$z > z_\alpha$ if we wish to reject when $\mu_x > \mu_y$ $z < -z_\alpha$ if we wish to reject when $\mu_x < \mu_y$ $\|z\| > z_{\alpha/2}$ if we wish to reject when $\mu_x \neq \mu_y$
2. $\mu_x = \mu_y$	Unknown σ_x and σ_y $\sigma_x = \sigma_y$	$t = \dfrac{\bar{x} - \bar{y}}{\sqrt{\dfrac{(n_x - 1)s_x^2 + (n_y - 1)s_y^2}{n_x + n_y - 2}}\sqrt{\dfrac{1}{n_x} + \dfrac{1}{n_y}}}$	Student's t—with $n - 1$ d.f.	$t > t_{\alpha;n_x+n_y-2}$ if we wish to reject when $\mu_x > \mu_y$ $t < -t_{\alpha;n_x+n_y-2}$ if we wish to reject when $\mu_x < \mu_y$ $\|t\| > t_{\alpha/2;n_x+n_y-2}$ if we wish to reject when $\mu_x \neq \mu_y$
3. $\mu_x = \mu_y$	Unknown σ_x and σ_y $\sigma_x \neq \sigma_y$	$t = \dfrac{\bar{x} - \bar{y}}{\sqrt{\dfrac{s_x^2}{n_x} + \dfrac{s_y^2}{n_y}}}$	Student's t—with ν d.f.	$t > t_{\alpha;\nu}$ if we wish to reject when $\mu_x > \mu_y$ $t < -t_{\alpha;\nu}$ if we wish to reject when $\mu_x < \mu_y$ $\|t\| > t_{\alpha/2;\nu}$ if we wish to reject when $\mu_x \neq \mu_y$ where d.f. ν is given by closest integer to $\nu = -2 + \dfrac{\left(\dfrac{s_x^2}{n_x} + \dfrac{s_y^2}{n_y}\right)^2}{\dfrac{\left(\dfrac{s_x^2}{n_x}\right)^2}{n_x + 1} + \dfrac{\left(\dfrac{s_y^2}{n_y}\right)^2}{n_y + 1}}$
4. $\mu_x = \mu_y$	Correlated pairs	$t = \dfrac{\bar{d}\sqrt{n}}{s_d}$ where $d_i = x_i - y_i$	Student's t—with $n - 1$ d.f.	$t > t_{\alpha;n-1}$ if we wish to reject when $\mu_x > \mu_y$ $t < -t_{\alpha;n-1}$ if we wish to reject when $\mu_x < \mu_y$ $\|t\| > t_{\alpha/2;n-1}$ if we wish to reject when $\mu_x \neq \mu_y$
5. $\sigma_x^2 = \sigma_y^2$		$F = \dfrac{s_x^2}{s_y^2}$ In a two-sided test, put larger mean square in the numerator	F with $n_x - 1$ and $n_y - 1$ d.f.	$F > F_{\alpha;n_x-1,n_y-1}$ if we wish to reject when $\sigma_x > \sigma_y$ $F > F_{\alpha/2;n_x-1,n_y-1}$ if $s_x^2 > s_y^2$ and we wish to reject when $\sigma_x \neq \sigma_y$ $F > F_{\alpha/2;n_y-1,n_x-1}$ if $s_x^2 < s_y^2$ and we wish to reject when $\sigma_x \neq \sigma_y$
6. $\theta_1 = \theta_2$	Large sample	$z = \dfrac{\dfrac{x_1}{n_1} - \dfrac{x_2}{n_2}}{\sqrt{\dfrac{\dfrac{x_1}{n_1}\left(1 - \dfrac{x_1}{n_1}\right)}{n_1} + \dfrac{\dfrac{x_2}{n_2}\left(1 - \dfrac{x_2}{n_2}\right)}{n_2}}}$ Continuity Correction: Replace x in numerator of formula with $x - \frac{1}{2}$ or $x + \frac{1}{2}$, whichever makes z numerically smallest.	Normal	$z > z_\alpha$ if we wish to reject when $\theta_1 > \theta_2$ $z < -z_\alpha$ if we wish to reject when $\theta_1 < \theta_2$ $\|z\| > z_{\alpha/2}$ if we wish to reject when $\theta_1 \neq \theta_2$

SUMMARY OF CONFIDENCE INTERVALS

Parameter	Conditions	Point Estimate	Confidence Interval
1. μ	Known σ	$\bar{x}$	$\bar{x} - z_{\alpha/2}\frac{\sigma}{\sqrt{n}} < \mu < \bar{x} + z_{\alpha/2}\frac{\sigma}{\sqrt{n}}$
2. μ	Unknown σ	$\bar{x}$	$\bar{x} - t_{\alpha/2}\frac{s}{\sqrt{n}} < \mu < \bar{x} + t_{\alpha/2}\frac{s}{\sqrt{n}}$
3. $\mu_x - \mu_y$	$\sigma_x = \sigma_y$ known	$\bar{x} - \bar{y}$	$\bar{x} - \bar{y} - z_{\alpha/2}\sqrt{\frac{\sigma_x^2}{n_x} + \frac{\sigma_y^2}{n_y}} < \mu_x - \mu_y < \bar{x} - \bar{y} + z_{\alpha/2}\sqrt{\frac{\sigma_x^2}{n_x} + \frac{\sigma_y^2}{n_y}}$
4. $\mu_x - \mu_y$	$\sigma_x = \sigma_y$ unknown	$\bar{x} - \bar{y}$	$\bar{x} - \bar{y} - t_{\alpha/2}\frac{\sqrt{(n_x - 1)s_x^2 + (n_y - 1)s_y^2}}{\sqrt{\frac{n_x n_y(n_x + n_y - 2)}{n_x + n_y}}} < \mu_x - \mu_y < \bar{x} - \bar{y} + t_{\alpha/2}\frac{\sqrt{(n_x - 1)s_x^2 + (n_y - 1)s_y^2}}{\sqrt{\frac{n_x n_y(n_x + n_y - 2)}{n_x + n_y}}}$
5. $\mu_d = \mu_x - \mu_y$	Correlated pairs σ_x and σ_y unknown	$\bar{d} = \bar{x} - \bar{y}$	$\bar{d} - t_{\alpha/2}\frac{s_d}{\sqrt{n}} < \mu_d < \bar{d} + t_{\alpha/2}\frac{s_d}{\sqrt{n}}$
6. σ		s	$\sqrt{\frac{(n-1)s^2}{\chi^2_{\alpha/2;n-1}}} < \sigma < \sqrt{\frac{(n-1)s^2}{\chi^2_{1-\alpha/2;n-1}}}$
7. $\frac{\sigma_x^2}{\sigma_y^2}$		$\frac{s_x^2}{s_y^2}$	$\frac{s_x^2}{s_y^2}\frac{1}{F_{\alpha/2;n_x-1,n_y-1}} < \frac{\sigma_x^2}{\sigma_y^2} < \frac{s_x^2}{s_y^2}\frac{1}{F_{1-\alpha/2;n_x-1,n_y-1}}$
8. θ	Large sample	$\frac{x}{n}$	$\frac{x}{n} - z_{\alpha/2}\sqrt{\frac{\frac{x}{n}\left(1 - \frac{x}{n}\right)}{n}} < \theta < \frac{x}{n} + z_{\alpha/2}\sqrt{\frac{\frac{x}{n}\left(1 - \frac{x}{n}\right)}{n}}$
9. $\theta_1 - \theta_2$	Large sample	$\frac{x_1}{n_1} - \frac{x_2}{n_2}$	$\frac{x_1}{n_1} - \frac{x_2}{n_2} - z_{\alpha/2}\sqrt{\frac{\frac{x_1}{n_1}\left(1 - \frac{x_1}{n_1}\right)}{n_1} + \frac{\frac{x_2}{n_2}\left(1 - \frac{x_2}{n_2}\right)}{n_2}} < \theta_1 - \theta_2 < \frac{x_1}{n_1} - \frac{x_2}{n_2} + z_{\alpha/2}\sqrt{\frac{\frac{x_1}{n_1}\left(1 - \frac{x_1}{n_1}\right)}{n_1} + \frac{\frac{x_2}{n_2}\left(1 - \frac{x_2}{n_2}\right)}{n_2}}$

ANALYSIS OF VARIANCE (ANOVA) TABLES

The analysis of variance (ANOVA) table containing the sum of squares, degrees of freedom, mean square, expectations, etc., present the initial analysis in a compact form. This kind of tabular representation is customarily used to set out the results of analysis of variance calculations. Appropriate ANOVA tables for various experimental design models are presented here. In the tables, the use of "dot notation" indicates a summing over all observations in the population, i.e., when summing over a suffix, that suffix is replaced by a dot. Small letters refer to observations, whereas capital letters refer to observation totals.

ANALYSIS OF VARIANCE AND EXPECTED MEAN SQUARES FOR THE ONE-WAY CLASSIFICATION

Model: $y_{ij} = \mu + \alpha_i + \epsilon_{ij} \quad (i = 1, 2, \ldots, k; j = 1, 2, \ldots, n_i)$

Source of variation	Degrees of freedom	Sum of squares	Mean square	Test statistic
Between groups	$k - 1$	$S_1 = \sum_i n_i(\bar{y}_{i\cdot} - \bar{y}_{\cdot\cdot})^2 = \sum_i \left(\frac{Y_{i\cdot}^2}{n_i}\right) - \frac{Y^2}{n}$	$s_1^2 = \frac{S_1}{k - 1}$	$F = \frac{s_1^2}{s_e^2}$
Within groups	$n - k$	$S_e = \sum_i \sum_j (\bar{y}_{ij} - \bar{y}_{i\cdot})^2 = \sum_i \sum_j y_{ij}^2 - \sum_i \left(\frac{Y_{i\cdot}^2}{n_i}\right)$	$s_e^2 = \frac{S_e}{n - k}$	
Total	$n - 1$	$S = \sum_i \sum_j (y_{ij} - \bar{y})^2 = \sum_i \sum_j y_{ij}^2 - \frac{Y^2}{n}$		

Source of variation	Degrees of freedom	Mean square	Expected mean square for: Fixed model	Random model
Between groups	$k - 1$	s_1^2	$\sigma^2 + \frac{\sum_i n_i\alpha_i^2}{k - 1}$	$\sigma^2 + \frac{1}{k - 1}\left(n - \frac{\sum n_i^2}{n}\right)\sigma_\alpha^2$
Within groups	$n - k$	s_e^2	σ^2	σ^2
Total	$n - 1$			

Notation:

$$Y_{i\cdot} = \sum_j y_{ij} \; ; \; Y = \sum_i \sum_j y_{ij} \; ; \; \bar{y}_{i\cdot} = \frac{1}{n_i} \sum_j y_{ij} = \frac{1}{n_i} Y_{i\cdot} \; ;$$

$$n = \sum_i n_i \; ; \; \bar{y} = \frac{1}{n} \sum_i \sum_j y_{ij} = \frac{Y}{n}$$

ANALYSIS OF VARIANCE AND EXPECTED MEAN SQUARES FOR THE TWO-WAY CLASSIFICATION WITH ONE OBSERVATION PER CELL

Model: $y_{ij} = \mu + \alpha_i + \beta_j + \epsilon_{ij} \quad (i = 1, 2, \ldots c; j = 1, 2, \ldots, r)$

Source of variation	Degrees of freedom	Sum of squares	Mean square	Test statistic
Column effects	$c - 1$	$SSC = \frac{\sum_i Y_{i.}^2}{r} - \frac{Y_{..}^2}{cr}$	$s_1^2 = \frac{SSC}{c - 1}$	$\frac{s_1^2}{s_e^2}$
Row effects	$r - 1$	$SSR = \frac{\sum_j Y_{.j}^2}{c} - \frac{Y_{..}^2}{cr}$	$s_2^2 = \frac{SSR}{r - 1}$	$\frac{s_2^2}{s_e^2}$
Error	$(c - 1)(r - 1)$	$SSE = SST - SSC - SSR$	$s_e^2 = \frac{SSE}{(c - 1)(r - 1)}$	
Total	$cr - 1$	$SST = \sum_i \sum_j y_{ij}^2 - \frac{Y_{..}^2}{cr}$		

Source of variation	Degrees of freedom	Mean square	Expected mean square for		
			Fixed model	Mixed model (α)	Random model
Column effects	$c - 1$	s_1^2	$\sigma^2 + r\left(\frac{\sum_i \alpha_i^2}{c - 1}\right)$	$\sigma^2 + r\left(\frac{\sum_i \alpha_i^2}{c - 1}\right)$	$\sigma^2 + r\sigma_\alpha^2$
Row effects	$r - 1$	s_2^2	$\sigma^2 + c\left(\frac{\sum_j \beta_j^2}{r - 1}\right)$	$\sigma^2 + c\sigma_\beta^2$	$\sigma^2 + c\sigma_\beta^2$
Error	$(c - 1)(r - 1)$	s_e^2	σ^2	σ^2	σ^2
Total	$cr - 1$				

ANALYSIS OF VARIANCE AND EXPECTED MEAN SQUARES FOR NESTED CLASSIFICATIONS WITH UNEQUAL SAMPLES

Model: $y_{iju} = \mu + \alpha_i + \delta_{ij} + \epsilon_{iju}$ $(i = 1, 2, \ldots, k; j = 1, 2, \ldots, n_i; u = 1, 2, \ldots, n_{ij})$

Source of variation	Degrees of freedom	Sum of squares	Mean square	Expected mean square for fixed model (α, δ)
Between main groups	$k - 1$	$S_1 = \sum_i \frac{Y_{i.}^2}{n_i} - \frac{Y^2}{n}$	$s_1^2 = \frac{S_1}{k-1}$	$\sigma^2 + \frac{\sum_i n_i \alpha_i^2}{k-1}$
Subgroups within main groups (experimental error)	$\sum_i n_i - k$	$S_2 = \sum_i \sum_j \frac{Y_{ij.}^2}{n_{ij}} - \sum_i \frac{Y_{i..}^2}{n_{i.}}$	$s_2^2 = \frac{S_2}{\sum_i n_i - k}$	$\sigma^2 + \frac{\sum_i \sum_j n_{ij}\delta_{ij}^2}{\sum_i n_i - k}$
Within subgroups (sampling error)	$n - \sum_i n_i$	$S_e = \sum_i \sum_j \sum_u y_{iju}^2 - \sum_i \sum_j \frac{Y_{ij.}^2}{n_{ij}}$	$s_e^2 = \frac{S_3}{n - \sum_i n_i}$	σ^2
Total	$n - 1$	$S = \sum_i \sum_j \sum_u y_{iju}^2 - \frac{Y^2}{n}$		

Source of variation	Degrees of freedom	Mean square	Expected mean square for		
			Mixed model (α)	Mixed model (δ)	Random model
Between main groups	$k - 1$	s_1^2	$\sigma^2 + b\sigma_\delta^2 + \frac{\sum_i n_i \alpha_i^2}{k-1}$	$\sigma^2 + c\delta_\alpha^2$	$\sigma^2 + b\sigma_\delta^2 + c\sigma_\alpha^2$
Experimental error	$\sum_i n_i - k$	s_2^2	$\sigma^2 + a\sigma_\delta^2$	$\sigma^2 + \frac{\sum_i \sum_j n_{ij}\delta_{ij}^2}{\sum_i n_i - k}$	$\sigma^2 + a\sigma_\delta^2$
Sampling error	$n - \sum_i n_i$	s_e^2	σ^2	σ^2	σ^2
Total	$n - 1$				

where

$$a = \frac{n - \sum_i \frac{\sum_j n_{ij}^2}{n_{i.}}}{\sum_i n_i - k}$$

$$b = \frac{\sum_i \frac{\sum_j n_{ij}^2}{n_i} - \frac{\sum_i \sum_j n_{ij}^2}{n}}{k - 1}$$

$$c = \frac{n - \frac{\sum_i n_i^2}{n}}{k - 1}$$

ANALYSIS OF VARIANCE AND EXPECTED MEAN SQUARES FOR NESTED CLASSIFICATIONS WITH EQUAL SAMPLES

Model: $y_{iju} = \mu + \alpha_i + \delta_{ij} + \epsilon_{iju}$ $(i = 1, 2, \ldots, k; j = 1, 2, \ldots, n; u = 1, 2, \ldots, r)$

Source of variation	Degrees of freedom	Sum of squares	Mean square	Expected mean square for fixed model (α, δ)
Between main groups	$k - 1$	$S_1 = \sum_i \frac{Y_i^2}{nr} - \frac{Y^2}{knr}$	$s_1^2 = \frac{S_1}{k - 1}$	$\sigma^2 + nr \frac{\sum_i \alpha_i^2}{k - 1}$
Experimental error	$k(n - 1)$	$S_2 = \frac{\sum_i \sum_j Y_{ij}^2}{r} - \frac{\sum_i Y_i^2}{nr}$	$s_2^2 = \frac{S_2}{k(n - 1)}$	$\sigma^2 + r \frac{\sum_i \sum_j \delta_{ij}^2}{k(n - 1)}$
Sampling error	$kn(r - 1)$	$S_e = \sum_i \sum_j \sum_u y_{iju}^2 - \frac{\sum_i \sum_j Y_{ij}^2}{r}$	$s_e^2 = \frac{S_e}{kn(r - 1)}$	σ^2
Total	$kn(r - 1)$	$S = \sum_i \sum_j \sum_u y_{iju}^2 - \frac{Y^2}{knr}$		

Source of variation	Degrees of freedom	Mean square	Expected mean square for		
			Mixed model (α)	Mixed model (δ)	Random model
Between main groups	$k - 1$	s_1^2	$\sigma^2 + r\sigma_\delta^2 + nr\left(\frac{\sum \alpha_i^2}{k - 1}\right)$	$\sigma^2 + nr\sigma_\alpha^2$	$\sigma^2 + r\sigma_\delta^2 + nr\sigma_\alpha^2$
Experimental error	$k(n - 1)$	s_2^2	$\sigma^2 + r\sigma_\delta^2$	$\sigma^2 + \frac{r \sum_i \sum_j \delta_{ij}^2}{k(n - 1)}$	$\sigma^2 + r\sigma_\delta^2$
Sampling error	$kn(r - 1)$	s_e^2	σ^2	σ^2	σ^2
Total	$knr - 1$				

where

$a = b = r$
$c = nr$

ANALYSIS OF VARIANCE AND EXPECTED MEAN SQUARES FOR A FIXED MODEL TWO-FACTOR FACTORIAL EXPERIMENT IN A ONE-WAY CLASSIFICATION DESIGN

Model: $y_{iju} = \mu + \alpha_i + \beta_j + (\alpha\beta)_{ij} + \epsilon_{iju}$
$(i = 1, 2, \ldots, c; j = 1, 2, \ldots, r; u = 1, 2, \ldots, n)$

Source of variation	Degrees of freedom	Sum of squares	Mean square	Expected mean square for fixed model $[\alpha, \beta, (\alpha\beta)]$
Treatment combinations	$cr - 1$	$SSTr$	$s_0^2 = \dfrac{SSTr}{cr - 1}$	$\sigma^2 + n\dfrac{\sum_i^c \sum_j^r (\mu_{ij} - \mu)^2}{cr - 1}$
Factor A	$c - 1$	SSA	$s_1^2 = \dfrac{SSA}{c - 1}$	$\sigma^2 + rn\dfrac{\sum_i^c \alpha_i^2}{c - 1}$
Factor B	$r - 1$	SSB	$s_2^2 = \dfrac{SSB}{r - 1}$	$\sigma^2 + cn\dfrac{\sum_j^r \beta_j^2}{r - 1}$
Interaction	$(c - 1)(r - 1)$	$SSAB = SSTr - SSA - SSB$	$s_3^2 = \dfrac{SSAB}{(c - 1)(r - 1)}$	$\sigma^2 + n\dfrac{\sum_i^c \sum_j^r (\alpha\beta)_{ij}^2}{(c - 1)(r - 1)}$
Within (error)	$cr(n - 1)$	$SSW = SST - SSTr$	$s_e^2 = \dfrac{SSW}{cr(n - 1)}$	σ^2
Total	$crn - 1$	SST		

where

$$SSTr = \frac{\sum_i^c \sum_j^r Y_{ij.}^2}{n} - \frac{Y_{...}^2}{crn} \qquad SSA = \frac{\sum_i^c Y_{i..}^2}{rn} - \frac{Y_{...}^2}{crn}$$

$$SSB = \frac{\sum_j^r Y_{.j.}^2}{cn} - \frac{Y_{...}^2}{crn} \qquad SST = \sum_i^c \sum_j^r \sum_u^n y_{iju}^2 - \frac{Y_{...}^2}{crn}$$

$$Y_{ij.} = \sum_u^n y_{iju} \qquad Y_{i..} = \sum_j^r \sum_u^n y_{iju} \qquad Y_{.j.} = \sum_i^c \sum_u^n y_{iju}$$

ANALYSIS OF VARIANCE AND EXPECTED MEAN SQUARES FOR A FIXED MODEL TWO-FACTOR FACTORIAL EXPERIMENT IN A ONE-WAY CLASSIFICATION DESIGN (continued)

Source of variation	Mean square	Expected mean square for	
		Random model	Mixed model (α)
Factor *A*	$s_1^2 = \frac{SSA}{c-1}$	$\sigma^2 + n\sigma_{\alpha\beta}^2 + rn\sigma_\alpha^2$	$\sigma^2 + n\sigma_{\alpha\beta}^2 + rn\frac{\sum_i \alpha_i^2}{c-1}$
Factor *B*	$s_2^2 = \frac{SSB}{r-1}$	$\sigma^2 + n\sigma_{\alpha\beta}^2 + cn\sigma_\beta^2$	$\sigma^2 + cn\sigma_\beta^2$
Interaction	$s_4^2 = \frac{SSAB}{(c-1)(r-1)}$	$\sigma^2 + n\sigma_{\alpha\beta}^2$	$\sigma^2 + n\sigma_{\alpha\beta}^2$
Within (error)	$s_e^2 = \frac{SSW}{cr(n-1)}$	σ^2	σ^2
Total	$s_5^2 = \frac{SST}{crn-1}$		

ANALYSIS OF VARIANCE AND EXPECTED MEAN SQUARES FOR A THREE-FACTOR FACTORIAL EXPERIMENT IN A COMPLETELY RANDOMIZED DESIGN

Model: $y_{ijku} = \mu + \alpha_i + \beta_j + \gamma_k + (\alpha\beta)_{ij} + (\alpha\gamma)_{ik} + (\beta\gamma)_{jk} + (\alpha\beta\gamma)_{ijk} + \epsilon_{ijku}$
$(i = 1, 2, \ldots, c;\ j = 1, 2, \ldots, r;\ k = 1, 2, \ldots, l;\ u = 1, 2, \ldots, n)$

Source of variation	Degrees of freedom	Sum of squares	Mean square	Expected mean square for *Fixed Model*
Factor *A*	$c - 1$	*SSA*	s_1^2	$\sigma^2 + rln\frac{\sum_i \alpha_i^2}{c-1}$
Factor *B*	$r - 1$	*SSB*	s_2^2	$\sigma^2 + cln\frac{\sum_j \beta_j^2}{r-1}$
Factor *C*	$l - 1$	*SSC*	s_3^2	$\sigma^2 + crn\frac{\sum_k \gamma_k^2}{l-1}$
Interaction $A \times B$	$(c-1)(r-1)$	*SSAB*	s_4^2	$\sigma^2 + ln\frac{\sum_i \sum_j (\alpha\beta)_{ij}^2}{(c-1)(r-1)}$

ANALYSIS OF VARIANCE AND EXPECTED MEAN SQUARES FOR A THREE-FACTOR FACTORIAL EXPERIMENT IN A COMPLETELY RANDOMIZED DESIGN (continued)

Source of variation	Degrees of freedom	Sum of squares	Mean square	Expected mean square for *Fixed Model*
Interaction $A \times C$	$(c-1)(l-1)$	*SSAC*	s_5^2	$\sigma^2 + rn\dfrac{\sum_i\sum_k(\alpha\beta)_{ik}^2}{(c-1)(l-1)}$
Interaction $B \times C$	$(r-1)(l-1)$	*SSBC*	s_6^2	$\sigma^2 + cn\dfrac{\sum_j\sum_k(\beta\gamma)_{jk}^2}{(r-1)(l-1)}$
Interaction $A \times B \times C$	$(c-1)(r-1)(l-1)$	*SSABC*	s_7^2	$\sigma^2 + n\dfrac{\sum_i\sum_j\sum_k(\alpha\beta\gamma)_{ijk}^2}{(c-1)(r-1)(l-1)}$
Within (error)	$crl(n-1)$	*SSE*	s_e^2	σ^2
Total	$crln - 1$	*SST*		

where

$$SST = \sum_i\sum_j\sum_k\sum_u y_{ijku}^2 - \frac{Y^2}{crln}$$

$$SSA = \frac{\sum_i Y_i^2}{rln} - \frac{Y^2}{crln}$$

$$SSB = \frac{\sum_j Y_{\cdot j}^2}{cln} - \frac{Y^2}{crln}$$

$$SSC = \frac{\sum_k Y_{\cdot\cdot k}^2}{crn} - \frac{Y^2}{crln}$$

$$SSTr(ABC) = \frac{\sum_i\sum_j\sum_k Y_{ijk}^2}{n} - \frac{Y^2}{crln}$$

$$SSTr(AB) = \frac{\sum_i\sum_j Y_{ij}^2}{ln} - \frac{Y^2}{crln}$$

ANALYSIS OF VARIANCE AND EXPECTED MEAN SQUARES FOR A THREE-FACTOR FACTORIAL EXPERIMENT IN A COMPLETELY RANDOMIZED DESIGN (continued)

$$SSTr(AC) = \frac{\sum_i \sum_k Y^2_{i.k.}}{rn} - \frac{Y^2_{....}}{crln}$$

$$SSTr(BC) = \frac{\sum_i \sum_k Y^2_{.jk.}}{cn} - \frac{Y^2_{....}}{crln}$$

$$SSAB = SSTr(AB) - SSA - SSB$$
$$SSAC = SSTr(AC) - SSA - SSC$$
$$SSBC = SSTr(BC) - SSB - SSC$$
$$SSABC = SSTr(ABC) - SSA - SSB - SSC - SSAB - SSAC - SSBC$$
$$SSE = SST - SSTr(ABC)$$

Source of variation	Mean square	Expected mean square for the Random model	Mixed model (α)	Mixed model (α,β)
Factor A	$s_1^2 = \frac{SSA}{c-1}$	$\sigma^2 + n\sigma^2_{\alpha\beta\gamma} + ln\sigma^2_{\alpha\beta} + rn\sigma^2_{\alpha\gamma} + rln\sigma^2_{\alpha}$	$\sigma^2 + n\sigma^2_{\alpha\beta\gamma} + ln\sigma^2_{\alpha\beta} + rn\sigma^2_{\alpha\gamma} + rln\frac{\sum \alpha_i^2}{c-1}$	$\sigma^2 + rn\sigma^2_{\alpha\gamma} + rln\frac{\sum_i \alpha_i^2}{c-1}$
Factor B	$s_2^2 = \frac{SSB}{r-1}$	$\sigma^2 + n\sigma^2_{\alpha\beta\gamma} + ln\sigma^2_{\alpha\beta} + cn\sigma^2_{\beta\gamma} + cln\sigma^2_{\beta}$	$\sigma^2 + cn\sigma^2_{\beta\gamma} + cln\sigma^2_{\beta}$	$\sigma^2 + cn\sigma^2_{\beta\gamma} + cln\frac{\sum_j \beta_j^2}{r-1}$
Factor C	$s_3^2 = \frac{SSC}{l-1}$	$\sigma^2 + n\sigma^2_{\alpha\beta\gamma} + rn\sigma^2_{\alpha\gamma} + cn\sigma^2_{\beta\gamma} + crn\sigma^2_{\gamma}$	$\sigma^2 + cn\sigma^2_{\beta\gamma} + crn\sigma^2_{\gamma}$	$\sigma^2 + crn\sigma^2_{\gamma}$
$A \times B$	$s_4^2 = \frac{SSAB}{(c-1)(r-1)}$	$\sigma^2 + n\sigma^2_{\alpha\beta\gamma} + ln\sigma^2_{\alpha\beta}$	$\sigma^2 + n\sigma^2_{\alpha\beta\gamma} + ln\sigma^2_{\alpha\beta}$	$\sigma^2 + n\sigma^2_{\alpha\beta\gamma} + ln\frac{\sum_i \sum_j (\alpha\beta)^2_{ij}}{(c-1)(r-1)}$
$A \times C$	$s_5^2 = \frac{SSAC}{(c-1)(l-1)}$	$\sigma^2 + n\sigma^2_{\alpha\beta\gamma} + rn\sigma^2_{\alpha\gamma}$	$\sigma^2 + n\sigma^2_{\alpha\beta\gamma} + rn\sigma^2_{\alpha\gamma}$	$\sigma^2 + rn\sigma^2_{\alpha\gamma}$
$B \times C$	$s_6^2 = \frac{SSBC}{(r-1)(l-1)}$	$\sigma^2 + n\sigma^2_{\alpha\beta\gamma} + cn\sigma^2_{\beta\gamma}$	$\sigma^2 + cn\sigma^2_{\beta\gamma}$	$\sigma^2 + cn\sigma^2_{\beta\gamma}$
$A \times B \times C$	$s_7^2 = \frac{SSABC}{(c-1)(r-1)(l-1)}$	$\sigma^2 + n\sigma^2_{\alpha\beta\gamma}$	$\sigma^2 + n\sigma^2_{\alpha\beta\gamma}$	$\sigma^2 + n\sigma^2_{\alpha\beta\gamma}$
Within (error)	$s_e^2 = \frac{SSE}{crl(n-1)}$	σ^2	σ^2	σ^2
Total	$s_0^2 = \frac{SST}{crln - 1}$			

ANALYSIS OF VARIANCE AND EXPECTED MEAN SQUARES FOR A $t \times t$ LATIN SQUARE

Model: $y_{ij(k)} = \mu + \alpha_i + \beta_j + \gamma_{(k)} + \epsilon_{ij(k)}$

$(i = 1, 2, \ldots, t; j = 1, 2, \ldots, t; k = 1, 2, \ldots, t)$

Source of variation	Degrees of freedom	Sum of squares	Mean square	Expected mean square for fixed model
Columns	$t - 1$	$SSC = \frac{\sum_i Y_{i..}^2}{t} - \frac{Y_{...}^2}{t^2}$	$s_1^2 = \frac{SSC}{t-1}$	$\sigma^2 + t\frac{\sum_i \alpha_i^2}{t-1}$
Rows	$t - 1$	$SSR = \frac{\sum_j Y_{.j.}^2}{t} - \frac{Y_{...}^2}{t^2}$	$s_2^2 = \frac{SSR}{t-1}$	$\sigma^2 + t\frac{\sum_j \beta_j^2}{t-1}$
Treatments	$t - 1$	$SSTr = \frac{\sum_k Y_{..(k)}^2}{t} - \frac{Y_{...}^2}{t^2}$	$s_3^2 = \frac{SSTr}{t-1}$	$\sigma^2 + t\frac{\sum_k \gamma_k^2}{t-1}$
Error	$(t-1)(t-2)$	$SSE = SST - SSC - SSR - SSTr$	$s_e^2 = \frac{SSE}{(t-1)(t-2)}$	σ^2
Total	$t^2 - 1$	$SST = \sum_i \sum_j y_{ij(k)}^2 - \frac{Y_{...}^2}{t^2}$		

Source of variation	Mean square	Expected mean square for: Random model	Mixed model (γ)	Mixed model (α, γ)
Columns	$s_1^2 = \frac{SSC}{t-1}$	$\sigma^2 + t\sigma_\alpha^2$	$\sigma^2 + t\sigma_\alpha^2$	$\sigma^2 + t\frac{\sum_i \alpha_i^2}{t-1}$
Rows	$s_2^2 = \frac{SSR}{t-1}$	$\sigma^2 + t\sigma_\beta^2$	$\sigma^2 + t\sigma_\beta^2$	$\sigma^2 + t\sigma_\beta^2$
Treatments	$s_3^2 = \frac{SSTr}{t-1}$	$\sigma^2 + t\sigma_\gamma^2$	$\sigma^2 + t\frac{\sum_k \gamma_k^2}{t-1}$	$\sigma^2 + t\frac{\sum_k \gamma_k^2}{t-1}$
Error	$s_e^2 = \frac{SSE}{(t-1)(t-2)}$	σ^2	σ^2	σ^2

ANALYSIS OF VARIANCE FOR A GRAECO-LATIN SQUARE

Model: $y_{ijuk} = \mu + \alpha_i + \beta_j + \gamma_u + \delta_k + \epsilon_{ijuk}$ $(i, j, u, k = 1, 2, \ldots, n)$

Source of variation	Degrees of freedom	Sum of squares	Mean square
Factor I (rows)	$n - 1$	$S_1 = \dfrac{\sum_i Y_{i\ldots}^2}{n} - \dfrac{Y_{\ldots\ldots}^2}{n^2}$	$s_1^2 = \dfrac{S_1}{n - 1}$
Factor II (columns)	$n - 1$	$S_2 = \dfrac{\sum_j Y_{.j..}^2}{n} - \dfrac{Y_{\ldots\ldots}^2}{n^2}$	$s_2^2 = \dfrac{S_2}{n - 1}$
Factor III (Latin letters)	$n - 1$	$S_3 = \dfrac{\sum_u Y_{..u.}^2}{n - 1} - \dfrac{Y_{\ldots\ldots}^2}{n^2}$	$s_3^2 = \dfrac{S_3}{n - 1}$
Factor IV (Greek letters)	$n - 1$	$S_4 = \dfrac{\sum_k Y_{\ldots k}^2}{n} - \dfrac{Y_{\ldots\ldots}^2}{n^2}$	$s_4^2 = \dfrac{S_4}{n - 1}$
Residual	$(n - 1)(n - 3)$	S_e = difference	$s_e^2 = \dfrac{S_e}{(n - 1)(n - 3)}$
Total	$n^2 - 1$	$S = \sum_i \sum_j y_{ijuk}^2 - \dfrac{Y_{\ldots\ldots}^2}{n^2}$	

ANALYSIS OF VARIANCE FOR A YOUDEN SQUARE

Model: $y_{iju} = \mu + \alpha_i + \beta_j + \gamma_u + \epsilon_{iju}$
$(i = 1, 2, \ldots, b; j = 1, 2, \ldots, t(= b); u = 1, 2, \ldots, k(<t))$

Source of variation	Degrees of freedom	Sum of squares	Mean square
Blocks (crude)		$S_1 = \sum_i \dfrac{Y_{i..}^2}{k} - \dfrac{Y_{\ldots}^2}{bk}$	
Treatments (adjusted)	$t - 1$	$S_2 = \dfrac{t - 1}{bk^2(k - 1)} \sum_j \left(kY_{.j.}^2 - \sum_{i(j)} Y_{i..}^2\right)$	$s_1^2 = \dfrac{S_2}{t - 1}$
Treatments (crude)		$S_3 = \sum_j \dfrac{Y_{.j.}^2}{r} - \dfrac{Y_{\ldots}^2}{tr}$	
Blocks (adjusted)	$b - 1$	$S_4 = \dfrac{b - 1}{bk^2(k - 1)} \sum_i \left(rY_{i..}^2 - \sum_{j(i)} Y_{.j.}^2\right)$	$s_2^2 = \dfrac{S_4}{b - 1}$
Factor II (γ)	$k - 1$	$S_5 = \dfrac{\sum_u Y_{..u}^2}{k} - \dfrac{Y_{\ldots}^2}{bk}$	$s_3^2 = \dfrac{S_5}{k - 1}$

ANALYSIS OF VARIANCE FOR A YOUDEN SQUARE (continued)

Source of variation	Degrees of freedom	Sum of squares	Mean square
Residual	$bk - t - b - k + 2$	$S_e = S - (S_1 + S_2 + S_5)$ $= S - (S_3 + S_4 + S_5)$	$s_e^2 = \dfrac{S_e}{bk - t - b - k + 2}$
Total	$bk - 1$	$S = \sum_i \sum_j y_{iju}^2 - \dfrac{Y^2}{bk}$	

(Note that $S_1 + S_2 = S_3 + S_4$)

ANALYSIS OF VARIANCE FOR BALANCED INCOMPLETE BLOCK (BIB)

Model: $y_{iju} = \mu + \alpha_i + \beta_j + \epsilon_{iju} \quad (i = 1, 2, \ldots, b; j = 1, 2, \ldots, t; u = n_{ij})$

Source of variation	Degrees of freedom	Sum of squares	Mean square
Blocks	$b - 1$	$S_1 = \dfrac{\sum_i Y_i^2}{k} - \dfrac{Y^2}{bk}$	$s_1^2 = \dfrac{S_1}{b - 1}$
Treatments (adjusted)	$t - 1$	$S_2 = \dfrac{t - 1}{bk^2(k - 1)} \sum_j \left[kY_j - \sum_{uij} Y_{i.}\right]^2$	$s_2^2 = \dfrac{S_2}{t - 1}$
Residual	$bk - t - b + 1$	S_e = difference	$s_e^2 = \dfrac{S_e}{bk - t - b + 1}$
Total	$bk - 1$	$S = \sum_i \sum_j y_{iju}^2 - \dfrac{Y^2}{bk}$	

where

t = number of treatment levels
b = number of blocks
k = number of treatment levels per block
r = number of replications of each treatment level
λ = number of blocks in which any given pair of treatment levels appear together
$bk = tr$
$r(k - 1) = \lambda(t - 1)$

GENERAL LINEAR MODEL

by Dr. Rolf E. Bargmann

1. NOTATION

A matrix will be denoted by bold-face capital letters, e.g., if **A** has m rows and n columns, we may often specify $\mathbf{A} = \mathbf{A}(m \times n)$

$$\mathbf{A} = \begin{bmatrix} a_{11} & a_{12} & \cdots & a_{1n} \\ a_{21} & a_{22} & \cdots & a_{2n} \\ \cdot & \cdot & \cdots & \cdot \\ a_{m1} & a_{m2} & \cdots & a_{mn} \end{bmatrix}.$$

$\mathbf{A}'$ denotes the transpose of **A**.
$(\mathbf{A})_{ij} = a_{ij}$ denotes the element in the i'th row and j'th column of **A**.
I denotes the identity matrix.
$\mathbf{D}_x$ denotes a diagonal matrix. The subscript indicates the terms in the diagonal.
$\tilde{\mathbf{T}}$, $\tilde{\mathbf{U}}$, i.e., any matrix with a tilde ($\tilde{}$) above it will denote a lower triangular matrix.

A column vector will be denoted in general, by a lower-case bold-face letter, e.g.,

$$\mathbf{x}, \mathbf{y}, \mathbf{j}, \boldsymbol{\beta}, \boldsymbol{\xi}; \mathbf{x} = \begin{bmatrix} x_1 \\ x_2 \\ \cdot \\ \cdot \\ \cdot \\ x_p \end{bmatrix}.$$

Occasionally, capital bold-face letters represent column vectors. Examples are as follows:

T (vector of treatment totals)
B (vector of Block totals).

A lower case letter with a prime denotes a row vector, e.g.,

$$\mathbf{x}' = [x_1 \quad x_2 \quad x_3 \quad \cdots \quad x_p] .$$

2. THE GENERAL LINEAR MODEL

2.1. The Simple Regression Model

$$y_i = \alpha + \beta x_i + e_i ,$$

where x_i is a fixed concomitant variable whose values are assumed to be known before an experiment is performed and is not subject to chance. Let E denote the expectation operator, var and cov the (population) variances and covariances, respectively.

$E(e_i) = 0$, var $(e_i) = \sigma^2$, cov $(e_i,e_j) = 0$, i.e., $E(y_i) = \alpha + \beta x_i$.

If we write

$$\begin{aligned} y_1 &= \alpha + \beta x_1 + e_1 \\ y_2 &= \alpha + \beta x_2 + e_2 \\ \cdot \quad & \quad \cdot \quad \cdot \quad \cdot \\ y_n &= \alpha + \beta x_n + e_n , \end{aligned}$$

we can write, in matrix form

$$\begin{bmatrix} y_1 \\ y_2 \\ y_3 \\ \cdot \\ y_n \end{bmatrix} = \begin{bmatrix} 1 & x_1 \\ 1 & x_2 \\ 1 & x_3 \\ \cdot & \cdot \\ 1 & x_n \end{bmatrix} \begin{bmatrix} \alpha \\ \beta \end{bmatrix} + \begin{bmatrix} e_1 \\ e_2 \\ e_3 \\ \cdot \\ e_n \end{bmatrix}$$

$$\mathbf{y} \quad = \quad \mathbf{A} \quad\; \boldsymbol{\xi} \;+\; \mathbf{e}\,,$$

where **A** is the design matrix and can be also written in the form

$$\mathbf{A} = [\underset{(1)}{\mathbf{j}}\,,\ \underset{(1)}{\mathbf{x}}](n).$$

The numbers in parentheses denote the order of the matrix.

j is a column vector containing all ones.
x is a column vector of all concomitant observations.

The simple regression model is frequently written in the form

$$y_i = \mu + \beta(x_i - \bar{x}) + e_i\,,$$

where $\mu = \alpha + \beta\bar{x}$.

This, too, can be written in the general linear model form

$$\begin{bmatrix} y_1 \\ y_2 \\ \cdot \\ \cdot \\ \cdot \\ y_n \end{bmatrix} = \begin{bmatrix} 1 & (x_1 - \bar{x}) \\ 1 & (x_2 - \bar{x}) \\ \cdot & \cdot \\ \cdot & \cdot \\ \cdot & \cdot \\ 1 & (x_n - \bar{x}) \end{bmatrix} \begin{bmatrix} \mu \\ \beta \end{bmatrix} + \begin{bmatrix} e_1 \\ e_2 \\ \cdot \\ \cdot \\ \cdot \\ e_n \end{bmatrix}$$

$$\mathbf{y} \quad = \quad \mathbf{A} \quad\quad \boldsymbol{\xi} \;+\; \mathbf{e}\,,$$

where $\mathbf{A} = [\mathbf{j}, (\mathbf{x} - \bar{x}\mathbf{j})]$.

2.2. Multiple Regression Model

$$y_i = \beta_0 + \beta_1 x_{1i} + \beta_2 x_{2i} + \beta_3 x_{3i} + \cdots \beta_k x_{ki} + e_i\,.$$

Assumption: $E(e_i) = 0$,

$$\text{var}\,(y_i) = \text{var}\,(e_i) = \sigma^2,$$
$$\text{cov}\,(y_i, y_j) = 0\,.$$

If we write

$$\begin{aligned} y_1 &= \beta_0 + \beta_1 x_{11} + \beta_2 x_{21} + \beta_3 x_{31} + \cdots \beta_k x_{k1} + e_1 \\ y_2 &= \beta_0 + \beta_1 x_{12} + \beta_2 x_{22} + \beta_3 x_{32} + \cdots \beta_k x_{k2} + e_2 \\ &\cdot \qquad \cdot \qquad \cdot \qquad \cdot \\ y_n &= \beta_0 + \beta_n x_{1n} + \beta_2 x_{2n} + \beta_3 x_{3n} + \cdots \beta_k x_{kn} + e_n\,, \end{aligned}$$

we can write

$$\begin{bmatrix} y_1 \\ y_2 \\ \cdot \\ y_n \end{bmatrix} = \begin{bmatrix} 1 & x_{11} & x_{21} & x_{31} & \cdots & x_{k1} \\ 1 & x_{12} & x_{22} & x_{32} & \cdots & x_{k2} \\ \cdot & \cdot & \cdot & \cdot & \cdots & \cdot \\ 1 & x_{1n} & x_{2n} & x_{3n} & \cdots & x_{kn} \end{bmatrix} \begin{bmatrix} \beta_0 \\ \beta_1 \\ \beta_2 \\ \beta_3 \\ \cdot \\ \beta_k \end{bmatrix} + \begin{bmatrix} e_1 \\ e_2 \\ e_3 \\ \cdot \\ e_n \end{bmatrix}$$

$$\mathbf{y} \quad = \quad \mathbf{A} \quad \boldsymbol{\xi} + e ,$$

where $\mathbf{A} = [\underset{(1)}{\mathbf{j}}, \underset{(k)}{\mathbf{X}}](n)$, and $\mathbf{X}$ denotes the matrix of all observations on all concomitant variables.

2.3. One-way Classification Analysis of Variance

Model

$$y_{ij} = \mu + \tau_i + e_{ij}$$

where μ = general effect
τ_i = treatment effects
e_{ij} = experimental error,
v treatments with effects $\tau_1, \tau_2, \ldots, \tau_v$; $j = 1, 2, 3, \ldots n_i$.

$$\begin{array}{lllll}
y_{11} = \mu + \tau_1 & & & + e_{11} \\
y_{12} = \mu + \tau_1 & & & + e_{12} \\
\cdot \quad \cdot & & & \cdot \\
y_{1n_1} = \mu + \tau_1 & & & + e_{1n_1} \\ \hline
y_{21} = \mu & + \tau_2 & & + e_{21} \\
\cdot \quad \cdot & \cdot & & \cdot \\
y_{2n_2} = \mu & + \tau_2 & & + e_{2n_2} \\ \hline
\cdot \quad \cdot & \cdot & & \cdot \\ \hline
y_{v1} = \mu & & + \tau_v & + e_{v1} \\
\cdot \quad \cdot & & \cdot & \cdot \\
y_{vn_v} = \mu & & + \tau_v & + e_{vn_v} .
\end{array}$$

We can again write this

$$\begin{bmatrix} y_{11} \\ y_{12} \\ \cdot \\ y_{1n_1} \\ y_{21} \\ \cdot \\ y_{2n_2} \\ \cdot \\ y_{v1} \\ y_{v2} \\ \cdot \\ y_{vn_v} \end{bmatrix} = \begin{bmatrix} 1 & 1 & 0 & 0 & \cdots & 0 & 0 \\ 1 & 1 & 0 & 0 & \cdots & 0 & 0 \\ \cdot & \cdot & \cdot & \cdot & \cdots & \cdot & \cdot \\ 1 & 1 & 0 & 0 & \cdots & 0 & 0 \\ \hline 1 & 0 & 1 & 0 & \cdots & 0 & 0 \\ \cdot & \cdot & \cdot & \cdot & \cdots & \cdot & \cdot \\ 1 & 0 & 1 & 0 & \cdots & 0 & 0 \\ \hline \cdot & \cdot & \cdot & \cdot & \cdots & \cdot & \cdot \\ \hline 1 & 0 & 0 & 0 & \cdots & 0 & 1 \\ 1 & 0 & 0 & 0 & \cdots & 0 & 1 \\ \cdot & \cdot & \cdot & \cdot & \cdots & \cdot & \cdot \\ 1 & 0 & 0 & 0 & & 0 & 1 \end{bmatrix} \begin{bmatrix} \mu \\ \tau_1 \\ \tau_2 \\ \cdot \\ \tau_v \end{bmatrix} + \mathbf{e}$$

$$\mathbf{y} \quad = \quad \mathbf{A} \quad \boldsymbol{\xi} + \mathbf{e} .$$

The design matrix **A** can be written

$$\mathbf{A} = [\underset{(1)}{\mathbf{j}}, \underset{(v)}{\mathbf{A}_\tau}](n),$$

where

$$\mathbf{A}_\tau = \begin{matrix}(n_1)\\(n_2)\\ \cdot \\ (n_v)\end{matrix}\begin{bmatrix}\mathbf{j} & 0 & 0 & \cdots & 0\\ 0 & \mathbf{j} & 0 & \cdots & 0\\ \cdot & \cdot & \cdot & \cdots & \cdot\\ 0 & 0 & 0 & \cdots & \mathbf{j}\end{bmatrix}$$

and the parameter vector can also be written

$$\boldsymbol{\xi} = \begin{bmatrix}\mu\\ \boldsymbol{\tau}\end{bmatrix}.$$

2.4. Two-way Classification (Two Factors Factorial)

Model

$$y_{ijk} = \mu + \alpha_i + \beta_j + \delta_{ij} + e_{ijk} \, ,$$

where μ = general effect
α_i = factor A effects (usually row effects)
β_j = factor B effects (usually column effects)
δ_{ij} = interaction effects.

For example:

$$\begin{bmatrix}\mathbf{y}_{11}\\ \mathbf{y}_{12}\\ \mathbf{y}_{13}\\ \mathbf{y}_{21}\\ \mathbf{y}_{22}\\ \mathbf{y}_{23}\end{bmatrix} = \begin{matrix}(n_{11})\\(n_{12})\\(n_{13})\\(n_{21})\\(n_{22})\\(n_{23})\end{matrix}\begin{bmatrix}\mathbf{j} & \mathbf{j} & 0 & \mathbf{j} & 0 & 0 & \mathbf{j} & 0 & 0 & 0 & 0 & 0\\ \mathbf{j} & \mathbf{j} & 0 & 0 & \mathbf{j} & 0 & 0 & \mathbf{j} & 0 & 0 & 0 & 0\\ \mathbf{j} & \mathbf{j} & 0 & 0 & 0 & \mathbf{j} & 0 & 0 & \mathbf{j} & 0 & 0 & 0\\ \mathbf{j} & 0 & \mathbf{j} & \mathbf{j} & 0 & 0 & 0 & 0 & 0 & \mathbf{j} & 0 & 0\\ \mathbf{j} & 0 & \mathbf{j} & 0 & \mathbf{j} & 0 & 0 & 0 & 0 & 0 & \mathbf{j} & 0\\ \mathbf{j} & 0 & \mathbf{j} & 0 & 0 & \mathbf{j} & 0 & 0 & 0 & 0 & 0 & \mathbf{j}\end{bmatrix}\begin{bmatrix}\mu\\ \alpha_1\\ \alpha_2\\ \beta_1\\ \beta_2\\ \beta_3\\ \delta_{11}\\ \delta_{12}\\ \delta_{13}\\ \delta_{21}\\ \delta_{22}\\ \delta_{23}\end{bmatrix} + \mathbf{e}$$

$$\mathbf{y} \quad = \quad \mathbf{A} \quad \boldsymbol{\xi} \quad + \mathbf{e} \, .$$

2.5. Analysis of Covariance

Analysis of covariance is equivalent to analysis of variance with one or more concomitant variables added.

For simplicity, let us take one-way classification and one concomitant variable.

Model

$$y_{ij} = \mu + \tau_i + \beta x_{ij} + e_{ij} \, .$$

As a vector equation, this model reads

$$
\begin{array}{lllllll}
y_{11} & = \mu & + \tau_1 & & & + \beta x_{11} & + e_{11} \\
y_{12} & = \mu & + \tau_1 & & & + \beta x_{12} & + e_{12} \\
\cdot & \cdot & \cdot & & & \cdot & \cdot \\
y_{1n_1} & = \mu & + \tau_1 & & & + \beta x_{1n_1} & + e_{1n_1} \\
\hline
y_{21} & = \mu & & + \tau_2 & & + \beta x_{21} & + e_{21} \\
\cdot & \cdot & & \cdot & & \cdot & \cdot \\
y_{2n_2} & = \mu & & + \tau_2 & & + \beta x_{2n_2} & + e_{2n_2} \\
\hline
y_{31} & = \mu & & & + \tau_3 & + \beta x_{31} & + e_{31} \\
\cdot & \cdot & & & \cdot & \cdot & \cdot \\
y_{3n_3} & = \mu & & & + \tau_3 & + \beta x_{3n_3} & + e_{3n_3}
\end{array}
$$

Let $\mathbf{x}_1$, $\mathbf{x}_2$, and $\mathbf{x}_3$ denote the concomitant observations in each group, then

$$
\begin{bmatrix} y_{11} \\ y_{12} \\ \cdot \\ \cdot \\ \cdot \\ y_{1n_1} \\ y_{21} \\ \cdot \\ \cdot \\ \cdot \\ y_{2n_2} \\ y_{31} \\ \cdot \\ \cdot \\ \cdot \\ y_{3n_3} \end{bmatrix}
=
\begin{bmatrix} \mathbf{j} & \mathbf{j} & \mathbf{0} & \mathbf{0} & \mathbf{x}_1 \\ \mathbf{j} & \mathbf{0} & \mathbf{j} & \mathbf{0} & \mathbf{x}_2 \\ \mathbf{j} & \mathbf{0} & \mathbf{0} & \mathbf{j} & \mathbf{x}_3 \end{bmatrix}
\begin{bmatrix} \mu \\ \tau_1 \\ \tau_2 \\ \tau_3 \\ \beta \end{bmatrix}
+ \mathbf{e}
$$

$$\mathbf{y} \quad = \quad \mathbf{A} \quad \boldsymbol{\xi} \; + \mathbf{e} \, .$$

With the above illustrations, it is clear that we can write a great variety of models in the general linear model form

$$\mathbf{y} = \mathbf{A}\boldsymbol{\xi} + \mathbf{e} \, .$$

3. SUMMARY OF RULES FOR MATRIX OPERATIONS

3.1. Let $E(\mathbf{y}) = \boldsymbol{\mu}$, var $(\mathbf{y}) = \boldsymbol{\Sigma}$, a symmetric matrix containing all possible variances and covariances. Then, $E(\mathbf{My}) = \mathbf{M}\boldsymbol{\mu}$, var $(\mathbf{My}) = \mathbf{M}\boldsymbol{\Sigma}\mathbf{M}'$, for any conforming matrix $\mathbf{M}$. $E(\mathbf{y}'\mathbf{M}) = \boldsymbol{\mu}'\mathbf{M}$, var $(\mathbf{y}'\mathbf{M}) = \mathbf{M}'\boldsymbol{\Sigma}\mathbf{M}$.

3.2. Partitioning of Determinants

$$
\begin{vmatrix} \mathbf{A} & \mathbf{B} \\ \mathbf{C} & \mathbf{D} \end{vmatrix} = |\mathbf{A}| \, |\mathbf{D} - \mathbf{C}\mathbf{A}^{-1}\mathbf{B}| \text{ if } \mathbf{A}^{-1} \text{ exists} \, .
$$

$$
= |\mathbf{D}| \, |\mathbf{A} - \mathbf{B}\mathbf{D}^{-1}\mathbf{C}| \text{ if } \mathbf{D}^{-1} \text{ exists} \, .
$$

3.3. Inverse of a Partitioned Matrix

$$\begin{bmatrix} \mathbf{A} & \mathbf{B} \\ \mathbf{C} & \mathbf{D} \end{bmatrix}^{-1} = \begin{bmatrix} \mathbf{X} & \mathbf{Y} \\ \mathbf{Z} & \mathbf{U} \end{bmatrix}$$

$$\begin{aligned} \text{where } \mathbf{X} &= [\mathbf{A} - \mathbf{B}\mathbf{D}^{-1}\mathbf{C}]^{-1} \\ \mathbf{U} &= [\mathbf{D} - \mathbf{C}\mathbf{A}^{-1}\mathbf{B}]^{-1} \\ \mathbf{Y} &= -\mathbf{A}^{-1}\mathbf{B}\mathbf{U} \\ \mathbf{Z} &= -\mathbf{D}^{-1}\mathbf{C}\mathbf{X}\ . \end{aligned}$$

3.3.1. *Symmetric Case*

$$\begin{bmatrix} \mathbf{A}_{11} & \mathbf{A}_{12} \\ \mathbf{A}_{12}' & \mathbf{A}_{22} \end{bmatrix}^{-1} = \begin{bmatrix} \mathbf{A}^{11} & \mathbf{A}^{12} \\ (\mathbf{A}^{12})' & \mathbf{A}^{22} \end{bmatrix}$$

$$\begin{aligned} \text{where } \mathbf{A}^{11} &= [\mathbf{A}_{11} - \mathbf{A}_{12}\mathbf{A}_{22}^{-1}\mathbf{A}_{12}']^{-1} \\ \mathbf{A}^{22} &= [\mathbf{A}_{22} - \mathbf{A}_{12}'\mathbf{A}_{11}^{-1}\mathbf{A}_{12}]^{-1} \\ \mathbf{A}^{12} &= -\mathbf{A}^{11}\mathbf{A}_{12}\mathbf{A}_{22}^{-1} \\ \text{or } \mathbf{A}^{12} &= -\mathbf{A}_{11}^{-1}\mathbf{A}_{12}\mathbf{A}^{22}\ . \end{aligned}$$

Computational steps: Order the sets in such a way that $\mathbf{A}_{22}$ is the smaller matrix.

a. Obtain $\mathbf{A}_{22}^{-1}$
b. Multiply $\mathbf{A}_{12}\mathbf{A}_{22}^{-1}$
c. Obtain $\mathbf{A}_{12}\mathbf{A}_{22}^{-1}\mathbf{A}_{12}'$
d. Obtain $\mathbf{A}_{11} - \mathbf{A}_{12}\mathbf{A}_{22}^{-1}\mathbf{A}_{12}'$
e. Invert the matrix in *d.*; thus obtain $\mathbf{A}^{11}$
f. Obtain $\mathbf{A}^{11}\mathbf{A}_{12}\mathbf{A}_{22}^{-1}$ by multiplying matrices from steps *e.* and *b.*
g. Change all signs in *f.*; thus obtain $\mathbf{A}^{12}$.
h. Obtain $(\mathbf{A}^{12})'$ by transposing *g.*
i. Obtain $\mathbf{A}_{12}'\mathbf{A}^{12}$, the latter factor from *g.*
j. Obtain $\mathbf{I} - \mathbf{A}_{12}'\mathbf{A}^{12}$, i.e., change all signs in off-diagonal elements of the matrix in step *i.* and complement diagonal elements to 1.
k. Obtain $\mathbf{A}_{22}^{-1}[\mathbf{I} - \mathbf{A}_{12}'\mathbf{A}^{12}]$, i.e., premultiply the matrix in *j.* by $\mathbf{A}_{22}^{-1}$ obtained in step *a.* This is $\mathbf{A}^{22}$.

3.4. Characteristic Roots

a. ch $(\mathbf{AB})$ = ch $(\mathbf{BA})$ except, possibly, for zero roots.
b. Corollary: tr $(\mathbf{AB})$ = tr $(\mathbf{BA})$.
c. If ch $(\mathbf{A}) = \lambda_i$, ch $(\mathbf{A}^{-1}) = 1/\lambda_i$, and ch $(\mathbf{I} \pm \mathbf{A}) = 1 \pm \lambda_i$.

3.5. Differentiation

3.5.1. *Definitions:*

Let f be a scalar function of $x_1, x_2, \ldots x_p$.

Then $\partial f/\partial \mathbf{x}$ denotes a column vector whose ith element is $\partial f/\partial x_i$.

Let f be a scalar function of $x_{11}, x_{12} \ldots x_{1q}, x_{21}, x_{22} \ldots x_{2q}, \ldots x_{p1}, x_{p2}, \ldots x_{pq}$. Then $\partial f/\partial \mathbf{X}$ denotes a matrix whose (i, j) element is $\partial f/\partial x_{ij}$. Note that, in this definition, x_{ij} denotes the element in the i'th row and j'th column of $\mathbf{X}$. If there are any functional relations between the elements of $\mathbf{X}$ (as, for instance, in a symmetric matrix) these relations will be *disregarded* in the above definition. In other words, x_{ij} denotes the variable in the i'th row and j'th column of $\mathbf{X}$, and x_{ji} denotes that in the j'th row and i'th column. If the two happen to be identical, a new symbol will be in order. For example, if $x_{ij} = x_{ji} = y_{ij}$, say, $\partial f/\partial y_{ij} = \partial f/\partial x_{ij} \cdot \partial x_{ij}/\partial y_{ij} + \partial f/\partial x_{ji} \cdot \partial x_{ji}/\partial y_{ij} = \partial f/\partial x_{ij} + \partial f/\partial x_{ji} = (\partial f/\partial \mathbf{X})_{ij} + (\partial f/\partial \mathbf{X})_{ji}$. Here, y_{ij} is the symbol for that distinct variable which occurs in two places in $\mathbf{X}$.

If $y_1, y_2, \ldots y_p$ are functions of x, $\partial \mathbf{y}'/\partial x$ denotes the row vector whose i'th element is $\partial y_i/\partial x$.

If $y_{11}, y_{12}, \ldots y_{1q}, y_{21}, \ldots y_{2q}, \ldots y_{p1}, \ldots y_{pq}$ are functions of x, $\partial \mathbf{Y}/\partial x$ denotes the matrix whose (i,j) element is $\partial y_{ij}/\partial x$.

If each of the quantities $y_1, y_2, \ldots y_q$ is a function of the variables $x_1, x_2, \ldots x_p$, $\partial \mathbf{y}'/\partial \mathbf{x}$ denotes a matrix of order (pxq) whose (i,j) element is $\partial y_j/\partial x_i$. *Note the interchange of subscripts.*

3.5.2. *Rules:*

1. $\partial(\mathbf{x}'\mathbf{x})/\partial \mathbf{x} = 2\mathbf{x}$
2. $\partial(\mathbf{x}'\mathbf{Q}\mathbf{x})/\partial \mathbf{x} = \mathbf{Q}\mathbf{x} + \mathbf{Q}'\mathbf{x}$
3. $\partial(\mathbf{x}'\mathbf{Q}\mathbf{x})/\partial \mathbf{x} = 2\mathbf{Q}\mathbf{x}$ if $\mathbf{Q}$ is symmetric.
4. $\partial(\mathbf{a}'\mathbf{x})/\partial \mathbf{x} = \mathbf{a}$
5. $\partial(\mathbf{a}'\mathbf{Q}\mathbf{x})/\partial \mathbf{x} = \mathbf{Q}'\mathbf{a}$
6. $\partial \text{ tr } (\mathbf{A}\mathbf{X})/\partial \mathbf{X} = \mathbf{A}'$
7. $\partial \text{ tr } (\mathbf{X}\mathbf{A})/\partial \mathbf{X} = \mathbf{A}'$
8. $\partial \log |\mathbf{X}|/\partial \mathbf{X} = (\mathbf{X}')^{-1}$, if $\mathbf{X}$ is square and nonsingular.
9. "Chain Rule No. 1": $\partial \mathbf{y}'/\partial \mathbf{x} = \partial \mathbf{z}'/\partial \mathbf{x} \cdot \partial \mathbf{y}'/\partial \mathbf{z}$.
10. $\partial(\mathbf{x}'\mathbf{A})/\partial \mathbf{x} = \mathbf{A}$
11. If $\mathbf{e} = \mathbf{b} - \mathbf{A}'\mathbf{x}$, $\partial(\mathbf{e}'\mathbf{e})/\partial \mathbf{x} = \partial \mathbf{e}'/\partial \mathbf{x} \cdot \partial(\mathbf{e}'\mathbf{e})/\partial \mathbf{e}$ (according to rule 9), $= -2\mathbf{A}'\mathbf{e}$ (by rules 10 and 1).
12. "Chain Rule No. 2": If the scalar z is related to a scalar x through variables y_{ij} ($i = 1, 2, \cdots p; j = 1, 2 \cdots q$),

$$\partial z/\partial x = \text{tr } [\partial z/\partial \mathbf{Y} \cdot \partial \mathbf{Y}'/\partial x]$$

or

$$\partial z/\partial x = \text{tr } [\partial z/\partial \mathbf{Y}' \cdot \partial \mathbf{Y}/\partial x]$$

This chain rule is correct regardless of any functional relationships which may exist between the elements of $\mathbf{Y}$.

3.6. Some Additional Definitions and Rules

$\mathbf{j}$ denotes a column vector, each element of which is 1. Hence $\mathbf{j}'\mathbf{A}$ is a row vector whose elements are the column sums of $\mathbf{A}$, and $\mathbf{A}\mathbf{j}$ denotes a column vector whose elements are the row sums of $\mathbf{A}$. $\mathbf{j}'\mathbf{A}\mathbf{j}$ denotes the sum of all elements in the matrix $\mathbf{A}$.

$\mathbf{I}$ denotes the identity matrix. If the order must be stated it will be added in parentheses. Hence $\mathbf{I}(p)$ denotes a $(p \times p)$ identity matrix.

If a tilde (˜) is placed above a matrix, the matrix is assumed to be triangular. For definiteness, the untransposed matrix

$$\tilde{\mathbf{T}} = \begin{bmatrix} t_{11} & 0 & 0 & \cdots & 0 \\ t_{21} & t_{22} & 0 & \cdots & 0 \\ t_{31} & t_{32} & t_{33} & \cdots & 0 \\ \cdot & \cdot & \cdot & \cdots & \cdot \\ t_{p1} & t_{p2} & t_{p3} & \cdots & t_{pp} \end{bmatrix}$$

is a "lower" triangular matrix, whereas the transposed matrix

$$\tilde{\mathbf{T}}' = \begin{bmatrix} t_{11} & t_{21} & t_{31} & \cdots & t_{p1} \\ 0 & t_{22} & t_{32} & \cdots & t_{p2} \\ 0 & 0 & t_{33} & \cdots & t_{p3} \\ \cdot & \cdot & \cdot & \cdots & \cdot \\ 0 & 0 & 0 & \cdots & t_{pp} \end{bmatrix}$$

is an "upper" triangular matrix.

If $\tilde{\mathbf{T}}$ is lower triangular, so is $\tilde{\mathbf{T}}^{-1}$.

If $\mathbf{Q}$ is a symmetric, positive-definite matrix, we can find, uniquely, a real matrix $\tilde{\mathbf{T}}$, such that $\mathbf{Q} = \tilde{\mathbf{T}}\tilde{\mathbf{T}}'$, provided we let the diagonal elements of $\tilde{\mathbf{T}}$ be positive. This matrix and its inverse can be readily obtained from the forward Doolittle solution. If, in each cycle, we divide each element of the next-to-last row (the row which is immediately above the one beginning with unity) by the square-root of the "leading" (first) element, we obtain $\tilde{\mathbf{T}}'$ on the left and $\tilde{\mathbf{T}}^{-1}$ on the right-hand side.

If $\mathbf{Q}$ is a $(p \times p)$, symmetric, positive-semidefinite matrix of rank r, the matrix $\tilde{\mathbf{T}}$ obtained in the above manner will have zeros to the right of the r'th column. $\mathbf{Q}$ can then be represented as

$$\mathbf{Q} = \begin{matrix} (r) \\ (p-r) \end{matrix} \overset{(r)}{\begin{bmatrix} \tilde{\mathbf{T}}_1 \\ \mathbf{T}_2 \end{bmatrix}} [\underset{(r)}{\tilde{\mathbf{T}}_1'} \quad , \quad \underset{(p-r)}{\mathbf{T}_2'}],$$

where, of course, only $\tilde{\mathbf{T}}_1$ is triangular. This is an important computational device in connection with rule 3.4.a. on characteristic roots. For, if the largest root of $\mathbf{AB}$ is desired, where both $\mathbf{A}$ and $\mathbf{B}$ are symmetric, but $\mathbf{A}$ is of low rank, we can obtain the representation

$$\mathbf{A} = \begin{matrix} (r) \\ (p-r) \end{matrix} \underset{(r)}{\begin{bmatrix} \tilde{\mathbf{T}}_1 \\ \mathbf{T}_2 \end{bmatrix}} [\tilde{\mathbf{T}}_1' \, , \, \mathbf{T}_2']$$

by the forward Doolittle solution. Then, by 3.4.a., $\text{ch}\,(\mathbf{AB}) = \text{ch}\left([\tilde{\mathbf{T}}_1' \, , \, \mathbf{T}_2']\mathbf{B}\begin{bmatrix} \tilde{\mathbf{T}}_1 \\ \mathbf{T}_2 \end{bmatrix}\right)$, and the matrix in parentheses is of small order and symmetric.

$\mathbf{D}_u$ denotes a diagonal matrix whose non-zero elements are $u_1, u_2 \cdots u_p$.

4. PRINCIPLE OF MINIMIZING QUADRATIC FORMS AND GAUSS MARKOV THEOREM

4.1. Some Remarks on Multivariate Distributions

In univariate situation, suppose we have a random variable x, such that

$$E(x) = \mu$$
$$\text{var}\,(x) = \sigma^2 .$$

If we want to find a random variable y, such that

$$E(y) = 0 \qquad \text{and} \qquad \text{var}\,(y) = 1 ,$$

i.e., we are to find y such that it has mean 0 and variance 1, we perform the "standardization"

$$y = \frac{x - \mu}{\sigma} .$$

We also recall that, if y is normally distributed,

$$y^2 = \frac{(x-\mu)^2}{\sigma^2} = \chi^2 \text{ with 1 d.f} .$$

In multivariate situations, we have random variables $\mathbf{x}$ such that

$$E(\mathbf{x}) = \boldsymbol{\mu} \qquad \text{and} \qquad \text{var}\,(\mathbf{x}) = \Sigma$$

and we wish to find $\mathbf{y}$ such that

$$E(\mathbf{y}) = \mathbf{0} \qquad \text{and} \qquad \text{var}\,(\mathbf{y}) = \mathbf{I} .$$

To obtain this, we will proceed as follows: Let

$$\mathbf{\Sigma} = \mathbf{\Gamma}\mathbf{\Gamma}',$$

where $\mathbf{\Gamma}$ is a lower triangular matrix, which, given $\mathbf{\Sigma}$, can be obtained conveniently as a by-product of the forward Doolittle analysis. Then,

$$\mathbf{\Sigma}^{-1} = (\mathbf{\Gamma}')^{-1}\mathbf{\Gamma}^{-1} .$$

Now, let

$$\begin{aligned} y &= \mathbf{\Gamma}^{-1}(\mathbf{x} - \boldsymbol{\mu}) \\ E(\mathbf{y}) &= \mathbf{\Gamma}^{-1}E(\mathbf{x} - \boldsymbol{\mu}) = \mathbf{0} \end{aligned}$$

and

$$\begin{aligned} \text{var}(\mathbf{y}) &= \mathbf{\Gamma}^{-1}\,\text{var}(\mathbf{x} - \boldsymbol{\mu})(\mathbf{\Gamma}')^{-1} \\ &= \mathbf{\Gamma}^{-1}\,\text{var}(\mathbf{x})(\mathbf{\Gamma}')^{-1} \\ &= \mathbf{\Gamma}^{-1}\Sigma(\mathbf{\Gamma}')^{-1} \\ &= \mathbf{\Gamma}^{-1}\mathbf{\Gamma}\mathbf{\Gamma}'(\mathbf{\Gamma}')^{-1} = \mathbf{I} . \end{aligned}$$

Hence $\mathbf{y}$ is of the desired standard form. Then

$$\begin{aligned} \mathbf{y}'\mathbf{y} &= (\mathbf{x}' - \boldsymbol{\mu}')(\Gamma^{-1})'\Gamma^{-1}(\mathbf{x} - \boldsymbol{\mu}) \\ &= (\mathbf{x}' - \boldsymbol{\mu}')\Sigma^{-1}(\mathbf{x} - \boldsymbol{\mu}) . \end{aligned}$$

This is called the "*Standard Quadratic Form*".

Since it is equal to the sum-of-squares of p standard variables, it will be distributed as χ^2 with p degrees of freedom, if $\mathbf{x}$ has the multivariate normal distribution.

4.2. The Principle of Least Squares

Recall that the General Linear Model is

$$\mathbf{y} = \mathbf{A}\boldsymbol{\xi} + \mathbf{e} .$$

On the assumption, for the time being that $\mathbf{A}$ is of full rank, the "least squares" approach tells us to estimate $\boldsymbol{\xi}$ in such a way that the sum of squares of errors is minimized. Then, $\mathbf{e}'\mathbf{e}$ is the desired sum of squares and

$$\begin{aligned} \mathbf{e} &= \mathbf{y} - \mathbf{A}\boldsymbol{\xi} \\ \mathbf{e}' &= \mathbf{y}' - \boldsymbol{\xi}'\mathbf{A}' \\ \mathbf{e}'\mathbf{e} &= (\mathbf{y}' - \boldsymbol{\xi}'\mathbf{A}')(\mathbf{y} - \mathbf{A}\boldsymbol{\xi}) \\ \frac{\partial(\mathbf{e}'\mathbf{e})}{\partial\boldsymbol{\xi}} &= -2\mathbf{A}'(\mathbf{y} - \mathbf{A}\boldsymbol{\xi}) . \end{aligned}$$

Setting this equal to zero, we obtain

$$\begin{aligned} \mathbf{A}'(\mathbf{y} - \mathbf{A}\hat{\boldsymbol{\xi}}) &= \mathbf{0} \\ (\mathbf{A}'\mathbf{A})\hat{\boldsymbol{\xi}} &= \mathbf{A}'\mathbf{y} . \end{aligned}$$

These are called the *Normal Equations* for the estimation of $\boldsymbol{\xi}$.

4.3. Minimum Variance Unbiased Estimates

The minimum variance, unbiased, linear estimate of $\boldsymbol{\xi}$ is obtained by the application of a very general form of the *Gauss Markov Theorem*:

Let

$$\begin{aligned} \mathbf{y} &= \mathbf{A}\boldsymbol{\xi} + \mathbf{e} \\ E(\mathbf{e}) &= \mathbf{0} \\ \text{var}(\mathbf{y}) &= \text{var}(\mathbf{e}) = \sigma^2\mathbf{V} \end{aligned}$$

where $\mathbf{V}$ is a matrix (square, symmetric, non-singular) of order $(n \times n)$ with known elements. That is to say that variances of y_i (regardless of i) and covariances between y_i and y_j are known except for an arbitrary scalar multiplier applied to all of them. Then the best linear estimate of an arbitrary linear function $\mathbf{l}'\boldsymbol{\xi}$ is equal to $\mathbf{l}'\hat{\boldsymbol{\xi}}$ where $\hat{\boldsymbol{\xi}}$ minimizes the quadratic form

$$\mathbf{e}'\mathbf{V}^{-1}\mathbf{e} \ .$$

Since

$$E(\mathbf{e}) = \mathbf{0}$$

and

$$\text{var}\ (\mathbf{e}) = \text{var}\ (\mathbf{y}) = \sigma^2\mathbf{V} \ ,$$

the standard quadratic form of **e** would be

$$\begin{aligned}(\mathbf{e}' - [E(\mathbf{e})'])[\text{var}\ (\mathbf{e})]^{-1}(\mathbf{e} - [E(\mathbf{e})]) &= (\mathbf{e}' - \mathbf{0}')[\sigma^2\mathbf{V}]^{-1}(\mathbf{e} - \mathbf{0}) \\ &= \frac{1}{\sigma^2}\,\mathbf{e}'\mathbf{V}^{-1}\mathbf{e} \ .\end{aligned}$$

Minimizing this expression is equivalent to minimizing

$$\mathbf{e}'\mathbf{V}^{-1}\mathbf{e} \ .$$

Hence, the statement, "The best linear estimate of an arbitrary function $\mathbf{l}'\boldsymbol{\xi}$ is equal to $\mathbf{l}'\hat{\boldsymbol{\xi}}$ where $\hat{\boldsymbol{\xi}}$ is obtained by minimizing the quadratic form $\mathbf{e}'\mathbf{V}^{-1}\mathbf{e}$", as made in the Gauss-Markov Theorem is, in fact, equivalent to the statement . . . where $\hat{\boldsymbol{\xi}}$ is obtained by minimizing the standard quadratic form due to error. The Normal Equations in this general case are $\mathbf{A}'\mathbf{V}^{-1}\mathbf{A}\hat{\boldsymbol{\xi}} = \mathbf{A}'\mathbf{V}^{-1}\mathbf{y}$.

5. GENERAL LINEAR HYPOTHESIS OF FULL RANK

In this section, we shall discuss, with illustrations, the problem of testing hypotheses about certain parameters and also derive some necessary distribution in connection with testing hypotheses.

5.1. Notation

In general, a null hypothesis will be stated as

$$\mathbf{C}\boldsymbol{\xi} = \mathbf{k} \ ,$$

where $\mathbf{C} = \mathbf{C}(n_h \times m)$, $(n_h \leq m)$, is called the hypothesis matrix and is of rank n_h.

$\boldsymbol{\xi}$ is an $(m \times 1)$ column vector of parameters as defined in the general linear model.

k is a vector of n_h known elements, usually equal to **0**.

n_h is called *degrees of freedom due to hypothesis*. Actually it is the number of rows in the hypothesis matrix **C**. In other words, it is the number of nonredundant statements embodied in the null hypothesis.

n_e is called the *degrees of freedom due to error* and is equal to the number of observations minus the effective number of parameters.

It is important to keep in mind that in stating a composite hypothesis, we should *never* make:

(1) contradicting statements such as,

$$H_0\colon \beta_1 = \beta_2 \quad \text{and} \quad \beta_1 = 2\beta_2 \text{ simultaneously}$$

(2) redundant statements such as,

$$H_0\colon \tau_1 = \tau_2 \quad \text{and} \quad 3\tau_1 = 3\tau_2 \ .$$

5.2. Simple Linear Regression

Model

$$y_i = \mu + \beta x_i + e_i$$

$$\text{parameter vector } \boldsymbol{\xi} = \begin{bmatrix} \mu \\ \beta \end{bmatrix}$$

EXAMPLE 1

$$H_0\colon \mu = 0$$
$$\text{Alt.}\colon \mu \neq 0$$

General linear hypothesis

$$[1,0] \begin{bmatrix} \mu \\ \beta \end{bmatrix} = 0$$
$$\mathbf{C} \quad \boldsymbol{\xi} \quad = 0\,, \qquad n_h = 1$$

EXAMPLE 2

$$H_0\colon \beta = 0$$
$$\text{Alt.}\colon \beta \neq 0$$
$$[0,1] \begin{bmatrix} \mu \\ \beta \end{bmatrix} = 0$$
$$\mathbf{C} \quad \boldsymbol{\xi} \quad = 0\,, \qquad n_h = 1$$

EXAMPLE 3

$$H_0\colon \mu = 0,\ \beta = 0 \text{ simultaneously}$$
$$\text{Alt.: At least one of the } \mu \text{ and } \beta \neq 0$$
$$\begin{bmatrix} 1 & 0 \\ 0 & 1 \end{bmatrix} \begin{bmatrix} \mu \\ \beta \end{bmatrix} = \begin{bmatrix} 0 \\ 0 \end{bmatrix}$$
$$\mathbf{C} \quad \boldsymbol{\xi} \quad = \quad \mathbf{0}\,, \qquad n_h = 2$$

EXAMPLE 4

$$H_0\colon \mu = \beta$$
$$\text{Alt.}\colon \mu \neq \beta$$
$$[1,-1] \begin{bmatrix} \mu \\ \beta \end{bmatrix} = 0\,, \qquad n_h = 1$$

5.3. Analysis of Variance, One-way Classification

$$y_{ij} = \mu + \tau_i + e_{ij} \qquad (i = 1, 2, 3 \cdots v)$$
$$\text{Parameter vector } \boldsymbol{\xi}' = [\mu, \tau_1, \tau_2, \tau_3, \ \ldots \ \tau_v]$$

EXAMPLE 1

$$H_0\colon \tau_1 = \tau_2 = \tau_3 = \cdots = \tau_v$$
$$\text{Alt.}\colon \tau_r \neq \tau_s \qquad \text{for at least one pair}$$

Keep in mind that we must not make redundant statements. Here we have $(v - 1)$ rows in the hypothesis matrix. i.e. $n_h = v - 1$

$$(v-1)\begin{bmatrix} 0 & 1 & -1 & 0 & 0 & \cdots & 0 \\ 0 & 1 & 0 & -1 & 0 & \cdots & 0 \\ 0 & 1 & 0 & 0 & -1 & \cdots & 0 \\ \cdot & & \cdot & & \cdot & & \cdot \\ 0 & 1 & 0 & 0 & 0 & \cdots & -1 \end{bmatrix} \begin{bmatrix} \mu \\ \tau_1 \\ \tau_2 \\ \tau_3 \\ \cdot \\ \cdot \\ \cdot \\ \tau_v \end{bmatrix} = \begin{bmatrix} 0 \\ 0 \\ 0 \\ 0 \\ \cdot \\ \cdot \\ \cdot \\ 0 \end{bmatrix} (v-1)$$
$$(v+1)$$
$$\mathbf{C} \qquad\qquad \boldsymbol{\xi} \quad = \quad \mathbf{0}$$

EXAMPLE 2

$$H_0: \tau_1 = \tau_2 = \tau_3 = \cdots = \tau_v = 0$$
$$\text{Alt.: At least one } \tau \neq 0$$

$$(v)\underbrace{\begin{bmatrix} 0 & 1 & 0 & 0 & 0 & \cdots & 0 \\ 0 & 0 & 1 & 0 & 0 & \cdots & 0 \\ 0 & 0 & 0 & 1 & 0 & \cdots & 0 \\ \cdot & \cdot & & \cdot & \cdot & \cdot\cdot\cdot & \cdot \\ 0 & 0 & 0 & 0 & 0 & \cdots & 1 \end{bmatrix}}_{(v+1)} \begin{bmatrix} \mu \\ \tau_1 \\ \tau_2 \\ \tau_3 \\ \cdot \\ \cdot \\ \cdot \\ \tau_v \end{bmatrix} = \begin{bmatrix} 0 \\ 0 \\ 0 \\ \cdot \\ \cdot \\ \cdot \\ 0 \end{bmatrix} (v)$$

$$\mathbf{C} \qquad \boldsymbol{\xi} = \mathbf{0}$$

n_h = number of rows in C and is equal to v .

EXAMPLE 3. For simplicity, let us take $i = 1, 2, 3, 4$

$$H_0: -\tau_1 + 2\tau_2 - \tau_3 = 0 \text{ (Quadratic contrast of three effects)}$$
$$\text{Alt.: Quadratic contrast} \neq 0$$

$$[0 \quad -1 \quad +2 \quad -1 \quad 0] \begin{bmatrix} \mu \\ \tau_1 \\ \tau_2 \\ \tau_3 \\ \tau_4 \end{bmatrix} = 0$$

$$\mathbf{C} \qquad \boldsymbol{\xi} = \mathbf{0}$$

5.4. Multiple Linear Regression

$$y_i = \mu + \beta_1 x_{1i} + \beta_2 x_{2i} + \beta_3 x_{3i} + \cdots \beta_k x_{ki} + e_i$$
$$\text{parameter vector } \boldsymbol{\xi}' = [\mu, \beta_1, \beta_2, \beta_3, \ldots \beta_k]$$

EXAMPLE 1

$$H_0: \beta_1 = 0$$
$$\text{Alt.: } \beta_1 \neq 0$$

$$[0,1,0,0 \cdots 0] \begin{bmatrix} \mu \\ \beta_1 \\ \beta_2 \\ \beta_3 \\ \cdot \\ \beta_k \end{bmatrix} = 0$$

$$\mathbf{C} \qquad \boldsymbol{\xi} = \mathbf{0}, \qquad n_h = 1.$$

EXAMPLE 2

$$H_0: \beta_1 = \beta_2 = \beta_3 = \cdots = \beta_k = 0$$
$$\text{Alt.: At least one } \beta \neq 0$$

$$(k)\underbrace{\begin{bmatrix} 0 & 1 & 0 & 0 & \cdots & 0 \\ 0 & 0 & 1 & 0 & \cdots & 0 \\ 0 & 0 & 0 & 1 & \cdots & 0 \\ \cdot & \cdot & \cdot & \cdot & & \cdot \\ 0 & 0 & 0 & 0 & \cdots & 1 \end{bmatrix}}_{(k+1)} \begin{bmatrix} \mu_1 \\ \beta_2 \\ \beta_3 \\ \beta_4 \\ \cdot \\ \cdot \\ \cdot \\ \beta_k \end{bmatrix} = \mathbf{0}$$

$$\mathbf{C} \qquad \boldsymbol{\xi} = \mathbf{0}, \qquad n_h = k.$$

EXAMPLE 3

H_0: $\beta_1 = 0$, $\beta_3 = 0$ simultaneously
Alt.: At least one of β_1 and $\beta_3 \neq 0$

$$\underset{\mathbf{C}}{\begin{bmatrix} 0 & 1 & 0 & 0 & \cdots & 0 \\ 0 & 0 & 0 & 1 & \cdots & 0 \end{bmatrix}} \underset{\boldsymbol{\xi}}{\begin{bmatrix} \mu \\ \beta_1 \\ \beta_2 \\ \beta_3 \\ \cdot \\ \cdot \\ \cdot \\ \beta_k \end{bmatrix}} = \underset{\mathbf{0}}{\begin{bmatrix} 0 \\ 0 \end{bmatrix}} ; \quad n_h = 2 .$$

5.5. Randomized Blocks

$$y_{ij} = \mu + \tau_i + \beta_j + e_{ij}$$

where μ is the general effect
τ_i are the treatment effects $(i = 1, 2, 3)$
β_j are the block effects $(j = 1, 2, 3, 4)$
e_{ij} is the experimental error

$$\text{parameter vector } \boldsymbol{\xi}' = [\mu, \tau_1, \tau_2, \tau_3, \beta_1, \beta_2, \beta_3, \beta_4]$$

EXAMPLE 1

H_0: $\tau_1 = \tau_2 = \tau_3$ (all treatments effects are equal)
Alt.: At least one pair $\tau_r \neq \tau_s$

$$\underset{\mathbf{C}}{\begin{bmatrix} 0 & 1 & -1 & 0 & 0 & 0 & 0 & 0 \\ 0 & 1 & 0 & -1 & 0 & 0 & 0 & 0 \end{bmatrix}} \underset{\boldsymbol{\xi}}{\begin{bmatrix} \mu \\ \tau_1 \\ \tau_2 \\ \tau_3 \\ \beta_1 \\ \beta_2 \\ \beta_3 \\ \beta_4 \end{bmatrix}} = \underset{\mathbf{0}}{\begin{bmatrix} 0 \\ 0 \end{bmatrix}} ; \quad n_h = 2 .$$

EXAMPLE 2

H_0: $-\tau_1 + 2\tau_2 - \tau_3 = 0$ (quadratic contrast)
Alt.: Quadratic contrast $\neq 0$

$$\underset{\mathbf{C}}{[0 \ \ -1 \ \ 2 \ \ -1 \ \ 0 \ \ 0 \ \ 0 \ \ 0]} \underset{\boldsymbol{\xi}}{\begin{bmatrix} \mu \\ \tau_1 \\ \tau_2 \\ \tau_3 \\ \beta_1 \\ \beta_2 \\ \beta_3 \\ \beta_4 \end{bmatrix}} = \mathbf{0} ; \quad n_h = 1 .$$

From the above illustrations, it can be seen that we can write a great variety of tests in the form of the General Linear Hypothesis provided that we make no redundant hypothesis statements.

5.6. Quadratic Form due to Hypothesis

So far we have discussed only the model of full rank. i.e., in the normal equations,

$$\mathbf{A'A\hat{\xi} = A'y} \ ,$$

(A′A) has an inverse. We shall continue to assume this model throughout this chapter. Recall the General Linear Model

$$\mathbf{y = A\xi + e}$$
$$E(\mathbf{y}) = \mathbf{A\xi} \quad \text{and} \quad \text{var}(\mathbf{y}) = \sigma^2\mathbf{I} \ .$$

We then have the normal equations,

$$\mathbf{A'A\hat{\xi} = A'y} \ .$$

The estimate of ξ is

$$\hat{\xi} = (\mathbf{A'A})^{-1}\mathbf{A'y} \ ,$$

and the variance of the estimate is

$$\begin{aligned} \text{var}(\hat{\xi}) &= (\mathbf{A'A})^{-1} \text{var}(\mathbf{A'y})(\mathbf{A'A})^{-1} \\ &= (\mathbf{A'A})^{-1}\mathbf{A'} \text{var}(\mathbf{y})\mathbf{A}(\mathbf{A'A})^{-1} \\ &= \sigma^2(\mathbf{A'A})^{-1}\mathbf{A'A}(\mathbf{A'A})^{-1} \\ &= \sigma^2(\mathbf{A'A})^{-1} \ . \end{aligned}$$

This is the expression for the variance-covariance matrix of the estimates of ξ. Now suppose that we have a null hypothesis

$$H_0\colon \mathbf{C\xi} = \mathbf{0} \ .$$

We have an unbiased estimate of $\mathbf{C\xi}$ namely $\mathbf{C\hat{\xi}}$, i.e., under the null hypothesis,

$$\begin{aligned} E(\mathbf{C\hat{\xi}}) &= \mathbf{C\xi} = \mathbf{0} \\ \text{var}(\mathbf{C\hat{\xi}}) &= \mathbf{C} \text{var}(\hat{\xi})\mathbf{C'} \\ &= \sigma^2\mathbf{C}(\mathbf{A'A})^{-1}\mathbf{C'}, \\ [\text{var}(\mathbf{C\hat{\xi}})]^{-1} &= \frac{1}{\sigma^2}[\mathbf{C}(\mathbf{A'A})^{-1}\mathbf{C'}]^{-1} \ . \end{aligned}$$

Thus, under the null hypothesis, the standard quadratic form is

$$\frac{1}{\sigma^2}\hat{\xi}'\mathbf{C'}[\mathbf{C}(\mathbf{A'A})^{-1}\mathbf{C'}]^{-1}\mathbf{C}\hat{\xi} \ .$$

The expression, $\hat{\xi}'\mathbf{C'}[\mathbf{C}(\mathbf{A'A})^{-1}\mathbf{C'}]^{-1}\mathbf{C}\hat{\xi}$, is called the *sum of squares due to hypothesis,* usually denoted by SSH. If $\mathbf{y}$ has the multivariate normal distribution, SSH/σ^2 is distributed as χ^2 with n_h degrees of freedom, since it is a standard quadratic form.

5.7. Sum of Squares due to Error

Recall the general linear model

$$\mathbf{y = A\xi + e} \ .$$

Let us define $\hat{\mathbf{e}} = \mathbf{y} - \mathbf{A}\hat{\xi}$, the error of estimation. Then, $\sum_{i=1}^{n} \hat{e}_i^2 = \hat{\mathbf{e}}'\hat{\mathbf{e}}$ is called the sum of squares of errors of estimation. It is customarily denoted by SSE

$$\begin{aligned} \text{SSE} = \hat{\mathbf{e}}'\hat{\mathbf{e}} &= (\mathbf{y'} - \hat{\xi}'\mathbf{A'})(\mathbf{y} - \mathbf{A}\hat{\xi}) \\ &= \mathbf{y'y} - \hat{\xi}'\mathbf{A'y} - \mathbf{y'A}\hat{\xi} + \hat{\xi}'\mathbf{A'A}\xi \\ &= \mathbf{y'y} - \hat{\xi}'\mathbf{A'y} - \mathbf{y'A}\hat{\xi} + \hat{\xi}'\mathbf{A'y} \\ &= \mathbf{y'y} - \mathbf{y'A}\hat{\xi} \ , \end{aligned}$$

where $\mathbf{y}'\mathbf{y}$ is the sum of squares over all observations.

$\mathbf{A}'\mathbf{y}$ is the column vector on the right hand side of the normal equations.

$\hat{\boldsymbol{\xi}}$ is a column vector whose elements are the estimates of $\boldsymbol{\xi}$.

In words, SSE is obtained by subtracting from the sum of squares of all observations, the scalar product of the vector of estimates of $\boldsymbol{\xi}$ and the vector on the right-hand side of the normal equations.

It should be noted that SSE can depend only on the model, and is determined once the model is stated; it is entirely independent of any hypothesis which may be stated or tested.

If $\mathbf{y}$ is normally distributed, SSE/σ^2 has the χ^2 distribution with n_e degrees of freedom. It is independent of any SSH.

5.8. Summary

We have the general linear model

$$\mathbf{y} = \mathbf{A}\boldsymbol{\xi} + \mathbf{e}$$
$$E(\mathbf{y}) = \mathbf{A}\boldsymbol{\xi} \ .$$

We assume that the model is of full rank, that is, $\mathbf{A}'\mathbf{A}$ is non-singular and thus has an inverse. If we further assume that

$$\text{var}\ (\mathbf{y}) = \sigma^2\mathbf{I} \ ,$$

that is, homoscedasticity plus independence, we will have the normal equations

$$(\mathbf{A}'\mathbf{A})\hat{\boldsymbol{\xi}} = \mathbf{A}'\mathbf{y}$$

and we can obtain the estimate of $\boldsymbol{\xi}$ by

$$\hat{\boldsymbol{\xi}} = (\mathbf{A}'\mathbf{A})^{-1}\mathbf{A}'\mathbf{y} \ .$$

Again, if we further assume that the elements of $\mathbf{y}$ are normally distributed, we may test the following hypothesis:

$$H_0\text{: } \mathbf{C}\boldsymbol{\xi} = \mathbf{0}$$
$$\text{Alt.: } \mathbf{C}\boldsymbol{\xi} = \mathbf{n} \qquad (\neq \mathbf{0})$$

This hypothesis matrix has n_h rows and, if we avoid inconsistency and redundancies in the statement of the hypothesis, n_h will be the "degrees of freedom due to hypothesis".

5.9. Computational Procedure for Testing a Hypothesis

In testing a hypothesis, proceed as follows:

(1) Obtain SSH, the so called "sum of squares due to hypothesis" from the formula

$$\text{SSH} = \hat{\boldsymbol{\xi}}'\mathbf{C}'[\mathbf{C}(\mathbf{A}'\mathbf{A})^{-1}\mathbf{C}']^{-1}\mathbf{C}\hat{\boldsymbol{\xi}} \ .$$

(2) Obtain SSE, the "sum of squares due to error" from

$$\text{SSE} = \sum_{\text{all}} y_i^2 - \mathbf{y}'\mathbf{A}\hat{\boldsymbol{\xi}} \ .$$

(3) Introduce n_e, the "degrees of freedom due to error" which equals n (sample size) minus effective number of parameters in the model.

(4) Then, if H_0 is true

$$\frac{\text{SSH}/n_h}{\text{SSE}/n_e} = F_{(n_h, n_e)} \ .$$

5.10. Regression Significance Test

Suppose that we have the general linear model

$$\mathbf{y} = \mathbf{A}\boldsymbol{\xi} + \mathbf{e}$$
$$E(\mathbf{y}) = \mathbf{A}\boldsymbol{\xi} \qquad \text{and} \qquad \text{var}(\mathbf{y}) = \sigma^2\mathbf{I} \; .$$

Under this model, we have the normal equations

$$\begin{aligned} \mathbf{A}'\mathbf{A}\hat{\boldsymbol{\xi}} &= \mathbf{A}'\mathbf{y} \\ \text{SSE} &= \mathbf{y}'\mathbf{y} - \mathbf{y}'\mathbf{A}\hat{\boldsymbol{\xi}} \\ \text{where } \hat{\boldsymbol{\xi}} &= (\mathbf{A}'\mathbf{A})^{-1}\mathbf{A}'\mathbf{y} \; . \end{aligned}$$

Now, suppose that our hypothesis is of such a nature that we can easily write the reduced model under the assumption that H_0 is true.

$$\mathbf{y} = \mathbf{A}\boldsymbol{\xi} + \mathbf{e}^*$$
$$\text{subject to the condition } \mathbf{C}\boldsymbol{\xi} = \mathbf{0} \; .$$

Analogously, after estimating $\boldsymbol{\xi}$ in the above model (reduced model) we may write

$$\text{SSE (reduced)} = \mathbf{y}'\mathbf{y} - \mathbf{y}'\mathbf{A}\hat{\boldsymbol{\xi}}$$

where $\hat{\boldsymbol{\xi}}$ is the estimate of $\boldsymbol{\xi}$ in the reduced model. We can then find the sum of squares due to that hypothesis by obtaining

SSE (reduced) and subtracting SSE (the original or general model), i.e.,

$$\text{SSH} = \text{SSE (reduced)} - \text{SSE}.$$

5.11. Alternate Form of the Distribution

$\dfrac{\text{SSE}}{\text{SSE} + \text{SSH}}$ has the Beta distribution with parameters $(n_{e/2}, n_{h/2})$.

The beta tests are *lower-tail* tests, i.e., we reject H_0 if the value of the observed ratio is *smaller* than the tabulated one, i.e.,

$$\text{rejection region } \beta < \text{constant}.$$

Actually in the tables, percentage points of β are stated as

$$\beta(a,b),$$

where $a = 2$ (second parameter)
$b = 2$ (first parameter).
Hence, read those tables simply as $\beta(n_h, n_e)$

$$\begin{aligned} \frac{\text{SSE}}{\text{SSE (reduced)}} &= \beta\left(\frac{n_e}{2}, \frac{n_h}{2}\right) && \text{(usual notation)} \\ &= \beta^*(n_h, n_e) && \text{(Tables for Beta percentage points)} \\ &= I\left(\frac{n_e}{2}, \frac{n_h}{2}\right) && \text{(Tables of the Incomplete Beta Function).} \end{aligned}$$

6. GENERAL LINEAR MODEL OF LESS THAN FULL RANK

So far we have restricted our discussion to models of full rank in the General Linear Model. In practice, many design models are not initially of this form. Models not of full rank are sometimes called singular models.

If, in the General Linear Model

$$\mathbf{y} = \mathbf{A}\boldsymbol{\xi} + \mathbf{e} \; ,$$

with normal equations

$$\mathbf{A}'\mathbf{A}\hat{\boldsymbol{\xi}} = \mathbf{A}'\mathbf{y}$$

the rank of the design matrix $\mathbf{A}$ is less than m ($r < m$) then ($\mathbf{A}'\mathbf{A}$) would be singular and has no inverse. We must examine the system to see whether a solution exists. We wish to find functions of the ξ_i's for which unbiased estimates exist.

6.1. Estimable Function and Estimability

Let us estimate a function $\mathbf{l}'\boldsymbol{\xi}$, i.e., find $\mathbf{c}'\mathbf{y} = \mathbf{l}'\hat{\boldsymbol{\xi}}$ such that the expectation

$$E(\mathbf{c}'\mathbf{y}) = \mathbf{l}'\boldsymbol{\xi} \text{ for all } \boldsymbol{\xi} ,$$

and var $(\mathbf{c}'\mathbf{y})$ = minimum, i.e., we would like to find a linear function of the y_i's such that

$$E(\mathbf{c}'\mathbf{y}) = \mathbf{l}'\boldsymbol{\xi} ,$$

where $\mathbf{l}'$ is a given vector of "weights". The constraints of unbiasedness are

$$\begin{aligned} E(\mathbf{c}'\mathbf{y}) &= \mathbf{l}'\boldsymbol{\xi} \\ \mathbf{c}'E(\mathbf{y}) &= \mathbf{l}'\boldsymbol{\xi} \\ \mathbf{c}'\mathbf{A}\boldsymbol{\xi} &= \mathbf{l}'\boldsymbol{\xi} \qquad \text{for all } \boldsymbol{\xi}, \text{ hence,} \\ \mathbf{c}'\mathbf{A} &= \mathbf{l}' \\ \mathbf{c}'\mathbf{A} - \mathbf{l}' &= \mathbf{0} . \end{aligned}$$

Hence, we are minimizing

$$\text{var } (\mathbf{c}'\mathbf{y}) \text{ subject to the constraints } \mathbf{c}'\mathbf{A} = \mathbf{l}'$$

where var $(\mathbf{c}'\mathbf{y}) = \sigma^2\mathbf{c}'\mathbf{c}$.

The criterion function Φ is then

$$\begin{aligned} \Phi &= \tfrac{1}{2}\mathbf{c}'\mathbf{c} - [\mathbf{c}'\mathbf{A} - \mathbf{l}']\boldsymbol{\lambda} \\ \frac{\partial\Phi}{\partial\mathbf{c}} &= \mathbf{c} - \mathbf{A}\boldsymbol{\lambda} . \end{aligned}$$

Setting the derivative equal to zero, we obtain

(6.1.1) $$\mathbf{A}\boldsymbol{\lambda} = \hat{\mathbf{c}}$$

Premultiplying by $\mathbf{A}'$, we have

$$\mathbf{A}'\mathbf{A}\boldsymbol{\lambda} = \mathbf{A}'\hat{\mathbf{c}} ,$$

which is equal to $\mathbf{l}$ under our constraints.

Hence,

(6.1.2) $$\mathbf{A}'\mathbf{A}\boldsymbol{\lambda} = \mathbf{l} .$$

(6.1.1) and (6.1.2) are called "conjugate normal equations". If $\mathbf{A}$ has rank r ($<m$) we can always select r columns which form a "basis" and take the remaining ($m - r$) columns as an extension. The latter columns are linear combinations of the former.

In the model

$$\mathbf{y} = \mathbf{A}\boldsymbol{\xi} + \mathbf{e}$$

let us order the elements in $\boldsymbol{\xi}$ as well as the columns in $\mathbf{A}$ in such a way that

$$\boldsymbol{\xi}' = [\underset{(r)}{\boldsymbol{\xi}_1'} \ , \ \underset{(m-r)}{\boldsymbol{\xi}_2'}]$$

and

$$\mathbf{A} = [\underset{(r)}{\mathbf{A}_1} \ , \ \underset{(m-r)}{\mathbf{A}_2}](r)$$

and that $\mathbf{A}_1$ is a basis of $\mathbf{A}$. The columns of $\mathbf{A}_2$ must then be linear combinations of those in $\mathbf{A}_1$. We may express this fact formally by saying there exists

$$\mathbf{Q}(r \times \overline{m-r}) \qquad \text{such that} \qquad \mathbf{A}_2 = \mathbf{A}_1\mathbf{Q} \ .$$

Suppose

$$\begin{aligned} \mathbf{A}_2 &= \mathbf{A}_1 Q \\ \mathbf{A}_1'\mathbf{A}_2 &= \mathbf{A}_1'\mathbf{A}_1 Q \\ \mathbf{Q} &= (\mathbf{A}_1'\mathbf{A}_1)^{-1}\mathbf{A}_1'\mathbf{A}_2 \ . \end{aligned}$$

This is one of the ways to determine $\mathbf{Q}$ when $\mathbf{A}_1$ and $\mathbf{A}_2$ are given. Usually, however, we would try to find $\mathbf{Q}$ by inspection.

Now,

$$\begin{aligned} \mathbf{A} &= \underset{(r)}{[\mathbf{A}_1} \ , \ \underset{(m-r)}{\mathbf{A}_2]}(r) \\ &= [\mathbf{A}_1, \mathbf{A}_1\mathbf{Q}] = \mathbf{A}_1\underset{(r)}{[\mathbf{I}} \quad \underset{(m-r)}{\mathbf{Q}]}(r) \end{aligned}$$

(6.1.2) can be written as

$$\begin{bmatrix} \mathbf{A}_1' \\ \mathbf{Q}'\mathbf{A}_1' \end{bmatrix} [\mathbf{A}_1 \ , \ \mathbf{A}_1\mathbf{Q}]\lambda = \begin{bmatrix} \mathbf{A}_1'\mathbf{A}_1 & \mathbf{A}_1'\mathbf{A}_1\mathbf{Q} \\ \mathbf{Q}'\mathbf{A}_1'\mathbf{A}_1 & \mathbf{Q}'\mathbf{A}_1'\mathbf{A}_1\mathbf{Q} \end{bmatrix} \lambda = \begin{bmatrix} \mathbf{l}_1 \\ \mathbf{l}_2 \end{bmatrix} \begin{matrix} (r) \\ (m-r) \end{matrix}$$

Expanding we have

$$(6.1.3) \qquad [\mathbf{A}_1'\mathbf{A}_1, \mathbf{A}_1'\mathbf{A}_1\mathbf{Q}]\lambda = \mathbf{l}_1$$

$$(6.1.4) \qquad [\mathbf{Q}'\mathbf{A}_1'\mathbf{A}_1, \mathbf{Q}'\mathbf{A}_1'\mathbf{A}_1\mathbf{Q}]\lambda = \mathbf{l}_2 \ .$$

Premultiply (6.1.3) by $\mathbf{Q}'$ and obtain

$$[\mathbf{Q}'\mathbf{A}_1'\mathbf{A}_1, \mathbf{Q}'\mathbf{A}_1'\mathbf{A}_1\mathbf{Q}]\lambda = \mathbf{Q}'\mathbf{l}_1 \ .$$

For consistency of the equation system, the condition

$$\mathbf{l}_2 = \mathbf{Q}'\mathbf{l}_1$$

must be met.

That is to say, in the function $\mathbf{l}'\xi$, $\mathbf{l}'$ cannot be chosen arbitrarily but must be of the form

$$\mathbf{l}' = \underset{(r)}{[\mathbf{l}_1'} \ , \ \underset{(m-r)}{\mathbf{l}_2']} \ , \quad \text{where}$$

$$(6.1.5) \qquad \mathbf{l}_2' = \mathbf{l}_1'\mathbf{Q} \ .$$

Only an $\mathbf{l}$ satisfying this relation can be used in the construction of a function which admits of a linear unbiased (and mathematically consistent) estimate.

(6.1.5) is called the condition of "estimability" of a linear function. Hence, we will call a function $\mathbf{l}'\xi$ *estimable* if $\mathbf{l}'$ can be written as

$$[\mathbf{l}_1', \mathbf{l}_2'] \ ,$$

where $\mathbf{l}_2'$ is related to $\mathbf{l}_1'$ in the same way as $\mathbf{A}_2$ to $\mathbf{A}_1$.

We may then define that a parametric function is said to be linearly *estimable* if there exists a linear combination of the observations whose expected value is equal to the function, i.e., if there exists an unbiased estimate.

Now, if the function $\mathbf{l}'\boldsymbol{\xi}$ is estimable, (6.1.3) can be written as

$$(\mathbf{A}_1'\mathbf{A}_1)[\mathbf{I},\mathbf{Q}]\boldsymbol{\lambda} = \mathbf{l}_1 \ .$$

Notice that $\mathbf{l}_2$ may be disregarded since it is determined by the relation $\mathbf{l}_2 = \mathbf{Q}'\mathbf{l}_1$, hence,

$$[\mathbf{I},\mathbf{Q}]\boldsymbol{\lambda} = (\mathbf{A}_1'\mathbf{A}_1)^{-1}\mathbf{l}_1 \ . \tag{6.1.6}$$

The first conjugate normal equations (6.1.1) stated

$$\mathbf{A}\boldsymbol{\lambda} = \hat{\mathbf{c}}$$

or,

$$[\mathbf{A}_1,\mathbf{A}_2]\boldsymbol{\lambda} = \hat{\mathbf{c}}$$
$$\mathbf{A}_1[\mathbf{I},\mathbf{Q}]\boldsymbol{\lambda} = \hat{\mathbf{c}} \ .$$

Inserting (6.1.6), we obtain

$$\mathbf{A}_1(\mathbf{A}_1'\mathbf{A}_1)^{-1}\mathbf{l}_1 = \hat{\mathbf{c}} \ .$$

Hence,

$$\hat{\mathbf{c}}'\mathbf{y} = \widehat{\mathbf{l}'\boldsymbol{\xi}} = \mathbf{l}_1'(\mathbf{A}_1'\mathbf{A}_1)^{-1}\mathbf{A}_1'\mathbf{y} \ ,$$

which is of the same form as in the non-singular case, except that $\mathbf{A}$ has been replaced by its basis $\mathbf{A}_1$ and in $\mathbf{l}$ we consider only the first r elements, i.e., $\mathbf{l}_1$.

Hence, the normal equations in the Least Squares approach, i.e.,

$$\mathbf{A}'\mathbf{A}\hat{\boldsymbol{\xi}} = \mathbf{A}'\mathbf{y}$$

can be used formally in the reduced statement

$$(\mathbf{A}_1'\mathbf{A}_1)\hat{\boldsymbol{\xi}}_1 = \mathbf{A}_1'\mathbf{y} \ .$$

6.2. General Linear Hypothesis Model of Less Than Full Rank

We have the general linear model

$$\begin{aligned}
\mathbf{y} &= \mathbf{A}\boldsymbol{\xi} + \mathbf{e} \\
&= [\mathbf{A}_1,\mathbf{A}_2]\begin{bmatrix}\boldsymbol{\xi}_1 \\ \boldsymbol{\xi}_2\end{bmatrix} + \mathbf{e} \\
&= [\mathbf{A}_1,\mathbf{A}_1\mathbf{Q}]\begin{bmatrix}\boldsymbol{\xi}_1 \\ \boldsymbol{\xi}_2\end{bmatrix} + \mathbf{e} \\
&= \mathbf{A}_1\boldsymbol{\xi}_1 + \mathbf{A}_1\mathbf{Q}\boldsymbol{\xi}_2 + \mathbf{e} \\
&= \mathbf{A}_1(\boldsymbol{\xi}_1 + \mathbf{Q}\boldsymbol{\xi}_2) + \mathbf{e} \ .
\end{aligned}$$

Hence, we may write the general linear model in the form $\mathbf{y} = \mathbf{A}_1\boldsymbol{\xi}^* + \mathbf{e}$, where $\boldsymbol{\xi}^* = \boldsymbol{\xi}_1 + \mathbf{Q}\boldsymbol{\xi}_2$.

6.2.1. *Sum of Squares Due to Error and Its Distribution*

Notice that $\mathbf{e}$ has not been changed in this model, hence we can set up the normal equations

$$(\mathbf{A}_1'\mathbf{A}_1)\hat{\boldsymbol{\xi}}^* = \mathbf{A}_1'\mathbf{y}.$$

$$\begin{aligned}
\text{SSE} = \mathbf{e}'\mathbf{e} &= \mathbf{y}'\mathbf{y} - \mathbf{y}'\mathbf{A}_1\hat{\boldsymbol{\xi}}^* \\
&= \mathbf{y}'\mathbf{y} - \mathbf{y}'\mathbf{A}_1(\mathbf{A}_1'\mathbf{A}_1)^{-1}\mathbf{A}_1'\mathbf{y}
\end{aligned}$$

Then, as before

$$\frac{\text{SSE}}{\sigma^2} = \chi^2(n - r) \qquad \text{where } r \text{ is the rank of } \mathbf{A},$$

and replaces m in the non-singular model. The "effective" number of parameters in the singular model is only r, the remaining $(m - r)$ parameters are determined in terms of the first r by the estimability condition.

6.2.2. *Sum of Squares Due to Hypothesis and Its Distribution*

Suppose that we wish to test

$$H_0\colon \mathbf{C}\boldsymbol{\xi} = \mathbf{0} ,$$

where $C = [\underset{(r)}{\mathbf{C}_1} \;,\; \underset{(m-r)}{\mathbf{C}_2}]$.

Then $\mathbf{C}\boldsymbol{\xi} = \mathbf{0}$ implies that

$$[\mathbf{C}_1,\mathbf{C}_2]\begin{bmatrix}\boldsymbol{\xi}_1\\ \boldsymbol{\xi}_2\end{bmatrix} = \begin{bmatrix}\mathbf{0}\\ \mathbf{0}\end{bmatrix}.$$

Each row on the left-hand side must represent an estimable function, hence, we must have

$$\mathbf{C}_2 = \mathbf{C}_1\mathbf{Q} .$$

This is called the condition of "testability", i.e., if

$$\mathbf{C} = \begin{bmatrix}\mathbf{c}_2'\\ \mathbf{c}_1'\\ \cdot\\ \cdot\\ \cdot\\ \mathbf{c}_{n_h}'\end{bmatrix},$$

where $(\mathbf{c}_i'\boldsymbol{\xi})$ is an estimable function $(i = 1, 2, \ldots, n_h)$. Then the null hypothesis

$$H_0\colon \mathbf{C}_1\boldsymbol{\xi}_1 + \mathbf{C}_2\boldsymbol{\xi}_2 = \mathbf{0}$$

can be written as

$$\mathbf{C}_1\boldsymbol{\xi}_1 + \mathbf{C}_1\mathbf{Q}\boldsymbol{\xi}_2 = \mathbf{0}$$

or simply $\mathbf{C}_1\boldsymbol{\xi}^* = \mathbf{0}$, where $\boldsymbol{\xi}^* = (\boldsymbol{\xi}_1 + \mathbf{Q}\boldsymbol{\xi}_2)$. Hence, we can formally state that a null hypothesis

$$H_0\colon \mathbf{C}\boldsymbol{\xi} = \mathbf{0}$$

is "*testable*" if $\mathbf{C}\boldsymbol{\xi}$ consists of n_h estimable functions, i.e., if $\mathbf{C}_2 = \mathbf{C}_1\mathbf{Q}$, where $\mathbf{C} = [\mathbf{C}_1,\mathbf{C}_2]$. Consequently,

$$\text{SSH} = \hat{\boldsymbol{\xi}}^{*\prime}\mathbf{C}_1'[\mathbf{C}_1(\mathbf{A}_1'\mathbf{A}_1)^{-1}\mathbf{C}_1']^{-1}\mathbf{C}_1\hat{\boldsymbol{\xi}}^* ,$$

where $\hat{\boldsymbol{\xi}}^* = (\mathbf{A}_1'\mathbf{A}_1)^{-1}\mathbf{A}_1\mathbf{y}$.

As before

$$\frac{\text{SSH}}{\sigma^2} = \chi^2_{(n_h)} .$$

Again, if the null-hypothesis is true, we have the test statistic F

$$\frac{\text{MSH}/n_h}{\text{MSE}/n_e} = \text{F}_{(n_h,n_e)} .$$

6.3. Constraints and Conditions

If the model is singular, of rank $r < m$, $(m - r)$ constraints on the $\hat{\xi}_i$'s (the estimates) may be arbitrarily introduced, for example:

$$\hat{\xi}_{r+1} = 0, \ldots, \hat{\xi}_m = 0 \tag{6.3.1}$$

or

$$\sum_{i=1}^{m} \hat{\xi}_i = 0, \sum_{i=1}^{m} n_i\hat{\xi}_i = 0 . \tag{6.3.2}$$

This is called *reparametrizing* the model. The constraining functions are fairly arbitrary, but they *must not be estimable* functions, otherwise the resulting model will still be singular.

In effect, this is done by deletion of the last $(m - r)$ rows and columns of $\mathbf{A'A}$ and the last $(m - r)$ elements of $\mathbf{A'y}$, for constraints of the type (6.3.1), or by adding a constant to all elements of $\mathbf{A'A}$, for constraints of the type (6.3.2). This has no effect on the value of estimable functions, or test statistics.

An entirely different situation prevails if we place conditions on the *parameters* of a model, especially on interactions. In the two-way classification model

$$E(y_{ijk}) = \mu + \alpha_i + \beta_j + \delta_{ij}$$

one usually specifies

$$\sum_i n_{ij}\delta_{ij} = 0 \qquad \text{for all } j\text{'s}$$

and

$$\sum_j n_{ij}\delta_{ij} = 0 \qquad \text{for all } i\text{'s} \ ,$$

where n_{ij} denotes the number of observations in the (i,j) cell. These are sometimes called *natural constraints* (they are neither *natural* nor *constraints*). They simply represent a set of *conditions* or *assumptions* on the interactions, minimizing this effect (making SSH for interaction a minimum). After introducing these conditions, one still has a singular model, which can be made nonsingular by introduction of the arbitrary constraints

$$\sum_i \hat{\alpha}_i = 0, \sum_j \hat{\beta}_j = 0 \ .$$

(Note the carets, for estimates). One could introduce the different assumptions,

$$\text{All } \alpha_i\text{'s} = 0$$
$$\text{All } \beta_j\text{'s} = 0$$

and would have a simple one-way classification model, quite different from the previous one. A classical example is the following. Suppose some organic substance is attacked by sulphuric acid or by sodium hydroxide.

		NaOH −	NaOH +
H_2SO_4	−	0	4
	+	6	0

Using, formally, the minimizing interaction conditions, one would obtain effect estimates as means of rows and columns

H_2SO_4	absent: 2	present: 3
NaOH	absent: 3	present: 2

and make the ridiculous inference that sodium hydroxide, by itself, has an inhibiting effect. The correct parametric model in this case would be

μ	$\mu + \beta$
$\mu + \alpha$	$\mu + \alpha + \beta + \delta$

,

i.e., interaction occurs only if both substances are present. This leads to the estimation

$$\begin{aligned}\hat{\mu} &= 0\\ \hat{\alpha} &= 6\\ \hat{\beta} &= 4\\ \hat{\delta} &= -10\ ,\end{aligned}$$

which is the appropriate neutralization model.

It is usually quite easy to decide whether a constraint or a condition is involved. The (model-changing) *conditions* are required whenever a hierarchy of effects is present (main effects, interactions, higher-order interactions), while constraints (with no effect on the model) can be introduced within the same kinds of effects (row effect estimates adding to zero, column effect estimates adding to zero). The sum of squares due to a given hypothesis is a good indicator of the situation. If it changes by the introduction of two different sets of combinations, they are *conditions*, and must be determined in accordance with plausibility of the physical model. If it stays the same, they are usually *constraints on the estimates*, and thus arbitrary, without effect on the model.

I.6 PLANS FOR DESIGN OF EXPERIMENTS

In this section, tables of combinatorial patterns usable as experimental designs are presented. No attempt is made to develop these patterns from first principles nor to discuss the choice of patterns or their applicability in experimental situations. These selected patterns are abridged from a more numerous set of patterns presented in the text *Experimental Designs* by Cochran and Cox (1957). The plan numbers refer to those in Cochran and Cox.

Plan 4.1 Selected latin squares

3 × 3

A	B	C
B	C	A
C	A	B

4 × 4

1

A	B	C	D
B	A	D	C
C	D	B	A
D	C	A	B

2

A	B	C	D
B	C	D	A
C	D	A	B
D	A	B	C

3

A	B	C	D
B	D	A	C
C	A	D	B
D	C	B	A

4

A	B	C	D
B	A	D	C
C	D	A	B
D	C	B	A

5 × 5

A	B	C	D	E
B	A	E	C	D
C	D	A	E	B
D	E	B	A	C
E	C	D	B	A

6 × 6

A	B	C	D	E	F
B	F	D	C	A	E
C	D	E	F	B	A
D	A	F	E	C	B
E	C	A	B	F	D
F	E	B	A	D	C

7 × 7

A	B	C	D	E	F	G
B	C	D	E	F	G	A
C	D	E	F	G	A	B
D	E	F	G	A	B	C
E	F	G	A	B	C	D
F	G	A	B	C	D	E
G	A	B	C	D	E	F

8 × 8

A	B	C	D	E	F	G	H
B	C	D	E	F	G	H	A
C	D	E	F	G	H	A	B
D	E	F	G	H	A	B	C
E	F	G	H	A	B	C	D
F	G	H	A	B	C	D	E
G	H	A	B	C	D	E	F
H	A	B	C	D	E	F	G

9 × 9

A	B	C	D	E	F	G	H	I
B	C	D	E	F	G	H	I	A
C	D	E	F	G	H	I	A	B
D	E	F	G	H	I	A	B	C
E	F	G	H	I	A	B	C	D
F	G	H	I	A	B	C	D	E
G	H	I	A	B	C	D	E	F
H	I	A	B	C	D	E	F	G
I	A	B	C	D	E	F	G	H

10 × 10

A	B	C	D	E	F	G	H	I	J
B	C	D	E	F	G	H	I	J	A
C	D	E	F	G	H	I	J	A	B
D	E	F	G	H	I	J	A	B	C
E	F	G	H	I	J	A	B	C	D
F	G	H	I	J	A	B	C	D	E
G	H	I	J	A	B	C	D	E	F
H	I	J	A	B	C	D	E	F	G
I	J	A	B	C	D	E	F	G	H
J	A	B	C	D	E	F	G	H	I

11 × 11

A	B	C	D	E	F	G	H	I	J	K
B	C	D	E	F	G	H	I	J	K	A
C	D	E	F	G	H	I	J	K	A	B
D	E	F	G	H	I	J	K	A	B	C
E	F	G	H	I	J	K	A	B	C	D
F	G	H	I	J	K	A	B	C	D	E
G	H	I	J	K	A	B	C	D	E	F
H	I	J	K	A	B	C	D	E	F	G
I	J	K	A	B	C	D	E	F	G	H
J	K	A	B	C	D	E	F	G	H	I
K	A	B	C	D	E	F	G	H	I	J

12 × 12

A	B	C	D	E	F	G	H	I	J	K	L
B	C	D	E	F	G	H	I	J	K	L	A
C	D	E	F	G	H	I	J	K	L	A	B
D	E	F	G	H	I	J	K	L	A	B	C
E	F	G	H	I	J	K	L	A	B	C	D
F	G	H	I	J	K	L	A	B	C	D	E
G	H	I	J	K	L	A	B	C	D	E	F
H	I	J	K	L	A	B	C	D	E	F	G
I	J	K	L	A	B	C	D	E	F	G	H
J	K	L	A	B	C	D	E	F	G	H	I
K	L	A	B	C	D	E	F	G	H	I	J
L	A	B	C	D	E	F	G	H	I	J	K

Plan 4.2 Graeco-latin squares

3 × 3

A_1	B_3	C_2
B_2	C_1	A_3
C_3	A_2	B_1

4 × 4

A_1	B_3	C_4	D_2
B_2	A_4	D_3	C_1
C_3	D_1	A_2	B_4
D_4	C_2	B_1	A_3

5 × 5

A_1	B_3	C_5	D_2	E_4
B_2	C_4	D_1	E_3	A_5
C_3	D_5	E_2	A_4	B_1
D_4	E_1	A_3	B_5	C_2
E_5	A_2	B_4	C_1	D_3

7 × 7

A_1	B_5	C_2	D_6	E_3	F_7	G_4
B_2	C_6	D_3	E_7	F_4	G_1	A_5
C_3	D_7	E_4	F_1	G_5	A_2	B_6
D_4	E_1	F_5	G_2	A_6	B_3	C_7
E_5	F_2	G_6	A_3	B_7	C_4	D_1
F_6	G_3	A_7	B_4	C_1	D_5	E_2
G_7	A_4	B_1	C_5	D_2	E_6	F_3

8 × 8

A_1	B_5	C_2	D_3	E_7	F_4	G_8	H_6
B_2	A_8	G_1	F_7	H_3	D_6	C_5	E_4
C_3	G_4	A_7	E_1	D_2	H_5	B_6	F_8
D_4	F_3	E_6	A_5	C_8	B_1	H_7	G_2
E_5	H_1	D_8	C_4	A_6	G_3	F_2	B_7
F_6	D_7	H_4	B_8	G_5	A_2	E_3	C_1
G_7	C_6	B_3	H_2	F_1	E_8	A_4	D_5
H_8	E_2	F_5	G_6	B_4	C_7	D_1	A_3

9 × 9

A_1	B_3	C_2	D_7	E_9	F_8	G_4	H_6	I_5
B_2	C_1	A_3	E_8	F_7	D_9	H_5	I_4	G_6
C_3	A_2	B_1	F_9	D_8	E_7	I_6	G_5	H_4
D_4	E_6	F_5	G_1	H_3	I_2	A_7	B_9	C_8
E_5	F_4	D_6	H_2	I_1	G_3	B_8	C_7	A_9
F_6	D_5	E_4	I_3	G_2	H_1	C_9	A_8	B_7
G_7	H_9	I_8	A_4	B_6	C_5	D_1	E_3	F_2
H_8	I_7	G_9	B_5	C_4	A_6	E_2	F_1	D_3
I_9	G_8	H_7	C_6	A_5	B_4	F_3	D_2	E_1

11 × 11

A_1	B_7	C_2	D_8	E_3	F_9	G_4	H_{10}	I_5	J_{11}	K_6
B_2	C_8	D_3	E_9	F_4	G_{10}	H_5	I_{11}	J_6	K_1	A_7
C_3	D_9	E_4	F_{10}	G_5	H_{11}	I_6	J_1	K_7	A_2	B_8
D_4	E_{10}	F_5	G_{11}	H_6	I_1	J_7	K_2	A_8	B_3	C_9
E_5	F_{11}	G_6	H_1	I_7	J_2	K_8	A_3	B_9	C_4	D_{10}
F_6	G_1	H_7	I_2	J_8	K_3	A_9	B_4	C_{10}	D_5	E_{11}
G_7	H_2	I_8	J_3	K_9	A_4	B_{10}	C_5	D_{11}	E_6	F_1
H_8	I_3	J_9	K_4	A_{10}	B_5	C_{11}	D_6	E_1	F_7	G_2
I_9	J_4	K_{10}	A_5	B_{11}	C_6	D_1	E_7	F_2	G_8	H_3
J_{10}	K_5	A_{11}	B_6	C_1	D_7	E_2	F_8	G_3	H_9	I_4
K_{11}	A_6	B_1	C_7	D_2	E_8	F_3	G_9	H_4	I_{10}	J_5

12 × 12

A_1	B_{12}	C_6	D_7	I_5	J_4	K_{10}	L_{11}	E_9	F_8	G_2	H_3
B_2	A_{11}	D_5	C_8	J_6	I_3	L_9	K_{12}	F_{10}	E_7	H_1	G_4
C_3	D_{10}	A_8	B_5	K_7	L_2	I_{12}	J_9	G_{11}	H_6	E_4	F_1
D_4	C_9	B_7	A_6	L_8	K_1	J_{11}	I_{10}	H_{12}	G_5	F_3	E_2
E_5	F_4	G_{10}	H_{11}	A_9	B_8	C_2	D_3	I_1	J_{12}	K_6	L_7
F_6	E_3	H_9	G_{12}	B_{10}	A_7	D_1	C_4	J_2	I_{11}	L_5	K_8
G_7	H_2	E_{12}	F_9	C_{11}	D_6	A_4	B_1	K_3	L_{10}	I_8	J_5
H_8	G_1	F_{11}	E_{10}	D_{12}	C_5	B_3	A_2	L_4	K_9	J_7	I_6
I_9	J_8	K_2	L_3	E_1	F_{12}	G_6	H_7	A_5	B_4	C_{10}	D_{11}
J_{10}	I_7	L_1	K_4	F_2	E_{11}	H_5	G_8	B_6	A_3	D_9	C_{12}
K_{11}	L_6	I_4	J_1	G_3	H_{10}	E_8	F_5	C_7	D_2	A_{12}	B_9
L_{12}	K_5	J_3	I_2	H_4	G_9	F_7	E_6	D_8	C_1	B_{11}	A_{10}

INDEX TO PLANS OF FACTORIAL EXPERIMENTS CONFOUNDED IN RANDOMIZED INCOMPLETE BLOCKS

a. Designs with which any number of replicates may be used

Type	Number of treat-ments	Number of units per block	Interactions confounded in a single replicate*	Plan
2^3	8	4	*ABC*	6.1
2^4	16	8	*ABCD*	6.2
2^4	16	4	*AB, ACD, BCD*	6.4
2^5	32	8	*ABC, ADE, BCDE*	6.5
2^6	64	16	*ABCD, ABEF, CDEF*	6.3
2^6	64	8	*ABC, CDE, ADF, BEF, ABDE, BCDF, ACEF*	6.6
3^3	27	9	*ABC* ($\frac{3}{4}$)	6.7
3^4	81	9	*ABC, ABD, ACD, BCD,* all ($\frac{3}{4}$)	6.8
4^2	16	4	*AB* ($\frac{2}{3}$)	6.12
4×2^2	16	8	*ABC* ($\frac{2}{3}$)	6.13

* The fractions in parentheses give the relative information on the comparisons which are confounded. Where no fraction is given, the comparison is completely confounded.

b. Balanced designs

Type	Number of treat-ments	Units per block	Number of replicates for a balanced design	Interactions confounded and relative information (in parentheses)*	Plan
2^4	16	4	6*n*†	All two-factor ($\frac{5}{6}$); all three factor ($\frac{1}{2}$)	6.4
2^5	32	8	5*n*	All three-factor ($\frac{4}{5}$); all four-factor ($\frac{4}{5}$)	6.5
2^6	64	8	10*n*	All three-factor ($\frac{4}{5}$); all four-factor ($\frac{4}{5}$)	6.6
3^3	27	9	4*n*	All three-factor ($\frac{3}{4}$)	6.7
3^4	81	9	4*n*	All three-factor ($\frac{3}{4}$)	6.8
3×2^2	12	6	3*n*‡	*BC* ($\frac{8}{9}$), *ABC* ($\frac{5}{9}$)	6.9
3×2^3	24	6	3*n*‡	*BC, BD, CD,* all ($\frac{8}{9}$); *ABC, ABD, ACD,* all ($\frac{5}{9}$)	6.10
$3^2 \times 2$	18	6	4*n*	*AB* ($\frac{7}{8}$), *ABC* ($\frac{5}{8}$)	6.11
4^2	16	4	3*n*	*AB* ($\frac{2}{3}$)	6.12
4×2^2	16	8	3*n*	*ABC* ($\frac{2}{3}$)	6.13
$4 \times 3 \times 2$	24	12	9*n*‡	*AC* ($\frac{26}{27}$), *ABC* ($\frac{23}{27}$)	6.14

* The factors *ABC* · · · are read from the left; thus the *BC* interaction in a 3×2^2 design is the interaction between the 2 factors at 2 levels.

† The symbol "6*n*" denotes that the number of replicates should be a multiple of 6.

‡ In these cases only the balanced design is recommended.

CONFOUNDED DESIGNS FOR OTHER FACTORIAL EXPERIMENTS

Type	Units per block	Number of replicates	Interactions confounded	Reference
$3^2 \times 2^2$	12	$2n$	AB ($\frac{7}{8}$); $ABCD$ ($\frac{5}{8}$)	6.6
$3^3 \times 2$	18	$2n$	ABC, $ABCD$	6.6
$3^3 \times 2$	6	$2n$	AB, AC, BC ($\frac{7}{8}$), ABD, ACD, BCD, ABC	6.1
4×3^2	12	$2n$	BC ($\frac{7}{8}$), ABC	6.6
$4^2 \times 2$	16	Any	ABC	6.6
$4^2 \times 3$	12	$3n$	AB ($\frac{26}{27}$), ABC	6.6
4^3	16	Any	ABC	6.7
4×2^3	8	$3n$	ABC, ABD, ACD	6.6
4^4	16	Any	ABC, ABD, ACD, BCD	6.7
5^2	5	$4n$	AB ($\frac{3}{4}$)	6.8
5×2^2	10	$5n$	BC ($\frac{24}{25}$), ABC	6.6
5^3	25	Any	ABC	6.8

Plan 6.1 2^3 factorial, blocks of 4 units

Rep. I, *ABC* confounded

abc	*ab*
a	*ac*
b	*bc*
c	(1)

Plan 6.2 2^4 factorial, blocks of 8 units

Rep. I, *ABCD* confounded

a	(1)
b	*ab*
c	*ac*
d	*bc*
abc	*ad*
abd	*bd*
acd	*cd*
bcd	*abcd*

Plan 6.3 2^6 factorial, blocks of 16 units

Rep. I, *ABCD*, *ABEF*, *CDEF* confounded

a	*c*	*ab*	*ac*
b	*d*	*cd*	*ad*
acd	*abc*	(1)	*bc*
bcd	*abd*	*abcd*	*bd*
ce	*ae*	*ace*	*abe*
de	*be*	*ade*	*cde*
abce	*acde*	*bce*	*e*
abde	*bcde*	*bde*	*abcde*
cf	*af*	*acf*	*abf*
df	*bf*	*adf*	*cdf*
abcf	*acdf*	*bcf*	*f*
abdf	*bcdf*	*bdf*	*abcdf*
aef	*cef*	*abef*	*acef*
bef	*def*	*cdef*	*adef*
acdef	*abcef*	*ef*	*bcef*
bcdef	*abdef*	*abcdef*	*bdef*

Plan 6.4 Balanced group of sets for 2^4 factorial, blocks of 4 units

Two-factor interactions are confounded in 1 replication and three-factor interactions are confounded in 3 replications. The columns are the blocks.

Rep. I, *AB, ACD, BCD* confounded

(1)	ab	a	b
abc	c	bc	ac
abd	d	bd	ad
cd	abcd	acd	bcd

Rep. II, *AC, ABD, BCD*

(1)	ac	a	c
abc	b	bc	ab
acd	d	cd	ad
bd	abcd	abd	bcd

Rep. III, *AD, ABC, BCD*

(1)	ad	a	d
abd	b	bd	ab
acd	c	cd	ac
bc	abcd	abc	bcd

Rep. IV, *BC, ABD, ACD*

(1)	bc	b	c
abc	a	ac	ab
bcd	d	cd	bd
ad	abcd	abd	acd

Rep. V, *BD, ABC, ACD*

(1)	bd	b	d
abd	a	ad	ab
bcd	c	cd	bc
ac	abcd	abc	acd

Rep. VI, *CD, ABC, ABD*

(1)	cd	c	d
acd	a	ad	ac
bcd	b	bd	bc
ab	abcd	abc	abd

Plan 6.5 Balanced group of sets for 2^5 factorial, blocks of 8 units

Three- and four-factor interactions are confounded in 1 replication.

Rep. I, *ABC, ADE, BCDE* confounded

(1)	ab	a	b
bc	ac	abc	c
abd	d	bd	ad
acd	bcd	be	abcd
abe	e	ce	ae
ace	bce	ade	abce
de	abde	abcde	bde
bcde	acde	cd	cde

Rep. II, *ABD, BCE, ACDE*

(1)	ab	a	b
ad	bd	d	abd
abc	c	bc	ac
bcd	acd	abcd	cd
abe	e	be	ae
bde	ade	abde	de
ce	abce	ace	bce
acde	bcde	cde	abcde

Rep. III, *ACE, BCD, ABDE*

(1)	ac	a	c
ae	ce	e	ace
abc	b	bc	ab
bce	abe	abce	be
acd	d	cd	ad
cde	ade	acde	de
bd	abcd	abd	bcd
abde	bcde	bde	abcde

Rep. IV, *ACD, BDE, ABCE*

(1)	ad	a	d
ac	cd	c	acd
abd	b	bd	ab
bcd	abc	abcd	bc
ade	e	de	ae
cde	ace	acde	ce
be	abde	abe	bde
abce	bcde	bce	abcde

Rep. V, *ABE, CDE, ABCD*

(1)	ae	a	e
ab	be	b	abe
ace	c	ce	ac
bce	abc	abce	bc
ade	d	de	ad
bde	abd	abde	bd
cd	acde	acd	cde
abcd	bcde	bcd	abcde

Plan 6.6 Balanced group of sets for 2^6 factorial, blocks of 8 units

All three- and four-factor interactions are confounded in 2 replications.

Rep. I, *ABC, CDE, ADF, BEF, ABDE, BCDF, ACEF* confounded

abc	a	b	(1)	bc	ac	c	ab
bd	cd	abcd	acd	abd	d	ad	bcd
ae	abce	ce	bce	e	abe	be	ace
cde	bde	ade	abde	acde	bcde	abcde	de
cf	bf	af	abf	acf	bcf	abcf	f
adf	abcdf	cdf	bcdf	df	abdf	bdf	acdf
bef	cef	abcef	acef	abef	ef	aef	bcef
abcdef	adef	bdef	def	bcdef	acdef	cdef	abdef

Rep. II, *ABD, DEF, BCF, ACE, ABEF, ACDF, BCDE*

abd	*b*	*a*	(1)	*ad*	*bd*	*d*	*ab*
cd	*ac*	*bc*	*abc*	*bcd*	*acd*	*abcd*	*c*
be	*abde*	*de*	*ade*	*e*	*abe*	*ae*	*bde*
ace	*cde*	*abcde*	*bcde*	*abce*	*ce*	*bce*	*acde*
af	*df*	*abdf*	*bdf*	*abf*	*f*	*bf*	*adf*
bcf	*abcdf*	*cdf*	*acdf*	*cf*	*abcf*	*acf*	*bcdf*
def	*aef*	*bef*	*abef*	*bdef*	*adef*	*abdef*	*ef*
abcdef	*bcef*	*acef*	*cef*	*acdef*	*bcdef*	*cdef*	*abcef*

Rep. III, *ABE, BDF, ACD, CEF, ADEF, BCDE, ABCF*

bc	*a*	*ac*	(1)	*abc*	*ab*	*b*	*c*
acd	*bd*	*bcd*	*abd*	*cd*	*d*	*ad*	*abcd*
abe	*ce*	*e*	*ace*	*be*	*bce*	*abce*	*ae*
de	*abcde*	*abde*	*bcde*	*ade*	*acde*	*cde*	*bde*
af	*bcf*	*bf*	*abcf*	*f*	*cf*	*acf*	*abf*
bdf	*acdf*	*adf*	*cdf*	*abdf*	*abcdf*	*bcdf*	*df*
cef	*abef*	*abcef*	*bef*	*acef*	*aef*	*ef*	*bcef*
abcdef	*def*	*cdef*	*adef*	*bcdef*	*bdef*	*abdef*	*acdef*

Rep. IV, *ABF, CDF, ADE, BCE, ABCD, BDEF, ACEF*

ac	*a*	*b*	(1)	*c*	*abc*	*bc*	*ab*
bd	*bcd*	*acd*	*abcd*	*abd*	*d*	*ad*	*cd*
bce	*be*	*ae*	*abe*	*abce*	*ce*	*ace*	*e*
ade	*acde*	*bcde*	*cde*	*de*	*abde*	*bde*	*abcde*
abf	*abcf*	*cf*	*bcf*	*bf*	*af*	*f*	*acf*
cdf	*df*	*abdf*	*adf*	*acdf*	*bcdf*	*abcdf*	*bdf*
ef	*cef*	*abcef*	*acef*	*aef*	*bef*	*abef*	*bcef*
abcdef	*abdef*	*def*	*bdef*	*bcdef*	*acdef*	*cdef*	*adef*

Rep. V, *ACF, BCD, ADE, BEF, ABDF, CDEF, ABCE*

ab	*a*	*bc*	(1)	*b*	*ac*	*c*	*abc*
bcd	*cd*	*abd*	*acd*	*abcd*	*d*	*ad*	*bd*
ce	*bce*	*ae*	*abce*	*ace*	*be*	*abe*	*e*
ade	*abde*	*cde*	*bde*	*de*	*abcde*	*bcde*	*acde*
acf	*abcf*	*f*	*bcf*	*cf*	*abf*	*bf*	*af*
df	*bdf*	*acdf*	*abdf*	*adf*	*bcdf*	*abcdf*	*cdf*
bef	*ef*	*abcef*	*aef*	*abef*	*cef*	*acef*	*bcef*
abcdef	*acdef*	*bdef*	*cdef*	*bcdef*	*adef*	*def*	*abdef*

Rep. VI, *ABC, BDE, ADF, CEF, ACDE, BCDF, ABEF*
Interchange *B* and *C* in replication I
Rep. VII, *ABF, DEF, BCD, ACE, ABDE, ACDF, BCEF*
Interchange *F* and *D* in replication II
Rep. VIII, *ABE, BDF, CDE, ACF, ADEF, ABCD, BCEF*
Interchange *A* and *E* in replication III
Rep. IX, *ABD, CDF, AEF, BCE, ABCF, BDEF, ACDE*
Interchange *F* and *D* in replication IV
Rep. X, *AEF, BDE, ACD, BCF, ABDF, CDEF, ABCE*
Interchange *E* and *C* in replication V

Plan 6.7 Balanced group of sets for 3^3 factorial, blocks of 9 units

ABC confounded

Rep. I, *ABC*(*W*)* *a*	*b*	*c*	Rep. II, *ABC*(*X*) *a*	*b*	*c*	Rep. III, *ABC*(*Y*) *a*	*b*	*c*	Rep. IV, *ABC*(*Z*) *a*	*b*	*c*
000	100	200	000	100	200	000	100	200	000	100	200
110	210	010	110	210	010	210	010	110	210	010	110
220	020	120	220	020	120	120	220	020	120	220	020
101	201	001	201	001	101	101	201	001	201	001	101
211	011	111	011	111	211	011	111	211	111	211	011
021	121	221	121	221	021	221	021	121	021	121	221
202	002	102	102	202	002	202	002	102	102	202	002
012	112	212	212	012	112	112	212	012	012	112	212
122	222	022	022	122	222	022	122	222	222	022	122

* Yates' notation.

Plan 6.8 Balanced group of sets for 3^4 factorial, blocks of 9 units

Three-factor interactions confounded

Rep. I, *ABC* I, *ABD* III, *ACD* IV, *BCD* II confounded

0000	0011	0022	0012	0020	0001	0021	0002	0010
1011	1022	1000	1020	1001	1012	1002	1010	1021
2022	2000	2011	2001	2012	2020	2010	2021	2002
0121	0102	0110	0100	0111	0122	0112	0120	0101
1102	1110	1121	1111	1122	1100	1120	1101	1112
2110	2121	2102	2122	2100	2111	2101	2112	2120
0212	0220	0201	0221	0202	0210	0200	0211	0222
1220	1201	1212	1202	1210	1221	1211	1222	1200
2201	2212	2220	2210	2221	2202	2222	2200	2211

Rep. II, *ABC* II, *ABD* IV, *ACD* I, *BCD* III

0000	0022	0011	0021	0010	0002	0012	0001	0020
1022	1011	1000	1010	1002	1021	1001	1020	1012
2011	2000	2022	2002	2021	2010	2020	2012	2001
0112	0101	0120	0100	0122	0111	0121	0110	0102
1101	1120	1112	1122	1111	1100	1110	1102	1121
2120	2112	2101	2111	2100	2122	2102	2121	2110
0221	0210	0202	0212	0201	0220	0200	0222	0211
1210	1202	1221	1201	1220	1212	1222	1211	1200
2202	2221	2210	2220	2212	2201	2211	2200	2222

Rep. III, *ABC* IV, *ABD* I, *ACD* II, *BCD* I

0000	0021	0012	0022	0010	0001	0011	0002	0020
1021	1012	1000	1010	1001	1022	1002	1020	1011
2012	2000	2021	2001	2022	2010	2020	2011	2002
0122	0110	0101	0111	0102	0120	0100	0121	0112
1110	1101	1122	1102	1120	1111	1121	1112	1100
2101	2122	2110	2120	2111	2102	2112	2100	2121
0211	0202	0220	0200	0221	0212	0222	0210	0201
1202	1220	1211	1221	1212	1200	1210	1201	1222
2220	2211	2202	2212	2200	2221	2201	2222	2210

Rep. IV, *ABC* III, *ABD* II, *ACD* III, *BCD* IV

0000	0012	0021	0011	0020	0002	0022	0001	0010
1012	1021	1000	1020	1002	1011	1001	1010	1022
2021	2000	2012	2002	2011	2020	2010	2022	2001
0111	0120	0102	0122	0101	0110	0100	0112	0121
1120	1102	1111	1101	1110	1122	1112	1121	1100
2102	2111	2120	2110	2122	2101	2121	2100	2112
0222	0201	0210	0200	0212	0221	0211	0220	0202
1201	1210	1222	1212	1221	1200	1220	1202	1211
2210	2222	2201	2221	2200	2212	2202	2211	2220

Plan 6.9 Balanced group of sets for 3 $\times$ 2^2 factorial, blocks of 6 units

BC, *ABC* confounded

Rep. I		Rep. II		Rep. III	
a	*b*	*a*	*b*	*a*	*b*
001	000	000	001	000	001
010	011	011	010	011	010
100	101	101	100	100	101
111	110	110	111	111	110
200	201	200	201	201	200
211	210	211	210	210	211

Plan 6.10 Balanced group of sets for 3 $\times$ 2^3 factorial, blocks of 6 units

BC, *BD*, *CD*
ABC, *ABD*, *ACD* confounded

Rep. I				Rep. II				Rep. III			
a	*b*	*c*	*d*	*a*	*b*	*c*	*d*	*a*	*b*	*c*	*d*
0100	0000	0001	0010	0010	0001	0000	0100	0001	0010	0100	0000
0011	0111	0110	0101	0101	0110	0111	0011	0110	0101	0011	0111
1010	1001	1000	1100	1001	1010	1100	1000	1100	1000	1001	1010
1101	1110	1111	1011	1110	1101	1011	1111	1011	1111	1110	1101
2001	2010	2100	2000	2100	2000	2001	2010	2010	2001	2000	2100
2110	2101	2011	2111	2011	2111	2110	2101	2101	2110	2111	2011

Plan 6.11 Balanced group of sets for 3^2 $\times$ 2 factorial, blocks of 6 units

AB, *ABC* confounded

Rep. I			Rep. II			Rep. III			Rep. IV		
a	*b*	*c*	*a*	*b*	*c*	*a*	*b*	*c*	*a*	*b*	*c*
100	200	000	200	000	100	100	200	000	200	000	100
210	010	110	010	110	210	010	110	210	110	210	010
020	120	220	120	220	020	220	020	120	020	120	220
201	001	101	101	201	001	201	001	101	101	201	001
011	111	211	211	011	111	111	211	011	011	111	211
121	221	021	021	121	221	021	121	221	221	021	121

Plan 6.12 Balanced group of sets for 4^2 factorial, blocks of 4 units

AB confounded

Rep. I				Rep. II				Rep. III			
a	*b*	*c*	*d*	*a*	*b*	*c*	*d*	*a*	*b*	*c*	*d*
33	32	31	30	33	30	32	31	33	31	32	30
22	23	20	21	21	22	20	23	20	22	21	23
10	11	12	13	12	11	13	10	11	13	10	12
01	00	03	02	00	03	01	02	02	00	03	01

Plan 6.13 Balanced group of sets for 4×2^2 factorial, blocks of 8 units

ABC confounded

Rep. I		Rep. II		Rep. III	
a	*b*	*a*	*b*	*a*	*b*
000	001	000	001	000	001
011	010	011	010	011	010
100	101	101	100	101	100
111	110	110	111	110	111
201	200	201	200	200	201
210	211	210	211	211	210
301	300	300	301	301	300
310	311	311	310	310	311

Plan 6.14 Balanced group of sets for $4 \times 3 \times 2$ factorial, blocks of 12 units

A'C, A'BC confounded

Rep. I		Rep. II		Rep. III	
a	*b*	*a*	*b*	*a*	*b*
000	001	001	000	001	000
011	010	010	011	011	010
021	020	021	020	020	021
100	101	101	100	101	100
111	110	110	111	111	110
121	120	121	120	120	121
201	200	200	201	200	201
210	211	211	210	210	211
220	221	220	221	221	220
301	300	300	301	300	301
310	311	311	310	310	311
320	321	320	321	321	320

A''C, A''BC

Rep. IV		Rep. V		Rep. VI	
a	*b*	*a*	*b*	*a*	*b*
001	000	000	001	000	001
010	011	011	010	010	011
020	021	020	021	021	020
100	101	101	100	101	100
111	110	110	111	111	110
121	120	121	120	120	121
200	201	201	200	201	200
211	210	210	211	211	210
221	220	221	220	220	221
301	300	300	301	300	301
310	311	311	310	310	311
320	321	320	321	321	320

$A' = a_3 + a_2 - a_1 - a_0$
$A'' = a_3 - a_2 - a_1 + a_0$
$A''' = a_3 - a_2 + a_1 - a_0$

A'''C, A'''BC

Rep. VII		Rep. VIII		Rep. IX	
a	*b*	*a*	*b*	*a*	*b*
000	001	001	000	001	000
011	010	010	011	011	010
021	020	021	020	020	021
101	100	100	101	100	101
110	111	111	110	110	111
120	121	120	121	121	120
200	201	201	200	201	200
211	210	210	211	211	210
221	220	221	220	220	221
301	300	300	301	300	301
310	311	311	310	310	311
320	321	320	321	321	320

INDEX TO PLANS FOR 2^n FACTORIALS IN FRACTIONAL REPLICATION

				Two-factor interactions		Error d.f.		
No. of factors	Fraction of a rep.	Size of expt.	Size of block	Total	Max. no. estimable	2-factors used as error	2-factors estimated	Plan no.
4	$\frac{1}{2}$	8	8	6	3*	3	0	6A.1‡
5	$\frac{1}{4}$	8	8	10	2*	2	0	6A.2‡
	$\frac{1}{2}$	16	16	10	10	10	0	6A.3‡
			8	10	9	9	0	6A.3‡
			4	10	7	7	0	6A.3‡
6	$\frac{1}{8}$	8	8	15	1*	1	0	6A.4‡
	$\frac{1}{4}$	16	16	15	7*	9	2	6A.5‡
			8	15	7*	8	1	6A.5‡
			4	15	6*	6	0	6A.5‡
	$\frac{1}{2}$	32	32	15	15	25	10	6A.6
			16	15	15	24	9	6A.6
			8	15	14	22	8	6A.6
			4	15	12	18	6	6A.6
7	$\frac{1}{16}$	8	8	21	0	0	0	6A.7‡
	$\frac{1}{8}$	16	16	21	7*	8	1	6A.9‡
			8	21	7*	7	0	6A.9‡
			4	21	4*	5	1	6A.8‡
	$\frac{1}{4}$	32	32	21	18†	24	6	6A.11
			16	21	18†	23	5	6A.11
			8	21	17†	21	4	6A.11
			4	21	14†	17	3	6A.10
	$\frac{1}{2}$	64	64	21	21	56	35	6A.13
			32	21	21	55	34	6A.13
			16	21	21	53	32	6A.13
			8	21	21	49	28	6A.13
			4	21	15	41	26	6A.12
8	$\frac{1}{16}$	16	16	28	7*	7	0	6A.14‡
			8	28	6*	6	0	6A.14‡
			4	28	4*	4	0	6A.14‡
	$\frac{1}{8}$	32	32	28	20†	23	3	6A.15‡
			16	28	19†	22	3	6A.15‡
			8	28	17†	20	3	6A.15‡
			4	28	13	16	3	6A.15‡
	$\frac{1}{4}$	64	64	28	28	55	27	6A.16
			32	28	28	54	26	6A.16
			16	28	28	52	24	6A.16
			8	28	26	48	22	6A.16
			4	28	21	40	19	6A.16
	$\frac{1}{2}$	128	128	28	28	119	91	6A.17
			64	28	28	118	90	6A.17
			32	28	28	116	88	6A.17
			16	28	28	112	84	6A.17
			8	28	26	104	78	6A.17

* All these interactions have other 2-factor interactions as aliases, and are estimable only if the aliases can be considered negligible. See plans for details.

† Some of the interactions have other 2-factor interactions as aliases. See plans for details.

‡ Except in unusual circumstances, only main effects can be estimated with this design.

Plan 6A.1 2^4 factorial in 8 units ($\frac{1}{2}$ replicate)

Defining contrast: *ABCD*

Estimable 2-factor interactions: $AB = CD$, $AC = BD$, $AD = BC$.

(1)
ab
ac
ad
bc
bd
cd
abcd

Effects	d.f.
Main	4
2-factor	3
Total	7

Plan 6A.2 2^5 factorial in 8 units ($\frac{1}{4}$ replicate)

Defining contrasts: *ABE*, *CDE*, *ABCD*

Main effects have 2-factors as aliases. The only estimable 2-factors are $AC = BD$ and $AD = BC$.

(1)
ab
cd
ace
bce
ade
bde
abcd

Effects	d.f.
Main	5
2-factor	2
Total	7

Plan 6A.3 2^5 factorial in 16 units ($\frac{1}{2}$ replicate)

Defining contrast: *ABCDE*

Blocks of 4 units

Estimable 2-factors: All except *CD*, *CE*, *DE* (confounded with blocks).

Blocks	(1)	(2)	(3)	(4)
	(1)	*ac*	*ae*	*ad*
	ab	*bc*	*be*	*bd*
	acde	*de*	*cd*	*ce*
	bcde	*abde*	*abcd*	*abce*

CD, *CE*, *DE* confounded.

Effects	d.f.
Block	3
Main	5
2-factor	7
Total	15

Blocks of 8 units

Estimable 2-factors: All except *DE*.

Combine blocks 1 and 2; and blocks 3 and 4. *DE* confounded.

Effects	d.f.
Block	1
Main	5
2-factor	9
Total	15

Blocks of 16 units

Estimable 2-factors: All.

Combine blocks 1–4.

Effects	d.f.
Main	5
2-factor	10
Total	15

Plan 6A.4 2^6 factorial in 8 units ($\frac{1}{8}$ replicate)

Defining contrasts: *ACE, ADF, BCF, BDE, ABCD, ABEF, CDEF*

Main effects have 2-factors as aliases. The only estimable 2-factor is the set $AB = CD = EF$.

(1)
acf
ade
bce
bdf
abcd
abef
cdef

Effects	d.f.
Main	6
2-factor ($AB = CD = EF$)	1
Total	7

Plan 6A.5 2^6 factorial in 16 units ($\frac{1}{4}$ replicate)

Defining contrasts: *ABCE, ABDF, CDEF*

Blocks of 4 units

Estimable 2-factors: The alias sets $AC = BE$, $AD = BF$, $AE = BC$, $AF = BD$, $CD = EF$, $CF = DE$.

Blocks (1)	(2)	(3)	(4)
(1)	*acd*	*ab*	*acf*
abce	*aef*	*ce*	*ade*
abdf	*bcf*	*df*	*bcd*
cdef	*bde*	*abcdef*	*bef*

AB, ACF, BCF confounded.

Effects	d.f.
Block	3
Main	6
2-factor	6
Total	15

Blocks of 8 units

Estimable 2-factors: Same as in blocks of 4 units, plus the set $AB = CE = DF$.

Combine blocks 1 and 2; and blocks 3 and 4. *ACF* confounded.

Effects	d.f.
Block	1
Main	6
2-factor	7
3-factor	1
Total	15

Blocks of 16 units

Estimable 2-factors: Same as in blocks of 8 units.

Combine blocks 1–4.

Effects	d.f.
Main	6
2-factor	7
3-factor	2
Total	15

Plan 6A.6 2^6 factorial in 32 units ($\frac{1}{2}$ replicate)

Defining contrast: *ABCDEF*

Blocks of 4 units

Estimable 2-factors: All except *AE, BF,* and *CD* (confounded with blocks).

Blocks (1)	(2)	(3)	(4)	(5)	(6)	(7)	(8)
(1)	*ab*	*ac*	*bc*	*ae*	*af*	*ad*	*bd*
abef	*ef*	*de*	*df*	*bf*	*be*	*ce*	*cf*
acde	*acdf*	*abdf*	*acef*	*cd*	*abcd*	*abcf*	*abce*
bcdf	*bcde*	*bcef*	*abde*	*abcdef*	*cdef*	*bdef*	*adef*

AE, BF, CD, ABC, ABD, ACF, ADF confounded.

Effects	d.f.
Block	7
Main	6
2-factor	12
Higher order	6
Total	31

Blocks of 8 units	*Blocks of 16 units*	*Blocks of 32 units*
Estimable 2-factors: All except *CD*.	Estimable 2-factors: All.	Estimable 2-factors: All.
Combine blocks 1 and 2; blocks 3 and 4; blocks 5 and 6; and blocks 7 and 8. *CD, ABC, ABD* confounded.	Estimable 3-factors: *ABC* = *DEF* is lost by confounding. The others are in alias pairs, e.g., *ABD* = *CEF*.	Estimable 3-factors: These are arranged in 10 alias pairs.
	Combine blocks 1–4; and blocks 5–8. *ABC* confounded.	Combine blocks 1–8.

Effects	d.f.
Block	3
Main	6
2-factor	14
Higher order	8
Total	31

Effects	d.f.
Block	1
Main	6
2-factor	15
3-factor	9
Total	31

Effects	d.f.
Main	6
2-factor	15
3-factor	10
Total	31

Plan 6A.7 2^7 factorial in 8 units ($\frac{1}{16}$ replicate)

Defining contrasts: *ABG, ACE, ADF, BCF, BDE, CDG, EFG, ABCD, ABEF, ACFG, ADEG, BCEG, BDFG, CDEF, ABCDEFG*

Main effects have 2-factors as aliases. No 2-factors are estimable.

(1)
abcd
abef
acfg
adeg
bceg
bdfg
cdef

Effects	d.f.
Main	7
Total	7

Plan 6A.8 2^7 factorial in 16 units ($\frac{1}{8}$ replicate)

Defining contrasts: *ABCD, ABEF, ACEG, ADFG, BCFG, BDEG, CDEF*

Blocks of 4 units

Estimable 2-factors: Only the alias sets *AE* = *BF* = *CG*; *AF* = *BE* = *DG*; *AG* = *CE* = *DF*; *BG* = *DE* = *CF*.

Blocks	(1)	(2)	(3)	(4)
	(1)	*abg*	*acf*	*ade*
	efg	*cdg*	*bdf*	*bce*
	abcd	*abef*	*aceg*	*adfg*
	abcdefg	*cdef*	*bdeg*	*bcfg*

AB = *CD* = *EF*,
AC = *BD* = *EG*,
AD = *BC* = *FG* confounded.

Effects	d.f.
Block	3
Main	7
2-factor	4
Higher order	1
Total	15

Plan 6A.9 2^7 factorial in 16 units ($\frac{1}{8}$ replicate)

Defining contrasts: *ABCD, ABEF, ACEG, ADFG, BCFG, BDEG, CDEF*

Blocks of 8 units

Estimable 2-factors: Same as in blocks of 4 units, plus the alias sets *AB* = *CD* = *EF*, *AC* = *BD* = *EG*, *AD* = *BC* = *FG*.

Blocks (1)	(2)
(1)	*abg*
abcd	*acf*
abef	*ade*
aceg	*bce*
adfg	*bdf*
bcfg	*cdg*
bdeg	*efg*
cdef	*abcdefg*

Effects	d.f.
Block	1
Main	7
2-factor	7
Total	15

ABG confounded.

Blocks of 16 units

Estimable 2-factors: Same as in blocks of 8 units.

Combine blocks 1 and 2 of the plan for blocks of 8 units.

Effects	d.f.
Main	7
2-factor	7
Higher order	1
Total	15

Plan 6A.10 2^7 factorial in 32 units ($\frac{1}{4}$ replicate)

Defining contrasts: *ABCDE, ABCFG, DEFG*

Blocks of 4 units

Estimable 2-factors: *AB, AC, BC*, and *DF* = *EG* are lost by confounding. All other 2-factors are estimable, except that *DE* = *FG* and *DG* = *EF*, so that members of these alias pairs cannot be separated.

Blocks (1)	(2)	(3)	(4)	(5)	(6)	(7)	(8)
(1)	*de*	*ab*	*cdg*	*ac*	*bdg*	*bc*	*adg*
defg	*fg*	*cdf*	*cef*	*bdf*	*bef*	*adf*	*aef*
abcdf	*abcdg*	*ceg*	*abde*	*beg*	*acde*	*aeg*	*bcfg*
abceg	*abcef*	*abdefg*	*abfg*	*acdefg*	*acfg*	*bcdefg*	*bcde*

Effects	d.f.
Block	7
Main	7
2-factor	14
Higher order	3
Total	31

AB, AC, BC, DF = *EG, ADG, BDG, CDG* confounded.

Plan 6A.11 2^7 factorial in 32 units ($\frac{1}{4}$ replicate)

Defining contrasts: *ABCDE, ABCFG, DEFG*

Blocks of 8 units

Estimable 2-factors: All except *DF* = *EG* (confounded with blocks). However, *DE* = *FG* and *DG* = *EF* are alias pairs which cannot be separated.

Blocks (1)	(2)	(3)	(4)
(1)	*bdg*	*ab*	*de*
bc	*bef*	*ac*	*fg*
adf	*cef*	*bdf*	*adg*
aeg	*abfg*	*beg*	*aef*
defg	*acfg*	*cdf*	*bcde*
abcdf	*abde*	*ceg*	*bcfg*
abceg	*acde*	*acdefg*	*abcdg*
bcdefg	*cdg*	*abdefg*	*abcef*

Effects	d.f.
Block	3
Main	7
2-factor	17
Higher order	4
Total	31

DF = *EG, ADE, AEF* confounded.

Blocks of 16 units

Estimable 2-factors: All, except that $DE = FG$, $DG = EF$, and $DF = EG$ are alias pairs.

Combine blocks 1 and 2; and blocks 3 and 4. AEF confounded.

Effects	d.f.
Block	1
Main	7
2-factor	18
Higher order	5
Total	31

Blocks of 32 units

Estimable 2-factors: Same as in blocks of 16 units.

Combine blocks 1–4.

Effects	d.f.
Main	7
2-factor	18
Higher order	6
Total	31

Plan 6A.12 2^7 factorial in 64 units ($\frac{1}{2}$ replicate)

Defining contrast: $ABCDEFG$

Blocks of 4 units

Estimable 2-factors: All except AB, AC, BC, EF, EG, and FG (confounded with blocks).

Blocks	(1)	(2)	(3)	(4)	(5)	(6)	(7)	(8)
	(1)	*ab*	*ac*	*bc*	*ae*	*be*	*ce*	*abce*
	abcd	*cd*	*bd*	*ad*	*bcde*	*acde*	*abde*	*de*
	defg	*abdefg*	*acdefg*	*bcdefg*	*adfg*	*bdfg*	*cdfg*	*abcdfg*
	abcefg	*cefg*	*befg*	*aefg*	*bcfg*	*acfg*	*abfg*	*fg*

Blocks	(9)	(10)	(11)	(12)	(13)	(14)	(15)	(16)
	af	*bf*	*cf*	*abcf*	*ef*	*abef*	*acef*	*bcef*
	bcdf	*acdf*	*abdf*	*df*	*abcdef*	*cdef*	*bdef*	*adef*
	adeg	*bdeg*	*cdeg*	*abcdeg*	*dg*	*abdg*	*acdg*	*bcdg*
	bceg	*aceg*	*abeg*	*eg*	*abcg*	*cg*	*bg*	*ag*

Effects	d.f.
Block	15
Main	7
2-factor	15
Higher order	26
Total	63

AB, AC, BC, EF, EG, FG, ADE, ADF, ADG, BDE, BDF, BDG, CDE, CDF, CDG confounded.

Plan 6A.13 2^7 factorial in 64 units ($\frac{1}{2}$ replicate)

Defining contrast: $ABCDEFG$

Blocks of 8 units

Estimable 2-factors: All.

Estimable 3-factors: All except ABC, ADE, AFG, BDF, BEG, CDG, CEF (confounded with blocks).

Blocks	(1)	(2)	(3)	(4)	(5)	(6)	(7)	(8)
	(1)	*bc*	*ac*	*ab*	*ag*	*af*	*ae*	*ad*
	abdg	*de*	*df*	*dg*	*bd*	*be*	*bf*	*bg*
	abef	*fg*	*eg*	*ef*	*ce*	*cd*	*cg*	*cf*
	acdf	*abdf*	*abde*	*acde*	*abcf*	*abcg*	*abcd*	*abce*
	aceg	*abeg*	*abfg*	*acfg*	*adef*	*adeg*	*adfg*	*aefg*
	bcde	*acdg*	*bcdg*	*bcdf*	*befg*	*bdfg*	*bdeg*	*bdef*
	bcfg	*acef*	*bcef*	*bceg*	*cdfg*	*cefg*	*cdef*	*cdeg*
	defg	*bcdefg*	*acdefg*	*abdefg*	*abcdeg*	*abcdef*	*abcefg*	*abcdfg*

Effects	d.f.
Block	7
Main	7
2-factor	21
3-factor	28
Total	63

Blocks of 16 units

Estimable 2-factors: All.

Estimable 3-factors: All except *ABC, ADE, AFG* (confounded).

Combine blocks 1 and 2; blocks 3 and 4; blocks 5 and 6; and blocks 7 and 8.

Effects	d.f.
Block	3
Main	7
2-factor	21
Higher order	32
Total	63

Blocks of 32 units

Estimable 2-factors: All.

Estimable 3-factors: All except *ABC* (confounded).

Combine blocks 1–4; and blocks 5–8.

Effects	d.f.
Block	1
Main	7
2-factor	21
3-factor	34
Total	63

Blocks of 64 units

Estimable 2-factors: All.

Estimable 3-factors: All.

Combine blocks 1–8.

Effects	d.f.
Main	7
2-factor	21
3-factor	35
Total	63

Plan 6A.14 2^8 factorial in 16 units ($\frac{1}{16}$ replicate)

Defining contrasts: *ABCD, ABEF, ABGH, ACEH, ACFG, ADEG, ADFH, BCEG, BCFH, BDEH, BDFG, CDEF, CDGH, EFGH, ABCDEFGH.*

Blocks of 4 units

Estimable 2-factors: Only the 4 alias sets $AE = BF = CH = DG$; $AF = BE = CG = DH$; $AG = BH = CF = DE$; $AH = BG = CE = DF$. Except in special circumstances, only main effects are estimable.

Blocks (1)	(2)	(3)	(4)
(1)	*abef*	*adeg*	*aceh*
abcd	*abgh*	*adfh*	*acfg*
efgh	*cdef*	*bceg*	*bdeh*
abcdefgh	*cdgh*	*bcfh*	*bdfg*

AB, AC, AD confounded.

Effects	d.f.
Block	3
Main	8
2-factor	4
Total	15

Blocks of 8 units

Estimable 2-factors: As in blocks of 4 units, plus the alias sets $AC = BD = EH = FG$; $AD = BC = EG = FH$.

Combine blocks 1 and 2; and blocks 3 and 4. *AB* confounded.

Effects	d.f.
Block	1
Main	8
2-factor	6
Total	15

Blocks of 16 units

Estimable 2-factors: As in blocks of 8 units, plus the alias set $AB = CD = EF = GH$.

Combine blocks 1–4.

Effects	d.f.
Main	8
2-factor	7
Total	15

Plan 6A.15 2^8 factorial in 32 units ($\frac{1}{8}$ replicate)

Defining contrasts: *BCDH, BDFG, CFGH, ABCEF, ABEGH, ACDEG, ADEFH*

Blocks of 4 units

Estimable 2-factors: All interactions of *A* and of *E*. All other 2-factors are lost by confounding.

Blocks (1)	(2)	(3)	(4)	(5)	(6)	(7)	(8)
(1)	*abd*	*dgh*	*cdf*	*afg*	*ach*	*bcg*	*bfh*
ae	*bde*	*abcf*	*abgh*	*efg*	*ceh*	*adfh*	*acdg*
abcdfgh	*cfgh*	*bcef*	*begh*	*bcdh*	*bdfg*	*defh*	*cdeg*
bcdefgh	*acefgh*	*adegh*	*acdef*	*abcdeh*	*abdefg*	*abceg*	*abefh*

BD, BF, BH, CF, DF, DH, FH and their aliases confounded.

Effects	d.f.
Block	7
Main	8
2-factor	13
Higher order	3
Total	31

Blocks of 8 units

Estimable 2-factors: All interactions of A and of E, and the alias pairs $BC = DH$, $BF = DG$, $BG = DF$, $BH = CD$.

Combine blocks 1 and 2; blocks 3 and 4; blocks 5 and 6; and blocks 7 and 8. BD, CF, FH confounded.

Effects	d.f.
Block	3
Main	8
2-factor	17
Higher order	3
Total	31

Blocks of 16 units

Estimable 2-factors: As in blocks of 8 units, plus the alias sets $CG = FH$, $BD = CH = FG$.

Combine blocks 1–4; and blocks 5–8. CF confounded.

Effects	d.f.
Block	1
Main	8
2-factor	19
Higher order	3
Total	31

Blocks of 32 units

Estimable 2-factors: All interactions of A and of E, plus the alias sets $BC = DH$, $BF = DG$, $BG = DF$, $BH = CD$, $CG = FH$, $CF = GH$, $BD = CH = FG$.

Combine blocks 1–8.

Effects	d.f.
Main	8
2-factor	20
Higher order	3
Total	31

Plan 6A.16 2^8 factorial in 64 units ($\frac{1}{4}$ replicate)

Defining contrasts: $ABCEG$, $ABDFH$, $CDEFGH$

Blocks of 4 units

Estimable 2-factors: All except AF, AH, BC, BG, CG, DE, FH (confounded with blocks).

Blocks	(1)	(2)	(3)	(4)	(5)	(6)	(7)	(8)
	(1)	adg	ach	beh	eg	fh	bef	acf
	adefh	abce	bfg	abdf	bcd	ade	abdh	bgh
	bcdeg	efgh	cdef	cdgh	adfgh	abcg	cdfg	cdeh
	abcfgh	bcdfh	abdegh	acefg	abcefh	bcdefgh	acegh	abdefg

(9)	(10)	(11)	(12)	(13)	(14)	(15)	(16)
ab	ce	afg	df	acd	cg	dh	agh
cfgh	bdg	bch	aeh	abeg	bde	aef	bcf
acdeg	acdfh	degh	bcefg	cefh	abfh	bcegh	defg
bdefh	abefgh	abcdef	abcdgh	bdfgh	acdefgh	abcdfg	abcdeh

Effects	d.f.
Block	15
Main	8
2-factor	21
Higher order	19
Total	63

AF, AH, BC, BG, CG, DE, FH, ACD, ADG, BEF, BEH, CDF, CEF, DFG, EFG confounded.

Blocks of 8 units

Estimable 2-factors: All except BC and FH (confounded with blocks).

Combine blocks 1 and 2; blocks 3 and 4; blocks 5 and 6; blocks 7 and 8; blocks 9 and 10; blocks 11 and 12; blocks 13 and 14; and blocks 15 and 16. BC, FH, ACD, BEF, BEH, CEF, DFG confounded.

Effects	d.f.
Block	7
Main	8
2-factor	26
Higher order	22
Total	63

Blocks of 16 units

Estimable 2-factors: All.

Combine blocks 1–4; blocks 5–8; blocks 9–12; and blocks 13–16. ACD, BEF, DFG confounded.

Effects	d.f.
Block	3
Main	8
2-factor	28
Higher order	24
Total	63

Blocks of 32 units

Estimable 2-factors: All.

Combine blocks 1–8; and blocks 9–16. *ACD* confounded.

Effects	d.f.
Block	1
Main	8
2-factor	28
Higher order	26
Total	63

Blocks of 64 units

Estimable 2-factors: All.

Combine blocks 1–16.

Effects	d.f.
Main	8
2-factor	28
Higher order	27
Total	63

Plan 6A.17 2^8 factorial in 128 units ($\frac{1}{2}$ replicate)

Defining contrast: *ABCDEFGH*

For blocks of 8 units, see end of plan.

Blocks of 16 units

Estimable 2-factors: All

Estimable 3-factors: All.

Blocks (1)	(2)	(3)	(4)	(5)	(6)	(7)	(8)
(1)	*acfh*	*fh*	*ac*	*af*	*ch*	*ah*	*cf*
abcd	*bdfh*	*abcdfh*	*bd*	*bcdf*	*abdh*	*bcdh*	*abdf*
adeg	*abefgh*	*abefgh*	*abeg*	*defg*	*begh*	*degh*	*befg*
bceg	*cdefgh*	*bcefgh*	*cdeg*	*abcefg*	*acdegh*	*abcegh*	*acdefg*
adfh	*ab*	*ad*	*abfh*	*dh*	*bf*	*df*	*bh*
bcfh	*cd*	*bc*	*cdfh*	*abch*	*acdf*	*abcf*	*acdh*
efgh	*aceg*	*eg*	*acefgh*	*aegh*	*cefg*	*aefg*	*cegh*
abcdefgh	*bdeg*	*abcdeg*	*bdefgh*	*bcdegh*	*abdefg*	*bcdefg*	*abdegh*
abgh	*ef*	*abfg*	*eh*	*bfgh*	*ae*	*bg*	*aefh*
aceh	*adfg*	*acef*	*adgh*	*cefh*	*dg*	*ce*	*dfgh*
bdeh	*bcfg*	*bdef*	*bcgh*	*abdefh*	*abcg*	*abde*	*abcfgh*
cdgh	*abcdef*	*cdfg*	*abcdeh*	*acdfgh*	*bcde*	*acdg*	*bcdefh*
abef	*gh*	*abeh*	*fg*	*be*	*afgh*	*befh*	*ag*
acfg	*adeh*	*acgh*	*adef*	*cg*	*defh*	*cfgh*	*de*
bdfg	*bceh*	*bdgh*	*bcef*	*abdg*	*abcefh*	*abdfgh*	*abce*
cdef	*abcdgh*	*cdeh*	*abcdfg*	*acde*	*bcdfgh*	*acdefh*	*bcdg*

ABCD, ABEF, ACFG, ADEG, BCEG, BDFG, CDEF confounded.

Effects	d.f.
Block	7
Main	8
2-factor	28
3-factor	56
Higher order	28
Total	127

Blocks of 32 units

Estimable 2-factors: All.

Estimable 3-factors: All.

Combine blocks 1 and 2; blocks 3 and 4; blocks 5 and 6; and blocks 7 and 8. *ABCD, ABEF, CDEF* confounded.

Effects	d.f.
Block	3
Main	8
2-factor	28
3-factor	56
Higher order	32
Total	127

Blocks of 64 units

Estimable 2-factors: All.

Estimable 3-factors: All.

Combine blocks 1–4; and blocks 5–8. *ABCD* confounded.

Effects	d.f.
Block	1
Main	8
2-factor	28
3-factor	56
Higher order	34
Total	127

Blocks of 128 units

Estimable 2-factors: All.

Estimable 3-factors: All.

Combine blocks 1–8.

Effects	d.f.
Main	8
2-factor	28
3-factor	56
Higher order	35
Total	127

Blocks of 8 units

Estimable 2-factors. All except *EG* and *FH* (confounded). Start with the plan for blocks of 32 units. The first 4 rows of blocks 1 and 2 form the first block of 8 units: i.e., this block contains 1, *abcd, adeg, bceg, acfh, bdfh, abefgh, cdefgh*. Similarly, rows 5–8 of blocks 1 and 2 give the second block, rows 9–12 the third and rows 13–16 the fourth. The remaining 12 blocks are formed likewise from blocks 3 and 4; blocks 5 and 6; and blocks 7 and 8.

Effects	d.f.
Block	15
Main	8
2-factor	26
Higher order	78
Total	127

Plan 6A.18 3^4 factorial in 27 units ($\frac{1}{3}$ replicate)

Defining contrasts: 2 d.f. from $ABCD$, equivalent to putting $D = ABC(Y)$

Blocks of 9 units

Estimable 2-factors: 16 of the 24 d.f. are clear. $CD(I)$ is lost by confounding. Also $AB(J) = CD(J)$; $AC(I) = BD(I)$; $AD(I) = BC(I)$.

Blocks (1)	(2)	(3)
0000	0021	0012
0122	0110	0101
0211	0202	0220
1022	1010	1001
1111	1102	1120
1200	1221	1212
2011	2002	2020
2100	2121	2112
2222	2210	2201

Effects	d.f.
Block	2
Main	8
2-factor	16
Total	26

If all interactions of D are negligible, the analysis may be written:

Effects	d.f.
Block	2
Main	8
AB, AC, BC	12
Error (from interactions of D)	4
Total	26

Blocks of 27 units

Estimable 2-factors: As in blocks of 9 units, plus $CD(I)$.

Combine blocks 1, 2, and 3. See section 6A.32 for analysis of variance.

Plan 6A.19 3^5 factorial in 81 units ($\frac{1}{3}$ replicate)

Defining contrasts: 2 d.f. from *ABCDE*

Blocks of 9 units

Estimable 2-factors: All except *AE*(*J*), which is confounded with blocks.

Blocks	(1)	(2)	(3)	(4)	(5)	(6)	(7)	(8)	(9)
ab	*cde*	*cde*	*cde*	*cde*	*cde*	*cde*	*cde*	*cde*	*cde*
00	000	201	102	120	021	222	111	012	210
10	122	020	221	212	110	011	200	101	002
20	211	112	010	001	202	100	022	220	121
01	110	011	212	200	101	002	221	122	020
11	202	100	001	022	220	121	010	211	112
21	021	222	120	111	012	210	102	000	201
02	220	121	022	010	211	112	001	202	100
12	012	210	111	102	000	201	120	021	222
22	101	002	200	221	122	020	212	110	011

Effects	d.f.
Block	8
Main	10
2-factor	38
Higher order	24
Total	80

Blocks of 27 units

Estimable 2-factors: All.

Combine blocks 1–3; blocks 4–6; blocks 7–9.

Effects	d.f.
Block	2
Main	10
2-factor	40
Higher order	28
Total	80

Blocks of 81 units

Estimable 2-factors: All.

Combine blocks 1–9.

Effects	d.f.
Main	10
2-factor	40
Higher order	30
Total	80

Plan 6A.20 4×2^4 factorial in 32 units ($\frac{1}{2}$ replicate)

Defining contrast: A''' *BCDE*

Blocks of 8 units

Estimable 2-factors: All except *DE* (confounded with blocks).

Blocks	(1)	(2)	(3)	(4)
ab	*cde*	*cde*	*cde*	*cde*
00	100	010	111	001
01	011	101	000	110
10	011	101	000	110
11	100	010	111	001
20	111	001	100	010
21	000	110	011	101
30	000	110	011	101
31	111	001	100	010

Effects	d.f.
Block	3
Main	7
2-factor	17
Higher order	4
Total	31

Blocks of 16 units

Estimable 2-factors: All.

Combine blocks 1, 2; and blocks 3, 4.

Effects	d.f.
Block	1
Main	7
2-factor	18
Higher order	5
Total	31

Blocks of 32 units

Estimable 2-factors: All.

Combine blocks 1, 2, 3, and 4.

Effects	d.f.
Main	7
2-factor	18
Higher order	6
Total	31

INDEX TO PLANS, INCOMPLETE BLOCK DESIGNS

t	k	r	b	λ†	E	Plan.	Type
4	2	3	6	1	.67	11.1	V
	3	3	4	2	.89	*	V
5	2	4	10	1	.62	11.2	V
	3	6	10	3	.83	11.1a	V
	4	4	5	3	.94	*	V
6	2	5	15	1	.60	11.3	I
	3	5	10	2	.80	11.4	III
	3	10	20	4	.80	11.5	I
	4	10	15	6	.90	11.6	II
	5	5	6	4	.96	*	V
7	2	6	21	1	.58	11.2a	II
	3	3	7	1	.78	11.7	V
	4	4	7	2	.88	11.8	V
	6	6	7	5	.97	*	V
8	2	7	28	1	.57	11.9	I
	4	7	14	3	.86	11.10	I
	7	7	8	6	.98	*	V
9	2	8	36	1	.56	11.3a	II
	4	8	18	3	.84	11.11	II
	5	10	18	5	.90	11.12	II
	6	8	12	5	.94	11.13	II
	8	8	9	7	.98	*	IV
10	2	9	45	1	.56	11.14	I
	3	9	30	2	.74	11.15	II
	4	6	15	2	.83	11.16	III
	5	9	18	4	.89	11.17	III
	6	9	15	5	.93	11.18	III
	9	9	10	8	.99	*	IV
11	2	10	55	1	.55	11.4a	II
	5	5	11	2	.88	11.19	IV
	6	6	11	3	.92	11.20	IV
	10	10	11	9	.99	*	IV
13	3	6	26	1	.72	11.21	II
	4	4	13	1	.81	11.22	IV
	9	9	13	6	.96	11.23	IV
15	3	7	35	1	.71	11.24	I
	7	7	15	3	.92	11.25	IV
	8	8	15	4	.94	11.26	IV
16	6	6	16	2	.89	11.27	IV
	6	9	24	3	.89	11.28	II
	10	10	16	6	.96	11.29	IV
19	3	9	57	1	.70	11.30	II
	9	9	19	4	.94	11.31	IV
	10	10	19	5	.95	11.32	IV
21	3	10	70	1	.70	11.33	I
	5	5	21	1	.84	11.34	IV
	7	10	30	3	.90	11.35	III
25	4	8	50	1	.78	11.36	II
	9	9	25	3	.93	11.37	IV
28	4	9	63	1	.78	11.38	I
	7	9	36	2	.89	11.39	III
31	6	6	31	1	.86	11.40	IV
	10	10	31	3	.93	11.41	IV
37	9	9	37	2	.91	11.42	IV
41	5	10	82	1	.82	11.43	II
57	8	8	57	1	.89	11.44	IV
73	9	9	73	1	.90	11.45	IV
91	10	10	91	1	.91	11.46	IV

† Number of times that two treatments appear together in the same block.

* These plans are constructed by forming all possible combinations of the t numbers in groups of size k. The number of blocks b serves as a check that no group has been missed.

Plan 11.1 $t = 4, k = 2, r = 3, b = 6, \lambda = 1, E = .67$, **Type V**

Block	Rep. I		Block	Rep. II		Block	Rep. III	
(1)	1	2	(3)	1	2	(5)	1	4
(2)	3	4	(4)	2	4	(6)	2	3

Plan 11.2 $t = 5, k = 2, r = 4, b = 10, \lambda = 1, E = .62$, **Type V**

Block	Reps. I and II		Block	Reps. III and IV	
(1)	1	2	(6)	1	4
(2)	3	4	(7)	2	3
(3)	2	5	(8)	3	5
(4)	1	3	(9)	1	5
(5)	4	5	(10)	2	4

Plan 11.1a $t = 5, k = 3, r = 6, b = 10, \lambda = 3, E = .83$, **Type V**

	Reps. I, II, and III				Reps. IV, V, and VI		
(1)	1	2	3	(6)	1	2	4
(2)	1	2	5	(7)	1	3	4
(3)	1	4	5	(8)	1	3	5
(4)	2	3	4	(9)	2	3	5
(5)	3	4	5	(10)	2	4	5

Plan 11.3 $t = 6, k = 2, r = 5, b = 15, \lambda = 1, E = .60$, **Type I**

Block	Rep. I			Rep. II			Rep. III			Rep. IV			Rep. V	
(1)	1	2	(4)	1	3	(7)	1	4	(10)	1	5	(13)	1	6
(2)	3	4	(5)	2	5	(8)	2	6	(11)	2	4	(14)	2	3
(3)	5	6	(6)	4	6	(9)	3	5	(12)	3	6	(15)	4	5

Plan 11.4 $t = 6, k = 3, r = 5, b = 10, \lambda = 2, E = .80$, **Type III**

Block							
(1)	1	2	5	(6)	2	3	4
(2)	1	2	6	(7)	2	3	5
(3)	1	3	4	(8)	2	4	6
(4)	1	3	6	(9)	3	5	6
(5)	1	4	5	(10)	4	5	6

Plan 11.5 $t = 6, k = 3, r = 10, b = 20, \lambda = 4, E = .80$, **Type I**

Block	Rep. I				Rep. II				Rep. III				Rep. IV				Rep. V		
(1)	1	2	3	(3)	1	2	4	(5)	1	2	5	(7)	1	2	6	(9)	1	3	4
(2)	4	5	6	(4)	3	5	6	(6)	3	4	6	(8)	3	4	5	(10)	2	5	6
	Rep. VI				Rep. VII				Rep. VIII				Rep. IX				Rep. X		
(11)	1	3	5	(13)	1	3	6	(15)	1	4	5	(17)	1	4	6	(19)	1	5	6
(12)	2	4	6	(14)	2	4	5	(16)	2	3	6	(18)	2	3	5	(20)	2	3	4

Plan 11.6 $t = 6, k = 4, r = 10, b = 15, \lambda = 6, E = .90$, **Type II**

Block	Reps. I and II		Reps. III and IV		Reps. V and VI		Reps. VII and VIII		Reps. IX and X
(1)	1 2 3 4	(4)	1 2 3 5	(7)	1 2 3 6	(10)	1 2 4 5	(13)	1 2 5 6
(2)	1 4 5 6	(5)	1 2 4 6	(8)	1 3 4 5	(11)	1 3 5 6	(14)	1 3 4 6
(3)	2 3 5 6	(6)	3 4 5 6	(9)	2 4 5 6	(12)	2 3 4 6	(15)	2 3 4 5

Plan 11.2a $t = 7, k = 2, r = 6, b = 21, \lambda = 1, E = .58$, **Type II**

Block	Reps. I and II		Reps. III and IV		Reps. V and VI
(1)	1 2	(8)	1 3	(15)	1 4
(2)	2 6	(9)	2 4	(16)	2 3
(3)	3 4	(10)	3 5	(17)	3 6
(4)	4 7	(11)	4 6	(18)	4 5
(5)	1 5	(12)	5 7	(19)	2 5
(6)	5 6	(13)	1 6	(20)	6 7
(7)	3 7	(14)	2 7	(21)	1 7

Plan 11.7 $t = 7, k = 3, r = 3, b = 7, \lambda = 1, E = .78$, **Type V**

Block							
(1)	1 2 4	(3)	3 4 6	(5)	5 6 1	(7)	7 1 3
(2)	2 3 5	(4)	4 5 7	(6)	6 7 2		

Plan 11.8 $t = 7, k = 4, r = 4, b = 7, \lambda = 2, E = .88$, **Type V**

Block							
(1)	3 5 6 7	(3)	1 2 5 7	(5)	2 3 4 7	(7)	2 4 5 6
(2)	1 4 6 7	(4)	1 2 3 6	(6)	1 3 4 5		

Plan 11.9 $t = 8, k = 2, r = 7, b = 28, \lambda = 1, E = .57$, **Type I**

Block	Rep. I		Rep. II		Rep. III		Rep. IV
(1)	1 2	(5)	1 3	(9)	1 4	(13)	1 5
(2)	3 4	(6)	2 8	(10)	2 7	(14)	2 3
(3)	5 6	(7)	4 5	(11)	3 6	(15)	4 7
(4)	7 8	(8)	6 7	(12)	5 8	(16)	6 8

Block	Rep. V		Rep. VI		Rep. VII
(17)	1 6	(21)	1 7	(25)	1 8
(18)	2 4	(22)	2 6	(26)	2 5
(19)	3 8	(23)	3 5	(27)	3 7
(20)	5 7	(24)	4 8	(28)	4 6

Plan 11.10 $t = 8, k = 4, r = 7, b = 14, \lambda = 3, E = .86$, **Type I**

Block	Rep. I		Rep. II		Rep. III		Rep. IV
(1)	1 2 3 4	(3)	1 2 7 8	(5)	1 3 6 8	(7)	1 4 6 7
(2)	5 6 7 8	(4)	3 4 5 6	(6)	2 4 5 7	(8)	2 3 5 8

Block	Rep. V		Rep. VI		Rep. VII
(9)	1 2 5 6	(11)	1 3 5 7	(13)	1 4 5 8
(10)	3 4 7 8	(12)	2 4 6 8	(14)	2 3 6 7

Plan 11.3a $t = 9, k = 2, r = 8, b = 36, \lambda = 1, E = .56$, **Type II**

Block	Reps. I and II		Block	Reps. III and IV		Block	Reps. V and VI		Block	Reps. VII and VIII	
(1)	1	2	(10)	1	3	(19)	1	4	(28)	1	5
(2)	2	8	(11)	2	5	(20)	2	6	(29)	2	4
(3)	3	4	(12)	3	6	(21)	2	3	(30)	3	8
(4)	4	7	(13)	4	9	(22)	4	5	(31)	4	6
(5)	5	6	(14)	5	8	(23)	5	7	(32)	3	5
(6)	1	6	(15)	6	7	(24)	6	8	(33)	6	9
(7)	3	7	(16)	1	7	(25)	7	9	(34)	2	7
(8)	8	9	(17)	4	8	(26)	1	8	(35)	7	8
(9)	5	9	(18)	2	9	(27)	3	9	(36)	1	9

Plan 11.11 $t = 9, k = 4, r = 8, b = 18, \lambda = 3, E = .84$, **Type II**

Block	Reps. I, II, III, and IV	Block	Reps. I, II, III, and IV	Block	Reps. V, VI, VII, and VIII	Block	Reps. V, VI, VII, and VIII
(1)	1 4 6 7	(6)	4 5 6 9	(10)	1 2 5 7	(15)	1 3 6 8
(2)	2 6 8 9	(7)	2 3 6 7	(11)	2 3 5 6	(16)	4 6 7 8
(3)	1 3 8 9	(8)	2 4 5 8	(12)	3 4 7 9	(17)	3 4 5 8
(4)	1 2 3 4	(9)	3 5 7 9	(13)	1 2 4 9	(18)	2 7 8 9
(5)	1 5 7 8			(14)	1 5 6 9		

Plan 11.12 $t = 9, k = 5, r = 10, b = 18, \lambda = 5, E = .90$, **Type II**

Block	Reps. I, II, III, IV, and V	Block	Reps. I, II, III, IV, and V	Block	Reps. VI, VII, VIII, IX, and X	Block	Reps. VI, VII, VIII, IX, and X
(1)	1 2 3 7 8	(6)	2 4 5 6 7	(10)	1 2 3 5 9	(15)	3 5 6 7 8
(2)	1 2 4 6 8	(7)	1 3 6 7 9	(11)	1 2 5 6 8	(16)	1 4 7 8 9
(3)	2 3 5 8 9	(8)	1 4 5 8 9	(12)	1 3 4 5 6	(17)	3 4 6 8 9
(4)	2 3 4 6 9	(9)	5 6 7 8 9	(13)	2 3 4 7 8	(18)	1 2 6 7 9
(5)	1 3 4 5 7			(14)	2 4 5 7 9		

Plan 11.13 $t = 9, k = 6, r = 8, b = 12, \lambda = 5, E = .94$, **Type II**

Block	Reps. I and II	Block	Reps. III and IV
(1)	1 2 4 5 7 8	(4)	1 2 5 6 7 9
(2)	2 3 5 6 8 9	(5)	1 3 4 5 8 9
(3)	1 3 4 6 7 9	(6)	2 3 4 6 7 8
	Reps. V and VI		**Reps. VII and VIII**
(7)	1 3 5 6 7 8	(10)	4 5 6 7 8 9
(8)	1 2 4 6 8 9	(11)	1 2 3 4 5 6
(9)	2 3 4 5 7 9	(12)	1 2 3 7 8 9

Plan 11.14 $t = 10, k = 2, r = 9, b = 45, \lambda = 1, E = .56$, **Type I**

Block	Rep. I		Block	Rep. II		Block	Rep. III		Block	Rep. IV		Block	Rep. V	
(1)	1	2	(6)	1	3	(11)	1	4	(16)	1	5	(21)	1	6
(2)	3	4	(7)	2	7	(12)	2	10	(17)	2	8	(22)	2	9
(3)	5	6	(8)	4	8	(13)	3	7	(18)	3	10	(23)	3	8
(4)	7	8	(9)	5	9	(14)	5	8	(19)	4	9	(24)	4	10
(5)	9	10	(10)	6	10	(15)	6	9	(20)	6	7	(25)	5	7

Rep. VI			Rep. VII			Rep. VIII			Rep. IX		
(26)	1	7	(31)	1	8	(36)	1	9	(41)	1	10
(27)	2	6	(32)	2	3	(37)	2	4	(42)	2	5
(28)	3	9	(33)	4	6	(38)	3	5	(43)	3	6
(29)	4	5	(34)	5	10	(39)	6	8	(44)	4	7
(30)	8	10	(35)	7	9	(40)	7	10	(45)	8	9

Plan 11.15 $t = 10, k = 3, r = 9, b = 30, \lambda = 2, E = .74$, **Type II**

Block	Reps. I, II, and III				Reps. IV, V, and VI				Reps. VII, VIII, and IX		
(1)	1	2	3	(11)	1	2	4	(21)	1	3	5
(2)	2	5	8	(12)	2	3	6	(22)	2	6	7
(3)	3	4	7	(13)	3	4	8	(23)	3	8	9
(4)	1	4	6	(14)	4	5	9	(24)	2	4	10
(5)	5	7	8	(15)	1	5	7	(25)	3	5	6
(6)	4	6	9	(16)	6	8	9	(26)	1	6	8
(7)	1	7	9	(17)	3	7	10	(27)	2	7	9
(8)	2	8	10	(18)	1	8	10	(28)	4	7	8
(9)	3	9	10	(19)	2	5	9	(29)	1	9	10
(10)	5	6	10	(20)	6	7	10	(30)	4	5	10

Plan 11.16 $t = 10, k = 4, r = 6, b = 15, \lambda = 2, E = .83$, **Type III**

Block														
(1)	1	2	3	4	(6)	1	6	8	10	(11)	3	5	9	10
(2)	1	2	5	6	(7)	2	3	6	9	(12)	3	6	7	10
(3)	1	3	7	8	(8)	2	4	7	10	(13)	3	4	5	8
(4)	1	4	9	10	(9)	2	5	8	10	(14)	4	5	6	7
(5)	1	5	7	9	(10)	2	7	8	9	(15)	4	6	8	9

Plan 11.17 $t = 10, k = 5, r = 9, b = 18, \lambda = 4, E = .89$, **Type III**

Block																	
(1)	1	2	3	4	5	(7)	1	4	5	6	10	(13)	2	5	6	8	10
(2)	1	2	3	6	7	(8)	1	4	8	9	10	(14)	2	6	7	9	10
(3)	1	2	4	6	9	(9)	1	5	7	9	10	(15)	3	4	6	7	10
(4)	1	2	5	7	8	(10)	2	3	4	8	10	(16)	3	4	5	7	9
(5)	1	3	6	8	9	(11)	2	3	5	9	10	(17)	3	5	6	8	9
(6)	1	3	7	8	10	(12)	2	4	7	8	9	(18)	4	5	6	7	8

Plan 11.18 $t = 10, k = 6, r = 9, b = 15, \lambda = 5, E = .93$, **Type III**

Block																				
(1)	1	2	4	5	8	9	(6)	2	3	4	6	8	10	(11)	1	4	5	7	8	10
(2)	5	6	7	8	9	10	(7)	1	2	6	7	9	10	(12)	1	2	3	5	7	10
(3)	2	4	5	6	9	10	(8)	1	3	5	6	8	9	(13)	2	3	5	6	7	8
(4)	1	2	4	6	7	8	(9)	1	2	3	8	9	10	(14)	1	3	4	5	6	10
(5)	3	4	7	8	9	10	(10)	2	3	4	5	7	9	(15)	1	3	4	6	7	9

Plan 11.4a $t = 11, k = 2, r = 10, b = 55, \lambda = 1, E = .55$, **Type II**

Block	Reps. I and II			Reps. III and IV			Reps. V and VI			Reps. VII and VIII			Reps. IX and X	
(1)	1	2	(12)	1	3	(23)	1	4	(34)	1	5	(45)	1	6
(2)	2	11	(13)	2	6	(24)	2	3	(35)	2	9	(46)	2	5
(3)	3	10	(14)	3	5	(25)	3	7	(36)	3	6	(47)	3	4
(4)	4	5	(15)	4	10	(26)	4	6	(37)	2	4	(48)	4	7
(5)	5	6	(16)	5	9	(27)	5	10	(38)	5	7	(49)	5	8
(6)	6	7	(17)	6	8	(28)	6	9	(39)	6	10	(50)	6	11
(7)	1	7	(18)	2	7	(29)	7	11	(40)	7	8	(51)	7	10
(8)	3	8	(19)	1	8	(30)	2	8	(41)	4	8	(52)	8	9
(9)	4	9	(20)	7	9	(31)	1	9	(42)	9	11	(53)	3	9
(10)	9	10	(21)	10	11	(32)	8	10	(43)	1	10	(54)	2	10
(11)	8	11	(22)	4	11	(33)	5	11	(44)	3	11	(55)	1	11

Plan 11.19 $t = 11, k = 5, r = 5, b = 11, \lambda = 2, E = .88$, **Type IV**

Block																	
(1)	1	2	3	5	8	(5)	5	6	7	9	1	(9)	9	10	11	2	5
(2)	2	3	4	6	9	(6)	6	7	8	10	2	(10)	10	11	1	3	6
(3)	3	4	5	7	10	(7)	7	8	9	11	3	(11)	11	1	2	4	7
(4)	4	5	6	8	11	(8)	8	9	10	1	4						

Plan 11.20 $t = 11, k = 6, r = 6, b = 11, \lambda = 3, E = .92$, **Type IV**

Block																				
(1)	4	6	7	9	10	11	(5)	2	3	4	8	10	11	(9)	1	3	4	6	7	8
(2)	1	5	7	8	10	11	(6)	1	3	4	5	9	11	(10)	2	4	5	7	8	9
(3)	1	2	6	8	9	11	(7)	1	2	4	5	6	10	(11)	3	5	6	8	9	10
(4)	1	2	3	7	9	10	(8)	2	3	5	6	7	11							

Plan 11.21 $t = 13, k = 3, r = 6, b = 26, \lambda = 1, E = .72$, **Type II**

Block	Reps. I, II, and III							Reps. IV, V, and VI						
(1)	1	3	9	(8)	3	8	10	(14)	2	5	6	(21)	9	12	13
(2)	2	4	10	(9)	4	9	11	(15)	3	6	7	(22)	1	10	13
(3)	3	5	11	(10)	5	10	12	(16)	4	7	8	(23)	1	2	11
(4)	4	6	12	(11)	6	11	13	(17)	5	8	9	(24)	2	3	12
(5)	5	7	13	(12)	1	7	12	(18)	6	9	10	(25)	3	4	13
(6)	1	6	8	(13)	2	8	13	(19)	7	10	11	(26)	1	4	5
(7)	2	7	9					(20)	8	11	12				

Plan 11.22 $t = 13, k = 4, r = 4, b = 13, \lambda = 1, E = .81$, **Type IV**

Block														
(1)	1	2	4	10	(6)	6	7	9	2	(11)	11	12	1	7
(2)	2	3	5	11	(7)	7	8	10	3	(12)	12	13	2	8
(3)	3	4	6	12	(8)	8	9	11	4	(13)	13	1	3	9
(4)	4	5	7	13	(9)	9	10	12	5					
(5)	5	6	8	1	(10)	10	11	13	6					

Plan 11.23 $t = 13, k = 9, r = 9, b = 13, \lambda = 6, E = .96$, **Type IV**

Block										Block									
(1)	3	5	6	7	8	9	11	12	13	(8)	1	2	3	5	6	7	10	12	13
(2)	1	4	6	7	8	9	10	12	13	(9)	1	2	3	4	6	7	8	11	13
(3)	1	2	5	7	8	9	10	11	13	(10)	1	2	3	4	5	7	8	9	12
(4)	1	2	3	6	8	9	10	11	12	(11)	2	3	4	5	6	8	9	10	13
(5)	2	3	4	7	9	10	11	12	13	(12)	1	3	4	5	6	7	9	10	11
(6)	1	3	4	5	8	10	11	12	13	(13)	2	4	5	6	7	8	10	11	12
(7)	1	2	4	5	6	9	11	12	13										

Plan 11.24 $t = 15, k = 3, r = 7, b = 35, \lambda = 1, E = .71$, **Type I**

Block	Rep. I				Rep. II				Rep. III				Rep. IV		
(1)	1	2	3	(6)	1	4	5	(11)	1	6	7	(16)	1	8	9
(2)	4	8	12	(7)	2	8	10	(12)	2	9	11	(17)	2	13	15
(3)	5	10	15	(8)	3	13	14	(13)	3	12	15	(18)	3	4	7
(4)	6	11	13	(9)	6	9	15	(14)	4	10	14	(19)	5	11	14
(5)	7	9	14	(10)	7	11	12	(15)	5	8	13	(20)	6	10	12

Block	Rep. V				Rep. VI				Rep. VII		
(21)	1	10	11	(26)	1	12	13	(31)	1	14	15
(22)	2	12	14	(27)	2	5	7	(32)	2	4	6
(23)	3	5	6	(28)	3	9	10	(33)	3	8	11
(24)	4	9	13	(29)	4	11	15	(34)	5	9	12
(25)	7	8	15	(30)	6	8	14	(35)	7	10	13

Plan 11.25 $t = 15, k = 7, r = 7, b = 15, \lambda = 3, E = .92$, **Type IV**

See incomplete latin squares Plan 13.7; randomize units in blocks ignoring replications.

Plan 11.26 $t = 15, k = 8, r = 8, b = 15, \lambda = 4, E = .94$, **Type IV**

See incomplete latin squares Plan 13.8; randomize units in blocks ignoring replications.

Plan 11.27 $t = 16, k = 6, r = 6, b = 16, \lambda = 2, E = .89$, **Type IV**

See incomplete latin squares Plan 13.9; randomize units in blocks ignoring replications.

Plan 11.28 $t = 16, k = 6, r = 9, b = 24, \lambda = 3, E = .89$, **Type II**

Block	Reps. I, II, and III							Reps. IV, V, and VI							Reps. VII, VIII, and IX					
(1)	1	2	5	6	11	12	(9)	1	3	6	8	13	15	(17)	1	4	5	8	10	11
(2)	3	4	7	8	9	10	(10)	2	4	5	7	14	16	(18)	2	3	6	7	9	12
(3)	5	6	9	10	13	14	(11)	5	7	9	11	13	15	(19)	5	8	9	12	13	16
(4)	7	8	11	12	15	16	(12)	6	8	10	12	14	16	(20)	1	4	6	7	13	16
(5)	1	2	9	10	15	16	(13)	2	4	6	8	9	11	(21)	1	4	9	12	14	15
(6)	3	4	11	12	13	14	(14)	1	3	5	7	10	12	(22)	6	7	10	11	14	15
(7)	1	2	7	8	13	14	(15)	2	4	10	12	13	15	(23)	2	3	10	11	13	16
(8)	3	4	5	6	15	16	(16)	1	3	9	11	14	16	(24)	2	3	5	8	14	15

Plan 11.29 $t = 16, k = 10, r = 10, b = 16, \lambda = 6, E = .96$, **Type IV**

See incomplete latin squares Plan 13.10; randomize units in blocks ignoring replications.

Plan 11.30 $t = 19, k = 3, r = 9, b = 57, \lambda = 1, E = .70$, **Type II**

See extended incomplete latin squares Plan 13.15a; randomize units in blocks ignoring replications.

Plan 11.31 $t = 19, k = 9, r = 9, b = 19, \lambda = 4, E = .94$, **Type IV**

See incomplete latin squares Plan 13.11; randomize units in blocks ignoring replications.

Plan 11.32 $t = 19, k = 10, r = 10, b = 19, \lambda = 5, E = .95$, **Type IV**

See incomplete latin squares Plan 13.12; randomize units in blocks ignoring replications.

Plan 11.33 $t = 21, k = 3, r = 10, b = 70, \lambda = 1, E = .70$, **Type I**

Block	Rep. I		Rep. II		Rep. III		Rep. IV		Rep. V
(1)	1 2 3	(8)	1 4 15	(15)	1 5 17	(22)	1 6 9	(29)	1 7 21
(2)	4 5 6	(9)	2 5 11	(16)	2 4 14	(23)	2 7 16	(30)	2 13 17
(3)	7 8 9	(10)	3 9 16	(17)	3 7 11	(24)	3 8 21	(31)	3 10 18
(4)	10 11 12	(11)	6 17 20	(18)	6 10 19	(25)	4 17 19	(32)	4 8 11
(5)	13 14 15	(12)	7 12 19	(19)	8 16 20	(26)	5 10 13	(33)	5 16 19
(6)	16 17 18	(13)	8 13 18	(20)	9 15 18	(27)	11 15 20	(34)	6 12 15
(7)	19 20 21	(14)	10 14 21	(21)	12 13 21	(28)	12 14 18	(35)	9 14 20
	Rep. VI		**Rep. VII**		**Rep. VIII**		**Rep. IX**		**Rep. X**
(36)	1 8 10	(43)	1 11 18	(50)	1 12 20	(57)	1 13 19	(64)	1 14 16
(37)	2 18 19	(44)	2 10 20	(51)	2 6 8	(58)	2 9 12	(65)	2 15 21
(38)	3 15 17	(45)	3 5 12	(52)	3 14 19	(59)	3 4 20	(66)	3 6 13
(39)	4 12 16	(46)	4 9 13	(53)	4 18 21	(60)	5 8 14	(67)	4 7 10
(40)	5 9 21	(47)	6 16 21	(54)	5 7 15	(61)	6 7 18	(68)	5 18 20
(41)	6 11 14	(48)	7 14 17	(55)	9 10 17	(62)	10 15 16	(69)	8 12 17
(42)	7 13 20	(49)	8 15 19	(56)	11 13 16	(63)	11 17 21	(70)	9 11 19

Plan 11.34 $t = 21, k = 5, r = 5, b = 21, \lambda = 1, E = .84$, **Type IV**

See incomplete latin squares Plan 13.13; randomize units in blocks ignoring replications.

Plan 11.35 $t = 21, k = 7, r = 10, b = 30, \lambda = 3, E = .90$, **Type III**

Block								Block							
(1)	2	5	10	11	17	19	20	(16)	2	7	10	13	18	20	21
(2)	3	6	11	12	18	20	21	(17)	3	1	11	14	19	21	15
(3)	4	7	12	13	19	21	15	(18)	4	2	12	8	20	15	16
(4)	5	1	13	14	20	15	16	(19)	5	3	13	9	21	16	17
(5)	6	2	14	8	21	16	17	(20)	6	4	14	10	15	17	18
(6)	7	3	8	9	15	17	18	(21)	7	5	8	11	16	18	19
(7)	1	4	9	10	16	18	19	(22)	1	2	4	8	9	11	21
(8)	3	4	8	13	17	19	20	(23)	2	3	5	9	10	12	15
(9)	4	5	9	14	18	20	21	(24)	3	4	6	10	11	13	16
(10)	5	6	10	8	19	21	15	(25)	4	5	7	11	12	14	17
(11)	6	7	11	9	20	15	16	(26)	5	6	1	12	13	8	18
(12)	7	1	12	10	21	16	17	(27)	6	7	2	13	14	9	19
(13)	1	2	13	11	15	17	18	(28)	7	1	3	14	8	10	20
(14)	2	3	14	12	16	18	19	(29)	1	2	3	4	5	6	7
(15)	1	6	9	12	17	19	20	(30)	8	9	10	11	12	13	14

Plan 11.36 $t = 25, k = 4, r = 8, b = 50, \lambda = 1, E = .78$, **Type II**

See extended incomplete latin squares Plan 13.16a; randomize units in blocks ignoring replications.

Plan 11.37 $t = 25, k = 9, r = 9, b = 25, \lambda = 3, E = .93$, **Type IV**

See incomplete latin squares Plan 13.1a; randomize units in blocks ignoring replications.

Plan 11.38 $t = 28, k = 4, r = 9, b = 63, \lambda = 1, E = .78$, **Type I**

Block	Rep. I				Block	Rep. II				Block	Rep. III			
(1)	28	1	10	19	(8)	28	2	11	20	(15)	28	3	12	21
(2)	2	9	13	16	(9)	3	1	14	17	(16)	4	2	15	18
(3)	3	8	11	18	(10)	4	9	12	10	(17)	5	1	13	11
(4)	4	7	23	24	(11)	5	8	24	25	(18)	6	9	25	26
(5)	5	6	20	27	(12)	6	7	21	19	(19)	7	8	22	20
(6)	12	17	22	25	(13)	13	18	23	26	(20)	14	10	24	27
(7)	14	15	21	26	(14)	15	16	22	27	(21)	16	17	23	19

Block	Rep. IV				Block	Rep. V				Block	Rep. VI			
(22)	28	4	13	22	(29)	28	5	14	23	(36)	28	6	15	24
(23)	5	3	16	10	(30)	6	4	17	11	(37)	7	5	18	12
(24)	6	2	14	12	(31)	7	3	15	13	(38)	8	4	16	14
(25)	7	1	26	27	(32)	8	2	27	19	(39)	9	3	19	20
(26)	8	9	23	21	(33)	9	1	24	22	(40)	1	2	25	23
(27)	15	11	25	19	(34)	16	12	26	20	(41)	17	13	27	21
(28)	17	18	24	20	(35)	18	10	25	21	(42)	10	11	26	22

Block	Rep. VII				Block	Rep. VIII				Block	Rep. IX			
(43)	28	7	16	25	(50)	28	8	17	26	(57)	28	9	18	27
(44)	8	6	10	13	(51)	9	7	11	14	(58)	1	8	12	15
(45)	9	5	17	15	(52)	1	6	18	16	(59)	2	7	10	17
(46)	1	4	20	21	(53)	2	5	21	22	(60)	3	6	22	23
(47)	2	3	26	24	(54)	3	4	27	25	(61)	4	5	19	26
(48)	18	14	19	22	(55)	10	15	20	23	(62)	11	16	21	24
(49)	11	12	27	23	(56)	12	13	19	24	(63)	13	14	20	25

Plan 11.39 $t = 28, k = 7, r = 9, b = 36, \lambda = 2, E = .89$, **Type III**

Block								Block							
(1)	4	7	8	9	14	23	28	(19)	4	8	11	17	19	21	25
(2)	1	5	9	10	11	15	24	(20)	1	13	14	18	23	25	26
(3)	6	8	13	15	16	18	21	(21)	2	4	5	6	16	22	23
(4)	7	12	13	17	22	24	25	(22)	3	4	10	11	12	14	18
(5)	4	10	16	17	20	26	27	(23)	1	9	14	16	17	19	22
(6)	2	11	18	19	22	26	28	(24)	1	2	4	13	20	24	28
(7)	1	3	6	12	19	23	27	(25)	3	5	8	17	23	24	26
(8)	2	3	5	14	20	21	25	(26)	5	6	7	10	19	25	28
(9)	1	2	8	10	12	16	25	(27)	1	6	7	8	11	20	26
(10)	2	3	6	9	11	13	17	(28)	9	10	13	19	20	21	23
(11)	4	5	12	13	15	19	26	(29)	2	8	14	15	19	24	27
(12)	3	7	16	18	19	20	24	(30)	3	9	15	16	25	26	28
(13)	6	10	14	21	22	24	26	(31)	5	8	9	12	18	20	22
(14)	11	15	20	22	23	25	27	(32)	11	12	16	21	23	24	28
(15)	1	5	17	18	21	27	28	(33)	1	3	4	7	15	21	22
(16)	2	7	9	12	21	26	27	(34)	5	7	11	13	14	16	27
(17)	3	8	10	13	22	27	28	(35)	4	6	9	18	24	25	27
(18)	6	12	14	15	17	20	28	(36)	2	7	10	15	17	18	23

Plan 11.40 $t = 31, k = 6, r = 6, b = 31, \lambda = 1, E = .86$, **Type IV**

See incomplete latin squares Plan 13.13; randomize units in blocks ignoring replications.

Plan 11.41 $t = 31, k = 10, r = 10, b = 31, \lambda = 3, E = .93$, **Type IV**

See incomplete latin squares Plan 13.2a; randomize units in blocks ignoring replications.

Plan 11.42 $t = 37, k = 9, r = 9, b = 37, \lambda = 2, E = .91$, **Type IV**

See incomplete latin squares Plan 13.15; randomize units in blocks ignoring replications.

Plan 11.43 $t = 41, k = 5, r = 10, b = 82, \lambda = 1, E = .82$, **Type III**

See extended latin squares Plan 13.17a; randomize units in blocks ignoring replications.

Plan 11.44 $t = 57, k = 8, r = 8, b = 57, \lambda = 1, E = .89$, **Type IV**

See incomplete latin squares Plan 13.3a; randomize units in blocks ignoring replications.

Plan 11.45 $t = 73, k = 9, r = 9, b = 73, \lambda = 1, E = .90$, **Type IV**

See incomplete latin squares Plan 13.4a; randomize units in blocks ignoring replications.

Plan 11.46 $t = 91, k = 10, r = 10, b = 91, \lambda = 1, E = .91$, **Type IV**

See incomplete latin squares Plan 13.5a; randomize units in blocks ignoring replications.

INDEX TO PLANS, INCOMPLETE LATIN SQUARES

t	k	r	b	λ	E	Plan	Type†
3	3	6	6	6	1.00	2LS	
	3	9	9	9	1.00	3LS	
	5	5	3	5	.96	13.16	III
	5	10	6	10	.96	13.16	IIa
	7	7	3	7	.98	13.17	IV
	8	8	3	8	.98	13.18	III
	10	10	3	10	.99	13.19	IV
4	3	3	4	2	.89	*	II
	3	6	8	4	.89	**	Ia
	3	9	12	6	.89	**	Ia
	4	8	8	8	1.00	2LS	
	5	5	4	5	.96	13.20	IV
	5	10	8	10	.96	13.20	IIa
	7	7	4	7	.98	13.21	III
	9	9	4	9	.99	13.22	IV
5	2	4	10	1	.67	13.6a	II
	3	6	10	3		13.7a	II
	4	4	5	3	.94	*	II
	4	8	10	6	.94	**	Ia
	5	10	10	10	1.00	2LS	
	6	6	5	6	.97	13.23	IV
	9	9	5	9	.99	13.24	III
6	5	5	6	4	.96	*	II
	5	10	12	8	.96	**	Ia
	7	7	6	7	.98	13.25	IV
7	2	6	21	1	.58	13.8a	V
	3	3	7	1	.78	13.1	II
	3	9	21	3	.78	13.1	Ia
	4	4	7	2	.88	13.2	II
	4	8	14	4	.88	13.2	Ia
	6	6	7	5	.97	*	II
	8	8	7	8	.98	13.26	IV
8	7	7	8	6	.98	*	II
9	2	8	36	1	.56	13.9a	V
	4	8	18	3	.84	13.10a	V
	5	10	18	5	.90	13.11a	V
	8	8	9	7	.98	*	II

t	k	r	b	λ	E	Plan	Type†
10	3	9	30	2	.74	13.12a	V
	9	9	10	8	.99	*	II
11	2	10	55	1	.55	13.13a	V
	5	5	11	2	.88	13.3	I
	6	6	11	3	.92	13.4	I
	10	10	11	9	.99	*	II
13	3	6	26	1	.72	13.14a	V
	4	4	13	1	.81	13.5	I
	9	9	13	6	.95	13.6	I
15	7	7	15	3	.92	13.7	I
	8	8	15	4	.94	13.8	I
16	6	6	16	2	.89	13.9	I
	10	10	16	6	.96	13.10	I
19	3	9	57	1	.70	13.15a	V
	9	9	19	4	.94	13.11	I
	10	10	19	5	.95	13.12	I
21	5	5	21	1	.84	13.13	I
25	4	8	50	1	.78	13.16a	V
	9	9	25	3	.93	13.1a	I
31	6	6	31	1	.86	13.14	I
	10	10	31	3	.93	13.2a	I
37	9	9	37	2	.91	13.15	I
41	5	10	82	1	.82	13.17a	V
57	8	8	57	1	.89	13.3a	I
73	9	9	73	1	.90	13.4a	I
91	10	10	91	1	.91	13.5a	I

* Constructed from a $t \times t$ latin square by omission of the last column.

** By repetition of the plan for $r = t - 1$, which is constructed by taking a $t \times t$ latin square and omitting the last column.

† This refers to the method of analysis. For types I, Ia, II, IIa, and V, see section 13.2; for types III and IV, see section 13.3.

Plan 13.1 $t = 7, k = 3, r = 3, b = 7, \lambda = 1, E = .78$, **Type II**

Block	Reps. I	II	III	Block	Reps. I	II	III
(1)	7	1	3	(5)	4	5	7
(2)	1	2	4	(6)	5	6	1
(3)	2	3	5	(7)	6	7	2
(4)	3	4	6				

Plan 13.2 $t = 7, k = 4, r = 4, b = 7, \lambda = 2, E = .88$, **Type II**

Block	Reps. I	II	III	IV	Block	Reps. I	II	III	IV
(1)	3	5	6	7	(5)	7	2	3	4
(2)	4	6	7	1	(6)	1	3	4	5
(3)	5	7	1	2	(7)	2	4	5	6
(4)	6	1	2	3					

Plan 13.3 $t = 11, k = 5, r = 5, b = 11, \lambda = 2, E = .88$, **Type I**

Block	I	II	III	IV	V
(1)	1	2	3	4	5
(2)	7	1	6	10	3
(3)	9	8	1	6	2
(4)	11	9	7	1	4
(5)	10	11	5	8	1
(6)	8	7	2	3	11
(7)	2	6	4	11	10
(8)	6	3	11	5	9
(9)	3	4	10	9	8
(10)	5	10	9	2	7
(11)	4	5	8	7	6

Plan 13.4 $t = 11, k = 6, r = 6, b = 11, \lambda = 3, E = .92$, **Type I**

Block	I	II	III	IV	V	VI
(1)	6	7	8	9	10	11
(2)	5	8	4	11	2	9
(3)	4	5	7	3	11	10
(4)	3	10	2	6	5	8
(5)	2	3	9	7	4	6
(6)	1	6	10	4	9	5
(7)	9	1	3	5	8	7
(8)	8	2	1	10	7	4
(9)	7	11	5	1	6	2
(10)	11	4	6	8	1	3
(11)	10	9	11	2	3	1

Plan 13.5 $t = 13, k = 4, r = 4, b = 13, \lambda = 1, E = .81$, **Type I**

Block	I	II	III	IV
(1)	13	1	3	9
(2)	1	2	4	10
(3)	2	3	5	11
(4)	3	4	6	12
(5)	4	5	7	13
(6)	5	6	8	1
(7)	6	7	9	2
(8)	7	8	10	3
(9)	8	9	11	4
(10)	9	10	12	5
(11)	10	11	13	6
(12)	11	12	1	7
(13)	12	13	2	8

Plan 13.6 $t = 13, k = 9, r = 9, b = 13, \lambda = 6, E = .95$, **Type I**

Block	I	II	III	IV	V	VI	VII	VIII	IX
(1)	2	5	6	7	9	10	11	12	13
(2)	3	6	7	8	10	11	12	13	1
(3)	4	7	8	9	11	12	13	1	2
(4)	5	8	9	10	12	13	1	2	3
(5)	6	9	10	11	13	1	2	3	4
(6)	7	10	11	12	1	2	3	4	5
(7)	8	11	12	13	2	3	4	5	6
(8)	9	12	13	1	3	4	5	6	7
(9)	10	13	1	2	4	5	6	7	8
(10)	11	1	2	3	5	6	7	8	9
(11)	12	2	3	4	6	7	8	9	10
(12)	13	3	4	5	7	8	9	10	11
(13)	1	4	5	6	8	9	10	11	12

Plan 13.7 $t = 15, k = 7, r = 7, b = 15, \lambda = 3, E = .92$, **Type I**

	Reps.								Reps.						
Block	I	II	III	IV	V	VI	VII		I	II	III	IV	V	VI	VII
(1)	13	8	12	6	7	1	9	(9)	8	6	4	15	10	13	2
(2)	5	14	10	7	12	2	8	(10)	10	4	5	11	1	12	13
(3)	15	12	11	5	8	3	6	(11)	9	13	14	10	6	5	3
(4)	12	11	6	9	2	4	14	(12)	14	7	13	3	4	8	11
(5)	4	5	8	1	14	9	15	(13)	7	15	9	12	3	10	4
(6)	11	9	7	2	13	15	5	(14)	3	1	2	8	9	11	10
(7)	1	2	3	4	5	6	7	(15)	6	10	15	14	11	7	1
(8)	2	3	1	13	15	14	12								

Plan 13.8 $t = 15, k = 8, r = 8, b = 15, \lambda = 4, E = .94$, **Type I**

	Reps.									Reps.							
Block	I	II	III	IV	V	VI	VII	VIII		I	II	III	IV	V	VI	VII	VIII
(1)	11	4	2	5	10	3	14	15	(9)	5	14	7	3	1	9	12	11
(2)	4	1	3	15	13	11	6	9	(10)	8	15	6	2	3	7	9	14
(3)	9	2	14	4	7	1	10	13	(11)	1	7	11	8	2	4	15	12
(4)	15	3	1	10	8	13	7	5	(12)	2	6	15	9	5	12	1	10
(5)	7	13	10	12	11	2	3	6	(13)	13	8	5	11	14	6	2	1
(6)	6	10	12	1	4	14	8	3	(14)	14	5	4	6	12	15	13	7
(7)	12	9	13	14	15	10	11	8	(15)	3	12	8	13	9	5	4	2
(8)	10	11	9	7	6	8	5	4									

Plan 13.9 $t = 16, k = 6, r = 6, b = 16, \lambda = 2, E = .89$, **Type I**

	Reps.							Reps.					
Block	I	II	III	IV	V	VI		I	II	III	IV	V	VI
(1)	1	2	3	4	5	6	(9)	9	15	11	5	13	2
(2)	2	7	8	9	10	1	(10)	10	11	6	12	2	14
(3)	3	1	13	7	11	12	(11)	11	4	16	3	9	10
(4)	4	8	1	11	14	15	(12)	12	3	10	15	8	5
(5)	5	12	14	1	16	9	(13)	13	6	9	14	3	8
(6)	6	10	15	13	1	16	(14)	14	13	5	10	7	4
(7)	7	14	2	16	15	3	(15)	15	9	4	6	12	7
(8)	8	16	12	2	4	13	(16)	16	5	7	8	6	11

Plan 13.10 $t = 16, k = 10, r = 10, b = 16, \lambda = 6, E = .96$, **Type I**

	Reps.									
Block	I	II	III	IV	V	VI	VII	VIII	IX	X
(1)	8	7	9	10	11	12	13	14	15	16
(2)	3	4	5	13	16	11	12	6	14	15
(3)	9	2	4	5	6	8	10	15	16	14
(4)	2	6	3	7	5	10	9	16	12	13
(5)	6	8	2	3	4	7	15	10	13	11
(6)	4	5	14	8	3	9	7	2	11	12
(7)	1	10	11	4	13	5	6	12	8	9
(8)	5	1	15	6	14	3	11	9	7	10
(9)	16	3	1	14	12	6	4	8	10	7
(10)	7	13	16	1	15	4	3	5	9	8
(11)	12	14	7	15	1	2	8	13	6	5
(12)	14	11	13	16	9	1	2	7	4	6
(13)	10	15	12	2	7	16	1	11	5	4
(14)	11	12	6	9	8	15	16	1	2	3
(15)	13	16	8	11	10	14	5	3	1	2
(16)	15	9	10	12	2	13	14	4	3	1

Plan 13.11 $t = 19, k = 9, r = 9, b = 19, \lambda = 4, E = .94$, **Type I**

	Reps.								
Block	I	II	III	IV	V	VI	VII	VIII	IX
(1)	1	2	3	4	5	6	7	8	9
(2)	14	1	2	3	4	12	11	10	13
(3)	17	16	1	2	15	10	6	5	11
(4)	12	13	16	1	2	7	18	15	8
(5)	9	10	12	16	1	3	17	19	7
(6)	8	11	13	19	17	1	3	6	18
(7)	7	18	11	14	16	19	1	4	5
(8)	6	9	17	12	14	18	15	1	4
(9)	5	8	9	10	13	15	19	14	1
(10)	13	5	14	9	18	2	16	3	17
(11)	10	6	7	15	19	14	2	18	3
(12)	18	17	5	8	12	4	10	2	19
(13)	19	4	15	7	9	17	13	11	2
(14)	2	19	6	11	8	9	14	16	12
(15)	3	15	10	18	11	8	4	9	16
(16)	4	3	19	5	6	16	12	13	15
(17)	15	7	8	17	3	11	5	12	14
(18)	16	14	4	6	7	13	8	17	10
(19)	11	12	18	13	10	5	9	7	6

Plan 13.12 $t = 19, k = 10, r = 10, b = 19, \lambda = 5, E = .95$, **Type I**

	Reps.									
Block	I	II	III	IV	V	VI	VII	VIII	IX	X
(1)	10	11	12	13	14	15	16	17	18	19
(2)	19	5	6	7	8	9	15	16	17	18
(3)	18	19	3	4	7	8	9	12	13	14
(4)	14	17	19	11	4	5	6	9	10	3
(5)	13	2	15	14	18	4	5	6	11	8
(6)	12	14	2	10	15	7	4	5	9	16
(7)	15	13	17	2	12	6	8	10	3	9
(8)	16	10	11	19	2	3	7	13	8	5
(9)	11	16	18	17	6	2	3	4	12	7
(10)	1	8	10	15	11	19	12	7	4	6
(11)	17	1	8	9	16	12	13	11	5	4
(12)	6	15	1	16	9	14	11	3	7	13
(13)	5	6	14	1	3	10	18	8	16	12
(14)	4	7	5	3	1	13	17	18	15	10
(15)	7	12	13	5	19	1	2	14	6	17
(16)	8	9	7	18	10	17	1	2	14	11
(17)	9	4	16	6	13	18	10	1	19	2
(18)	3	18	9	12	5	11	19	15	2	1
(19)	2	3	4	8	17	16	14	19	1	15

Plan 13.13 $t = 21, k = 5, r = 5, b = 21, \lambda = 1, E = .84$, **Type I**

	Reps.				
Block	I	II	III	IV	V
(1)	21	1	4	14	16
(2)	1	2	5	15	17
(3)	2	3	6	16	18
(4)	3	4	7	17	19
(5)	4	5	8	18	20
(6)	5	6	9	19	21
(7)	6	7	10	20	1
(8)	7	8	11	21	2
(9)	8	9	12	1	3
(10)	9	10	13	2	4
(11)	10	11	14	3	5

	Reps.				
	I	II	III	IV	V
(12)	11	12	15	4	6
(13)	12	13	16	5	7
(14)	13	14	17	6	8
(15)	14	15	18	7	9
(16)	15	16	19	8	10
(17)	16	17	20	9	11
(18)	17	18	21	10	12
(19)	18	19	1	11	13
(20)	19	20	2	12	14
(21)	20	21	3	13	15

Plan 13.1a $t = 25, k = 9, r = 9, b = 25, \lambda = 3, E = .93$, **Type I**

	Reps.								
Block	I	II	III	IV	V	VI	VII	VIII	IX
(1)	1	2	3	4	5	6	7	8	9
(2)	2	4	9	10	24	17	15	22	12
(3)	3	24	8	23	18	21	13	4	10
(4)	4	22	25	8	20	12	11	3	19
(5)	5	15	17	18	8	11	2	13	20
(6)	6	8	12	13	1	14	24	25	15
(7)	7	16	5	22	3	10	25	15	13
(8)	8	10	11	16	6	22	23	1	17
(9)	9	13	20	5	12	23	1	21	22
(10)	10	19	14	12	16	2	8	5	21
(11)	11	18	19	24	10	1	5	9	25
(12)	12	6	10	25	7	18	20	2	23
(13)	13	11	4	9	23	25	14	16	2
(14)	14	3	7	17	11	5	12	23	24
(15)	15	20	21	1	14	7	10	11	4
(16)	16	17	18	7	13	19	4	12	1
(17)	17	14	13	20	19	3	9	10	6
(18)	18	9	22	14	25	8	21	17	7
(19)	19	7	23	15	9	20	16	24	8
(20)	20	5	16	6	4	24	22	14	18
(21)	21	12	6	11	15	9	3	18	16
(22)	22	21	24	19	2	13	6	7	11
(23)	23	1	2	3	22	15	18	19	14
(24)	24	25	1	2	21	16	17	20	3
(25)	25	23	15	21	17	4	19	6	5

Plan 13.14 $t = 31, k = 6, r = 6, b = 31, \lambda = 1, E = .86$, **Type I**

	Reps.							Reps.					
Block	I	II	III	IV	V	VI		I	II	III	IV	V	VI
(1)	31	1	3	8	12	18	(17)	16	17	19	24	28	3
(2)	1	2	4	9	13	19	(18)	17	18	20	25	29	4
(3)	2	3	5	10	14	20	(19)	18	19	21	26	30	5
(4)	3	4	6	11	15	21	(20)	19	20	22	27	31	6
(5)	4	5	7	12	16	22	(21)	20	21	23	28	1	7
(6)	5	6	8	13	17	23	(22)	21	22	24	29	2	8
(7)	6	7	9	14	18	24	(23)	22	23	25	30	3	9
(8)	7	8	10	15	19	25	(24)	23	24	26	31	4	10
(9)	8	9	11	16	20	26	(25)	24	25	27	1	5	11
(10)	9	10	12	17	21	27	(26)	25	26	28	2	6	12
(11)	10	11	13	18	22	28	(27)	26	27	29	3	7	13
(12)	11	12	14	19	23	29	(28)	27	28	30	4	8	14
(13)	12	13	15	20	24	30	(29)	28	29	31	5	9	15
(14)	13	14	16	21	25	31	(30)	29	30	1	6	10	16
(15)	14	15	17	22	26	1	(31)	30	31	2	7	11	17
(16)	15	16	18	23	27	2							

Plan 13.2a $t = 31, k = 10, r = 10, b = 31, \lambda = 3, E = .93$, **Type I**

	Reps.									
Block	I	II	III	IV	V	VI	VII	VIII	IX	X
(1)	1	2	4	8	9	11	15	16	18	28
(2)	2	3	12	9	10	17	16	19	5	22
(3)	3	4	20	10	17	13	6	18	11	23
(4)	4	5	7	11	12	21	18	14	19	24
(5)	5	6	1	12	13	8	19	20	15	25
(6)	6	7	13	16	14	9	20	21	2	26
(7)	7	1	15	14	8	10	21	17	3	27
(8)	8	11	17	25	16	23	29	7	26	5
(9)	9	12	24	29	27	18	1	26	17	6
(10)	10	13	18	19	29	25	2	27	28	7
(11)	11	14	22	26	19	20	3	28	29	1
(12)	12	8	27	23	20	29	4	22	21	2
(13)	13	9	29	28	21	15	5	23	24	3
(14)	14	10	25	22	15	16	24	29	6	4
(15)	15	24	26	5	2	27	11	10	30	20
(16)	16	25	6	30	3	28	12	11	27	21
(17)	17	26	28	7	30	22	13	12	4	15
(18)	18	27	23	1	5	30	14	13	22	16
(19)	19	28	30	2	6	14	8	24	23	17
(20)	20	22	8	3	7	24	9	30	25	18
(21)	21	23	10	4	1	26	30	25	9	19
(22)	22	21	11	17	24	1	25	2	31	13
(23)	23	15	3	18	25	2	26	31	12	14
(24)	24	16	19	31	26	3	27	4	13	8
(25)	25	17	14	27	31	4	28	5	20	9
(26)	26	18	5	21	28	31	22	6	8	10
(27)	27	19	31	15	22	6	23	9	7	11
(28)	28	20	16	24	23	7	31	1	10	12
(29)	29	30	2	6	4	5	7	3	1	31
(30)	30	31	9	13	11	12	10	8	14	29
(31)	31	29	21	20	18	19	17	15	16	30

Plan 13.16 $t = 3, k = 5, r = 5, b = 3, \lambda = 5, E = .96$, **Type III**

	Reps.				
Block	I	II	III	IV	V
(1)	1	2	3	2	3
(2)	2	3	1	1	2
(3)	3	1	2	3	1

Plan 13.17 $t = 3, k = 7, r = 7, b = 3, \lambda = 7, E = .98$, **Type IV**

	Reps.						
Block	I	II	III	IV	V	VI	VII
(1)	1	2	3	1	2	3	1
(2)	2	3	1	3	1	2	2
(3)	3	1	2	2	3	1	3

Plan 13.18 $t = 3, k = 8, r = 8, b = 3, \lambda = 8, E = .98$, **Type III**

	Reps.							
Block	I	II	III	IV	V	VI	VII	VIII
(1)	1	2	3	1	2	3	1	2
(2)	2	3	1	3	1	2	2	3
(3)	3	1	2	2	3	1	3	1

Plan 13.19 $t = 3, k = 10, r = 10, b = 3, \lambda = 10, E = .99$, **Type IV**

	Reps.									
Block	I	II	III	IV	V	VI	VII	VIII	IX	X
(1)	1	2	3	1	2	3	1	2	3	1
(2)	2	3	1	3	1	2	2	3	1	3
(3)	3	1	2	2	3	1	3	1	2	2

Plan 13.20 $t = 4, k = 5, r = 5, b = 4, \lambda = 5, E = .96$, **Type IV**

	Reps.				
Block	I	II	III	IV	V
(1)	1	2	3	4	1
(2)	2	3	4	1	4
(3)	3	4	1	2	3
(4)	4	1	2	3	2

Plan 13.21 $t = 4, k = 7, r = 7, b = 4, \lambda = 7, E = .98$, **Type III**

	Reps.						
Block	I	II	III	IV	V	VI	VII
(1)	1	2	3	4	1	2	3
(2)	2	1	4	3	3	4	1
(3)	3	4	1	2	4	3	2
(4)	4	3	2	1	2	1	4

Plan 13.22 $t = 4, k = 9, r = 9, b = 4, \lambda = 9, E = .99$, **Type IV**

	Reps.							
Block	I	II	III	IV	V	VI	VII	VIII	IX
(1)	1	2	3	4	1	2	3	4	1
(2)	2	1	4	3	3	4	1	2	4
(3)	3	4	1	2	4	3	2	1	2
(4)	4	3	2	1	2	1	4	3	3

Plan 13.23 $t = 5, k = 6, r = 6, b = 5, \lambda = 6, E = .97$, **Type IV**

	Reps.					
Block	I	II	III	IV	V	VI
(1)	1	2	3	4	5	1
(2)	2	4	5	3	1	3
(3)	3	1	2	5	4	4
(4)	4	5	1	2	3	2
(5)	5	3	4	1	2	5

Plan 13.24 $t = 5, k = 9, r = 9, b = 5, \lambda = 9, E = .99$, **Type III**

	Reps.								
Block	I	II	III	IV	V	VI	VII	VIII	IX
(1)	1	2	3	4	5	1	2	3	4
(2)	2	3	4	5	1	4	5	1	2
(3)	3	4	5	1	2	2	3	4	5
(4)	4	5	1	2	3	5	1	2	3
(5)	5	1	2	3	4	3	4	5	1

Plan 13.25 $t = 6, k = 7, r = 7, b = 6, \lambda = 7, E = .98$, **Type IV**

Block	I	II	III	IV	V	VI	VII
(1)	1	2	3	4	5	6	1
(2)	2	3	6	1	4	5	3
(3)	3	6	2	5	1	4	5
(4)	4	5	1	2	6	3	4
(5)	5	1	4	6	3	2	6
(6)	6	4	5	3	2	1	2

Plan 13.26 $t = 7, k = 8, r = 8, b = 7, \lambda = 8, E = .98$, **Type IV**

Block	I	II	III	IV	V	VI	VII	VIII
(1)	1	2	3	4	5	6	7	1
(2)	2	5	1	7	6	4	3	3
(3)	3	6	7	2	4	1	5	7
(4)	4	7	5	6	3	2	1	6
(5)	5	4	2	3	1	7	6	5
(6)	6	3	4	1	7	5	2	4
(7)	7	1	6	5	2	3	4	2

EXTENDED INCOMPLETE LATIN SQUARES

Plan 13.6a $t = 5, k = 2, r = 4, b = 10, \lambda = 1, E = .67$, **Type II**

Block	I	II
(1)	1	2
(2)	2	5
(3)	3	4
(4)	4	1
(5)	5	3

Block	III	IV
(6)	1	3
(7)	2	4
(8)	3	2
(9)	4	5
(10)	5	1

Plan 13.7a $t = 5, k = 3, r = 6, b = 10, \lambda = 3, E = .83$, **Type II**

Block	I	II	III
(1)	1	2	3
(2)	2	1	5
(3)	3	4	2
(4)	4	5	1
(5)	5	3	4

Block	IV	V	VI
(6)	1	2	4
(7)	2	3	5
(8)	3	4	1
(9)	4	5	2
(10)	5	1	3

Plan 13.8a $t = 7, k = 2, r = 6, b = 21, \lambda = 1, E = .58$, **Type V**

Block	I	II	Block	III	IV	Block	V	VI
(1)	1	2	(8)	1	3	(15)	1	4
(2)	2	6	(9)	2	4	(16)	2	3
(3)	3	4	(10)	3	5	(17)	3	6
(4)	4	7	(11)	4	6	(18)	4	5
(5)	5	1	(12)	5	7	(19)	5	2
(6)	6	5	(13)	6	1	(20)	6	7
(7)	7	3	(14)	7	2	(21)	7	1

Plan 13.9a $t = 9, k = 2, r = 8, b = 36, \lambda = 1, E = .56$, **Type V**

Block	I	II	Block	III	IV	Block	V	VI	Block	VII	VIII
(1)	1	2	(10)	1	3	(19)	1	4	(28)	1	5
(2)	2	8	(11)	2	5	(20)	2	6	(29)	2	4
(3)	3	4	(12)	3	6	(21)	3	2	(30)	3	8
(4)	4	7	(13)	4	9	(22)	4	5	(31)	4	6
(5)	5	6	(14)	5	8	(23)	5	7	(32)	5	3
(6)	6	1	(15)	6	7	(24)	6	8	(33)	6	9
(7)	7	3	(16)	7	1	(25)	7	9	(34)	7	2
(8)	8	9	(17)	8	4	(26)	8	1	(35)	8	7
(9)	9	5	(18)	9	2	(27)	9	3	(36)	9	1

Plan 13.10a $t = 9, k = 4, r = 8, b = 18, \lambda = 3, E = .84$, **Type V**

Block	I	II	III	IV		V	VI	VII	VIII
(1)	1	4	6	7	(10)	1	2	5	7
(2)	2	6	8	9	(11)	2	3	6	5
(3)	3	8	9	1	(12)	3	4	7	9
(4)	4	1	3	2	(13)	4	9	2	1
(5)	5	7	1	8	(14)	5	1	9	6
(6)	6	9	4	5	(15)	6	8	1	3
(7)	7	3	2	6	(16)	7	6	4	8
(8)	8	2	5	4	(17)	8	5	3	4
(9)	9	5	7	3	(18)	9	7	8	2

Plan 13.11a $t = 9, k = 5, r = 10, b = 18, \lambda = 5, E = .90$, **Type V**

Block	I	II	III	IV	V		VI	VII	VIII	IX	X
(1)	1	2	3	7	8	(10)	1	2	3	5	9
(2)	2	6	8	4	1	(11)	2	6	5	1	8
(3)	3	8	5	9	2	(12)	3	5	1	4	6
(4)	4	3	9	2	6	(13)	4	3	2	8	7
(5)	5	1	7	3	4	(14)	5	7	9	2	4
(6)	6	4	2	5	7	(15)	6	8	7	3	5
(7)	7	9	1	6	3	(16)	7	4	8	9	1
(8)	8	5	4	1	9	(17)	8	9	4	6	3
(9)	9	7	6	8	5	(18)	9	1	6	7	2

Plan 13.12a $t = 10, k = 3, r = 9, b = 30, \lambda = 2, E = .74$, **Type V**

Block	I	II	III		IV	V	VI		VII	VIII	IX
(1)	1	2	3	(11)	1	2	4	(21)	1	3	5
(2)	2	5	8	(12)	2	3	6	(22)	2	7	6
(3)	3	7	4	(13)	3	4	8	(23)	3	8	9
(4)	4	1	6	(14)	4	9	5	(24)	4	2	10
(5)	5	8	7	(15)	5	7	1	(25)	5	6	3
(6)	6	4	9	(16)	6	8	9	(26)	6	1	8
(7)	7	9	1	(17)	7	10	3	(27)	7	9	2
(8)	8	10	2	(18)	8	1	10	(28)	8	4	7
(9)	9	3	10	(19)	9	5	2	(29)	9	10	1
(10)	10	6	5	(20)	10	6	7	(30)	10	5	4

Plan 13.13a $t = 11, k = 2, r = 10, b = 55, \lambda = 1, E = .55$, **Type V**

Block	Reps. I	II	Block	Reps. III	IV	Block	Reps. V	VI
(1)	1	2	(12)	1	3	(23)	1	4
(2)	2	11	(13)	2	6	(24)	2	3
(3)	3	10	(14)	3	5	(25)	3	7
(4)	4	5	(15)	4	10	(26)	4	6
(5)	5	6	(16)	5	9	(27)	5	10
(6)	6	7	(17)	6	8	(28)	6	9
(7)	7	1	(18)	7	2	(29)	7	11
(8)	8	3	(19)	8	1	(30)	8	2
(9)	9	4	(20)	9	7	(31)	9	1
(10)	10	9	(21)	10	11	(32)	10	8
(11)	11	8	(22)	11	4	(33)	11	5

Block	Reps. VII	VIII	Block	Reps. IX	X
(34)	1	5	(45)	1	6
(35)	2	9	(46)	2	5
(36)	3	6	(47)	3	4
(37)	4	2	(48)	4	7
(38)	5	7	(49)	5	8
(39)	6	10	(50)	6	11
(40)	7	8	(51)	7	10
(41)	8	4	(52)	8	9
(42)	9	11	(53)	9	3
(43)	10	1	(54)	10	2
(44)	11	3	(55)	11	1

Plan 13.14a $t = 13, k = 3, r = 6, b = 26, \lambda = 1, E = .72$, **Type V**

Block	Reps. I	II	III	Block	Reps. I	II	III
(1)	1	3	9	(8)	8	10	3
(2)	2	4	10	(9)	9	11	4
(3)	3	5	11	(10)	10	12	5
(4)	4	6	12	(11)	11	13	6
(5)	5	7	13	(12)	12	1	7
(6)	6	8	1	(13)	13	2	8
(7)	7	9	2				

Block	Reps. IV	V	VI	Block	Reps. IV	V	VI
(14)	2	6	5	(21)	9	13	12
(15)	3	7	6	(22)	10	1	13
(16)	4	8	7	(23)	11	2	1
(17)	5	9	8	(24)	12	3	2
(18)	6	10	9	(25)	13	4	3
(19)	7	11	10	(26)	1	5	4
(20)	8	12	11				

Plan 13.15a $t = 19, k = 3, r = 9, b = 57, \lambda = 1, E = .70$, **Type V**

Block	Reps. I	II	III
(1)	1	7	11
(2)	2	8	12
(3)	3	9	13
(4)	4	10	14
(5)	5	11	15
(6)	6	12	16
(7)	7	13	17
(8)	8	14	18
(9)	9	15	19
(10)	10	16	1
(11)	11	17	2
(12)	12	18	3
(13)	13	19	4
(14)	14	1	5
(15)	15	2	6
(16)	16	3	7
(17)	17	4	8
(18)	18	5	9
(19)	19	6	10

	Reps. IV	V	VI
(20)	2	3	14
(21)	3	4	15
(22)	4	5	16
(23)	5	6	17
(24)	6	7	18
(25)	7	8	19
(26)	8	9	1
(27)	9	10	2
(28)	10	11	3
(29)	11	12	4
(30)	12	13	5
(31)	13	14	6
(32)	14	15	7
(33)	15	16	8
(34)	16	17	9
(35)	17	18	10
(36)	18	19	11
(37)	19	1	12
(38)	1	2	13

	Reps. VII	VIII	IX
(39)	4	6	9
(40)	5	7	10
(41)	6	8	11
(42)	7	9	12
(43)	8	10	13
(44)	9	11	14
(45)	10	12	15
(46)	11	13	16
(47)	12	14	17
(48)	13	15	18
(49)	14	16	19
(50)	15	17	1
(51)	16	18	2
(52)	17	19	3
(53)	18	1	4
(54)	19	2	5
(55)	1	3	6
(56)	2	4	7
(57)	3	5	8

Plan 13.16a $t = 25, k = 4, r = 8, b = 50, \lambda = 1, E = .78$, **Type V**

Block	Reps. I	II	III	IV
(1)	1	2	6	25
(2)	2	3	7	21
(3)	3	4	8	22
(4)	4	5	9	23
(5)	5	1	10	24
(6)	6	7	11	5
(7)	7	8	12	1
(8)	8	9	13	2
(9)	9	10	14	3
(10)	10	6	15	4
(11)	11	12	16	10
(12)	12	13	17	6
(13)	13	14	18	7
(14)	14	15	19	8
(15)	15	11	20	9
(16)	16	17	21	15
(17)	17	18	22	11
(18)	18	19	23	12
(19)	19	20	24	13
(20)	20	16	25	14
(21)	21	22	1	20
(22)	22	23	2	16
(23)	23	24	3	17
(24)	24	25	4	18
(25)	25	21	5	19

	Reps. V	VI	VII	VIII
(26)	1	3	11	19
(27)	2	4	12	20
(28)	3	5	13	16
(29)	4	1	14	17
(30)	5	2	15	18
(31)	6	8	16	24
(32)	7	9	17	25
(33)	8	10	18	21
(34)	9	6	19	22
(35)	10	7	20	23
(36)	11	13	21	4
(37)	12	14	22	5
(38)	13	15	23	1
(39)	14	11	24	2
(40)	15	12	25	3
(41)	16	18	1	9
(42)	17	19	2	10
(43)	18	20	3	6
(44)	19	16	4	7
(45)	20	17	5	8
(46)	21	23	6	14
(47)	22	24	7	15
(48)	23	25	8	11
(49)	24	21	9	12
(50)	25	22	10	13

MAIN EFFECT AND INTERACTIONS IN 2^2, 2^3, 2^4, 2^5, AND 2^6 FACTORIAL DESIGNS

TREATMENT COMBINATIONS / EFFECT	T (2^2)	A (2^2)	B (2^2)	AB (2^2)	C (2^3)	AC (2^3)	BC (2^3)	ABC (2^3)	D (2^4)	AD (2^4)	BD (2^4)	ABD (2^4)	CD (2^4)	ACD (2^4)	BCD (2^4)	ABCD (2^4)	E (2^5)	AE (2^5)	BE (2^5)	ABE (2^5)	CE (2^5)	ACE (2^5)	BCE (2^5)	ABCE (2^5)	DE (2^5)	ADE (2^5)	BDE (2^5)	ABDE (2^5)	CDE (2^5)	ACDE (2^5)	BCDE (2^5)	ABCDE (2^5)
(1)	+	−	−	+	−	+	+	−	−	+	+	−	+	−	−	+	−	+	+	−	+	−	−	+	+	−	−	+	−	+	+	−
a	+	+	−	−	−	−	+	+	−	−	+	+	+	+	−	−	−	−	+	+	+	+	−	−	+	+	−	−	−	−	+	+
b	+	−	+	−	−	+	−	+	−	+	−	+	+	−	+	−	−	+	−	+	+	−	+	−	+	−	+	−	−	+	−	+
ab	+	+	+	+	−	−	−	−	−	−	−	−	+	+	+	+	−	−	−	−	+	+	+	+	+	+	+	+	−	−	−	−
c	+	−	−	+	+	−	−	+	−	+	+	−	−	+	+	−	−	+	+	−	−	+	+	−	+	−	−	+	+	−	−	+
ac	+	+	−	−	+	+	−	−	−	−	+	+	−	−	+	+	−	−	+	+	−	−	+	+	+	+	−	−	+	+	−	−
bc	+	−	+	−	+	−	+	−	−	+	−	+	−	+	−	+	−	+	−	+	−	+	−	+	+	−	+	−	+	−	+	−
abc	+	+	+	+	+	+	+	+	−	−	−	−	−	−	−	−	−	−	−	−	−	−	−	−	+	+	+	+	+	+	+	+
d	+	−	−	+	−	+	+	−	+	−	−	+	−	+	+	−	−	+	+	−	+	−	−	+	−	+	+	−	+	−	−	+
ad	+	+	−	−	−	−	+	+	+	+	−	−	−	−	+	+	−	−	+	+	+	+	−	−	−	−	+	+	+	+	−	−
bd	+	−	+	−	−	+	−	+	+	−	+	−	−	+	−	+	−	+	−	+	+	−	+	−	−	+	−	+	+	−	+	−
abd	+	+	+	+	−	−	−	−	+	+	+	+	−	−	−	−	−	−	−	−	+	+	+	+	−	−	−	−	+	+	+	+
cd	+	−	−	+	+	−	−	+	+	−	−	+	+	−	−	+	−	+	+	−	−	+	+	−	−	+	+	−	−	+	+	−
acd	+	+	−	−	+	+	−	−	+	+	−	−	+	+	−	−	−	−	+	+	−	−	+	+	−	−	+	+	−	−	+	+
bcd	+	−	+	−	+	−	+	−	+	−	+	−	+	−	+	−	−	+	−	+	−	+	−	+	−	+	−	+	−	+	−	+
abcd	+	+	+	+	+	+	+	+	+	+	+	+	+	+	+	+	−	−	−	−	−	−	−	−	−	−	−	−	−	−	−	−
e	+	−	−	+	−	+	+	−	−	+	+	−	+	−	−	+	+	−	−	+	−	+	+	−	−	+	+	−	+	−	−	+
ae	+	+	−	−	−	−	+	+	−	−	+	+	+	+	−	−	+	+	−	−	−	−	+	+	−	−	+	+	+	+	−	−
be	+	−	+	−	−	+	−	+	−	+	−	+	+	−	+	−	+	−	+	−	−	+	−	+	−	+	−	+	+	−	+	−
abe	+	+	+	+	−	−	−	−	−	−	−	−	+	+	+	+	+	+	+	+	−	−	−	−	−	−	−	−	+	+	+	+
ce	+	−	−	+	+	−	−	+	−	+	+	−	−	+	+	−	+	−	−	+	+	−	−	+	−	+	+	−	−	+	+	−
ace	+	+	−	−	+	+	−	−	−	−	+	+	−	−	+	+	+	+	−	−	+	+	−	−	−	−	+	+	−	−	+	+
bce	+	−	+	−	+	−	+	−	−	+	−	+	−	+	−	+	+	−	+	−	+	−	+	−	−	+	−	+	−	+	−	+
abce	+	+	+	+	+	+	+	+	−	−	−	−	−	−	−	−	+	+	+	+	+	+	+	+	−	−	−	−	−	−	−	−
de	+	−	−	+	−	+	+	−	+	−	−	+	−	+	+	−	+	−	−	+	−	+	+	−	+	−	−	+	−	+	+	−
ade	+	+	−	−	−	−	+	+	+	+	−	−	−	−	+	+	+	+	−	−	−	−	+	+	+	+	−	−	−	−	+	+
bde	+	−	+	−	−	+	−	+	+	−	+	−	−	+	−	+	+	−	+	−	−	+	−	+	+	−	+	−	−	+	−	+
abde	+	+	+	+	−	−	−	−	+	+	+	+	−	−	−	−	+	+	+	+	−	−	−	−	+	+	+	+	−	−	−	−
cde	+	−	−	+	+	−	−	+	+	−	−	+	+	−	−	+	+	−	−	+	+	−	−	+	+	−	−	+	+	−	−	+
acde	+	+	−	−	+	+	−	−	+	+	−	−	+	+	−	−	+	+	−	−	+	+	−	−	+	+	−	−	+	+	−	−
bcde	+	−	+	−	+	−	+	−	+	−	+	−	+	−	+	−	+	−	+	−	+	−	+	−	+	−	+	−	+	−	+	−
abcde	+	+	+	+	+	+	+	+	+	+	+	+	+	+	+	+	+	+	+	+	+	+	+	+	+	+	+	+	+	+	+	+

MAIN EFFECT AND INTERACTIONS IN 2^2, 2^3, 2^4, 2^5, AND 2^6 FACTORIAL DESIGNS

2^6

F, AF, BF, ABF	CF, ACF, BCF, ABCF	DF, ADF, BDF, ABDF	CDF, ACDF, BCDF, ABCDF	EF, AEF, BEF, ABEF	CEF, ACEF, BCEF, ABCEF	DEF, ADEF, BDEF, ABDEF	CDEF, ACDEF, BCDEF, ABCDEF
− + + −	+ − − +	+ − − +	− + + −	+ − − +	− + + −	− + + −	+ − − +
− − + +	+ + − −	+ + − −	− − + +	+ + − −	− − + +	− − + +	+ + − −
− + − +	+ − + −	+ − + −	− + − +	+ − + −	− + − +	− + − +	+ − + −
− − − −	+ + + +	+ + + +	− − − −	+ + + +	− − − −	− − − −	+ + + +
− + + −	− + + −	+ − − +	+ − − +	+ − − +	+ − − +	− + + −	− + + −
− − + +	− − + +	+ + − −	+ + − −	+ + − −	+ + − −	− − + +	− − + +
− + − +	− + − +	+ − + −	+ − + −	+ − + −	+ − + −	− + − +	− + − +
− − − −	− − − −	+ + + +	+ + + +	+ + + +	+ + + +	− − − −	− − − −
− + + −	+ − − +	− + + −	+ − − +	+ − − +	− + + −	+ − − +	− + + −
− − + +	+ + − −	− − + +	+ + − −	+ + − −	− − + +	+ + − −	− − + +
− + − +	+ − + −	− + − +	+ − + −	+ − + −	− + − +	+ − + −	− + − +
− − − −	+ + + +	− − − −	+ + + +	+ + + +	− − − −	+ + + +	− − − −
− + + −	− + + −	− + + −	− + + −	+ − − +	+ − − +	+ − − +	+ − − +
− − + +	− − + +	− − + +	− − + +	+ + − −	+ + − −	+ + − −	+ + − −
− + − +	− + − +	− + − +	− + − +	+ − + −	+ − + −	+ − + −	+ − + −
− − − −	− − − −	− − − −	− − − −	+ + + +	+ + + +	+ + + +	+ + + +
− + + −	+ − − +	+ − − +	− + + −	− + + −	+ − − +	+ − − +	− + + −
− − + +	+ + − −	+ + − −	− − + +	− − + +	+ + − −	+ + − −	− − + +
− + − +	+ − + −	+ − + −	− + − +	− + − +	+ − + −	+ − + −	− + − +
− − − −	+ + + +	+ + + +	− − − −	− − − −	+ + + +	+ + + +	− − − −
− + + −	− + + −	+ − − +	+ − − +	− + + −	− + + −	+ − − +	+ − − +
− − + +	− − + +	+ + − −	+ + − −	− − + +	− − + +	+ + − −	+ + − −
− + − +	− + − +	+ − + −	+ − + −	− + − +	− + − +	+ − + −	+ − + −
− − − −	− − − −	+ + + +	+ + + +	− − − −	− − − −	+ + + +	+ + + +
− + + −	+ − − +	− + + −	+ − − +	− + + −	+ − − +	− + + −	+ − − +
− − + +	+ + − −	− − + +	+ + − −	− − + +	+ + − −	− − + +	+ + − −
− + − +	+ − + −	− + − +	+ − + −	− + − +	+ − + −	− + − +	+ − + −
− − − −	+ + + +	− − − −	+ + + +	− − − −	+ + + +	− − − −	+ + + +
− + + −	− + + −	− + + −	− + + −	− + + −	− + + −	− + + −	− + + −
− − + +	− − + +	− − + +	− − + +	− − + +	− − + +	− − + +	− − + +
− + − +	− + − +	− + − +	− + − +	− + − +	− + − +	− + − +	− + − +
− − − −	− − − −	− − − −	− − − −	− − − −	− − − −	− − − −	− − − −

MAIN EFFECT AND INTERACTIONS IN 2^2, 2^3, 2^4, 2^5, AND 2^6 FACTORIAL DESIGNS

EFFECT		2^2				2^3								2^4																2^5		
TREATMENT COMBINATIONS	T	A	B	AB	C	AC	BC	ABC	D	AD	BD	ABD	CD	ACD	BCD	ABCD	E	AE	BE	ABE	CE	ACE	BCE	ABCE	DE	ADE	BDE	ABDE	CDE	ACDE	BCDE	ABCDE
f	+	−	−	+	−	+	+	−	−	+	+	−	+	−	−	+	−	+	+	−	+	−	−	+	+	−	−	+	−	+	+	−
af	+	+	−	−	−	−	+	+	−	−	+	+	+	+	−	−	−	−	+	+	+	+	−	−	+	+	−	−	−	−	+	+
bf	+	−	+	−	−	+	−	+	−	+	−	+	+	−	+	−	−	+	−	+	+	−	+	−	+	−	+	−	−	+	−	+
abf	+	+	+	+	−	−	−		−	−	−	−	+	+	+	+	−	−	−	−	+	+	+	+	+	+	+	+	−	−	−	−
cf	+	−	−	+	+	−	−	+	−	+	+	−	−	+	+	−	−	+	+	−	−	+	+	−	+	−	−	+	+	−	−	+
acf	+	+	−	−	+	+	−	−	−	−	+	+	−	−	+	+	−	−	+	+	−	−	+	+	+	+	−	−	+	+	−	−
bcf	+	−	+	−	+	−	+	−	−	+	−	+	−	+	−	+	−	+	−	+	−	+	−	+	+	−	+	−	+	−	+	−
abcf	+	+	+	+	+	+	+	+	−	−	−	−	−	−	−	−	−	−	−	−	−	−	−	−	+	+	+	+	+	+	+	+
df	+	−	−	+	−	+	+	−	+	−	−	+	−	+	+	−	−	+	+	−	+	−	−	+	−	+	+	−	+	−	−	+
adf	+	+	−	−	−	−	+	+	+	+	−	−	−	−	+	+	−	−	+	+	+	+	−	−	−	−	+	+	+	+	−	−
bdf	+	−	+	−	−	+	−	+	+	−	+	−	−	+	−	+	−	+	−	+	+	−	+	−	−	+	−	+	+	−	+	−
abdf	+	+	+	+	−	−	−	−	+	+	+	+	−	−	−	−	−	−	−	−	+	+	+	+	−	−	−	−	+	+	+	+
cdf	+	−	−	+	+	−	−	+	+	−	−	+	+	−	−	+	−	+	+	−	−	+	+	−	−	+	+	−	−	+	+	−
acdf	+	+	−	−	+	+	−	−	+	+	−	−	+	+	−	−	−	−	+	+	−	−	+	+	−	−	+	+	−	−	+	+
bcdf	+	−	+	−	+	−	+	−	+	−	+	−	+	−	+	−	−	+	−	+	−	+	−	+	−	+	−	+	−	+	−	+
abcdf	+	+	+	+	+	+	+	+	+	+	+	+	+	+	+	+	−	−	−	−	−	−	−	−	−	−	−	−	−	−	−	−
ef	+	−	−	+	−	+	+	−	−	+	+	−	+	−	−	+	+	−	−	+	−	+	+	−	−	+	+	−	+	−	−	+
acf	+	+	−	−	−	−	+	+	−	−	+	+	+	+	−	−	+	+	−	−	−	−	+	+	−	−	+	+	+	+	−	−
bef	+	−	+	−	−	+	−	+	−	+	−	+	+	−	+	−	+	−	+	−	−	+	−	+	−	+	−	+	+	−	+	−
abef	+	+	+	+	−	−	−	−	−	−	−	−	+	+	+	+	+	+	+	+	−	−	−	−	−	−	−	−	+	+	+	+
cef	+	−	−	+	+	−	−	+	−	+	+	−	−	+	+	−	+	−	−	+	+	−	−	+	−	+	+	−	−	+	+	−
acef	+	+	−	−	+	+	−	−	−	−	+	+	−	−	+	+	+	+	−	−	+	+	−	−	−	−	+	+	−	−	+	+
bcef	+	−	+	−	+	−	+	−	−	+	−	+	−	+	−	+	+	−	+	−	+	−	+	−	−	+	−	+	−	+	−	+
abcef	+	+	+	+	+	+	+	+	−	−	−	−	−	−	−	−	+	+	+	+	+	+	+	+	−	−	−	−	−	−	−	−
def	+	−	−	+	−	+	+	−	+	−	−	+	−	+	+	−	+	−	−	+	−	+	+	−	+	−	−	+	−	+	+	−
adef	+	+	−	−	−	−	+	+	+	+	−	−	−	−	+	+	+	+	−	−	−	−	+	+	+	+	−	−	−	−	+	+
bdef	+	−	+	−	−	+	−	+	+	−	+	−	−	+	−	+	+	−	+	−	−	+	−	+	+	−	+	−	−	+	−	+
abdef	+	+	+	+	−	−	−	−	+	+	+	+	−	−	−	−	+	+	+	+	−	−	−	−	+	+	+	+	−	−	−	−
cdef	+	−	−	+	+	−	−	+	+	−	−	+	+	−	−	+	+	−	−	+	+	−	−	+	+	−	−	+	+	−	−	+
acdef	+	+	−	−	+	+	−	−	+	+	−	−	+	+	−	−	+	+	−	−	+	+	−	−	+	+	−	−	+	+	−	−
bcdef	+	−	+	−	+	−	+	−	+	−	+	−	+	−	+	−	+	−	+	−	+	−	+	−	+	−	+	−	+	−	+	−
abcdef	+	+	+	+	+	+	+	+	+	+	+	+	+	+	+	+	+	+	+	+	+	+	+	+	+	+	+	+	+	+	+	+

MAIN EFFECT AND INTERACTIONS IN 2^2, 2^3, 2^4, 2^5, AND 2^6 FACTORIAL DESIGNS

2^6

F AF BF ABF	CF ACF BCF ABCF	DF ADF BDF ABDF	CDF ACDF BCDF ABCDF	EF AEF BEF ABEF	CEF ACEF BCEF ABCEF	DEF ADEF BDEF ABDEF	CDEF ACDEF BCDEF ABCDEF
+−−+	−++−	−++−	+−−+	−++−	+−−+	+−−+	−++−
++−−	−−++	−−++	++−−	−−++	++−−	++−−	−−++
+−+−	−+−+	−+−+	+−+−	−+−+	+−+−	+−+−	−+−+
++++	−−−−	−−−−	++++	−−−−	++++	++++	−−−−
+−−+	+−−+	−++−	−++−	−++−	−++−	+−−+	+−−+
++−−	++−−	−−++	−−++	−−++	−−++	++−−	++−−
+−+−	+−+−	−+−+	−+−+	−+−+	−+−+	+−+−	+−+−
++++	++++	−−−−	−−−−	−−−−	−−−−	++++	++++
+−−+	−++−	+−−+	−++−	−++−	+−−+	−++−	+−−+
++−−	−−++	++−−	−−++	−−++	++−−	−−++	++−−
+−+−	−+−+	+−+−	−+−+	−+−+	+−+−	−+−+	+−+−
++++	−−−−	++++	−−−−	−−−−	++++	−−−−	++++
+−−+	+−−+	+−−+	+−−+	−++−	−++−	−++−	−++−
++−−	++−−	++−−	++−−	−−++	−−++	−−++	−−++
+−+−	+−+−	+−+−	+−+−	−+−+	−+−+	−+−+	−+−+
++++	++++	++++	++++	−−−−	−−−−	−−−−	−−−−
+−−+	−++−	−++−	+−−+	+−−+	−++−	−++−	+−−+
++−−	−−++	−−++	++−−	++−−	−−++	−−++	++−−
+−+−	−+−+	−+−+	+−+−	+−+−	−+−+	−+−+	+−+−
++++	−−−−	−−−−	++++	++++	−−−−	−−−−	++++
+−−+	+−−+	−++−	−++−	+−−+	+−−+	−++−	−++−
++−−	++−−	−−++	−−++	++−−	++−−	−−++	−−++
+−+−	+−+−	−+−+	−+−+	+−+−	+−+−	−+−+	−+−+
++++	++++	−−−−	−−−−	++++	++++	−−−−	−−−−
+−−+	−++−	+−−+	−++−	+−−+	−++−	+−−+	−++−
++−−	−−++	++−−	−−++	++−−	−−++	++−−	−−++
+−+−	−+−+	+−+−	−+−+	+−+−	−+−+	+−+−	−+−+
++++	−−−−	++++	−−−−	++++	−−−−	++++	−−−−
+−−+	+−−+	+−−+	+−−+	+−−+	+−−+	+−−+	+−−+
++−−	++−−	++−−	++−−	++−−	++−−	++−−	++−−
+−+−	+−+−	+−+−	+−+−	+−+−	+−+−	+−+−	+−+−
++++	++++	++++	++++	++++	++++	++++	++++

II. NORMAL DISTRIBUTION

II.1 THE NORMAL PROBABILITY FUNCTION AND RELATED FUNCTIONS

This table gives values of:

a) $f(x)$ = the probability density of a standardized random variable

$$= \frac{1}{\sqrt{2\pi}} e^{-\frac{1}{2}x^2}$$

For negative values of x, one uses the fact that $f(-x) = f(x)$.

b) $F(x)$ = the cumulative distribution function of a standardized normal random variable

$$= \int_{-\infty}^{x} \frac{1}{\sqrt{2\pi}} e^{-\frac{1}{2}t^2}\, dt$$

For negative values of x, one uses the relationship $F(-x) = 1 - F(x)$. Values of x corresponding to a few special values of $F(x)$ are given in a separate table following the main table. (See page 115.)

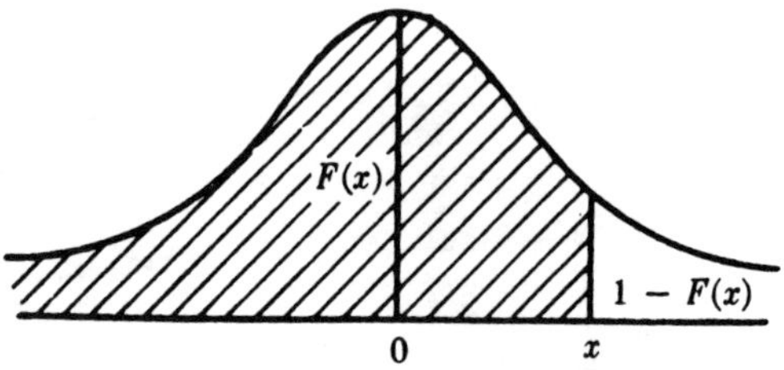

c) $f'(x)$ = the first derivative of $f(x)$ with respect to x

$$= -\frac{x}{\sqrt{2\pi}} e^{-\frac{1}{2}x^2} = -xf(x)$$

d) $f''(x)$ = the second derivative of $f(x)$ with respect to x

$$= \frac{(x^2 - 1)}{\sqrt{2\pi}} e^{-\frac{1}{2}x^2} = (x^2 - 1)f(x)$$

e) $f'''(x)$ = the third derivative of $f(x)$ with respect to x

$$= \frac{3x - x^3}{\sqrt{2\pi}} e^{-\frac{1}{2}x^2} = (3x - x^3)f(x)$$

f) $f^{\text{iv}}(x)$ = the fourth derivative of $f(x)$ with respect to x

$$= \frac{x^4 - 6x^2 + 3}{\sqrt{2\pi}} e^{-\frac{1}{2}x^2} = (x^4 - 6x^2 + 3)f(x)$$

It should be noted that other probability integrals can be evaluated by the use of these tables. For example,

$$\int_0^x f(t)dt = \tfrac{1}{2} \operatorname{erf}\left(\frac{x}{\sqrt{2}}\right),$$

where $\operatorname{erf}\left(\frac{x}{\sqrt{2}}\right)$ represents the error function associated with the normal curve.

To evaluate erf (2.3) one proceeds as follows: Since $\frac{x}{\sqrt{2}} = 2.3$, one finds $x = (2.3)(\sqrt{2}) = 3.25$. In the entry opposite $x = 3.25$, the value 0.9994 is given. Subtracting 0.5000 from the tabular value, one finds the value 0.4994. Thus erf (2.3) = 2(0.4994) = 0.9988.

NORMAL DISTRIBUTION AND RELATED FUNCTIONS

x	$F(x)$	$1 - F(x)$	$f(x)$	$f'(x)$	$f''(x)$	$f'''(x)$	$f^{\text{iv}}(x)$
.00	.5000	.5000	.3989	−.0000	−.3989	.0000	1.1968
.01	.5040	.4960	.3989	−.0040	−.3989	.0120	1.1965
.02	.5080	.4920	.3989	−.0080	−.3987	.0239	1.1956
.03	.5120	.4880	.3988	−.0120	−.3984	.0359	1.1941
.04	.5160	.4840	.3986	−.0159	−.3980	.0478	1.1920
.05	.5199	.4801	.3984	−.0199	−.3975	.0597	1.1894
.06	.5239	.4761	.3982	−.0239	−.3968	.0716	1.1861
.07	.5279	.4721	.3980	−.0279	−.3960	.0834	1.1822
.08	.5319	.4681	.3977	−.0318	−.3951	.0952	1.1778
.09	.5359	.4641	.3973	−.0358	−.3941	.1070	1.1727
.10	.5398	.4602	.3970	−.0397	−.3930	.1187	1.1671
.11	.5438	.4562	.3965	−.0436	−.3917	.1303	1.1609
.12	.5478	.4522	.3961	−.0475	−.3904	.1419	1.1541
.13	.5517	.4483	.3956	−.0514	−.3889	.1534	1.1468
.14	.5557	.4443	.3951	−.0553	−.3873	.1648	1.1389
.15	.5596	.4404	.3945	−.0592	−.3856	.1762	1.1304
.16	.5636	.4364	.3939	−.0630	−.3838	.1874	1.1214
.17	.5675	.4325	.3932	−.0668	−.3819	.1986	1.1118
.18	.5714	.4286	.3925	−.0707	−.3798	.2097	1.1017
.19	.5753	.4247	.3918	−.0744	−.3777	.2206	1.0911
.20	.5793	.4207	.3910	−.0782	−.3754	.2315	1.0799
.21	.5832	.4168	.3902	−.0820	−.3730	.2422	1.0682
.22	.5871	.4129	.3894	−.0857	−.3706	.2529	1.0560
.23	.5910	.4090	.3885	−.0894	−.3680	.2634	1.0434
.24	.5948	.4052	.3876	−.0930	−.3653	.2737	1.0302
.25	.5987	.4013	.3867	−.0967	−.3625	.2840	1.0165
.26	.6026	.3974	.3857	−.1003	−.3596	.2941	1.0024
.27	.6064	.3936	.3847	−.1039	−.3566	.3040	0.9878
.28	.6103	.3897	.3836	−.1074	−.3535	.3138	0.9727
.29	.6141	.3859	.3825	−.1109	−.3504	.3235	0.9572
.30	.6179	.3821	.3814	−.1144	−.3471	.3330	0.9413
.31	.6217	.3783	.3802	−.1179	−.3437	.3423	0.9250
.32	.6255	.3745	.3790	−.1213	−.3402	.3515	0.9082
.33	.6293	.3707	.3778	−.1247	−.3367	.3605	0.8910
.34	.6331	.3669	.3765	−.1280	−.3330	.3693	0.8735
.35	.6368	.3632	.3752	−.1313	−.3293	.3779	0.8556
.36	.6406	.3594	.3739	−.1346	−.3255	.3864	0.8373
.37	.6443	.3557	.3725	−.1378	−.3216	.3947	0.8186
.38	.6480	.3520	.3712	−.1410	−.3176	.4028	0.7996
.39	.6517	.3483	.3697	−.1442	−.3135	.4107	0.7803
.40	.6554	.3446	.3683	−.1473	−.3094	.4184	0.7607
.41	.6591	.3409	.3668	−.1504	−.3051	.4259	0.7408
.42	.6628	.3372	.3653	−.1534	−.3008	.4332	0.7206
.43	.6664	.3336	.3637	−.1564	−.2965	.4403	0.7001
.44	.6700	.3300	.3621	−.1593	−.2920	.4472	0.6793
.45	.6736	.3264	.3605	−.1622	−.2875	.4539	0.6583
.46	.6772	.3228	.3589	−.1651	−.2830	.4603	0.6371
.47	.6808	.3192	.3572	−.1679	−.2783	.4666	0.6156
.48	.6844	.3156	.3555	−.1707	−.2736	.4727	0.5940
.49	.6879	.3121	.3538	−.1734	−.2689	.4785	0.5721
.50	.6915	.3085	.3521	−.1760	−.2641	.4841	0.5501

NORMAL DISTRIBUTION AND RELATED FUNCTIONS

x	$F(x)$	$1 - F(x)$	$f(x)$	$f'(x)$	$f''(x)$	$f'''(x)$	$f^{iv}(x)$
.50	.6915	.3085	.3521	−.1760	−.2641	.4841	.5501
.51	.6950	.3050	.3503	−.1787	−.2592	.4895	.5279
.52	.6985	.3015	.3485	−.1812	−.2543	.4947	.5056
.53	.7019	.2981	.3467	−.1837	−.2493	.4996	.4831
.54	.7054	.2946	.3448	−.1862	−.2443	.5043	.4605
.55	.7088	.2912	.3429	−.1886	−.2392	.5088	.4378
.56	.7123	.2877	.3410	−.1920	−.2341	.5131	.4150
.57	.7157	.2843	.3391	−.1933	−.2289	.5171	.3921
.58	.7190	.2810	.3372	−.1956	−.2238	.5209	.3691
.59	.7224	.2776	.3352	−.1978	−.2185	.5245	.3461
.60	.7257	.2743	.3332	−.1999	−.2133	.5278	.3231
.61	.7291	.2709	.3312	−.2020	−.2080	.5309	.3000
.62	.7324	.2676	.3292	−.2041	−.2027	.5338	.2770
.63	.7357	.2643	.3271	−.2061	−.1973	.5365	.2539
.64	.7389	.2611	.3251	−.2080	−.1919	.5389	.2309
.65	.7422	.2578	.3230	−.2099	−.1865	.5411	.2078
.66	.7454	.2546	.3209	−.2118	−.1811	.5431	.1849
.67	.7486	.2514	.3187	−.2136	−.1757	.5448	.1620
.68	.7517	.2483	.3166	−.2153	−.1702	.5463	.1391
.69	.7549	.2451	.3144	−.2170	−.1647	.5476	.1164
.70	.7580	.2420	.3123	−.2186	−.1593	.5486	.0937
.71	.7611	.2389	.3101	−.2201	−.1538	.5495	.0712
.72	.7642	.2358	.3079	−.2217	−.1483	.5501	.0487
.73	.7673	.2327	.3056	−.2231	−.1428	.5504	.0265
.74	.7704	.2296	.3034	−.2245	−.1373	.5506	.0043
.75	.7734	.2266	.3011	−.2259	−.1318	.5505	−.0176
.76	.7764	.2236	.2989	−.2271	−.1262	.5502	−.0394
.77	.7794	.2206	.2966	−.2284	−.1207	.5497	−.0611
.78	.7823	.2177	.2943	−.2296	−.1153	.5490	−.0825
.79	.7852	.2148	.2920	−.2307	−.1098	.5481	−.1037
.80	.7881	.2119	.2897	−.2318	−.1043	.5469	−.1247
.81	.7910	.2090	.2874	−.2328	−.0988	.5456	−.1455
.82	.7939	.2061	.2850	−.2337	−.0934	.5440	−.1660
.83	.7967	.2033	.2827	−.2346	−.0880	.5423	−.1862
.84	.7995	.2005	.2803	−.2355	−.0825	.5403	−.2063
.85	.8023	.1977	.2780	−.2363	−.0771	.5381	−.2260
.86	.8051	.1949	.2756	−.2370	−.0718	.5358	−.2455
.87	.8078	.1922	.2732	−.2377	−.0664	.5332	−.2646
.88	.8106	.1894	.2709	−.2384	−.0611	.5305	−.2835
.89	.8133	.1867	.2685	−.2389	−.0558	.5276	−.3021
.90	.8159	.1841	.2661	−.2395	−.0506	.5245	−.3203
.91	.8186	.1814	.2637	−.2400	−.0453	.5212	−.3383
.92	.8212	.1788	.2613	−.2404	−.0401	.5177	−.3559
.93	.8238	.1762	.2589	−.2408	−.0350	.5140	−.3731
.94	.8264	.1736	.2565	−.2411	−.0299	.5102	−.3901
.95	.8289	.1711	.2541	−.2414	−.0248	.5062	−.4066
.96	.8315	.1685	.2516	−.2416	−.0197	.5021	−.4228
.97	.8340	.1660	.2492	−.2417	−.0147	.4978	−.4387
.98	.8365	.1635	.2468	−.2419	−.0098	.4933	−.4541
.99	.8389	.1611	.2444	−.2420	−.0049	.4887	−.4692
1.00	.8413	.1587	.2420	−.2420	.0000	.4839	−.4839

NORMAL DISTRIBUTION AND RELATED FUNCTIONS

x	$F(x)$	$1 - F(x)$	$f(x)$	$f'(x)$	$f''(x)$	$f'''(x)$	$f^{iv}(x)$
1.00	.8413	.1587	.2420	−.2420	.0000	.4839	−.4839
1.01	.8438	.1562	.2396	−.2420	.0048	.4790	−.4983
1.02	.8461	.1539	.2371	−.2419	.0096	.4740	−.5122
1.03	.8485	.1515	.2347	−.2418	.0143	.4688	−.5257
1.04	.8508	.1492	.2323	−.2416	.0190	.4635	−.5389
1.05	.8531	.1469	.2299	−.2414	.0236	.4580	−.5516
1.06	.8554	.1446	.2275	−.2411	.0281	.4524	−.5639
1.07	.8577	.1423	.2251	−.2408	.0326	.4467	−.5758
1.08	.8599	.1401	.2227	−.2405	.0371	.4409	−.5873
1.09	.8621	.1379	.2203	−.2401	.0414	.4350	−.5984
1.10	.8643	.1357	.2179	−.2396	.0458	.4290	−.6091
1.11	.8665	.1335	.2155	−.2392	.0500	.4228	−.6193
1.12	.8686	.1314	.2131	−.2386	.0542	.4166	−.6292
1.13	.8708	.1292	.2107	−.2381	.0583	.4102	−.6386
1.14	.8729	.1271	.2083	−.2375	.0624	.4038	−.6476
1.15	.8749	.1251	.2059	−.2368	.0664	.3973	−.6561
1.16	.8770	.1230	.2036	−.2361	.0704	.3907	−.6643
1.17	.8790	.1210	.2012	−.2354	.0742	.3840	−.6720
1.18	.8810	.1190	.1989	−.2347	.0780	.3772	−.6792
1.19	.8830	.1170	.1965	−.2339	.0818	.3704	−.6861
1.20	.8849	.1151	.1942	−.2330	.0854	.3635	−.6926
1.21	.8869	.1131	.1919	−.2322	.0890	.3566	−.6986
1.22	.8888	.1112	.1895	−.2312	.0926	.3496	−.7042
1.23	.8907	.1093	.1872	−.2303	.0960	.3425	−.7094
1.24	.8925	.1075	.1849	−.2293	.0994	.3354	−.7141
1.25	.8944	.1056	.1826	−.2283	.1027	.3282	−.7185
1.26	.8962	.1038	.1804	−.2273	.1060	.3210	−.7224
1.27	.8980	.1020	.1781	−.2262	.1092	.3138	−.7259
1.28	.8997	.1003	.1758	−.2251	.1123	.3065	−.7291
1.29	.9015	.0985	.1736	−.2240	.1153	.2992	−.7318
1.30	.9032	.0968	.1714	−.2228	.1182	.2918	−.7341
1.31	.9049	.0951	.1691	−.2216	.1211	.2845	−.7361
1.32	.9066	.0934	.1669	−.2204	.1239	.2771	−.7376
1.33	.9082	.0918	.1647	−.2191	.1267	.2697	−.7388
1.34	.9099	.0901	.1626	−.2178	.1293	.2624	−.7395
1.35	.9115	.0885	.1604	−.2165	.1319	.2550	−.7399
1.36	.9131	.0869	.1582	−.2152	.1344	.2476	−.7400
1.37	.9147	.0853	.1561	−.2138	.1369	.2402	−.7396
1.38	.9162	.0838	.1539	−.2125	.1392	.2328	−.7389
1.39	.9177	.0823	.1518	−.2110	.1415	.2254	−.7378
1.40	.9192	.0808	.1497	−.2096	.1437	.2180	−.7364
1.41	.9207	.0793	.1476	−.2082	.1459	.2107	−.7347
1.42	.9222	.0778	.1456	−.2067	.1480	.2033	−.7326
1.43	.9236	.0764	.1435	−.2052	.1500	.1960	−.7301
1.44	.9251	.0749	.1415	−.2037	.1519	.1887	−.7274
1.45	.9265	.0735	.1394	−.2022	.1537	.1815	−.7243
1.46	.9279	.0721	.1374	−.2006	.1555	.1742	−.7209
1.47	.9292	.0708	.1354	−.1991	.1572	.1670	−.7172
1.48	.9306	.0694	.1334	−.1975	.1588	.1599	−.7132
1.49	.9319	.0681	.1315	−.1959	.1604	.1528	−.7089
1.50	.9332	.0668	.1295	−.1943	.1619	.1457	−.7043

NORMAL DISTRIBUTION AND RELATED FUNCTIONS

x	$F(x)$	$1 - F(x)$	$f(x)$	$f'(x)$	$f''(x)$	$f'''(x)$	$f^{iv}(x)$
1.50	.9332	.0668	.1295	−.1943	.1619	.1457	−.7043
1.51	.9345	.0655	.1276	−.1927	.1633	.1387	−.6994
1.52	.9357	.0643	.1257	−.1910	.1647	.1317	−.6942
1.53	.9370	.0630	.1238	−.1894	.1660	.1248	−.6888
1.54	.9382	.0618	.1219	−.1877	.1672	.1180	−.6831
1.55	.9394	.0606	.1200	−.1860	.1683	.1111	−.6772
1.56	.9406	.0594	.1182	−.1843	.1694	.1044	−.6710
1.57	.9418	.0582	.1163	−.1826	.1704	.0977	−.6646
1.58	.9429	.0571	.1145	−.1809	.1714	.0911	−.6580
1.59	.9441	.0559	.1127	−.1792	.1722	.0846	−.6511
1.60	.9452	.0548	.1109	−.1775	.1730	.0781	−.6441
1.61	.9463	.0537	.1092	−.1757	.1738	.0717	−.6368
1.62	.9474	.0526	.1074	−.1740	.1745	.0654	−.6293
1.63	.9484	.0516	.1057	−.1723	.1751	.0591	−.6216
1.64	.9495	.0505	.1040	−.1705	.1757	.0529	−.6138
1.65	.9505	.0495	.1023	−.1687	.1762	.0468	−.6057
1.66	.9515	.0485	.1006	−.1670	.1766	.0408	−.5975
1.67	.9525	.0475	.0989	−.1652	.1770	.0349	−.5891
1.68	.9535	.0465	.0973	−.1634	.1773	.0290	−.5806
1.69	.9545	.0455	.0957	−.1617	.1776	.0233	−.5720
1.70	.9554	.0446	.0940	−.1599	.1778	.0176	−.5632
1.71	.9564	.0436	.0925	−.1581	.1779	.0120	−.5542
1.72	.9573	.0427	.0909	−.1563	.1780	.0065	−.5452
1.73	.9582	.0418	.0893	−.1546	.1780	.0011	−.5360
1.74	.9591	.0409	.0878	−.1528	.1780	−.0042	−.5267
1.75	.9599	.0401	.0863	−.1510	.1780	−.0094	−.5173
1.76	.9608	.0392	.0848	−.1492	.1778	−.0146	−.5079
1.77	.9616	.0384	.0833	−.1474	.1777	−.0196	−.4983
1.78	.9625	.0375	.0818	−.1457	.1774	−.0245	−.4887
1.79	.9633	.0367	.0804	−.1439	.1772	−.0294	−.4789
1.80	.9641	.0359	.0790	−.1421	.1769	−.0341	−.4692
1.81	.9649	.0351	.0775	−.1403	.1765	−.0388	−.4593
1.82	.9656	.0344	.0761	−.1386	.1761	−.0433	−.4494
1.83	.9664	.0336	.0748	−.1368	.1756	−.0477	−.4395
1.84	.9671	.0329	.0734	−.1351	.1751	−.0521	−.4295
1.85	.9678	.0322	.0721	−.1333	.1746	−.0563	−.4195
1.86	.9686	.0314	.0707	−.1316	.1740	−.0605	−.4095
1.87	.9693	.0307	.0694	−.1298	.1734	−.0645	−.3995
1.88	.9699	.0301	.0681	−.1281	.1727	−.0685	−.3894
1.89	.9706	.0294	.0669	−.1264	.1720	−.0723	−.3793
1.90	.9713	.0287	.0656	−.1247	.1713	−.0761	−.3693
1.91	.9719	.0281	.0644	−.1230	.1705	−.0797	−.3592
1.92	.9726	.0274	.0632	−.1213	.1697	−.0832	−.3492
1.93	.9732	.0268	.0620	−.1196	.1688	−.0867	−.3392
1.94	.9738	.0262	.0608	−.1179	.1679	−.0900	−.3292
1.95	.9744	.0256	.0596	−.1162	.1670	−.0933	−.3192
1.96	.9750	.0250	.0584	−.1145	.1661	−.0964	−.3093
1.97	.9756	.0244	.0573	−.1129	.1651	−.0994	−.2994
1.98	.9761	.0239	.0562	−.1112	.1641	−.1024	−.2895
1.99	.9767	.0233	.0551	−.1096	.1630	−.1052	−.2797
2.00	.9772	.0228	.0540	−.1080	.1620	−.1080	−.2700

NORMAL DISTRIBUTION AND RELATED FUNCTIONS

x	$F(x)$	$1 - F(x)$	$f(x)$	$f'(x)$	$f''(x)$	$f'''(x)$	$f^{iv}(x)$
2.00	.9773	.0227	.0540	−.1080	.1620	−.1080	−.2700
2.01	.9778	.0222	.0529	−.1064	.1609	−.1106	−.2603
2.02	.9783	.0217	.0519	−.1048	.1598	−.1132	−.2506
2.03	.9788	.0212	.0508	−.1032	.1586	−.1157	−.2411
2.04	.9793	.0207	.0498	−.1016	.1575	−.1180	−.2316
2.05	.9798	.0202	.0488	−.1000	.1563	−.1203	−.2222
2.06	.9803	.0197	.0478	−.0985	.1550	−.1225	−.2129
2.07	.9808	.0192	.0468	−.0969	.1538	−.1245	−.2036
2.08	.9812	.0188	.0459	−.0954	.1526	−.1265	−.1945
2.09	.9817	.0183	.0449	−.0939	.1513	−.1284	−.1854
2.10	.9821	.0179	.0440	−.0924	.1500	−.1302	−.1765
2.11	.9826	.0174	.0431	−.0909	.1487	−.1320	−.1676
2.12	.9830	.0170	.0422	−.0894	.1474	−.1336	−.1588
2.13	.9834	.0166	.0413	−.0879	.1460	−.1351	−.1502
2.14	.9838	.0162	.0404	−.0865	.1446	−.1366	−.1416
2.15	.9842	.0158	.0396	−.0850	.1433	−.1380	−.1332
2.16	.9846	.0154	.0387	−.0836	.1419	−.1393	−.1249
2.17	.9850	.0150	.0379	−.0822	.1405	−.1405	−.1167
2.18	.9854	.0146	.0371	−.0808	.1391	−.1416	−.1086
2.19	.9857	.0143	.0363	−.0794	.1377	−.1426	−.1006
2.20	.9861	.0139	.0355	−.0780	.1362	−.1436	−.0927
2.21	.9864	.0136	.0347	−.0767	.1348	−.1445	−.0850
2.22	.9868	.0132	.0339	−.0754	.1333	−.1453	−.0774
2.23	.9871	.0129	.0332	−.0740	.1319	−.1460	−.0700
2.24	.9875	.0125	.0325	−.0727	.1304	−.1467	−.0626
2.25	.9878	.0122	.0317	−.0714	.1289	−.1473	−.0554
2.26	.9881	.0119	.0310	−.0701	.1275	−.1478	−.0484
2.27	.9884	.0116	.0303	−.0689	.1260	−.1483	−.0414
2.28	.9887	.0113	.0297	−.0676	.1245	−.1486	−.0346
2.29	.9890	.0110	.0290	−.0664	.1230	−.1490	−.0279
2.30	.9893	.0107	.0283	−.0652	.1215	−.1492	−.0214
2.31	.9896	.0104	.0277	−.0639	.1200	−.1494	−.0150
2.32	.9898	.0102	.0270	−.0628	.1185	−.1495	−.0088
2.33	.9901	.0099	.0264	−.0616	.1170	−.1496	−.0027
2.34	.9904	.0096	.0258	−.0604	.1155	−.1496	.0033
2.35	.9906	.0094	.0252	−.0593	.1141	−.1495	.0092
2.36	.9909	.0091	.0246	−.0581	.1126	−.1494	.0149
2.37	.9911	.0089	.0241	−.0570	.1111	−.1492	.0204
2.38	.9913	.0087	.0235	−.0559	.1096	−.1490	.0258
2.39	.9916	.0084	.0229	−.0548	.1081	−.1487	.0311
2.40	.9918	.0082	.0224	−.0538	.1066	−.1483	.0362
2.41	.9920	.0080	.0219	−.0527	.1051	−.1480	.0412
2.42	.9922	.0078	.0213	−.0516	.1036	−.1475	.0461
2.43	.9925	.0075	.0208	−.0506	.1022	−.1470	.0508
2.44	.9927	.0073	.0203	−.0496	.1007	−.1465	.0554
2.45	.9929	.0071	.0198	−.0486	.0992	−.1459	.0598
2.46	.9931	.0069	.0194	−.0476	.0978	−.1453	.0641
2.47	.9932	.0068	.0189	−.0467	.0963	−.1446	.0683
2.48	.9934	.0066	.0184	−.0457	.0949	−.1439	.0723
2.49	.9936	.0064	.0180	−.0448	.0935	−.1432	.0762
2.50	.9938	.0062	.0175	−.0438	.0920	−.1424	.0800

NORMAL DISTRIBUTION AND RELATED FUNCTIONS

x	$F(x)$	$1 - F(x)$	$f(x)$	$f'(x)$	$f''(x)$	$f'''(x)$	$f^{iv}(x)$
2.50	.9938	.0062	.0175	−.0438	.0920	−.1424	.0800
2.51	.9940	.0060	.0171	−.0429	.0906	−.1416	.0836
2.52	.9941	.0059	.0167	−.0420	.0892	−.1408	.0871
2.53	.9943	.0057	.0163	−.0411	.0878	−.1399	.0905
2.54	.9945	.0055	.0158	−.0403	.0864	−.1389	.0937
2.55	.9946	.0054	.0155	−.0394	.0850	−.1380	.0968
2.56	.9948	.0052	.0151	−.0386	.0836	−.1370	.0998
2.57	.9949	.0051	.0147	−.0377	.0823	−.1360	.1027
2.58	.9951	.0049	.0143	−.0369	.0809	−.1350	.1054
2.59	.9952	.0048	.0139	−.0361	.0796	−.1339	.1080
2.60	.9953	.0047	.0136	−.0353	.0782	−.1328	.1105
2.61	.9955	.0045	.0132	−.0345	.0769	−.1317	.1129
2.62	.9956	.0044	.0129	−.0338	.0756	−.1305	.1152
2.63	.9957	.0043	.0126	−.0330	.0743	−.1294	.1173
2.64	.9959	.0041	.0122	−.0323	.0730	−.1282	.1194
2.65	.9960	.0040	.0119	−.0316	.0717	−.1270	.1213
2.66	.9961	.0039	.0116	−.0309	.0705	−.1258	.1231
2.67	.9962	.0038	.0113	−.0302	.0692	−.1245	.1248
2.68	.9963	.0037	.0110	−.0295	.0680	−.1233	.1264
2.69	.9964	.0036	.0107	−.0288	.0668	−.1220	.1279
2.70	.9965	.0035	.0104	−.0281	.0656	−.1207	.1293
2.71	.9966	.0034	.0101	−.0275	.0644	−.1194	.1306
2.72	.9967	.0033	.0099	−.0269	.0632	−.1181	.1317
2.73	.9968	.0032	.0096	−.0262	.0620	−.1168	.1328
2.74	.9969	.0031	.0093	−.0256	.0608	−.1154	.1338
2.75	.9970	.0030	.0091	−.0250	.0597	−.1141	.1347
2.76	.9971	.0029	.0088	−.0244	.0585	−.1127	.1356
2.77	.9972	.0028	.0086	−.0238	.0574	−.1114	.1363
2.78	.9973	.0027	.0084	−.0233	.0563	−.1100	.1369
2.79	.9974	.0026	.0081	−.0227	.0552	−.1087	.1375
2.80	.9974	.0026	.0079	−.0222	.0541	−.1073	.1379
2.81	.9975	.0025	.0077	−.0216	.0531	−.1059	.1383
2.82	.9976	.0024	.0075	−.0211	.0520	−.1045	.1386
2.83	.9977	.0023	.0073	−.0206	.0510	−.1031	.1389
2.84	.9977	.0023	.0071	−.0201	.0500	−.1017	.1390
2.85	.9978	.0022	.0069	−.0196	.0490	−.1003	.1391
2.86	.9979	.0021	.0067	−.0191	.0480	−.0990	.1391
2.87	.9979	.0021	.0065	−.0186	.0470	−.0976	.1391
2.88	.9980	.0020	.0063	−.0182	.0460	−.0962	.1389
2.89	.9981	.0019	.0061	−.0177	.0451	−.0948	.1388
2.90	.9981	.0019	.0060	−.0173	.0441	−.0934	.1385
2.91	.9982	.0018	.0058	−.0168	.0432	−.0920	.1382
2.92	.9982	.0018	.0056	−.0164	.0423	−.0906	.1378
2.93	.9983	.0017	.0055	−.0160	.0414	−.0893	.1374
2.94	.9984	.0016	.0053	−.0156	.0405	−.0879	.1369
2.95	.9984	.0016	.0051	−.0152	.0396	−.0865	.1364
2.96	.9985	.0015	.0050	−.0148	.0388	−.0852	.1358
2.97	.9985	.0015	.0048	−.0144	.0379	−.0838	.1352
2.98	.9986	.0014	.0047	−.0140	.0371	−.0825	.1345
2.99	.9986	.0014	.0046	−.0137	.0363	−.0811	.1337
3.00	.9987	.0013	.0044	−.0133	.0355	−.0798	.1330

NORMAL DISTRIBUTION AND RELATED FUNCTIONS

x	$F(x)$	$1 - F(x)$	$f(x)$	$f'(x)$	$f''(x)$	$f'''(x)$	$f^{iv}(x)$
3.00	.9987	.0013	.0044	–.0133	.0355	–.0798	.1330
3.01	.9987	.0013	.0043	–.0130	.0347	–.0785	.1321
3.02	.9987	.0013	.0042	–.0126	.0339	–.0771	.1313
3.03	.9988	.0012	.0040	–.0123	.0331	–.0758	.1304
3.04	.9988	.0012	.0039	–.0119	.0324	–.0745	.1294
3.05	.9989	.0011	.0038	–.0116	.0316	–.0732	.1285
3.06	.9989	.0011	.0037	–.0113	.0309	–.0720	.1275
3.07	.9989	.0011	.0036	–.0110	.0302	–.0707	.1264
3.08	.9990	.0010	.0035	–.0107	.0295	–.0694	.1254
3.09	.9990	.0010	.0034	–.0104	.0288	–.0682	.1243
3.10	.9990	.0010	.0033	–.0101	.0281	–.0669	.1231
3.11	.9991	.0009	.0032	–.0099	.0275	–.0657	.1220
3.12	.9991	.0009	.0031	–.0096	.0268	–.0645	.1208
3.13	.9991	.0009	.0030	–.0093	.0262	–.0633	.1196
3.14	.9992	.0008	.0029	–.0091	.0256	–.0621	.1184
3.15	.9992	.0008	.0028	–.0088	.0249	–.0609	.1171
3.16	.9992	.0008	.0027	–.0086	.0243	–.0598	.1159
3.17	.9992	.0008	.0026	–.0083	.0237	–.0586	.1146
3.18	.9993	.0007	.0025	–.0081	.0232	–.0575	.1133
3.19	.9993	.0007	.0025	–.0079	.0226	–.0564	.1120
3.20	.9993	.0007	.0024	–.0076	.0220	–.0552	.1107
3.21	.9993	.0007	.0023	–.0074	.0215	–.0541	.1093
3.22	.9994	.0006	.0022	–.0072	.0210	–.0531	.1080
3.23	.9994	.0006	.0022	–.0070	.0204	–.0520	.1066
3.24	.9994	.0006	.0021	–.0068	.0199	–.0509	.1053
3.25	.9994	.0006	.0020	–.0066	.0194	–.0499	.1039
3.26	.9994	.0006	.0020	–.0064	.0189	–.0488	.1025
3.27	.9995	.0005	.0019	–.0062	.0184	–.0478	.1011
3.28	.9995	.0005	.0018	–.0060	.0180	–.0468	.0997
3.29	.9995	.0005	.0018	–.0059	.0175	–.0458	.0983
3.30	.9995	.0005	.0017	–.0057	.0170	–.0449	.0969
3.31	.9995	.0005	.0017	–.0055	.0166	–.0439	.0955
3.32	.9995	.0005	.0016	–.0054	.0162	–.0429	.0941
3.33	.9996	.0004	.0016	–.0052	.0157	–.0420	.0927
3.34	.9996	.0004	.0015	–.0050	.0153	–.0411	.0913
3.35	.9996	.0004	.0015	–.0049	.0149	–.0402	.0899
3.36	.9996	.0004	.0014	–.0047	.0145	–.0393	.0885
3.37	.9996	.0004	.0014	–.0046	.0141	–.0384	.0871
3.38	.9996	.0004	.0013	–.0045	.0138	–.0376	.0857
3.39	.9997	.0003	.0013	–.0043	.0134	–.0367	.0843
3.40	.9997	.0003	.0012	–.0042	.0130	–.0359	.0829
3.41	.9997	.0003	.0012	–.0041	.0127	–.0350	.0815
3.42	.9997	.0003	.0012	–.0039	.0123	–.0342	.0801
3.43	.9997	.0003	.0011	–.0038	.0120	–.0334	.0788
3.44	.9997	.0003	.0011	–.0037	.0116	–.0327	.0774
3.45	.9997	.0003	.0010	–.0036	.0113	–.0319	.0761
3.46	.9997	.0003	.0010	–.0035	.0110	–.0311	.0747
3.47	.9997	.0003	.0010	–.0034	.0107	–.0304	.0734
3.48	.9997	.0003	.0009	–.0033	.0104	–.0297	.0721
3.49	.9998	.0002	.0009	–.0032	.0101	–.0290	.0707
3.50	.9998	.0002	.0009	–.0031	.0098	–.0283	.0694

NORMAL DISTRIBUTION AND RELATED FUNCTIONS

x	$F(x)$	$1 - F(x)$	$f(x)$	$f'(x)$	$f''(x)$	$f'''(x)$	$f^{iv}(x)$
3.50	.9998	.0002	.0009	−.0031	.0098	−.0283	.0694
3.51	.9998	.0002	.0008	−.0030	.0095	−.0276	.0681
3.52	.9998	.0002	.0008	−.0029	.0093	−.0269	.0669
3.53	.9998	.0002	.0008	−.0028	.0090	−.0262	.0656
3.54	.9998	.0002	.0008	−.0027	.0087	−.0256	.0643
3.55	.9998	.0002	.0007	−.0026	.0085	−.0249	.0631
3.56	.9998	.0002	.0007	−.0025	.0082	−.0243	.0618
3.57	.9998	.0002	.0007	−.0024	.0080	−.0237	.0606
3.58	.9998	.0002	.0007	−.0024	.0078	−.0231	.0594
3.59	.9998	.0002	.0006	−.0023	.0075	−.0225	.0582
3.60	.9998	.0002	.0006	−.0022	.0073	−.0219	.0570
3.61	.9998	.0002	.0006	−.0021	.0071	−.0214	.0559
3.62	.9999	.0001	.0006	−.0021	.0069	−.0208	.0547
3.63	.9999	.0001	.0005	−.0020	.0067	−.0203	.0536
3.64	.9999	.0001	.0005	−.0019	.0065	−.0198	.0524
3.65	.9999	.0001	.0005	−.0019	.0063	−.0192	.0513
3.66	.9999	.0001	.0005	−.0018	.0061	−.0187	.0502
3.67	.9999	.0001	.0005	−.0017	.0059	−.0182	.0492
3.68	.9999	.0001	.0005	−.0017	.0057	−.0177	.0481
3.69	.9999	.0001	.0004	−.0016	.0056	−.0173	.0470
3.70	.9999	.0001	.0004	−.0016	.0054	−.0168	.0460
3.71	.9999	.0001	.0004	−.0015	.0052	−.0164	.0450
3.72	.9999	.0001	.0004	−.0015	.0051	−.0159	.0440
3.73	.9999	.0001	.0004	−.0014	.0049	−.0155	.0430
3.74	.9999	.0001	.0004	−.0014	.0048	−.0150	.0420
3.75	.9999	.0001	.0004	−.0013	.0046	−.0146	.0410
3.76	.9999	.0001	.0003	−.0013	.0045	−.0142	.0401
3.77	.9999	.0001	.0003	−.0012	.0043	−.0138	.0392
3.78	.9999	.0001	.0003	−.0012	.0042	−.0134	.0382
3.79	.9999	.0001	.0003	−.0012	.0041	−.0131	.0373
3.80	.9999	.0001	.0003	−.0011	.0039	−.0127	.0365
3.81	.9999	.0001	.0003	−.0011	.0038	−.0123	.0356
3.82	.9999	.0001	.0003	−.0010	.0037	−.0120	.0347
3.83	.9999	.0001	.0003	−.0010	.0036	−.0116	.0339
3.84	.9999	.0001	.0003	−.0010	.0034	−.0113	.0331
3.85	.9999	.0001	.0002	−.0009	.0033	−.0110	.0323
3.86	.9999	.0001	.0002	−.0009	.0032	−.0107	.0315
3.87	.9999	.0001	.0002	−.0009	.0031	−.0104	.0307
3.88	.9999	.0001	.0002	−.0008	.0030	−.0100	.0299
3.89	1.0000	.0000	.0002	−.0008	.0029	−.0098	.0292
3.90	1.0000	.0000	.0002	−.0008	.0028	−.0095	.0284
3.91	1.0000	.0000	.0002	−.0008	.0027	−.0092	.0277
3.92	1.0000	.0000	.0002	−.0007	.0026	−.0089	.0270
3.93	1.0000	.0000	.0002	−.0007	.0026	−.0086	.0263
3.94	1.0000	.0000	.0002	−.0007	.0025	−.0084	.0256
3.95	1.0000	.0000	.0002	−.0006	.0024	−.0081	.0250
3.96	1.0000	.0000	.0002	−.0006	.0023	−.0079	.0243
3.97	1.0000	.0000	.0002	−.0006	.0022	−.0076	.0237
3.98	1.0000	.0000	.0001	−.0006	.0022	−.0074	.0230
3.99	1.0000	.0000	.0001	−.0006	.0021	−.0072	.0224
4.00	1.0000	.0000	.0001	−.0005	.0020	−.0070	.0218

x	1.282	1.645	1.960	2.326	2.576	3.090
$F(x)$	.90	.95	.975	.99	.995	.999
$2[1 - F(x)]$	.20	.10	.05	.02	.01	.002

II.2 TOLERANCE FACTORS FOR NORMAL DISTRIBUTIONS

This table gives factors K such that the probability is γ that at least a proportion P of the distribution will be included between $\bar{x} - Ks$ and $\bar{x} + Ks$, where $\bar{x}$ and s are estimates of the mean and standard deviation computed from a sample of size N. Values of K are given for $P = 0.75, 0.90, 0.95, 0.99, 0.999$ and $\gamma = 0.75, 0.90, 0.95, 0.99$ and for various values of N. For example, if $\bar{x} = 10.0$ and $s = 1.0$, $N = 16$, the interval $\bar{x} \pm Ks = 10.0 \pm 3.812(1.0) = 10.0 \pm 3.812$, or the interval 6.188 to 13.812 will contain 99% of the population with confidence coefficient 0.95. The values of K are computed assuming that the observations are from normal populations.

TOLERANCE FACTORS FOR NORMAL DISTRIBUTIONS

λ = 0.75

N \ P	0.75	0.90	0.95	0.99	0.999	N \ P	0.75	0.90	0.95	0.99	0.999
2	4.498	6.301	7.414	9.531	11.920	55	1.249	1.785	2.127	2.795	3.571
3	2.501	3.538	4.187	5.431	6.844	60	1.243	1.778	2.118	2.784	3.556
4	2.035	2.892	3.431	4.471	5.657	65	1.239	1.771	2.110	2.773	3.543
5	1.825	2.599	3.088	4.033	5.117	70	1.235	1.765	2.104	2.764	3.531
6	1.704	2.429	2.889	3.779	4.802	75	1.231	1.760	2.098	2.757	3.521
7	1.624	2.318	2.757	3.611	4.593	80	1.228	1.756	2.092	2.749	3.512
8	1.568	2.238	2.663	3.491	4.444	85	1.225	1.752	2.087	2.743	3.504
9	1.525	2.178	2.593	3.400	4.330	90	1.223	1.748	2.083	2.737	3.497
10	1.492	2.131	2.537	3.328	4.241	95	1.220	1.745	2.079	2.732	3.490
11	1.465	2.093	2.493	3.271	4.169	100	1.218	1.742	2.075	2.727	3.484
12	1.443	2.062	2.456	3.223	4.110	110	1.214	1.736	2.069	2.719	3.473
13	1.425	2.036	2.424	3.183	4.059	120	1.211	1.732	2.063	2.712	3.464
14	1.409	2.013	2.398	3.148	4.016	130	1.208	1.728	2.059	2.705	3.456
15	1.395	1.994	2.375	3.118	3.979	140	1.206	1.724	2.054	2.700	3.449
16	1.383	1.977	2.355	3.092	3.946	150	1.204	1.721	2.051	2.695	3.443
17	1.372	1.962	2.337	3.069	3.917	160	1.202	1.718	2.047	2.691	3.437
18	1.363	1.948	2.321	3.048	3.891	170	1.200	1.716	2.044	2.687	3.432
19	1.355	1.936	2.307	3.030	3.867	180	1.198	1.713	2.042	2.683	3.427
20	1.347	1.925	2.294	3.013	3.846	190	1.197	1.711	2.039	2.680	3.423
21	1.340	1.915	2.282	2.998	3.827	200	1.195	1.709	2.037	2.677	3.419
22	1.334	1.906	2.271	2.984	3.809	250	1.190	1.702	2.028	2.665	3.404
23	1.328	1.898	2.261	2.971	3.793	300	1.186	1.696	2.021	2.656	3.393
24	1.322	1.891	2.252	2.959	3.778	400	1.181	1.688	2.012	2.644	3.378
25	1.317	1.883	2.244	2.948	3.764	500	1.177	1.683	2.006	2.636	3.368
26	1.313	1.877	2.236	2.938	3.751	600	1.175	1.680	2.002	2.631	3.360
27	1.309	1.871	2.229	2.929	3.740	700	1.173	1.677	1.998	2.626	3.355
30	1.297	1.855	2.210	2.904	3.708	800	1.171	1.675	1.996	2.623	3.350
35	1.283	1.834	2.185	2.871	3.667	900	1.170	1.673	1.993	2.620	3.347
40	1.271	1.818	2.166	2.846	3.635	1000	1.169	1.671	1.992	2.617	3.344
45	1.262	1.805	2.150	2.826	3.609	∞	1.150	1.645	1.960	2.576	3.291
50	1.255	1.794	2.138	2.809	3.588						

TOLERANCE FACTORS FOR NORMAL DISTRIBUTIONS

	$\lambda = 0.90$										
N \ P	0.75	0.90	0.95	0.99	0.999	N \ P	0.75	0.90	0.95	0.99	0.999
2	11.407	15.978	18.800	24.167	30.227	55	1.329	1.901	2.265	2.976	3.801
3	4.132	5.847	6.919	8.974	11.309	60	1.320	1.887	2.248	2.955	3.774
4	2.932	4.166	4.943	6.440	8.149	65	1.312	1.875	2.235	2.937	3.751
5	2.454	3.494	4.152	5.423	6.879	70	1.304	1.865	2.222	2.920	3.730
6	2.196	3.131	3.723	4.870	6.188	75	1.298	1.856	2.211	2.906	3.712
7	2.034	2.902	3.452	4.521	5.750	80	1.292	1.848	2.202	2.894	3.696
8	1.921	2.743	3.264	4.278	5.446	85	1.287	1.841	2.193	2.882	3.682
9	1.839	2.626	3.125	4.098	5.220	90	1.283	1.834	2.185	2.872	3.669
10	1.775	2.535	3.018	3.959	5.046	95	1.278	1.828	2.178	2.863	3.657
11	1.724	2.463	2.933	3.849	4.906	100	1.275	1.822	2.172	2.854	3.646
12	1.683	2.404	2.863	3.758	4.792	110	1.268	1.813	2.160	2.839	3.626
13	1.648	2.355	2.805	3.682	4.697	120	1.262	1.804	2.150	2.826	3.610
14	1.619	2.314	2.756	3.618	4.615	130	1.257	1.797	2.141	2.814	3.595
15	1.594	2.278	2.713	3.562	4.545	140	1.252	1.791	2.134	2.804	3.582
16	1.572	2.246	2.676	3.514	4.484	150	1.248	1.785	2.127	2.795	3.571
17	1.552	2.219	2.643	3.471	4.430	160	1.245	1.780	2.121	2.787	3.561
18	1.535	2.194	2.614	3.433	4.382	170	1.242	1.775	2.116	2.780	3.552
19	1.520	2.172	2.588	3.399	4.339	180	1.239	1.771	2.111	2.774	3.543
20	1.506	2.152	2.564	3.368	4.300	190	1.236	1.767	2.106	2.768	3.536
21	1.493	2.135	2.543	3.340	4.264	200	1.234	1.764	2.102	2.762	3.429
22	1.482	2.118	2.524	3.315	4.232	250	1.224	1.750	2.085	2.740	3.501
23	1.471	2.103	2.506	3.292	4.203	300	1.217	1.740	2.073	2.725	3.481
24	1.462	2.089	2.489	3.270	4.176	400	1.207	1.726	2.057	2.703	3.453
25	1.453	2.077	2.474	3.251	4.151	500	1.201	1.717	2.046	2.689	3.434
26	1.444	2.065	2.460	3.232	4.127	600	1.196	1.710	2.038	2.678	3.421
27	1.437	2.054	2.447	3.215	4.106	700	1.192	1.705	2.032	2.670	3.411
30	1.417	2.025	2.413	3.170	4.049	800	1.189	1.701	2.027	2.663	3.402
35	1.390	1.988	2.368	3.112	3.974	900	1.187	1.697	2.023	2.658	3.396
40	1.370	1.959	2.334	3.066	3.917	1000	1.185	1.695	2.019	2.654	3.390
45	1.354	1.935	2.306	3.030	3.871	∞	1.150	1.645	1.960	2.576	3.291
50	1.340	1.916	2.284	3.001	3.833						

TOLERANCE FACTORS FOR NORMAL DISTRIBUTIONS

	λ = 0.95										
N \ P	0.75	0.90	0.95	0.99	0.999	N \ P	0.75	0.90	0.95	0.99	0.999
2	22.858	32.019	37.674	48.430	60.573	55	1.382	1.976	2.354	3.094	3.951
3	5.922	8.380	9.916	12.861	16.208	60	1.369	1.958	2.333	3.066	3.916
4	3.779	5.369	6.370	8.299	10.502	65	1.359	1.943	2.315	3.042	3.886
5	3.002	4.275	5.079	6.634	8.415	70	1.349	1.929	2.299	3.021	3.859
6	2.604	3.712	4.414	5.775	7.337	75	1.341	1.917	2.285	3.002	3.835
7	2.361	3.369	4.007	5.248	6.676	80	1.334	1.907	2.272	2.986	3.814
8	2.197	3.136	3.732	4.891	6.226	85	1.327	1.897	2.261	2.971	3.795
9	2.078	2.967	3.532	4.631	5.899	90	1.321	1.889	2.251	2.958	3.778
10	1.987	2.839	3.379	4.433	5.649	95	1.315	1.881	2.241	2.945	3.763
11	1.916	2.737	3.259	4.277	5.452	100	1.311	1.874	2.233	2.934	3.748
12	1.858	2.655	3.162	4.150	5.291	110	1.302	1.861	2.218	2.915	3.723
13	1.810	2.587	3.081	4.044	5.158	120	1.294	1.850	2.205	2.898	3.702
14	1.770	2.529	3.012	3.955	5.045	130	1.288	1.841	2.194	2.883	3.683
15	1.735	2.480	2.954	3.878	4.949	140	1.282	1.833	2.184	2.870	3.666
16	1.705	2.437	2.903	3.812	4.865	150	1.277	1.825	1.175	2.859	3.652
17	1.679	2.400	2.858	3.754	4.791	160	1.272	1.819	2.167	2.848	3.638
18	1.655	2.366	2.819	3.702	4.725	170	1.268	1.813	2.160	2.839	3.627
19	1.635	2.337	2.784	3.656	4.667	180	1.264	1.808	2.154	2.831	3.616
20	1.616	2.310	2.752	3.615	4.614	190	1.261	1.803	2.148	2.823	3.606
21	1.599	2.286	2.723	3.577	4.567	200	1.258	1.798	2.143	2.816	3.597
22	1.584	2.264	2.697	3.543	4.523	250	1.245	1.780	2.121	2.788	3.561
23	1.570	2.244	2.673	3.512	4.484	300	1.236	1.767	2.106	2.767	3.535
24	1.557	2.225	2.651	3.483	4.447	400	1.223	1.749	2.084	2.739	3.499
25	1.545	2.208	2.631	3.457	4.413	500	1.215	1.737	2.070	2.721	3.475
26	1.534	2.193	2.612	3.432	4.382	600	1.209	1.729	2.060	2.707	3.458
27	1.523	2.178	2.595	3.409	4.353	700	1.204	1.722	2.052	2.697	3.445
30	1.497	2.140	2.549	3.350	4.278	800	1.201	1.717	2.046	2.688	3.434
35	1.462	2.090	2.490	3.272	4.179	900	1.198	1.712	2.040	2.682	3.426
40	1.435	2.052	2.445	3.213	4.104	1000	1.195	1.709	2.036	2.676	3.418
45	1.414	2.021	2.408	3.165	4.042	∞	1.150	1.645	1.960	2.576	3.291
50	1.396	1.996	2.379	3.126	3.993						

TOLERANCE FACTORS FOR NORMAL DISTRIBUTIONS

$\lambda = 0.99$

N \ P	0.75	0.90	0.95	0.99	0.999	N \ P	0.75	0.90	0.95	0.99	0.999
2	114.363	160.193	188.491	242.300	303.054	55	1.490	2.130	2.538	3.335	4.260
3	13.378	18.930	22.401	29.055	36.616	60	1.471	2.103	2.506	3.293	4.206
4	6.614	9.398	11.150	14.527	18.383	65	1.455	2.080	2.478	3.257	4.160
5	4.643	6.612	7.855	10.260	13.015	70	1.440	2.060	2.454	3.225	4.120
6	3.743	5.337	6.345	8.301	10.548	75	1.428	2.042	2.433	3.197	4.084
7	3.233	4.613	5.488	7.187	9.142	80	1.417	2.026	2.414	3.173	4.053
8	2.905	4.147	4.936	6.468	8.234	85	1.407	2.012	2.397	3.150	4.024
9	2.677	3.822	4.550	5.966	7.600	90	1.398	1.999	2.382	3.130	3.999
10	2.508	3.582	4.265	5.594	7.129	95	1.390	1.987	2.368	3.112	3.976
11	2.378	3.397	4.045	5.308	6.766	100	1.383	1.977	2.355	3.096	3.954
12	2.274	3.250	3.870	5.079	6.477	110	1.369	1.958	2.333	3.066	3.917
13	2.190	3.130	3.727	4.893	6.240	120	1.358	1.942	2.314	3.041	3.885
14	2.120	3.029	3.608	4.737	6.043	130	1.349	1.928	2.298	3.019	3.857
15	2.060	2.945	3.507	4.605	5.876	140	1.340	1.916	2.283	3.000	3.833
16	2.009	2.872	3.421	4.492	5.732	150	1.332	1.905	2.270	2.983	3.811
17	1.965	2.808	3.345	4.393	5.607	160	1.326	1.896	2.259	2.968	3.792
18	1.926	2.753	3.279	4.307	5.497	170	1.320	1.887	2.248	2.955	3.774
19	1.891	2.703	3.221	4.230	5.399	180	1.314	1.879	2.239	2.942	3.759
20	1.860	2.659	3.168	4.161	5.312	190	1.309	1.872	2.230	2.931	3.744
21	1.833	2.620	3.121	4.100	5.234	200	1.304	1.865	2.222	2.921	3.731
22	1.808	2.584	3.078	4.044	5.163	250	1.286	1.839	2.191	2.880	3.678
23	1.785	2.551	3.040	3.993	5.098	300	1.273	1.820	2.169	2.850	3.641
24	1.764	2.522	3.004	3.947	5.039	400	1.255	1.794	2.138	2.809	3.589
25	1.745	2.494	2.972	3.904	4.985	500	1.243	1.777	2.117	2.783	3.555
26	1.727	2.469	2.941	3.865	4.935	600	1.234	1.764	2.102	2.763	3.530
27	1.711	2.446	2.914	3.828	4.888	700	1.227	1.755	2.091	2.748	3.511
30	1.668	2.385	2.841	3.733	4.768	800	1.222	1.747	2.082	2.736	3.495
35	1.613	2.306	2.748	3.611	4.611	900	1.218	1.741	2.075	2.726	3.483
40	1.571	2.247	2.677	3.518	4.493	1000	1.214	1.736	2.068	2.718	3.472
45	1.539	2.200	2.621	3.444	4.399	∞	1.150	1.645	1.960	2.576	3.291
50	1.512	2.162	2.576	3.385	4.323						

II.3 FACTORS FOR COMPUTING PROBABLE ERRORS

The probable error of a series of n measures $a_1, a_2, a_3 \cdots a_n$, the mean of which is m, is given by the expression,

$$e = \frac{0.6745}{\sqrt{n-1}} \sqrt{(m-a_1)^2 + (m-a_2)^2 + \cdots + (m-a_n)^2}\ .$$

The probable error of the mean is,

$$E = \frac{0.6745}{\sqrt{n(n-1)}} \sqrt{(m-a_1)^2 + (m-a_2)^2 + \cdots + (m-a_n)^2}$$

The following approximate equations are convenient forms for computation,

$$e = 0.8453 \frac{\Sigma d}{\sqrt{n(n-1)}}$$

$$E = 0.8453 \frac{\Sigma d}{n\sqrt{n-1}}\ .$$

The symbol Σd represents the arithmetical sum of the deviations.

For convenience in computing the probable error the value of several of the factors involved is given for values of n from 2 to 100.

FACTORS FOR COMPUTING PROBABLE ERRORS

n	$\frac{1}{\sqrt{n}}$	$\frac{1}{\sqrt{n(n-1)}}$	$\frac{.6745}{\sqrt{n-1}}$	$\frac{.6745}{\sqrt{n(n-1)}}$	$\frac{.8453}{n\sqrt{n-1}}$	$\frac{.8453}{\sqrt{n(n-1)}}$
2	.707107	.707107	.6745	.4769	.4227	.5978
3	.577350	.408248	.4769	.2754	.1993	.3451
4	.500000	.288675	.3894	.1947	.1220	.2440
5	.447214	.223607	.3372	.1508	.0845	.1890
6	.408248	.182574	.3016	.1231	.0630	.1543
7	.377964	.154303	.2754	.1041	.0493	.1304
8	.353553	.133631	.2549	.0901	.0399	.1130
9	.333333	.117851	.2385	.0795	.0332	.0996
10	.316228	.105409	.2248	.0711	.0282	.0891
11	.301511	.095346	.2133	.0643	.0243	.0806
12	.288675	.087039	.2034	.0587	.0212	.0736
13	.277350	.080064	.1947	.0540	.0188	.0677
14	.267261	.074125	.1871	.0500	.0167	.0627
15	.258199	.069007	.1803	.0465	.0151	.0583
16	.250000	.064550	.1742	.0435	.0136	.0546
17	.242536	.060634	.1686	.0409	.0124	.0513
18	.235702	.057166	.1636	.0386	.0114	.0483
19	.229416	.054074	.1590	.0365	.0105	.0457
20	.223607	.051299	.1547	.0346	.0097	.0434
21	.218218	.048795	.1508	.0329	.0090	.0412
22	.213201	.046524	.1472	.0314	.0084	.0393
23	.208514	.044455	.1438	.0300	.0078	.0376
24	.204124	.042563	.1406	.0287	.0073	.0360
25	.200000	.040825	.1377	.0275	.0069	.0345
26	.196116	.039223	.1349	.0265	.0065	.0332
27	.192450	.037743	.1323	.0255	.0061	.0319
28	.188982	.036370	.1298	.0245	.0058	.0307
29	.185695	.035093	.1275	.0237	.0055	.0297
30	.182574	.033903	.1252	.0229	.0052	.0287
31	.179605	.032791	.1231	.0221	.0050	.0277
32	.176777	.031750	.1211	.0214	.0047	.0268
33	.174078	.030773	.1192	.0208	.0045	.0260
34	.171499	.029854	.1174	.0201	.0043	.0252
35	.169031	.028989	.1157	.0196	.0041	.0245
36	.166667	.028172	.1140	.0190	.0040	.0238
37	.164399	.027400	.1124	.0185	.0038	.0232
38	.162221	.026669	.1109	.0180	.0037	.0225
39	.160128	.025976	.1094	.0175	.0035	.0220
40	.158114	.025318	.1080	.0171	.0034	.0214
41	.156174	.024693	.1066	.0167	.0033	.0209
42	.154303	.024098	.1053	.0163	.0031	.0204
43	.152499	.023531	.1041	.0159	.0030	.0199
44	.150756	.022990	.1029	.0155	.0029	.0194
45	.149071	.022473	.1017	.0152	.0028	.0190
46	.147442	.021979	.1005	.0148	.0027	.0186
47	.145865	.021507	.0994	.0145	.0027	.0182
48	.144338	.021054	.0984	.0142	.0026	.0178
49	.142857	.020620	.0974	.0139	.0025	.0174
50	.141421	.020203	.0964	.0136	.0024	.0171

FACTORS FOR COMPUTING PROBABLE ERRORS

n	$\frac{1}{\sqrt{n}}$	$\frac{1}{\sqrt{n(n-1)}}$	$\frac{.6745}{\sqrt{n-1}}$	$\frac{.6745}{\sqrt{n(n-1)}}$	$\frac{.8453}{n\sqrt{n-1}}$	$\frac{.8453}{\sqrt{n(n-1)}}$
50	.141421	.020203	.0964	.0136	.0024	.0171
51	.140028	.019803	.0954	.0134	.0023	.0167
52	.138675	.019418	.0945	.0131	.0023	.0164
53	.137361	.019048	.0935	.0129	.0022	.0161
54	.136083	.018692	.0927	.0126	.0022	.0158
55	.134840	.018349	.0918	.0124	.0021	.0155
56	.133631	.018019	.0910	.0122	.0020	.0152
57	.132453	.017700	.0901	.0119	.0020	.0150
58	.131306	.017392	.0893	.0117	.0019	.0147
59	.130189	.017095	.0886	.0115	.0019	.0145
60	.129099	.016807	.0878	.0113	.0018	.0142
61	.128037	.016529	.0871	.0112	.0018	.0140
62	.127000	.016261	.0864	.0110	.0018	.0138
63	.125988	.016001	.0857	.0108	.0017	.0135
64	.125000	.015749	.0850	.0106	.0017	.0133
65	.124035	.015504	.0843	.0105	.0016	.0131
66	.123091	.015268	.0837	.0103	.0016	.0129
67	.122169	.015038	.0830	.0101	.0016	.0127
68	.121268	.014815	.0824	.0100	.0015	.0125
69	.120386	.014599	.0818	.0099	.0015	.0123
70	.119523	.014389	.0812	.0097	.0015	.0122
71	.118678	.014185	.0806	.0096	.0014	.0120
72	.117851	.013986	.0801	.0094	.0014	.0118
73	.117041	.013793	.0795	.0093	.0014	.0117
74	.116248	.013606	.0789	.0092	.0013	.0115
75	.115470	.013423	.0784	.0091	.0013	.0113
76	.114708	.013245	.0779	.0089	.0013	.0112
77	.113961	.013072	.0773	.0088	.0013	.0111
78	.113228	.012904	.0769	.0087	.0012	.0109
79	.112509	.012739	.0764	.0086	.0012	.0108
80	.111803	.012579	.0759	.0085	.0012	.0106
81	.111111	.012423	.0754	.0084	.0012	.0105
82	.110432	.012270	.0749	.0083	.0012	.0104
83	.109764	.012121	.0745	.0082	.0011	.0103
84	.109109	.011976	.0740	.0081	.0011	.0101
85	.108465	.011835	.0736	.0080	.0011	.0100
86	.107833	.011696	.0732	.0079	.0011	.0099
87	.107211	.011561	.0727	.0078	.0011	.0098
88	.106600	.011429	.0723	.0077	.0010	.0097
89	.106000	.011300	.0719	.0076	.0010	.0096
90	.105409	.011173	.0715	.0075	.0010	.0094
91	.104828	.011050	.0711	.0075	.0010	.0093
92	.104257	.010929	.0707	.0074	.0010	.0092
93	.103695	.010811	.0703	.0073	.0010	.0091
94	.103142	.010695	.0699	.0072	.0009	.0090
95	.102598	.010582	.0696	.0071	.0009	.0089
96	.102062	.010471	.0692	.0071	.0009	.0089
97	.101535	.010363	.0688	.0070	.0009	.0088
98	.101015	.010257	.0685	.0069	.0009	.0087
99	.100504	.010152	.0681	.0069	.0009	.0086
100	.100000	.010050	.0678	.0068	.0008	.0085

II.4 PROBABILITY OF OCCURRENCE OF DEVIATIONS

The significance of deviations is indicated by this table. The probability of occurrence of deviations as great as or greater than any specific value is given for various ratios of deviation to probable error and also with respect to the standard deviation. The probability of occurrence is stated in per cent or chances in 100. The odds against occurrence are also stated. The probable error is 0.6745 × the standard deviation.

Ratio, dev. to P.E.	Probable occurrence %	Odds against, to 1	Ratio dev. to std. dev.	Probable occurrence %	Odds against, to 1
1.0	50.00	1.00	0.67449	50.00	1.00
1.1	45.81	1.18	0.7	48.39	1.07
1.2	41.83	1.39	0.8	42.37	1.36
1.3	38.06	1.63	0.9	36.81	1.72
1.4	34.50	1.90	1.0	31.73	2.15
1.5	31.17	2.21	1.1	27.13	2.69
1.6	28.05	2.57	1.2	23.01	3.35
1.7	25.15	2.98	1.3	19.36	4.17
1.8	22.47	3.45	1.4	16.15	5.19
1.9	20.00	4.00	1.5	13.36	6.48
2.0	17.73	4.64	1.6	10.96	8.12
2.1	15.67	5.38	1.7	8.91	10.22
2.2	13.78	6.25	1.8	7.19	12.92
2.3	12.08	7.28	1.9	5.74	16.41
2.4	10.55	8.48	2.0	4.55	20.98
2.5	9.18	9.90	2.1	3.57	26.99
2.6	7.95	11.58	2.2	2.78	34.96
2.7	6.86	13.58	2.3	2.14	45.62
2.8	5.89	15.96	2.4	1.64	59.99
2.9	5.05	18.82	2.5	1.24	79.52
3.0	4.30	22.24	2.6	.932	106.3
3.1	3.65	26.37	2.7	.693	143.2
3.2	3.09	31.36	2.8	.511	194.7
3.3	2.60	37.42	2.9	.373	267.0
3.4	2.18	44.80	3.0	.270	369.4
3.5	1.82	53.82	3.1	.194	515.7
3.6	1.52	64.89	3.2	.137	726.7
3.7	1.26	78.53	3.3	.0967	1033.
3.8	1.04	95.38	3.4	.0674	1483.
3.9	.853	116.3	3.5	.0465	2149.
4.0	.698	142.3	3.6	.0318	3142.
4.1	.569	174.9	3.7	.0216	4637.
4.2	.461	215.8	3.8	.0145	6915.
4.3	.373	267.2	3.9	.00962	10394.
4.4	.300	332.4	4.0	.00634	15772.
4.5	.240	415.0	5.0	5.73×10^{-5}	1.744×10^{6}
4.6	.192	520.4	6.0	2.0×10^{-7}	5.0×10^{8}
4.7	.152	655.3	7.0	2.6×10^{-10}	3.9×10^{11}
4.8	.121	828.3			
4.9	.0950	1052.			
5.0	.0745	1341.			
6.0	.0052	19300.			
7.0	.00023	4.27×10^{5}			
8.0	6.8×10^{-6}	1.47×10^{7}			
9.0	1.3×10^{-7}	7.30×10^{8}			
10.0	1.5×10^{-9}	6.5×10^{10}			

Valid for samples of size 30 or greater.

II.5 OPERATING CHARACTERISTIC (OC) CURVES FOR A TEST ON THE MEAN OF A NORMAL DISTRIBUTION WITH KNOWN STANDARD DEVIATION

The OC curves give the sample sizes needed for given values of $\alpha = P$ (Type I error) and $\beta = P$ (Type II error) for a test of the hypothesis Ho: $\mu = \mu_0$ where the standard deviation is known. The statistic used is $z = \dfrac{(\bar{x} - \mu_0)\sqrt{n}}{\sigma}$ which is distributed as the standard normal distribution. The required sample size is obtained by entering the appropriate set of curves for given α and β for various values of $\Delta = \dfrac{|\mu_1 - \mu_0|}{\sigma}$ for both one-sided and two-sided tests.

The OC curves can also be used to give the sample sizes for a test of the hypothesis H_0: $\mu_x = \mu_y$, where the standard deviations σ_x and σ_y are known. The statistic used is $z = \dfrac{\bar{x} - \bar{y}}{\sqrt{\dfrac{\sigma_x^2}{n_x} + \dfrac{\sigma_y^2}{n_y}}}$. The required sample size is obtained by entering the appropriate set of curves for given α and β for various values of $\Delta = \dfrac{|\mu_x - \mu_y|}{\sqrt{\sigma_x^2 + \sigma_y^2}}$ for both one-sided and two-sided tests.

OC CURVES FOR A TEST ON THE MEAN OF A NORMAL DISTRIBUTION WITH KNOWN STANDARD DEVIATION

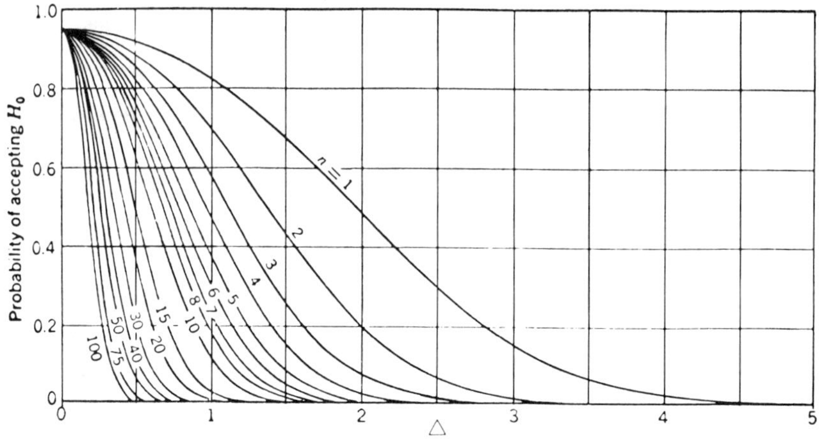

a) OC curves for different values of n for the two-sided normal test for a level of significance $\alpha = 0.05$.

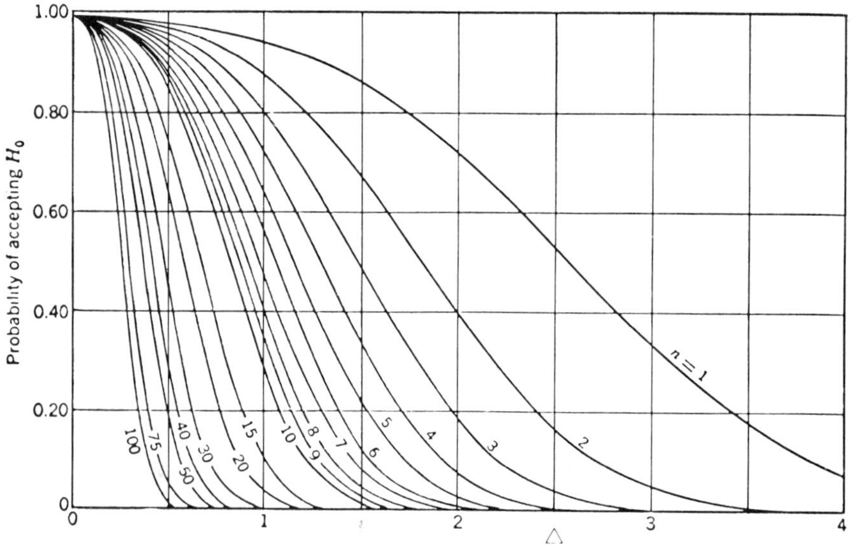

b) OC curves for different values of n for the two-sided normal test for a level of significance $\alpha = 0.01$.

OC CURVES FOR A TEST ON THE MEAN OF A NORMAL DISTRIBUTION WITH KNOWN STANDARD DEVIATION

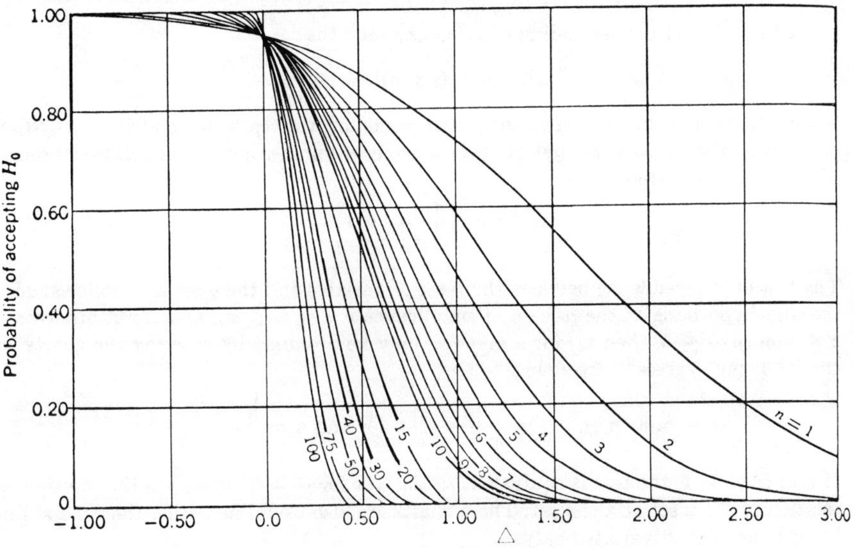

c) OC curves for different values of n for the one-sided normal test for a level of significance $\alpha = 0.05$.

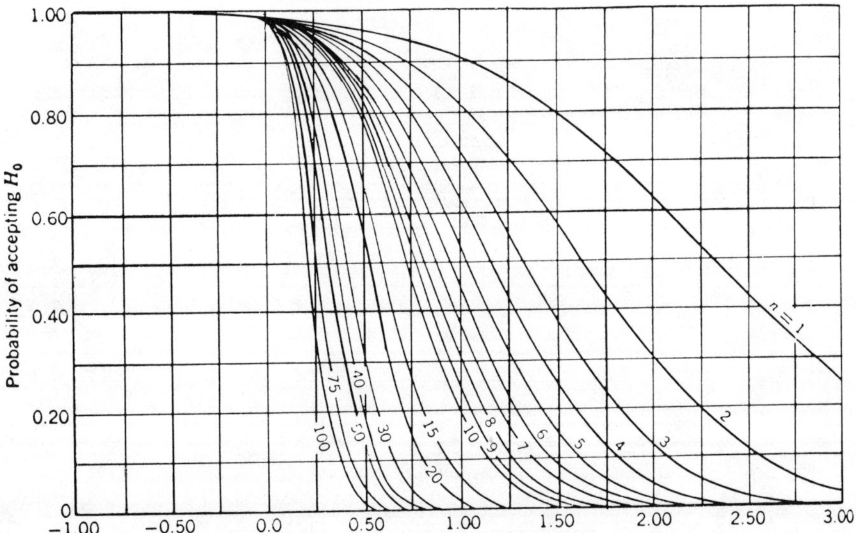

d) OC curves for different values of n for the one-sided normal test for a level of significance $\alpha = 0.01$.

II.6 CHARTS OF THE UPPER 1%, 2.5%, AND 5% POINTS OF THE DISTRIBUTION OF THE LARGEST CHARACTERISTIC ROOT

Charts I–XII enable finding of $x_\alpha(s,m,n)$ such that

$$P[\theta_s \leq x_\alpha(s,m,n)] = 1 - \alpha,$$

where θ_s is the largest of s non-zero roots of the $(p \times p)$ matrix $S_{12}S_{22}^{-1}S_{12}'S_{11}^{-1}$, and where the covariance matrix from a $(p + q)$-variate normal population based on $N - 1$ degrees of freedom is

$$S = \begin{bmatrix} S_{11} & S_{12} \\ S_{12}' & S_{22} \end{bmatrix}.$$

The test of independence between the p-set of variates and the q-set is as follows: accept the null hypothesis at the α-level of significance if $c = \theta_s \leq x_\alpha$, and reject otherwise. If $2 \leq \min(p,q) \leq 5$, then x_α, for a given α, may be obtained by entering the charts with the following degrees of freedom:

$$s = \min(p,q), \qquad m = \frac{|p - q| - 1}{2}, \text{ and } n = \frac{N - p - q - 2}{2}.$$

If $\min(p,q) = 1$, the test is equivalent to the test for $\rho^2 = 0$ where ρ is the multiple correlation of the p set on the q set. These charts are also useful in testing the general linear hypothesis in multivariate analysis.

CHART I

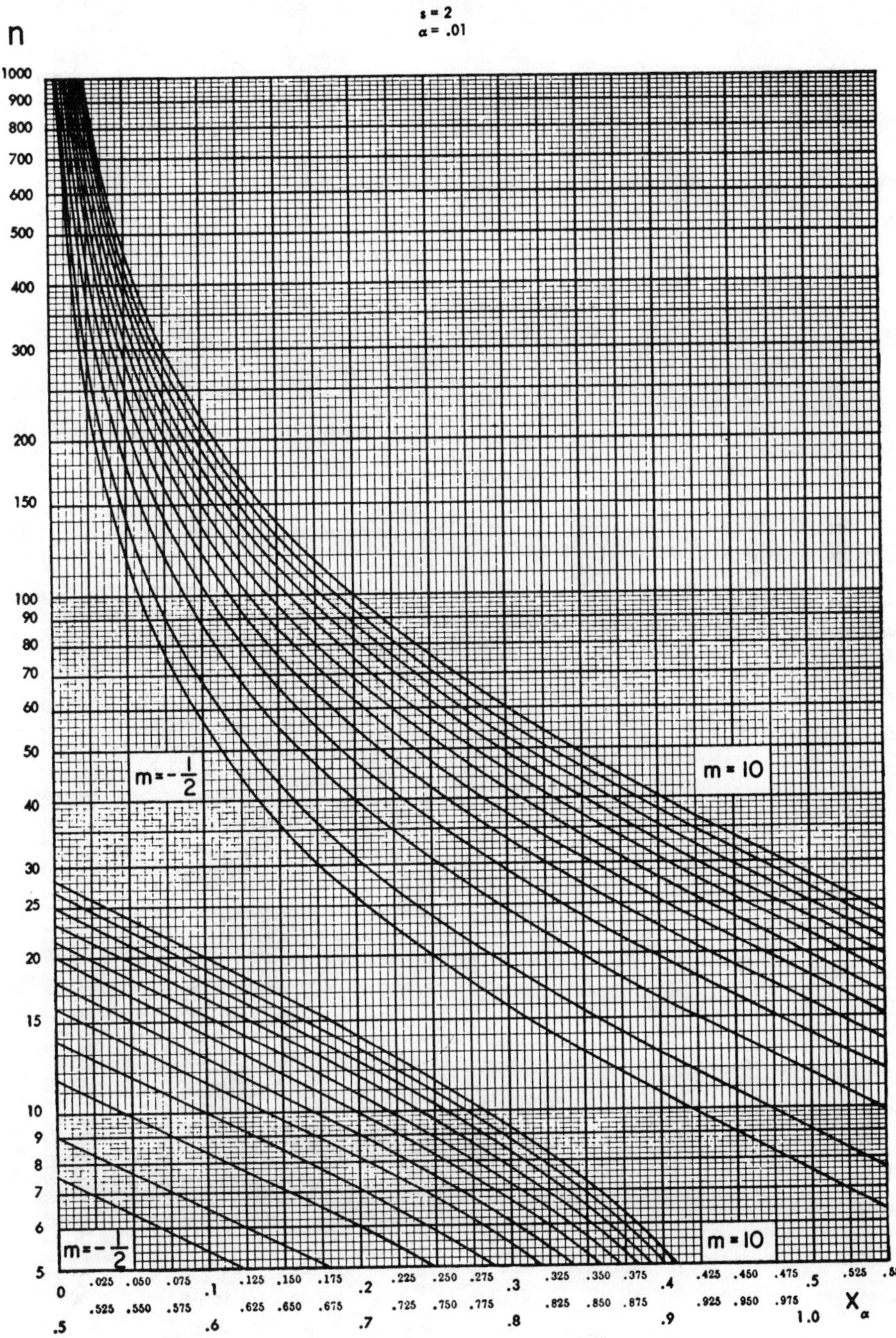
s = 2
α = .01
n
1000
900
800
700
600
500
400
300
200
150
100
90
80
70
60
50
40
30
25
20
15
10
9
8
7
6
5
m = -1/2
m = 10
m = -1/2
m = 10
0 .025 .050 .075 .1 .125 .150 .175 .2 .225 .250 .275 .3 .325 .350 .375 .4 .425 .450 .475 .5 .525 .550
.525 .550 .575 .625 .650 .675 .725 .750 .775 .825 .850 .875 .925 .950 .975
.5 .6 .7 .8 .9 1.0
X_α

CHART II

s = 2

α = .025

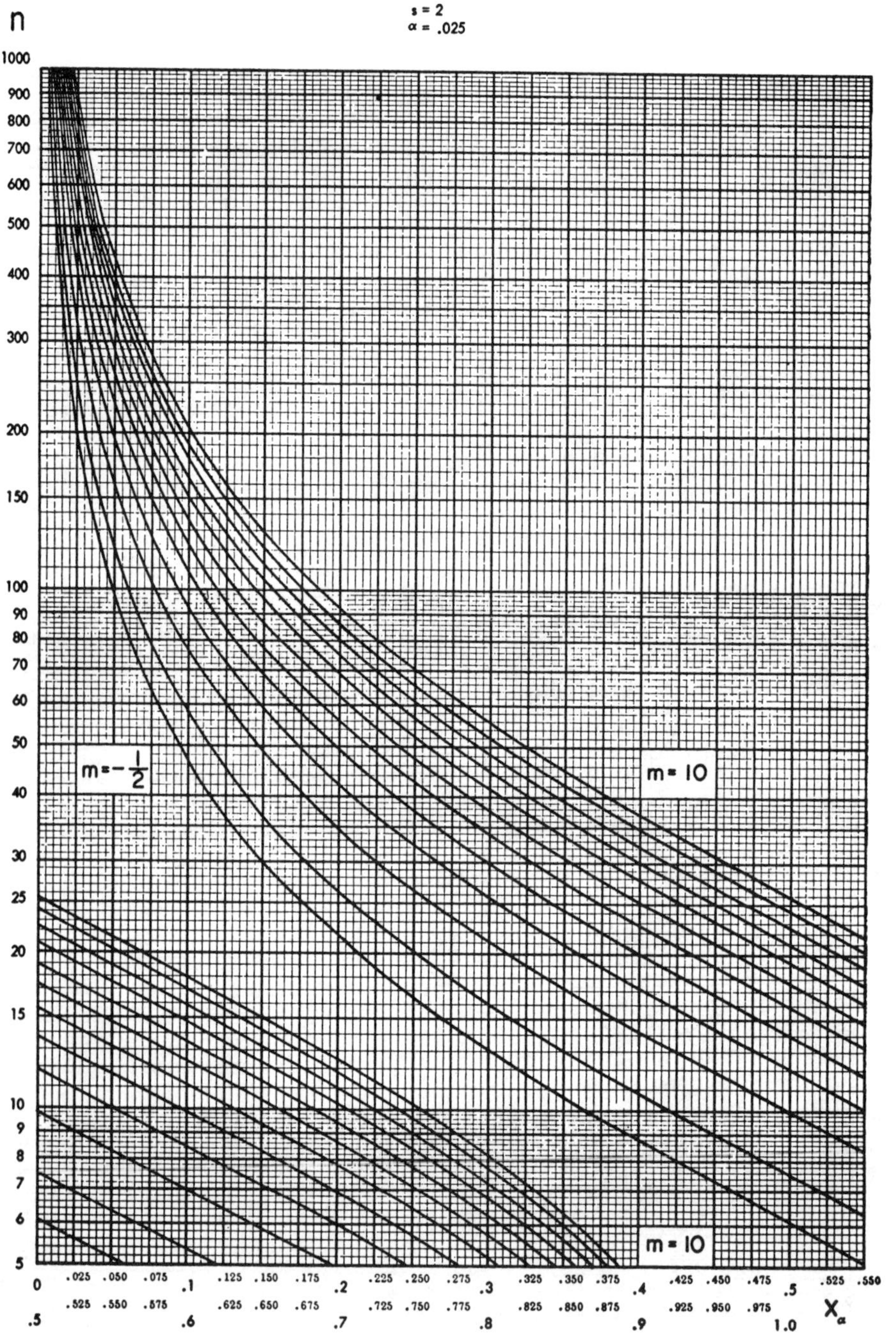

CHART III

$s = 2$
$\alpha = .05$

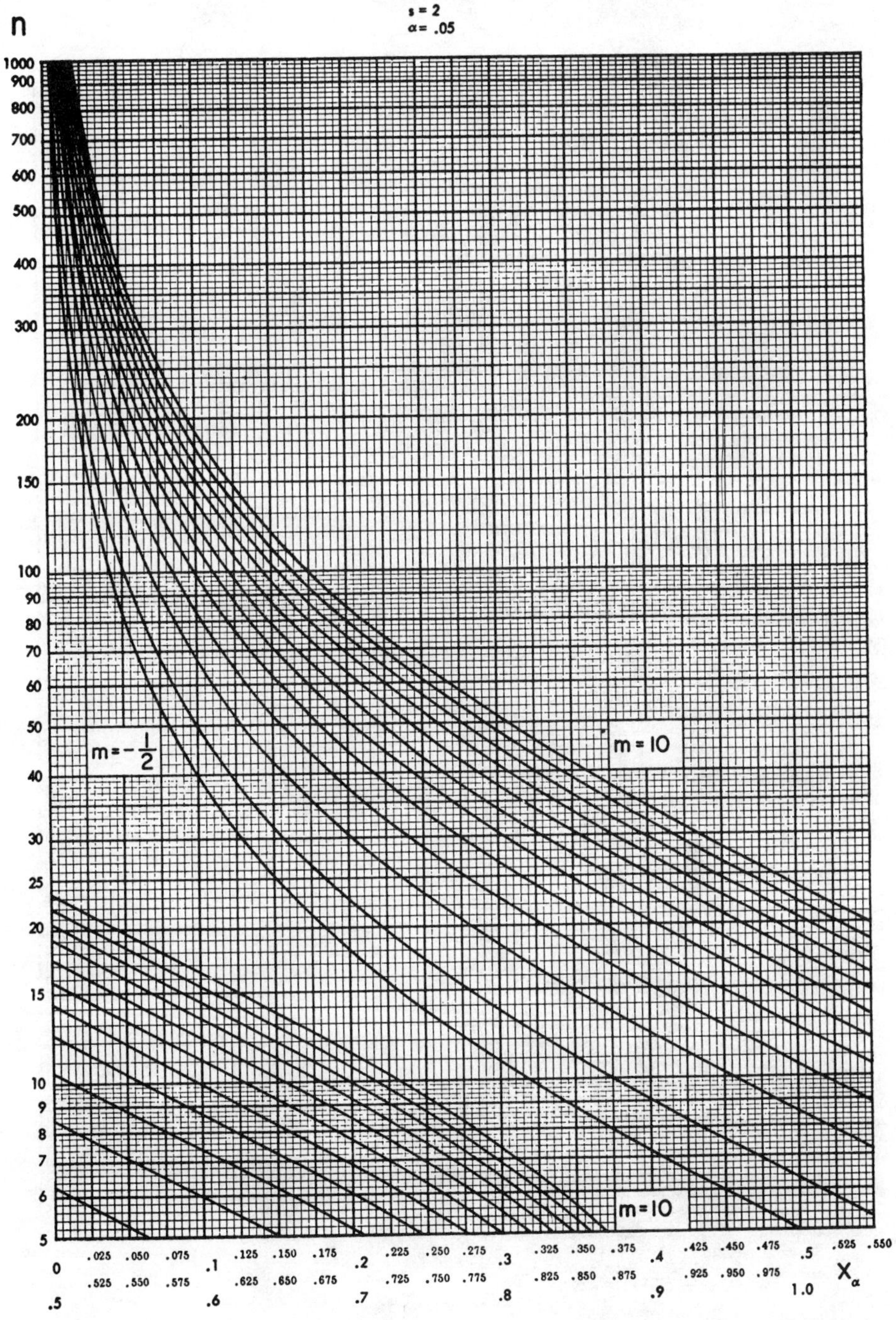

CHART IV

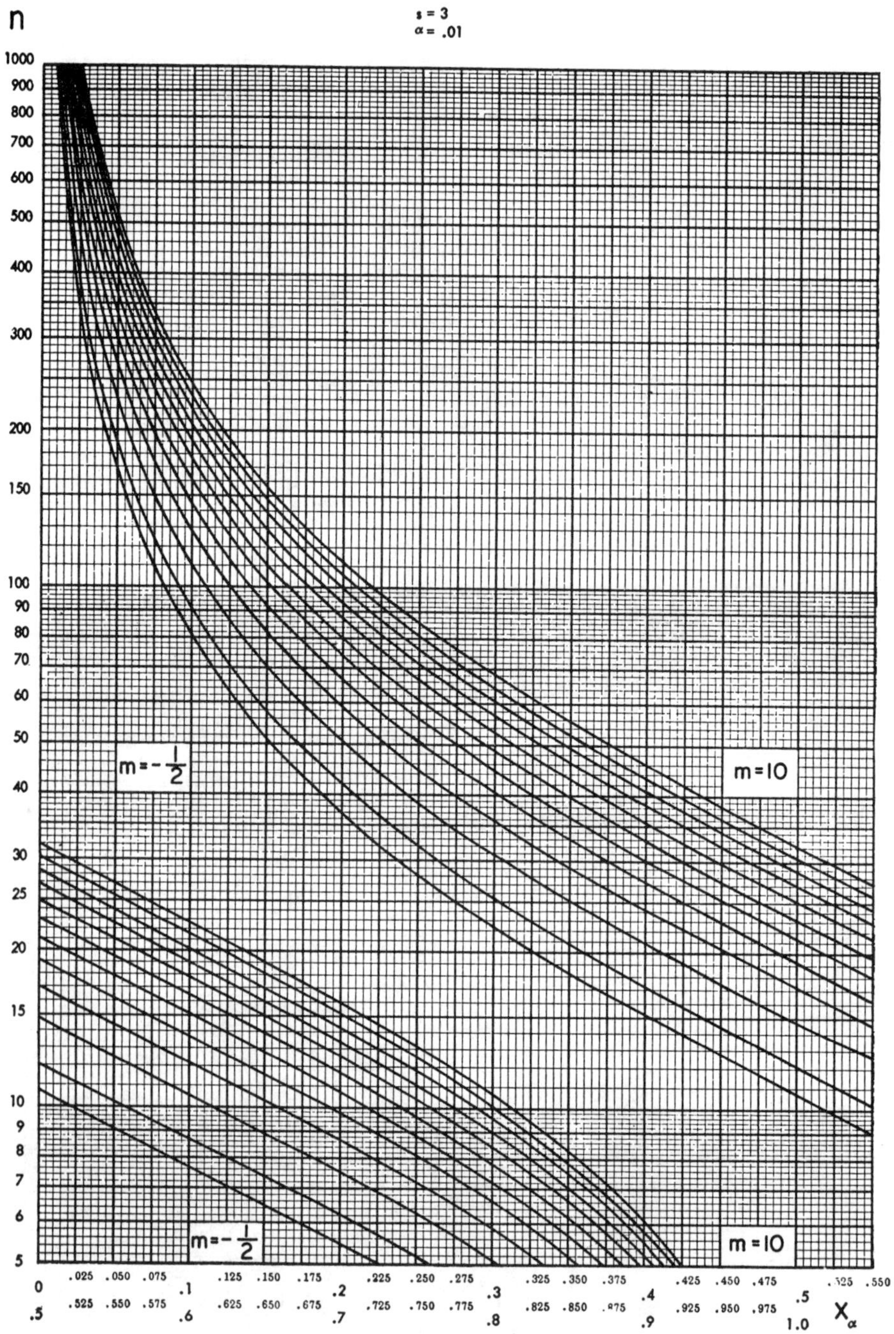
n
s = 3
α = .01
1000
900
800
700
600
500
400
300
200
150
100
90
80
70
60
50
40
30
25
20
15
10
9
8
7
6
5
m = - 1/2
m = 10
m = - 1/2
m = 10
0 .025 .050 .075 .1 .125 .150 .175 .2 .225 .250 .275 .3 .325 .350 .375 .4 .425 .450 .475 .5 .525 .550
.5 .525 .550 .575 .6 .625 .650 .675 .7 .725 .750 .775 .8 .825 .850 .875 .9 .925 .950 .975 1.0
X_α

CHART V

$s = 3$
$\alpha = .025$

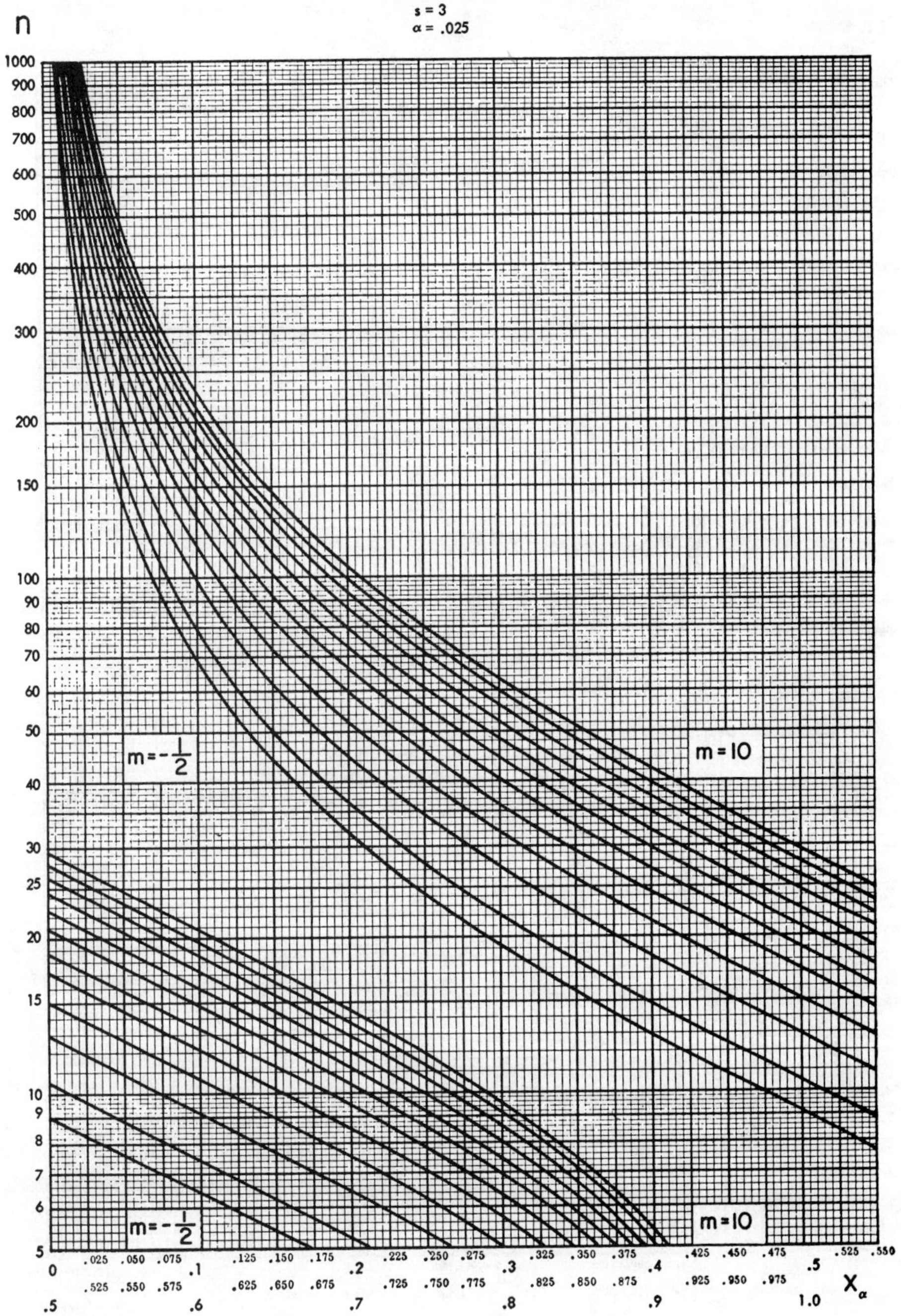

CHART VI

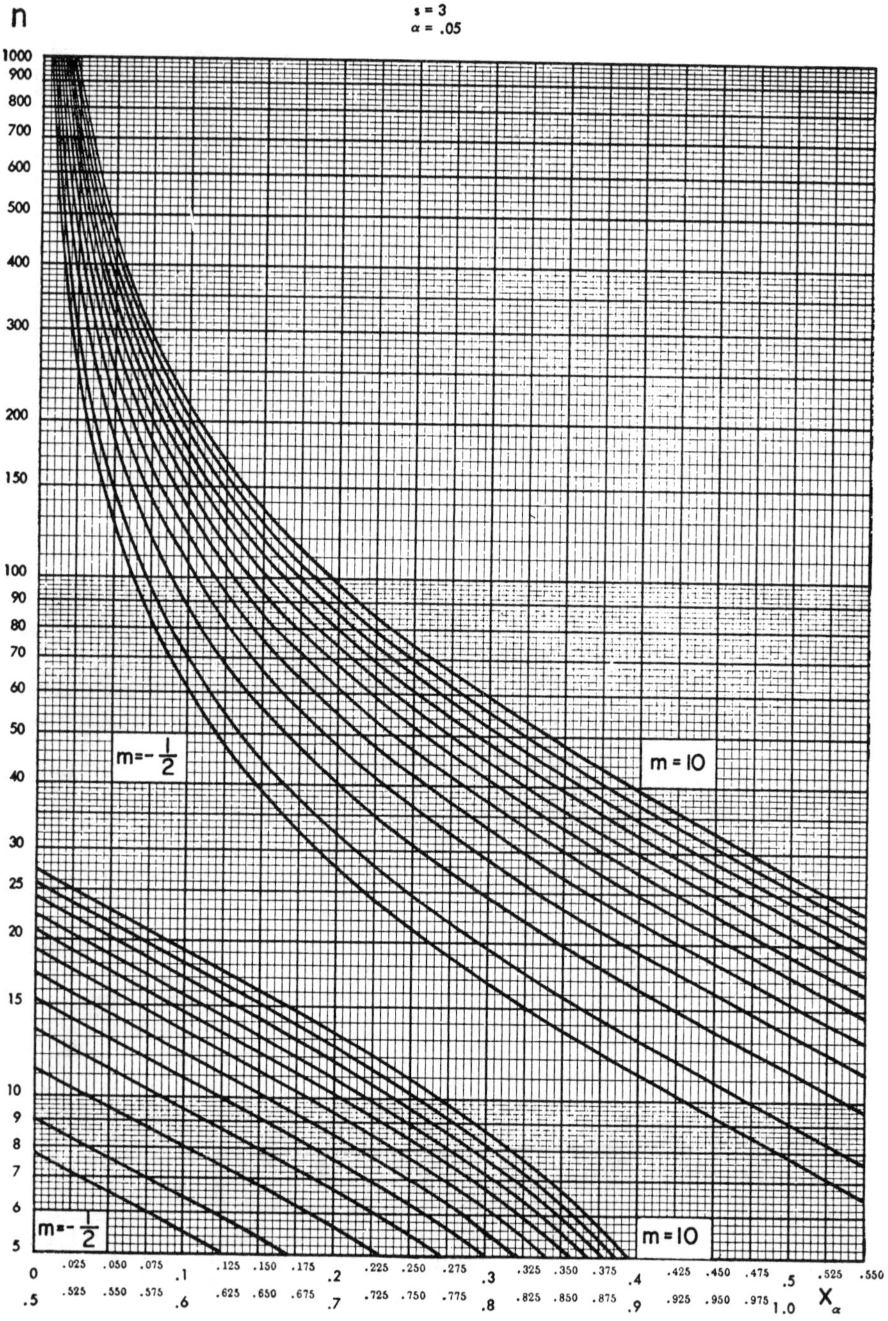
s = 3
α = .05
n
1000
900
800
700
600
500
400
300
200
150
100
90
80
70
60
50
40
30
25
20
15
10
9
8
7
6
5
m = -1/2
m = 10
m = -1/2
m = 10
0 .025 .050 .075 .1 .125 .150 .175 .2 .225 .250 .275 .3 .325 .350 .375 .4 .425 .450 .475 .5 .525 .550
.5 .525 .550 .575 .6 .625 .650 .675 .7 .725 .750 .775 .8 .825 .850 .875 .9 .925 .950 .975 1.0
X_α

CHART VII

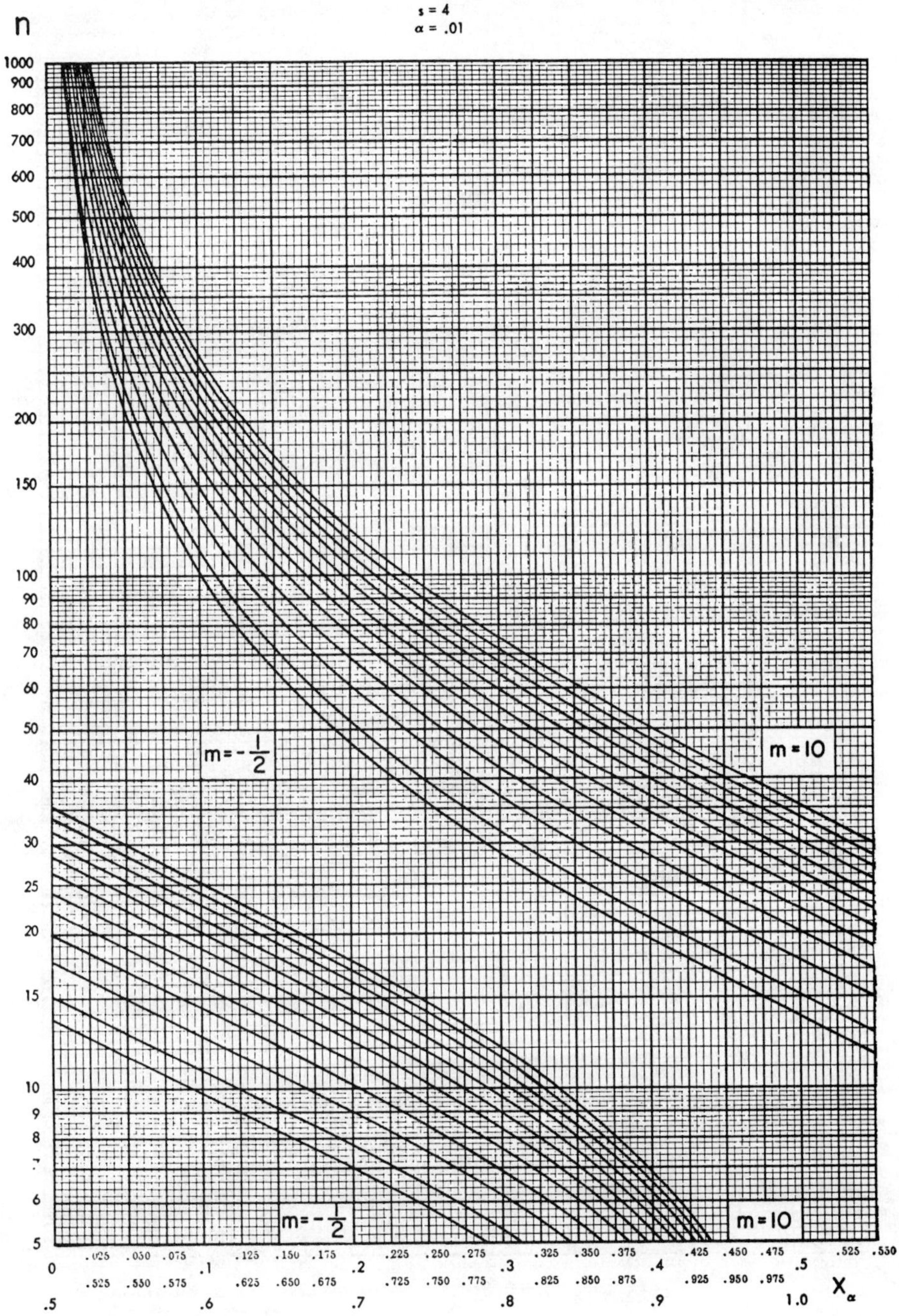
s = 4
α = .01
n
1000
900
800
700
600
500
400
300
200
150
100
90
80
70
60
50
40
30
25
20
15
10
9
8
6
5
m = −1/2
m = 10
m = −1/2
m = 10
0
.025 .050 .075
.1
.125 .150 .175
.2
.225 .250 .275
.3
.325 .350 .375
.4
.425 .450 .475
.5
.525 .550
.525 .550 .575
.625 .650 .675
.725 .750 .775
.825 .850 .875
.925 .950 .975
.5
.6
.7
.8
.9
1.0
Xα

CHART VIII

$s = 4$
$\alpha = .025$

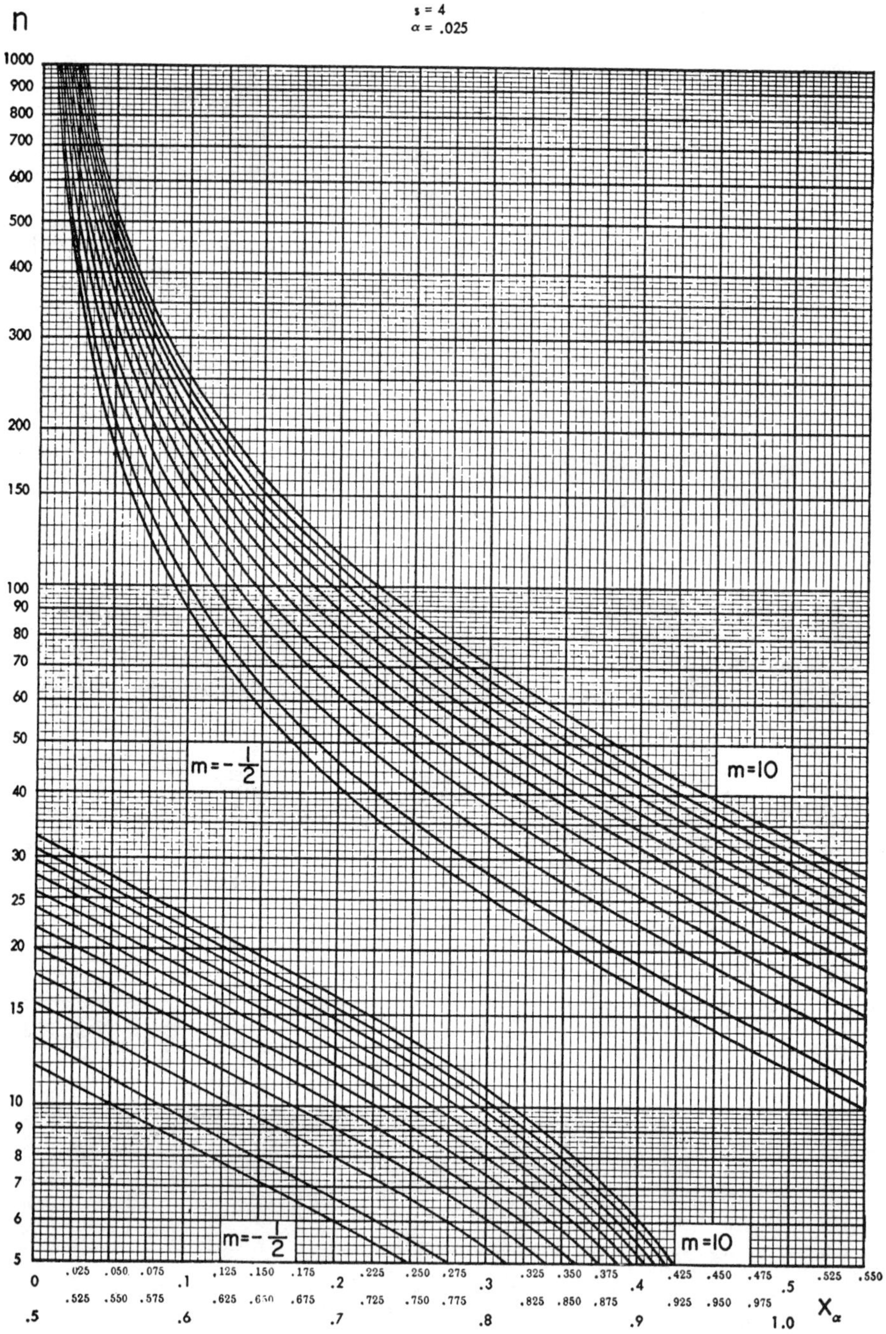

CHART IX

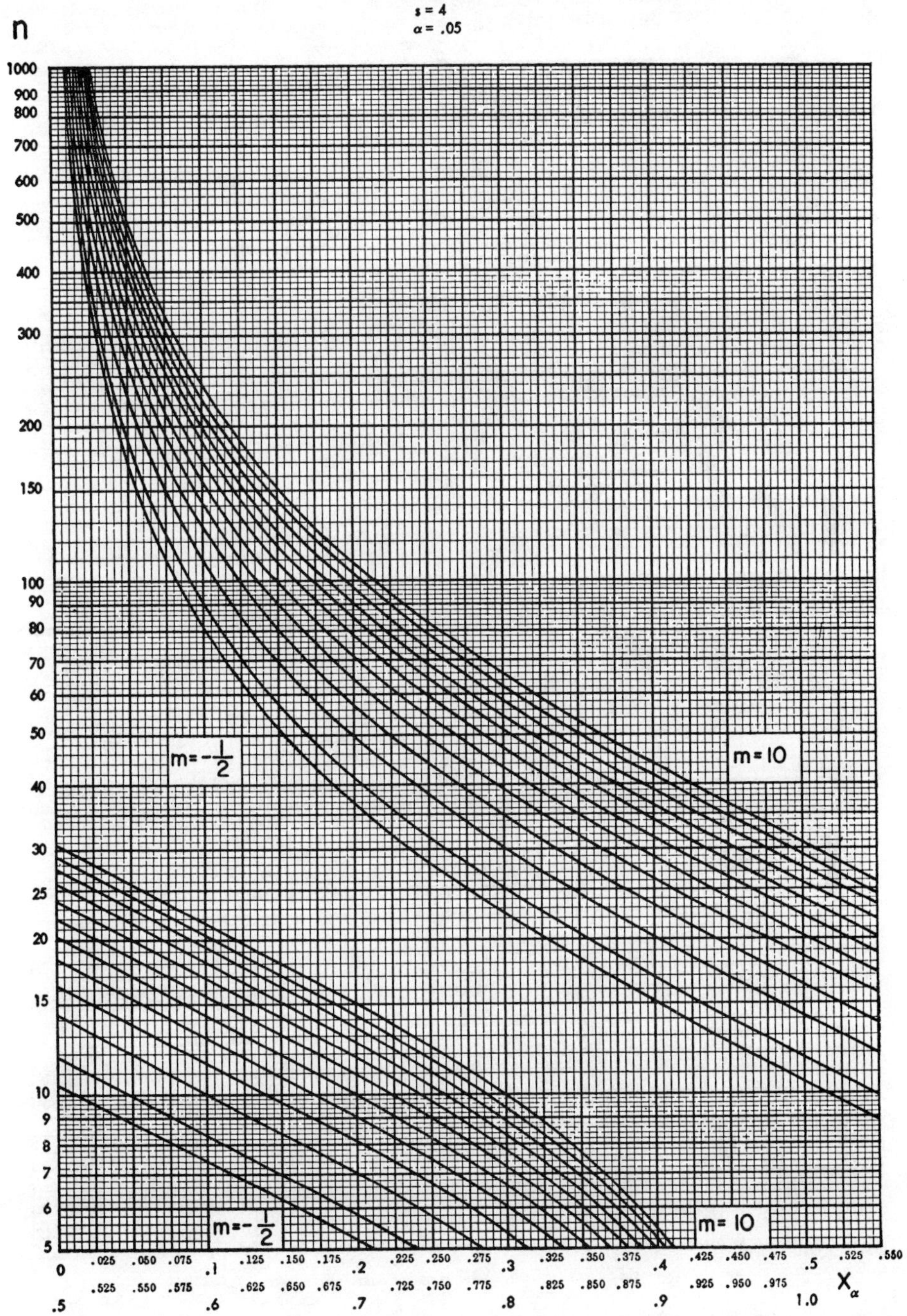
s = 4
α = .05
n
1000
900
800
700
600
500
400
300
200
150
100
90
80
70
60
50
40
30
25
20
15
10
9
8
7
6
5
m=-1/2
m=10
m=-1/2
m=10
0 .025 .050 .075 .1 .125 .150 .175 .2 .225 .250 .275 .3 .325 .350 .375 .4 .425 .450 .475 .5 .525 .550
.5 .525 .550 .575 .6 .625 .650 .675 .7 .725 .750 .775 .8 .825 .850 .875 .9 .925 .950 .975 1.0
X_α

CHART X

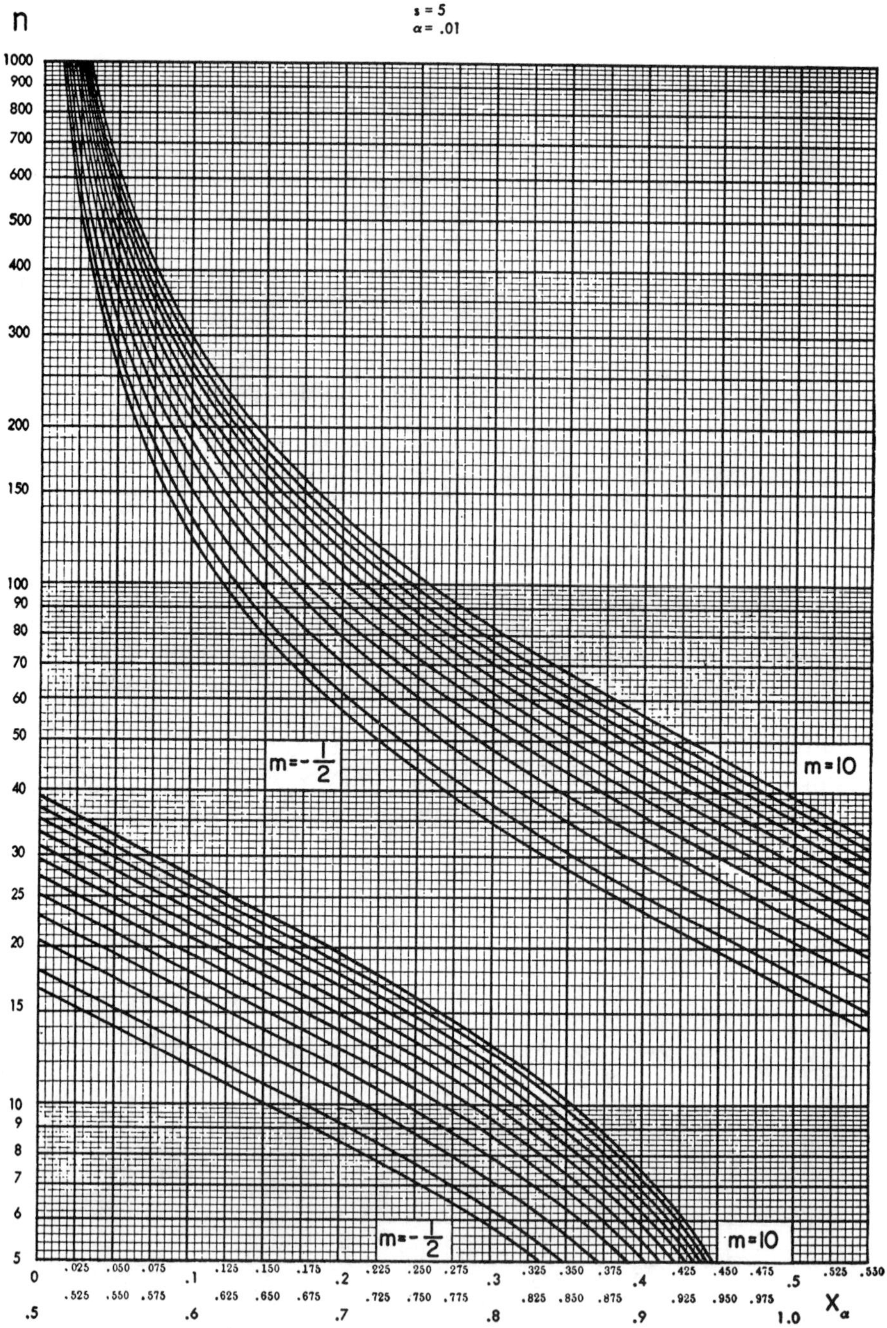
s = 5
α = .01
n
1000
900
800
700
600
500
400
300
200
150
100
90
80
70
60
50
40
30
25
20
15
10
9
8
7
6
5
m=-1/2
m=10
m=-1/2
m=10
0
.025
.050
.075
.1
.125
.150
.175
.2
.225
.250
.275
.3
.325
.350
.375
.4
.425
.450
.475
.5
.525
.550
.5
.525
.550
.575
.6
.625
.650
.675
.7
.725
.750
.775
.8
.825
.850
.875
.9
.925
.950
.975
1.0
X_α

CHART XI

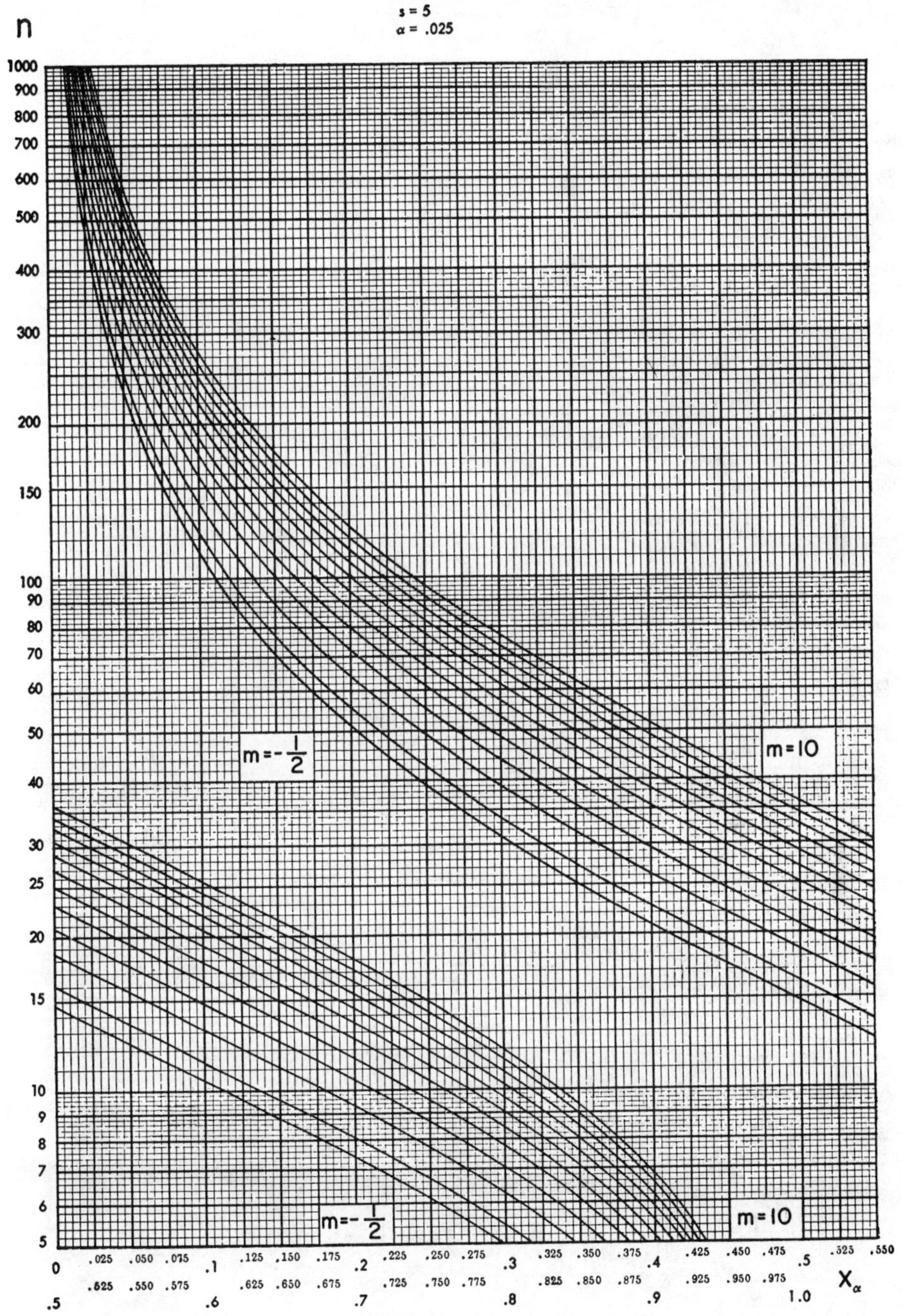
n
s = 5
α = .025
1000
900
800
700
600
500
400
300
200
150
100
90
80
70
60
50
40
30
25
20
15
10
9
8
7
6
5
m = -1/2
m = 10
m = -1/2
m = 10
0 .025 .050 .075 .1 .125 .150 .175 .2 .225 .250 .275 .3 .325 .350 .375 .4 .425 .450 .475 .5 .525 .550
.5 .525 .550 .575 .6 .625 .650 .675 .7 .725 .750 .775 .8 .825 .850 .875 .9 .925 .950 .975 1.0
X_α

CHART XII

$s = 5$
$\alpha = .05$

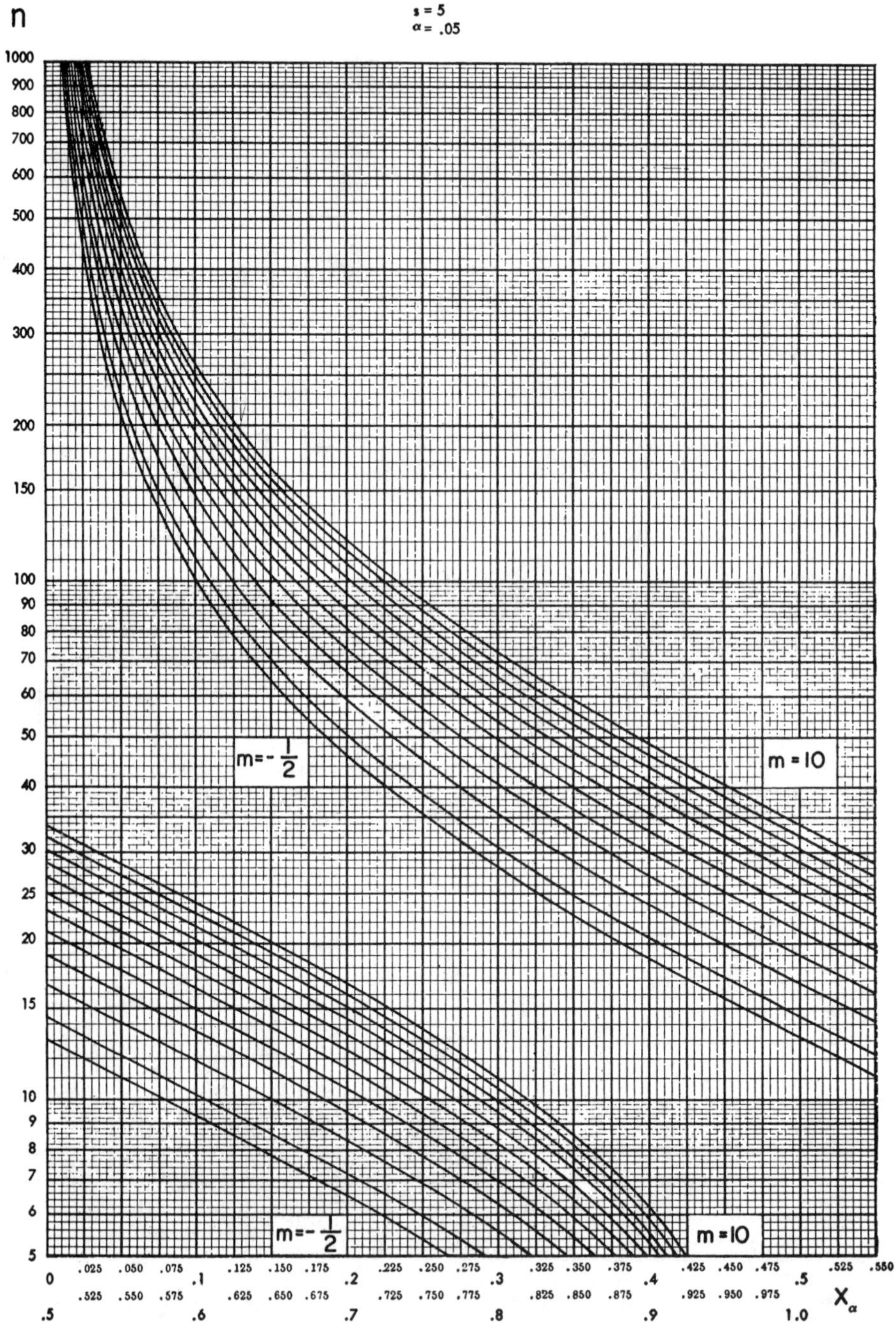

III. BINOMIAL, POISSON, HYPERGEOMETRIC, AND NEGATIVE BINOMIAL DISTRIBUTIONS

III.1 CUMULATIVE TERMS, BINOMIAL DISTRIBUTION FUNCTION

$$B(x;n,p) = \sum_{k=0}^{x} \binom{n}{k} p^k(1 - p)^{n-k}$$

		p									
n	***x***	**0.05**	**0.10**	**0.15**	**0.20**	**0.25**	**0.30**	**0.35**	**0.40**	**0.45**	**0.50**
2	0	0.9025	0.8100	0.7225	0.6400	0.5625	0.4900	0.4225	0.3600	0.3025	0.2500
	1	0.9975	0.9900	0.9775	0.9600	0.9375	0.9100	0.8755	0.8400	0.7975	0.7500
3	0	0.8574	0.7290	0.6141	0.5120	0.4219	0.3430	0.2746	0.2160	0.1664	0.1250
	1	0.9928	0.9720	0.9392	0.8960	0.8438	0.7840	0.7182	0.6480	0.5748	0.5000
	2	0.9999	0.9990	0.9966	0.9920	0.9844	0.9730	0.9571	0.9360	0.9089	0.8750
4	0	0.8145	0.6561	0.5220	0.4096	0.3164	0.2401	0.1785	0.1296	0.0915	0.0625
	1	0.9860	0.9477	0.8905	0.8192	0.7383	0.6517	0.5630	0.4752	0.3910	0.3125
	2	0.9995	0.9963	0.9880	0.9728	0.9492	0.9163	0.8735	0.8208	0.7585	0.6875
	3	1.0000	0.9999	0.9995	0.9984	0.9961	0.9919	0.9850	0.9744	0.9590	0.9375
5	0	0.7738	0.5905	0.4437	0.3277	0.2373	0.1681	0.1160	0.0778	0.0503	0.0312
	1	0.9774	0.9185	0.8352	0.7373	0.6328	0.5282	0.4284	0.3370	0.2562	0.1875
	2	0.9988	0.9914	0.9734	0.9421	0.8965	0.8369	0.7648	0.6826	0.5931	0.5000
	3	1.0000	0.9995	0.9978	0.9933	0.9844	0.9692	0.9460	0.9130	0.8688	0.8125
	4	1.0000	1.0000	0.9999	0.9997	0.9990	0.9976	0.9947	0.9898	0.9815	0.9688
6	0	0.7351	0.5314	0.3771	0.2621	0.1780	0.1176	0.0754	0.0467	0.0277	0.0156
	1	0.9672	0.8857	0.7765	0.6554	0.5339	0.4202	0.3191	0.2333	0.1636	0.1094
	2	0.9978	0.9842	0.9527	0.9011	0.8306	0.7443	0.6471	0.5443	0.4415	0.3438
	3	0.9999	0.9987	0.9941	0.9830	0.9624	0.9295	0.8826	0.8208	0.7447	0.6562
	4	1.0000	0.9999	0.9996	0.9984	0.9954	0.9891	0.9777	0.9590	0.9308	0.8906
	5	1.0000	1.0000	1.0000	0.9999	0.9998	0.9993	0.9982	0.9959	0.9917	0.9844
7	0	0.6983	0.4783	0.3206	0.2097	0.1335	0.0824	0.0490	0.0280	0.0152	0.0078
	1	0.9556	0.8503	0.7166	0.5767	0.4449	0.3294	0.2338	0.1586	0.1024	0.0625
	2	0.9962	0.9743	0.9262	0.8520	0.7564	0.6471	0.5323	0.4199	0.3164	0.2266
	3	0.9998	0.9973	0.9879	0.9667	0.9294	0.8740	0.8002	0.7102	0.6083	0.5000
	4	1.0000	0.9998	0.9988	0.9953	0.9871	0.9712	0.9444	0.9037	0.8471	0.7734
	5	1.0000	1.0000	0.9999	0.9996	0.9987	0.9962	0.9910	0.9812	0.9643	0.9375
	6	1.0000	1.0000	1.0000	1.0000	0.9999	0.9998	0.9994	0.9984	0.9963	0.9922
8	0	0.6634	0.4305	0.2725	0.1678	0.1001	0.0576	0.0319	0.0168	0.0084	0.0039
	1	0.9428	0.8131	0.6572	0.5033	0.3671	0.2553	0.1691	0.1064	0.0632	0.0352
	2	0.9942	0.9619	0.8948	0.7969	0.6785	0.5518	0.4278	0.3154	0.2201	0.1445
	3	0.9996	0.9950	0.9786	0.9437	0.8862	0.8059	0.7064	0.5941	0.4770	0.3633
	4	1.0000	0.9996	0.9971	0.9896	0.9727	0.9420	0.8939	0.8263	0.7396	0.6367
	5	1.0000	1.0000	0.9998	0.9988	0.9958	0.9887	0.9747	0.9502	0.9115	0.8555
	6	1.0000	1.0000	1.0000	0.9999	0.9996	0.9987	0.9964	0.9915	0.9819	0.9648
	7	1.0000	1.0000	1.0000	1.0000	1.0000	0.9999	0.9998	0.9993	0.9983	0.9961
9	0	0.6302	0.3874	0.2316	0.1342	0.0751	0.0404	0.0207	0.0101	0.0046	0.0020
	1	0.9288	0.7748	0.5995	0.4362	0.3003	0.1960	0.1211	0.0705	0.0385	0.0195
	2	0.9916	0.9470	0.8591	0.7382	0.6007	0.4628	0.3373	0.2318	0.1495	0.0898
	3	0.9994	0.9917	0.9661	0.9144	0.8343	0.7297	0.6089	0.4826	0.3614	0.2539
	4	1.0000	0.9991	0.9944	0.9804	0.9511	0.9012	0.8283	0.7334	0.6214	0.5000
	5	1.0000	0.9999	0.9994	0.9969	0.9900	0.9747	0.9464	0.9006	0.8342	0.7461
	6	1.0000	1.0000	1.0000	0.9997	0.9987	0.9957	0.9888	0.9750	0.9502	0.9102
	7	1.0000	1.0000	1.0000	1.0000	0.9999	0.9996	0.9986	0.9962	0.9909	0.9805
	8	1.0000	1.0000	1.0000	1.0000	1.0000	1.0000	0.9999	0.9997	0.9992	0.9980

III.1 CUMULATIVE TERMS, BINOMIAL DISTRIBUTION FUNCTION (continued)

		p									
n	*x*	0.05	0.10	0.15	0.20	0.25	0.30	0.35	0.40	0.45	0.50
10	0	0.5987	0.3487	0.1969	0.1074	0.0563	0.0282	0.0135	0.0060	0.0025	0.0010
	1	0.9139	0.7361	0.5443	0.3758	0.2440	0.1493	0.0860	0.0464	0.0232	0.0107
	2	0.9885	0.9298	0.8202	0.6778	0.5256	0.3828	0.2616	0.1673	0.0996	0.0547
	3	0.9990	0.9872	0.9500	0.8791	0.7759	0.6496	0.5138	0.3823	0.2660	0.1719
	4	0.9999	0.9984	0.9901	0.9672	0.9219	0.8497	0.7515	0.6331	0.5044	0.3770
	5	1.0000	0.9999	0.9986	0.9936	0.9803	0.9527	0.9051	0.8338	0.7384	0.6230
	6	1.0000	1.0000	0.9999	0.9991	0.9965	0.9894	0.9740	0.9452	0.8980	0.8281
	7	1.0000	1.0000	1.0000	0.9999	0.9996	0.9984	0.9952	0.9877	0.9726	0.9453
	8	1.0000	1.0000	1.0000	1.0000	1.0000	0.9999	0.9995	0.9983	0.9955	0.9893
	9	1.0000	1.0000	1.0000	1.0000	1.0000	1.0000	1.0000	0.9999	0.9997	0.9990
11	0	0.5688	0.3138	0.1673	0.0859	0.0422	0.0198	0.0088	0.0036	0.0014	0.0005
	1	0.8981	0.6974	0.4922	0.3221	0.1971	0.1130	0.0606	0.0302	0.0139	0.0059
	2	0.9848	0.9104	0.7788	0.6174	0.4552	0.3127	0.2001	0.1189	0.0652	0.0327
	3	0.9984	0.9815	0.9306	0.8389	0.7133	0.5696	0.4256	0.2963	0.1911	0.1133
	4	0.9999	0.9972	0.9841	0.9496	0.8854	0.7897	0.6683	0.5328	0.3971	0.2744
	5	1.0000	0.9997	0.9973	0.9883	0.9657	0.9218	0.8513	0.7535	0.6331	0.5000
	6	1.0000	1.0000	0.9997	0.9980	0.9924	0.9784	0.9499	0.9006	0.8262	0.7256
	7	1.0000	1.0000	1.0000	0.9998	0.9988	0.9957	0.9878	0.9707	0.9390	0.8867
	8	1.0000	1.0000	1.0000	1.0000	0.9999	0.9994	0.9980	0.9941	0.9852	0.9673
	9	1.0000	1.0000	1.0000	1.0000	1.0000	1.0000	0.9998	0.9993	0.9978	0.9941
	10	1.0000	1.0000	1.0000	1.0000	1.0000	1.0000	1.0000	1.0000	0.9998	0.9995
12	0	0.5404	0.2824	0.1422	0.0687	0.0317	0.0138	0.0057	0.0022	0.0008	0.0002
	1	0.8816	0.6590	0.4435	0.2749	0.1584	0.0850	0.0424	0.0196	0.0083	0.0032
	2	0.9804	0.8891	0.7358	0.5583	0.3907	0.2528	0.1513	0.0834	0.0421	0.0193
	3	0.9978	0.9744	0.9078	0.7946	0.6488	0.4925	0.3467	0.2253	0.1345	0.0730
	4	0.9998	0.9957	0.9761	0.9274	0.8424	0.7237	0.5833	0.4382	0.3044	0.1938
	5	1.0000	0.9995	0.9954	0.9806	0.9456	0.8822	0.7873	0.6652	0.5269	0.3872
	6	1.0000	0.9999	0.9993	0.9961	0.9857	0.9614	0.9154	0.8418	0.7393	0.6128
	7	1.0000	1.0000	0.9999	0.9994	0.9972	0.9905	0.9745	0.9427	0.8883	0.8062
	8	1.0000	1.0000	1.0000	0.9999	0.9996	0.9983	0.9944	0.9847	0.9644	0.9270
	9	1.0000	1.0000	1.0000	1.0000	1.0000	0.9998	0.9992	0.9972	0.9921	0.9807
	10	1.0000	1.0000	1.0000	1.0000	1.0000	1.0000	0.9999	0.9997	0.9989	0.9968
	11	1.0000	1.0000	1.0000	1.0000	1.0000	1.0000	1.0000	1.0000	0.9999	0.9998
13	0	0.5133	0.2542	0.1209	0.0550	0.0238	0.0097	0.0037	0.0013	0.0004	0.0001
	1	0.8646	0.6213	0.3983	0.2336	0.1267	0.0637	0.0296	0.0126	0.0049	0.0017
	2	0.9755	0.8661	0.6920	0.5017	0.3326	0.2025	0.1132	0.0579	0.0269	0.0112
	3	0.9969	0.9658	0.8820	0.7437	0.5843	0.4206	0.2783	0.1686	0.0929	0.0461
	4	0.9997	0.9935	0.9658	0.9009	0.7940	0.6543	0.5005	0.3530	0.2279	0.1334
	5	1.0000	0.9991	0.9925	0.9700	0.9198	0.8346	0.7159	0.5744	0.4268	0.2905
	6	1.0000	0.9999	0.9987	0.9930	0.9757	0.9376	0.8705	0.7712	0.6437	0.5000
	7	1.0000	1.0000	0.9998	0.9988	0.9944	0.9818	0.9538	0.9023	0.8212	0.7095
	8	1.0000	1.0000	1.0000	0.9998	0.9990	0.9960	0.9874	0.9679	0.9302	0.8666
	9	1.0000	1.0000	1.0000	1.0000	0.9999	0.9993	0.9975	0.9922	0.9797	0.9539
	10	1.0000	1.0000	1.0000	1.0000	1.0000	0.9999	0.9997	0.9987	0.9959	0.9888
	11	1.0000	1.0000	1.0000	1.0000	1.0000	1.0000	1.0000	0.9999	0.9995	0.9983
	12	1.0000	1.0000	1.0000	1.0000	1.0000	1.0000	1.0000	1.0000	1.0000	0.9999

III.1 CUMULATIVE TERMS, BINOMIAL DISTRIBUTION FUNCTION (continued)

		p									
n	*x*	**0.05**	**0.10**	**0.15**	**0.20**	**0.25**	**0.30**	**0.35**	**0.40**	**0.45**	**0.50**
14	0	0.4877	0.2288	0.1028	0.0440	0.0178	0.0068	0.0024	0.0008	0.0002	0.0001
	1	0.8470	0.5846	0.3567	0.1979	0.1010	0.0475	0.0205	0.0081	0.0029	0.0009
	2	0.9699	0.8416	0.6479	0.4481	0.2811	0.1608	0.0839	0.0398	0.0170	0.0065
	3	0.9958	0.9559	0.8535	0.6982	0.5213	0.3552	0.2205	0.1243	0.0632	0.0287
	4	0.9996	0.9908	0.9533	0.8702	0.7415	0.5842	0.4227	0.2793	0.1672	0.0898
	5	1.0000	0.9985	0.9885	0.9561	0.8883	0.7805	0.6405	0.4859	0.3373	0.2120
	6	1.0000	0.9998	0.9978	0.9884	0.9617	0.9067	0.8164	0.6925	0.5461	0.3953
	7	1.0000	1.0000	0.9997	0.9976	0.9897	0.9685	0.9247	0.8499	0.7414	0.6074
	8	1.0000	1.0000	1.0000	0.9996	0.9978	0.9917	0.9757	0.9417	0.8811	0.7880
	9	1.0000	1.0000	1.0000	1.0000	0.9997	0.9983	0.9940	0.9825	0.9574	0.9102
	10	1.0000	1.0000	1.0000	1.0000	1.0000	0.9989	0.9989	0.9961	0.9886	0.9713
	11	1.0000	1.0000	1.0000	1.0000	1.0000	1.0000	0.9999	0.9994	0.9978	0.9935
	12	1.0000	1.0000	1.0000	1.0000	1.0000	1.0000	1.0000	0.9999	0.9997	0.9991
	13	1.0000	1.0000	1.0000	1.0000	1.0000	1.0000	1.0000	1.0000	1.0000	0.9999
15	0	0.4633	0.2059	0.0874	0.0352	0.0134	0.0047	0.0016	0.0005	0.0001	0.0000
	1	0.8290	0.5490	0.3186	0.1671	0.0802	0.0353	0.0142	0.0052	0.0017	0.0005
	2	0.9638	0.8159	0.6042	0.3980	0.2361	0.1268	0.0617	0.0271	0.0107	0.0037
	3	0.9945	0.9444	0.8227	0.6482	0.4613	0.2969	0.1727	0.0905	0.0424	0.0176
	4	0.9994	0.9873	0.9383	0.8358	0.6865	0.5155	0.3519	0.2173	0.1204	0.0592
	5	0.9999	0.9978	0.9832	0.9389	0.8516	0.7216	0.5643	0.4032	0.2608	0.1509
	6	1.0000	0.9997	0.9964	0.9819	0.9434	0.8689	0.7548	0.6098	0.4522	0.3036
	7	1.0000	1.0000	0.9996	0.9958	0.9827	0.9500	0.8868	0.7869	0.6535	0.5000
	8	1.0000	1.0000	0.9999	0.9992	0.9958	0.9848	0.9578	0.9050	0.8182	0.6964
	9	1.0000	1.0000	1.0000	0.9999	0.9992	0.9963	0.9876	0.9662	0.9231	0.8491
	10	1.0000	1.0000	1.0000	1.0000	0.9999	0.9993	0.9972	0.9907	0.9745	0.9408
	11	1.0000	1.0000	1.0000	1.0000	1.0000	0.9999	0.9995	0.9981	0.9937	0.9824
	12	1.0000	1.0000	1.0000	1.0000	1.0000	1.0000	0.9999	0.9997	0.9989	0.9963
	13	1.0000	1.0000	1.0000	1.0000	1.0000	1.0000	1.0000	1.0000	0.9999	0.9995
	14	1.0000	1.0000	1.0000	1.0000	1.0000	1.0000	1.0000	1.0000	1.0000	1.0000
16	0	0.4401	0.1853	0.0743	0.0281	0.0100	0.0033	0.0010	0.0003	0.0001	0.0000
	1	0.8108	0.5147	0.2839	0.1407	0.0635	0.0261	0.0098	0.0033	0.0010	0.0003
	2	0.9571	0.7892	0.5614	0.3518	0.1971	0.0994	0.0451	0.0183	0.0066	0.0021
	3	0.9930	0.9316	0.7899	0.5981	0.4050	0.2459	0.1339	0.0651	0.0281	0.0106
	4	0.9991	0.9830	0.9209	0.7982	0.6302	0.4499	0.2892	0.1666	0.0853	0.0384
	5	0.9999	0.9967	0.9765	0.9183	0.8103	0.6598	0.4900	0.3288	0.1976	0.1051
	6	1.0000	0.9995	0.9944	0.9733	0.9204	0.8247	0.6881	0.5272	0.3660	0.2272
	7	1.0000	0.9999	0.9989	0.9930	0.9729	0.9256	0.8406	0.7161	0.5629	0.4018
	8	1.0000	1.0000	0.9998	0.9985	0.9925	0.9743	0.9329	0.8577	0.7441	0.5982
	9	1.0000	1.0000	1.0000	0.9998	0.9984	0.9929	0.9771	0.9417	0.8759	0.7728
	10	1.0000	1.0000	1.0000	1.0000	0.9997	0.9984	0.9938	0.9809	0.9514	0.8949
	11	1.0000	1.0000	1.0000	1.0000	1.0000	0.9997	0.9987	0.9951	0.9851	0.9616
	12	1.0000	1.0000	1.0000	1.0000	1.0000	1.0000	0.9998	0.9991	0.9965	0.9894
	13	1.0000	1.0000	1.0000	1.0000	1.0000	1.0000	1.0000	0.9999	0.9994	0.9979
	14	1.0000	1.0000	1.0000	1.0000	1.0000	1.0000	1.0000	1.0000	1.0000	0.9997
	15	1.0000	1.0000	1.0000	1.0000	1.0000	1.0000	1.0000	1.0000	1.0000	1.0000

III.1 CUMULATIVE TERMS, BINOMIAL DISTRIBUTION FUNCTION (continued)

		p									
n	*x*	0.05	0.10	0.15	0.20	0.25	0.30	0.35	0.40	0.45	0.50
17	0	0.4181	0.1668	0.0631	0.0225	0.0075	0.0023	0.0007	0.0002	0.0000	0.0000
	1	0.7922	0.4818	0.2525	0.1182	0.0501	0.0193	0.0067	0.0021	0.0006	0.0001
	2	0.9497	0.7618	0.5198	0.3096	0.1637	0.0774	0.0327	0.0123	0.0041	0.0012
	3	0.9912	0.9174	0.7556	0.5489	0.3530	0.2019	0.1028	0.0464	0.0184	0.0063
	4	0.9988	0.9779	0.9013	0.7582	0.5739	0.3887	0.2348	0.1260	0.0596	0.0245
	5	0.9999	0.9953	0.9681	0.8943	0.7653	0.5968	0.4197	0.2639	0.1471	0.0717
	6	1.0000	0.9992	0.9917	0.9623	0.8929	0.7752	0.6188	0.4478	0.2902	0.1662
	7	1.0000	0.9999	0.9983	0.9891	0.9598	0.8954	0.7872	0.6405	0.4743	0.3145
	8	1.0000	1.0000	0.9997	0.9974	0.9876	0.9597	0.9006	0.8011	0.6626	0.5000
	9	1.0000	1.0000	1.0000	0.9995	0.9969	0.9873	0.9617	0.9081	0.8166	0.6855
	10	1.0000	1.0000	1.0000	0.9999	0.9994	0.9968	0.9880	0.9652	0.9174	0.8338
	11	1.0000	1.0000	1.0000	1.0000	0.9999	0.9993	0.9970	0.9894	0.9699	0.9283
	12	1.0000	1.0000	1.0000	1.0000	1.0000	0.9999	0.9994	0.9975	0.9914	0.9755
	13	1.0000	1.0000	1.0000	1.0000	1.0000	1.0000	0.9999	0.9995	0.9981	0.9936
	14	1.0000	1.0000	1.0000	1.0000	1.0000	1.0000	1.0000	0.9999	0.9997	0.9988
	15	1.0000	1.0000	1.0000	1.0000	1.0000	1.0000	1.0000	1.0000	1.0000	0.9999
	16	1.0000	1.0000	1.0000	1.0000	1.0000	1.0000	1.0000	1.0000	1.0000	1.0000
18	0	0.3972	0.1501	0.0536	0.0180	0.0056	0.0016	0.0004	0.0001	0.0000	0.0000
	1	0.7735	0.4503	0.2241	0.0991	0.0395	0.0142	0.0046	0.0013	0.0003	0.0001
	2	0.9419	0.7338	0.4797	0.2713	0.1353	0.0600	0.0236	0.0082	0.0025	0.0007
	3	0.9891	0.9018	0.7202	0.5010	0.3057	0.1646	0.0783	0.0328	0.0120	0.0038
	4	0.9985	0.9718	0.8794	0.7164	0.5187	0.3327	0.1886	0.0942	0.0411	0.0154
	5	0.9998	0.9936	0.9581	0.8671	0.7175	0.5344	0.3550	0.2088	0.1077	0.0481
	6	1.0000	0.9988	0.9882	0.9487	0.8610	0.7217	0.5491	0.3743	0.2258	0.1189
	7	1.0000	0.9998	0.9973	0.9837	0.9431	0.8593	0.7283	0.5634	0.3915	0.2403
	8	1.0000	1.0000	0.9995	0.9957	0.9807	0.9404	0.8609	0.7368	0.5778	0.4073
	9	1.0000	1.0000	0.9999	0.9991	0.9946	0.9790	0.9403	0.8653	0.7473	0.5927
	10	1.0000	1.0000	1.0000	0.9998	0.9988	0.9939	0.9788	0.9424	0.8720	0.7597
	11	1.0000	1.0000	1.0000	1.0000	0.9998	0.9986	0.9938	0.9797	0.9463	0.8811
	12	1.0000	1.0000	1.0000	1.0000	1.0000	0.9997	0.9986	0.9942	0.9817	0.9519
	13	1.0000	1.0000	1.0000	1.0000	1.0000	1.0000	0.9997	0.9987	0.9951	0.9846
	14	1.0000	1.0000	1.0000	1.0000	1.0000	1.0000	1.0000	0.9998	0.9990	0.9962
	15	1.0000	1.0000	1.0000	1.0000	1.0000	1.0000	1.0000	1.0000	0.9999	0.9993
	16	1.0000	1.0000	1.0000	1.0000	1.0000	1.0000	1.0000	1.0000	1.0000	0.9999
19	0	0.3774	0.1351	0.0456	0.0144	0.0042	0.0011	0.0003	0.0001	0.0000	0.0000
	1	0.7547	0.4203	0.1985	0.0829	0.0310	0.0104	0.0031	0.0008	0.0002	0.0000
	2	0.9335	0.7054	0.4413	0.2369	0.1113	0.0462	0.0170	0.0055	0.0015	0.0004
	3	0.9868	0.8850	0.6841	0.4551	0.2630	0.1332	0.0591	0.0230	0.0077	0.0022
	4	0.9980	0.9648	0.8556	0.6733	0.4654	0.2822	0.1500	0.0696	0.0280	0.0096
	5	0.9998	0.9914	0.9463	0.8369	0.6678	0.4739	0.2968	0.1629	0.0777	0.0318
	6	1.0000	0.9983	0.9837	0.9324	0.8251	0.6655	0.4812	0.3081	0.1727	0.0835
	7	1.0000	0.9997	0.9959	0.9767	0.9225	0.8180	0.6656	0.4878	0.3169	0.1796
	8	1.0000	1.0000	0.9992	0.9933	0.9713	0.9161	0.8145	0.6675	0.4940	0.3238
	9	1.0000	1.0000	0.9999	0.9984	0.9911	0.9674	0.9125	0.8139	0.6710	0.5000
	10	1.0000	1.0000	1.0000	0.9997	0.9977	0.9895	0.9653	0.9115	0.8159	0.6762
	11	1.0000	1.0000	1.0000	1.0000	0.9995	0.9972	0.9886	0.9648	0.9129	0.8204
	12	1.0000	1.0000	1.0000	1.0000	0.9999	0.9994	0.9969	0.9884	0.9658	0.9165
	13	1.0000	1.0000	1.0000	1.0000	1.0000	0.9999	0.9993	0.9969	0.9891	0.9682
	14	1.0000	1.0000	1.0000	1.0000	1.0000	1.0000	0.9999	0.9994	0.9972	0.9904
	15	1.0000	1.0000	1.0000	1.0000	1.0000	1.0000	1.0000	0.9999	0.9995	0.9978
	16	1.0000	1.0000	1.0000	1.0000	1.0000	1.0000	1.0000	1.0000	0.9999	0.9996
	17	1.0000	1.0000	1.0000	1.0000	1.0000	1.0000	1.0000	1.0000	1.0000	1.0000

III.1 CUMULATIVE TERMS, BINOMIAL DISTRIBUTION FUNCTION (continued)

		p									
n	*x*	**0.05**	**0.10**	**0.15**	**0.20**	**0.25**	**0.30**	**0.35**	**0.40**	**0.45**	**0.50**
20	0	0.3585	0.1216	0.0388	0.0115	0.0032	0.0008	0.0002	0.0000	0.0000	0.0000
	1	0.7358	0.3917	0.1756	0.0692	0.0243	0.0076	0.0021	0.0005	0.0001	0.0000
	2	0.9245	0.6769	0.4049	0.2061	0.0913	0.0355	0.0121	0.0036	0.0009	0.0002
	3	0.9841	0.8670	0.6477	0.4114	0.2252	0.1071	0.0444	0.0160	0.0049	0.0013
	4	0.9974	0.9568	0.8298	0.6296	0.4148	0.2375	0.1182	0.0510	0.0189	0.0059
	5	0.9997	0.9987	0.9327	0.8042	0.6172	0.4164	0.2454	0.1256	0.0553	0.0207
	6	1.0000	0.9976	0.9781	0.9133	0.7858	0.6080	0.4166	0.2500	0.1299	0.0577
	7	1.0000	0.9996	0.9941	0.9679	0.8982	0.7723	0.6010	0.4159	0.2520	0.1316
	8	1.0000	0.9999	0.9987	0.9900	0.9591	0.8867	0.7624	0.5956	0.4143	0.2517
	9	1.0000	1.0000	0.9998	0.9974	0.9861	0.9520	0.8782	0.7553	0.5914	0.4119
	10	1.0000	1.0000	1.0000	0.9994	0.9961	0.9829	0.9468	0.8725	0.7507	0.5881
	11	1.0000	1.0000	1.0000	0.9999	0.9991	0.9949	0.9804	0.9435	0.8692	0.7483
	12	1.0000	1.0000	1.0000	1.0000	0.9998	0.9987	0.9940	0.9790	0.9420	0.8684
	13	1.0000	1.0000	1.0000	1.0000	1.0000	0.9997	0.9985	0.9935	0.9786	0.9423
	14	1.0000	1.0000	1.0000	1.0000	1.0000	1.0000	0.9997	0.9984	0.9936	0.9793
	15	1.0000	1.0000	1.0000	1.0000	1.0000	1.0000	1.0000	0.9997	0.9985	0.9941
	16	1.0000	1.0000	1.0000	1.0000	1.0000	1.0000	1.0000	1.0000	0.9997	0.9987
	17	1.0000	1.0000	1.0000	1.0000	1.0000	1.0000	1.0000	1.0000	1.0000	0.9998
	18	1.0000	1.0000	1.0000	1.0000	1.0000	1.0000	1.0000	1.0000	1.0000	1.0000

III.2. CUMULATIVE TERMS, POISSON DISTRIBUTION FUNCTION

$$F(x{:}\lambda) = \sum_{k=0}^{x} e^{-\lambda} \frac{\lambda^k}{k!}$$

λ \ x	0	1	2	3	4	5	6	7	8	9
0.02	0.980	1.000								
0.04	0.961	0.999	1.000							
0.06	0.942	0.998	1.000							
0.08	0.923	0.997	1.000							
0.10	0.905	0.995	1.000							
0.15	0.861	0.990	0.999	1.000						
0.20	0.819	0.982	0.999	1.000						
0.25	0.779	0.974	0.998	1.000						
0.30	0.741	0.963	0.996	1.000						
0.35	0.705	0.951	0.994	1.000						
0.40	0.670	0.938	0.992	0.999	1.000					
0.45	0.638	0.925	0.989	0.999	1.000					
0.50	0.607	0.910	0.986	0.998	1.000					
0.55	0.577	0.894	0.982	0.998	1.000					
0.60	0.549	0.878	0.997	0.977	1.000					
0.65	0.522	0.861	0.972	0.996	0.999	1.000				
0.70	0.497	0.844	0.966	0.994	0.999	1.000				
0.75	0.472	0.827	0.959	0.993	0.999	1.000				
0.80	0.449	0.809	0.953	0.991	0.999	1.000				
0.85	0.427	0.791	0.945	0.989	0.998	1.000				
0.90	0.407	0.772	0.937	0.987	0.998	1.000				
0.95	0.387	0.754	0.929	0.984	0.997	1.000				
1.00	0.368	0.736	0.920	0.981	0.996	0.999	1.000			
1.1	0.333	0.699	0.900	0.974	0.995	0.999	1.000			
1.2	0.301	0.663	0.879	0.966	0.992	0.998	1.000			
1.3	0.273	0.627	0.857	0.957	0.989	0.998	1.000			
1.4	0.247	0.592	0.833	0.946	0.986	0.997	0.999	1.000		
1.5	0.223	0.558	0.809	0.934	0.981	0.996	0.999	1.000		
1.6	0.202	0.525	0.783	0.921	0.976	0.994	0.999	1.000		
1.7	0.183	0.493	0.757	0.907	0.970	0.992	0.998	1.000		
1.8	0.165	0.463	0.731	0.891	0.964	0.990	0.997	0.999	1.000	
1.9	0.150	0.434	0.704	0.875	0.956	0.987	0.997	0.999	1.000	
2.0	0.135	0.406	0.677	0.857	0.947	0.983	0.995	0.999	1.000	
2.2	0.111	0.355	0.623	0.819	0.928	0.975	0.993	0.998	1.000	
2.4	0.091	0.308	0.570	0.779	0.904	0.964	0.988	0.997	0.999	1.000
2.6	0.074	0.267	0.518	0.736	0.877	0.951	0.983	0.995	0.999	1.000
2.8	0.061	0.231	0.469	0.692	0.848	0.935	0.976	0.992	0.998	0.999
3.0	0.050	0.199	0.423	0.647	0.815	0.916	0.966	0.988	0.996	0.999
3.2	0.041	0.171	0.380	0.603	0.781	0.895	0.955	0.983	0.994	0.998
3.4	0.033	0.147	0.340	0.558	0.744	0.871	0.942	0.977	0.992	0.997
3.6	0.027	0.126	0.303	0.515	0.706	0.844	0.927	0.969	0.988	0.996
3.8	0.022	0.107	0.269	0.473	0.668	0.816	0.909	0.960	0.984	0.994
4.0	0.018	0.092	0.238	0.433	0.629	0.785	0.889	0.949	0.979	0.992

III.2. CUMULATIVE TERMS, POISSON DISTRIBUTION FUNCTION (continued)

λ \ x	0	1	2	3	4	5	6	7	8	9
4.2	0.015	0.078	0.210	0.395	0.590	0.753	0.867	0.936	0.972	0.989
4.4	0.012	0.066	0.185	0.359	0.551	0.720	0.844	0.921	0.964	0.985
4.6	0.010	0.056	0.163	0.326	0.513	0.686	0.818	0.905	0.955	0.980
4.8	0.008	0.048	0.143	0.294	0.476	0.651	0.791	0.887	0.944	0.975
5.0	0.007	0.040	0.125	0.265	0.440	0.616	0.762	0.867	0.932	0.968
5.2	0.006	0.034	0.109	0.238	0.406	0.581	0.732	0.845	0.918	0.960
5.4	0.005	0.029	0.095	0.213	0.373	0.546	0.702	0.822	0.903	0.951
5.6	0.004	0.024	0.082	0.191	0.342	0.512	0.670	0.797	0.886	0.941
5.8	0.003	0.021	0.072	0.170	0.313	0.478	0.638	0.771	0.867	0.929
6.0	0.002	0.017	0.062	0.151	0.285	0.446	0.606	0.744	0.847	0.916

	10	11	12	13	14	15	16
2.8	1.000						
3.0	1.000						
3.2	1.000						
3.4	0.999	1.000					
3.6	0.999	1.000					
3.8	0.998	0.999	1.000				
4.0	0.997	0.999	1.000				
4.2	0.996	0.999	1.000				
4.4	0.994	0.998	0.999	1.000			
4.6	0.992	0.997	0.999	1.000			
4.8	0.990	0.996	0.999	1.000			
5.0	0.986	0.995	0.998	0.999	1.000		
5.2	0.982	0.993	0.997	0.999	1.000		
5.4	0.977	0.990	0.996	0.999	1.000		
5.6	0.972	0.988	0.995	0.998	0.999	1.000	
5.8	0.965	0.984	0.993	0.997	0.999	1.000	
6.0	0.957	0.980	0.991	0.996	0.999	0.999	1.000

λ \ x	0	1	2	3	4	5	6	7	8	9
6.2	0.002	0.015	0.054	0.134	0.259	0.414	0.574	0.716	0.826	0.902
6.4	0.002	0.012	0.046	0.119	0.235	0.384	0.542	0.687	0.803	0.886
6.6	0.001	0.010	0.040	0.105	0.213	0.355	0.511	0.658	0.780	0.869
6.8	0.001	0.009	0.034	0.093	0.192	0.327	0.480	0.628	0.755	0.850
7.0	0.001	0.007	0.030	0.082	0.173	0.301	0.450	0.599	0.729	0.830
7.2	0.001	0.006	0.025	0.072	0.156	0.276	0.420	0.569	0.703	0.810
7.4	0.001	0.005	0.022	0.063	0.140	0.253	0.392	0.539	0.676	0.788
7.6	0.001	0.004	0.019	0.055	0.125	0.231	0.365	0.510	0.648	0.765
7.8	0.000	0.004	0.016	0.048	0.112	0.210	0.338	0.481	0.620	0.741
8.0	0.000	0.003	0.014	0.042	0.100	0.191	0.313	0.453	0.593	0.717

III.2. CUMULATIVE TERMS, POISSON DISTRIBUTION FUNCTION (continued)

λ x	0	1	2	3	4	5	6	7	8	9
8.5	0.000	0.002	0.009	0.030	0.074	0.150	0.256	0.386	0.523	0.653
9.0	0.000	0.001	0.006	0.021	0.055	0.116	0.207	0.324	0.456	0.587
9.5	0.000	0.001	0.004	0.015	0.040	0.089	0.165	0.269	0.392	0.522
10.0	0.000	0.000	0.003	0.010	0.029	0.067	0.130	0.220	0.333	0.458

	10	11	12	13	14	15	16	17	18	19
6.2	0.949	0.975	0.989	0.995	0.998	0.999	1.000			
6.4	0.939	0.969	0.986	0.994	0.997	0.999	1.000			
6.6	0.927	0.963	0.982	0.992	0.997	0.999	0.999	1.000		
6.8	0.915	0.955	0.978	0.990	0.996	0.998	0.999	1.000		
7.0	0.901	0.947	0.973	0.987	0.994	0.998	0.999	1.000		
7.2	0.887	0.937	0.967	0.984	0.993	0.997	0.999	0.999	1.000	
7.4	0.871	0.926	0.961	0.980	0.991	0.996	0.998	0.999	1.000	
7.6	0.854	0.915	0.954	0.976	0.989	0.995	0.998	0.999	1.000	
7.8	0.835	0.902	0.945	0.971	0.986	0.993	0.997	0.999	1.000	
8.0	0.816	0.888	0.936	0.966	0.983	0.992	0.996	0.998	0.999	1.000
8.5	0.763	0.849	0.909	0.949	0.973	0.986	0.993	0.997	0.999	1.999
9.0	0.706	0.803	0.876	0.926	0.959	0.978	0.989	0.995	0.998	0.999
9.5	0.645	0.752	0.836	0.898	0.940	0.967	0.982	0.991	0.996	0.998
10.0	0.583	0.697	0.792	0.864	0.917	0.951	0.973	0.986	0.993	0.997

	20	21	22
8.5	1.000		
9.0	1.000		
9.5	0.999	1.000	
10.0	0.998	0.999	1.000

λ x	0	1	2	3	4	5	6	7	8	9
10.5	0.000	0.000	0.002	0.007	0.021	0.050	0.102	0.179	0.279	0.397
11.0	0.000	0.000	0.001	0.005	0.015	0.038	0.079	0.143	0.232	0.341
11.5	0.000	0.000	0.001	0.003	0.011	0.028	0.060	0.114	0.191	0.289
12.0	0.000	0.000	0.001	0.002	0.008	0.020	0.046	0.090	0.155	0.242
12.5	0.000	0.000	0.000	0.002	0.005	0.015	0.035	0.070	0.125	0.201
13.0	0.000	0.000	0.000	0.001	0.004	0.011	0.026	0.054	0.100	0.166
13.5	0.000	0.000	0.000	0.001	0.003	0.008	0.019	0.041	0.079	0.135
14.0	0.000	0.000	0.000	0.000	0.002	0.006	0.014	0.032	0.062	0.109
14.5	0.000	0.000	0.000	0.000	0.001	0.004	0.010	0.024	0.048	0.088
15.0	0.000	0.000	0.000	0.000	0.001	0.003	0.008	0.018	0.037	0.070

III.2. CUMULATIVE TERMS, POISSON DISTRIBUTION FUNCTION (continued)

	10	11	12	13	14	15	16	17	18	19
10.5	0.521	0.639	0.742	0.825	0.888	0.932	0.960	0.978	0.988	0.994
11.0	0.460	0.579	0.689	0.781	0.854	0.907	0.944	0.968	0.982	0.991
11.5	0.402	0.520	0.633	0.733	0.815	0.878	0.924	0.954	0.974	0.986
12.0	0.347	0.462	0.576	0.682	0.772	0.844	0.899	0.937	0.963	0.979
12.5	0.297	0.406	0.519	0.628	0.725	0.806	0.869	0.916	0.948	0.969
13.0	0.252	0.353	0.463	0.573	0.675	0.764	0.835	0.890	0.930	0.957
13.5	0.211	0.304	0.409	0.518	0.623	0.718	0.798	0.861	0.908	0.942
14.0	0.176	0.260	0.358	0.464	0.570	0.669	0.756	0.827	0.883	0.923
14.5	0.145	0.220	0.311	0.413	0.518	0.619	0.711	0.790	0.853	0.901
15.0	0.118	0.185	0.268	0.363	0.466	0.568	0.664	0.749	0.819	0.875

	20	21	22	23	24	25	26	27	28	29
10.5	0.997	0.999	1.999	1.000						
11.0	0.995	0.998	0.999	1.000						
11.5	0.992	0.996	0.998	0.999	1.000					
12.0	0.988	0.994	0.997	0.999	0.999	1.000				
12.5	0.983	0.991	0.995	0.998	0.999	0.999	1.000			
13.0	0.975	0.986	0.992	0.996	0.998	0.999	1.000			
13.5	0.965	0.980	0.989	0.994	0.997	0.998	0.999	1.000		
14.0	0.952	0.971	0.983	0.991	0.995	0.997	0.999	0.999	1.000	
14.5	0.936	0.960	0.976	0.986	0.992	0.996	0.998	0.999	0.999	1.000
15.0	0.917	0.947	0.967	0.981	0.989	0.994	0.997	0.998	0.999	1.000

λ \ x	4	5	6	7	8	9	10	11	12	13
16	0.000	0.001	0.004	0.010	0.022	0.043	0.077	0.127	0.193	0.275
17	0.000	0.001	0.002	0.005	0.013	0.026	0.049	0.085	0.135	0.201
18	0.000	0.000	0.001	0.003	0.007	0.015	0.030	0.055	0.092	0.143
19	0.000	0.000	0.001	0.002	0.004	0.009	0.018	0.035	0.061	0.098
20	0.000	0.000	0.000	0.001	0.002	0.005	0.011	0.021	0.039	0.066
21	0.000	0.000	0.000	0.000	0.001	0.003	0.006	0.013	0.025	0.043
22	0.000	0.000	0.000	0.000	0.001	0.002	0.004	0.008	0.015	0.028
23	0.000	0.000	0.000	0.000	0.000	0.001	0.002	0.004	0.009	0.017
24	0.000	0.000	0.000	0.000	0.000	0.000	0.001	0.003	0.005	0.011
25	0.000	0.000	0.000	0.000	0.000	0.000	0.001	0.001	0.003	0.006

	14	15	16	17	18	19	20	21	22	23
16	0.368	0.467	0.566	0.659	0.742	0.812	0.868	0.911	0.942	0.963
17	0.281	0.371	0.468	0.564	0.655	0.736	0.805	0.861	0.905	0.937
18	0.208	0.287	0.375	0.469	0.562	0.651	0.731	0.799	0.855	0.899
19	0.150	0.215	0.292	0.378	0.469	0.561	0.647	0.725	0.793	0.849
20	0.105	0.157	0.221	0.297	0.381	0.470	0.559	0.644	0.721	0.787
21	0.072	0.111	0.163	0.227	0.302	0.384	0.471	0.558	0.640	0.716

III.2. CUMULATIVE TERMS, POISSON DISTRIBUTION FUNCTION (continued)

	14	**15**	**16**	**17**	**18**	**19**	**20**	**21**	**22**	**23**
22	0.048	0.077	0.117	0.169	0.232	0.306	0.387	0.472	0.556	0.637
23	0.031	0.052	0.082	0.123	0.175	0.238	0.310	0.389	0.472	0.555
24	0.020	0.034	0.056	0.087	0.128	0.180	0.243	0.314	0.392	0.473
25	0.012	0.022	0.038	0.060	0.092	0.134	0.185	0.247	0.318	0.394

	24	**25**	**26**	**27**	**28**	**29**	**30**	**31**	**32**	**33**
16	0.978	0.987	0.993	0.996	0.998	0.999	0.999	1.000		
17	0.959	0.975	0.985	0.991	0.995	0.997	0.999	0.999	1.000	
18	0.932	0.955	0.972	0.983	0.990	0.994	0.997	0.998	0.999	1.000
19	0.893	0.927	0.951	0.969	0.980	0.988	0.993	0.996	0.998	0.999
20	0.843	0.888	0.922	0.948	0.966	0.978	0.987	0.992	0.995	0.997
21	0.782	0.838	0.883	0.917	0.944	0.963	0.976	0.985	0.991	0.994
22	0.712	0.777	0.832	0.877	0.913	0.940	0.959	0.973	0.983	0.989
23	0.635	0.708	0.772	0.827	0.873	0.908	0.936	0.956	0.971	0.981
24	0.554	0.632	0.704	0.768	0.823	0.868	0.904	0.932	0.953	0.969
25	0.473	0.553	0.629	0.700	0.763	0.818	0.863	0.900	0.929	0.950

	34	**35**	**36**	**37**	**38**	**39**	**40**	**41**	**42**	**43**
19	0.909	1.000								
20	0.999	0.999	1.000							
21	0.997	0.998	0.999	1.999	1.000					
22	0.994	0.996	0.998	0.999	0.999	1.000				
23	0.998	0.993	0.996	0.997	0.999	0.999	1.000			
24	0.979	0.987	0.992	0.995	0.997	0.998	0.999	0.999		
25	0.966	0.978	0.985	0.991	0.994	0.997	0.998	0.999	1.000	

III.3 CONFIDENCE LIMITS FOR PROPORTIONS

The general term of the binomial expansion is given by

$$f(x;n,\theta) = \binom{n}{x}\theta^x(1-\theta)^{n-x}, \qquad x = 0, 1, 2, \ldots, n.$$

For known n, and for a given value of x', the values of the confidence limits θ_a and θ_b, $(\theta_a < \theta_b)$ are defined by

$$\sum_{x=x'}^{n} f(x;n,\theta_a) = \alpha \qquad \text{and} \qquad \sum_{x=0}^{x'} f(x;n,\theta_b) = \alpha,$$

where the cumulative sums may be evaluated conveniently from the cumulative binomial distribution tables.

The charts show confidence limits for θ for

$$1 - 2\alpha = .95, \text{ and } .99$$

or

$$\alpha = .025, \text{ and } .005$$

and for $n = 8, 10, 12, 16, 20, 24, 30, 40, 60, 100, 200, 400, 1000$.

The tables show confidence limits for θ for

$$1 - 2\alpha = .95, \text{ and } .99$$

or

$$\alpha = .025, \text{ and } .005.$$

Example: Observed relative frequency 8/30 = 0.267. The 95 per cent confidence limits for θ are 0.123 and 0.459.

Example: Observed relative frequency 8/30 = 0.267. The 99 per cent confidence limits for θ are 0.093 and 0.516.

CONFIDENCE LIMITS FOR PROPORTIONS
(CONFIDENCE COEFFICIENT 0.95)

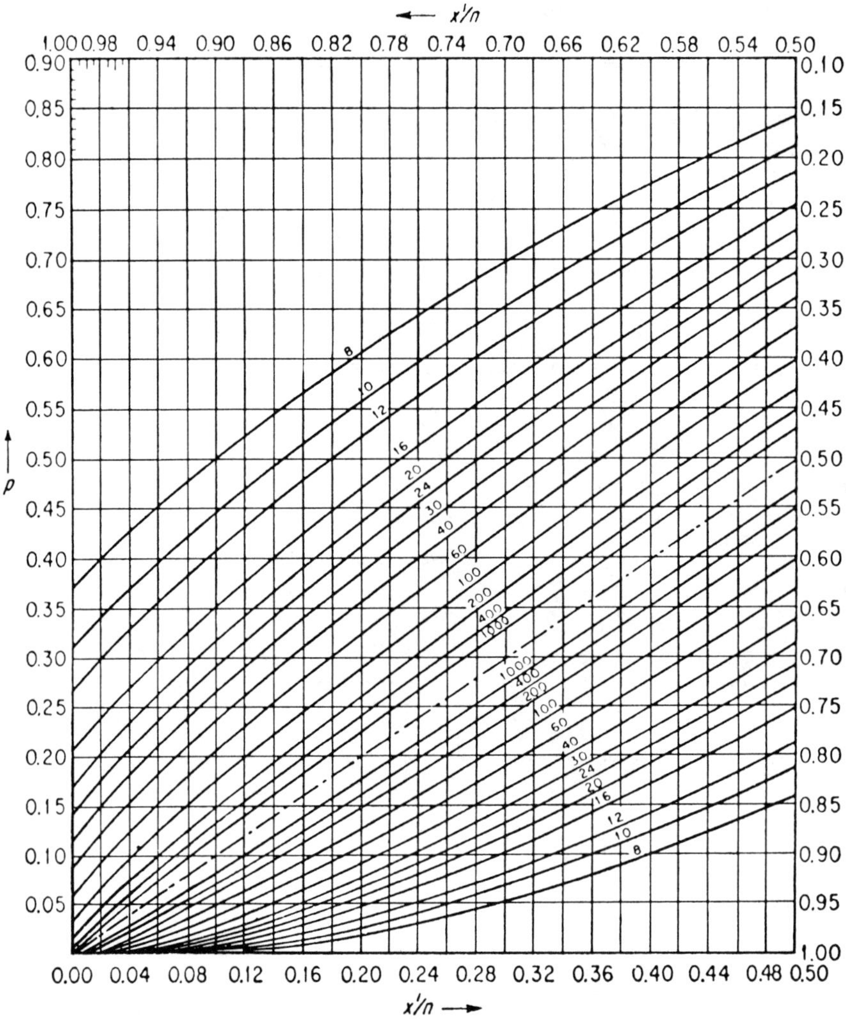

CONFIDENCE LIMITS FOR PROPORTIONS
(CONFIDENCE COEFFICIENT 0.99)

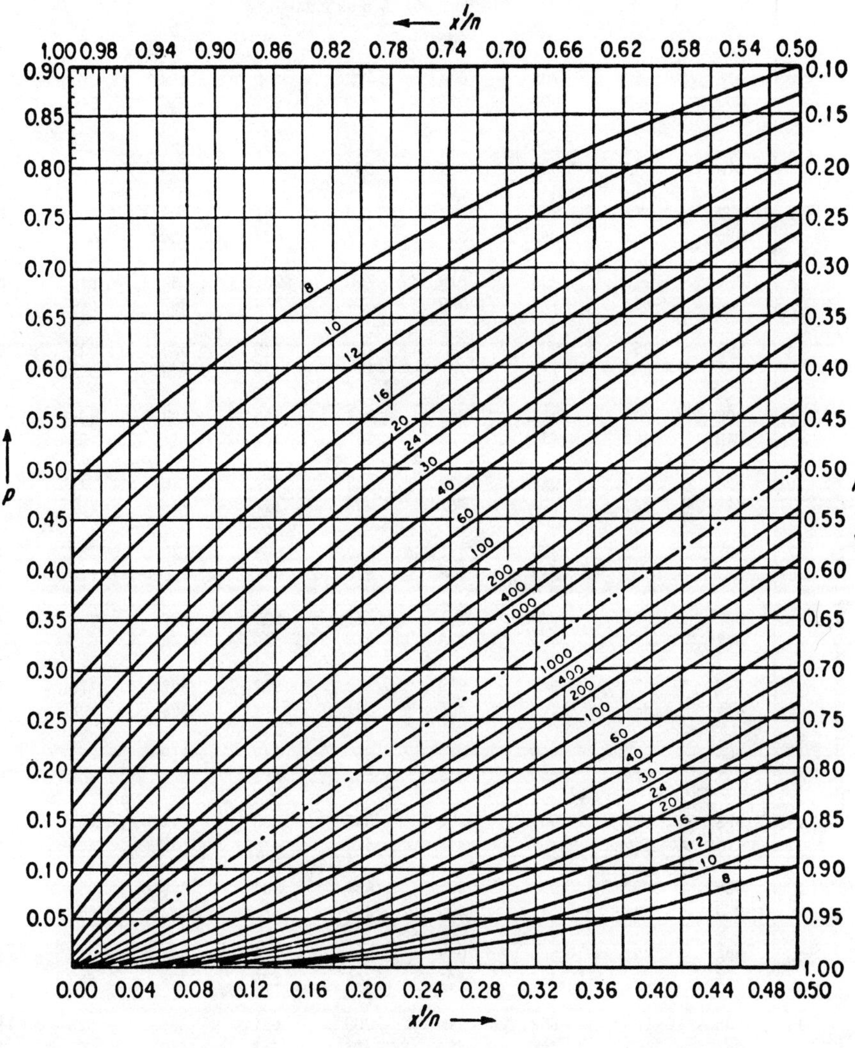

CONFIDENCE LIMITS FOR PROPORTIONS (CONFIDENCE COEFFICIENT .95)

x Denotes the Numerator and n the Denominator of the Relative Frequency

x (Numerator of the Relative Frequency) \ $n-x$ (Denominator Minus Numerator)	1	2	3	4	5	6	7	8	9
0	975	842	708	602	522	459	410	369	336
	000	*000*	*000*	*000*	*000*	*000*	*000*	*000*	*000*
1	987	906	806	716	641	579	527	483	445
	013	*008*	*006*	*005*	*004*	*004*	*003*	*003*	*003*
2	992	932	853	777	710	651	600	556	518
	094	*068*	*053*	*043*	*037*	*032*	*028*	*025*	*023*
3	994	947	882	816	755	701	652	610	572
	194	*147*	*118*	*099*	*085*	*075*	*067*	*060*	*055*
4	995	957	901	843	788	738	692	651	614
	284	*223*	*184*	*157*	*137*	*122*	*109*	*099*	*091*
5	996	963	915	863	813	766	723	684	649
	359	*290*	*245*	*212*	*187*	*167*	*151*	*139*	*128*
6	996	968	925	878	833	789	749	711	677
	421	*349*	*299*	*262*	*234*	*211*	*192*	*177*	*163*
7	997	972	933	891	849	808	770	734	701
	473	*400*	*348*	*308*	*277*	*251*	*230*	*213*	*198*
8	997	975	940	901	861	823	787	753	722
	517	*444*	*390*	*349*	*316*	*289*	*266*	*247*	*230*
9	997	977	945	909	872	837	802	770	740
	555	*482*	*428*	*386*	*351*	*323*	*299*	*278*	*260*
10	998	979	950	916	882	848	816	785	756
	587	*516*	*462*	*419*	*384*	*354*	*329*	*308*	*289*
11	998	981	953	922	890	858	827	797	769
	615	*546*	*492*	*449*	*413*	*383*	*357*	*335*	*315*
12	998	982	957	927	897	867	837	809	782
	640	*572*	*519*	*476*	*440*	*410*	*384*	*361*	*340*
13	998	983	960	932	903	874	846	819	793
	661	*595*	*544*	*501*	*465*	*435*	*408*	*384*	*364*
14	998	984	962	936	909	881	854	828	803
	681	*617*	*566*	*524*	*488*	*457*	*430*	*407*	*385*
15	998	985	964	939	913	887	861	836	812
	698	*636*	*586*	*544*	*509*	*478*	*451*	*427*	*406*
16	999	986	966	943	918	893	868	844	820
	713	*653*	*604*	*563*	*529*	*498*	*471*	*447*	*425*
17	999	987	968	946	922	898	874	851	828
	727	*669*	*621*	*581*	*547*	*516*	*488*	*465*	*443*

CONFIDENCE LIMITS FOR PROPORTIONS (CONFIDENCE COEFFICIENT .95)

x DENOTES THE NUMERATOR AND n THE DENOMINATOR OF THE RELATIVE FREQUENCY

$n-x$ / x (Numerator of the Relative Frequency)	Denominator minus Numerator								
	1	2	3	4	5	6	7	8	9
18	999	988	970	948	925	902	879	857	835
	740	*683*	*637*	*597*	*564*	*533*	*506*	*482*	*460*
19	999	988	971	950	929	906	884	862	841
	751	*696*	*651*	*612*	*579*	*549*	*522*	*498*	*476*
20	999	989	972	953	932	910	889	868	847
	762	*708*	*664*	*626*	*593*	*564*	*537*	*513*	*492*
22	999	990	975	956	937	917	897	877	858
	781	*730*	*688*	*651*	*619*	*590*	*565*	*541*	*519*
24	999	991	976	960	942	923	904	885	867
	797	*749*	*708*	*673*	*642*	*614*	*589*	*566*	*545*
26	999	991	978	962	945	928	910	893	875
	810	*765*	*726*	*693*	*663*	*636*	*611*	*588*	*567*
28	999	992	980	965	949	932	916	899	882
	822	*779*	*743*	*710*	*681*	*655*	*631*	*609*	*588*
30	999	992	981	967	952	936	920	904	889
	833	*792*	*757*	*725*	*697*	*672*	*649*	*627*	*607*
35	999	993	983	971	958	944	930	916	902
	855	*818*	*786*	*758*	*732*	*708*	*686*	*666*	*647*
40	999	994	985	975	963	951	938	925	912
	871	*838*	*809*	*783*	*759*	*737*	*717*	*698*	*679*
45	999	995	987	977	967	956	944	933	921
	885	*855*	*828*	*804*	*782*	*761*	*742*	*724*	*707*
50	1000	995	988	979	970	960	949	939	928
	896	*868*	*843*	*821*	*800*	*781*	*763*	*746*	*730*
60	1000	996	990	983	975	966	957	948	939
	912	*888*	*867*	*848*	*830*	*813*	*797*	*782*	*767*
80	1000	997	992	987	981	974	967	960	953
	933	*915*	*898*	*882*	*868*	*855*	*842*	*829*	*816*
100	1000	998	994	989	984	979	973	967	962
	946	*931*	*917*	*904*	*892*	*881*	*870*	*859*	*849*
200	1000	999	997	995	992	989	986	983	980
	973	*965*	*957*	*951*	*944*	*938*	*932*	*926*	*920*
500	1000	1000	999	998	997	996	995	993	992
	989	*986*	*983*	*980*	*977*	*974*	*972*	*969*	*967*
∞	1000	1000	1000	1000	1000	1000	1000	1000	1000
	1000	*1000*	*1000*	*1000*	*1000*	*1000*	*1000*	*1000*	*1000*

CONFIDENCE LIMITS FOR PROPORTIONS (CONFIDENCE COEFFICIENT .95)

x Denotes the Numerator and n the Denominator of the Relative Frequency

x (Numerator of the Relative Frequency) \ $n-x$ (Denominator minus Numerator)	10	11	12	13	14	15	16	17	18
0	308	285	265	247	232	218	206	195	185
	000	*000*	*000*	*000*	*000*	*000*	*000*	*000*	*000*
1	413	385	360	339	319	302	287	273	260
	002	*002*	*002*	*002*	*002*	*002*	*001*	*001*	*001*
2	484	454	428	405	383	364	347	331	317
	021	*019*	*018*	*017*	*016*	*015*	*014*	*013*	*012*
3	538	508	481	456	434	414	396	379	363
	050	*047*	*043*	*040*	*038*	*036*	*034*	*032*	*030*
4	581	551	524	499	476	456	437	419	403
	084	*078*	*073*	*068*	*064*	*061*	*057*	*054*	*052*
5	616	587	560	535	512	491	471	453	436
	118	*110*	*103*	*097*	*091*	*087*	*082*	*078*	*075*
6	646	617	590	565	543	522	502	484	467
	152	*142*	*133*	*126*	*119*	*113*	*107*	*102*	*098*
7	671	643	616	592	570	549	529	512	494
	184	*173*	*163*	*154*	*146*	*139*	*132*	*126*	*121*
8	692	665	639	616	593	573	553	535	518
	215	*203*	*191*	*181*	*172*	*164*	*156*	*149*	*143*
9	711	685	660	636	615	594	575	557	540
	244	*231*	*218*	*207*	*197*	*188*	*180*	*172*	*165*
10	728	702	678	655	634	614	595	577	560
	272	*257*	*244*	*232*	*221*	*211*	*202*	*194*	*186*
11	743	718	694	672	651	631	612	594	578
	298	*282*	*268*	*256*	*244*	*234*	*224*	*215*	*207*
12	756	732	709	687	666	647	628	611	594
	322	*306*	*291*	*278*	*266*	*255*	*245*	*235*	*227*
13	768	744	722	701	680	661	643	626	609
	345	*328*	*313*	*299*	*287*	*275*	*264*	*255*	*245*
14	779	756	734	713	694	675	657	640	624
	366	*349*	*334*	*320*	*306*	*295*	*283*	*273*	*264*
15	789	766	745	725	705	687	669	653	637
	386	*369*	*353*	*339*	*325*	*313*	*302*	*291*	*281*
16	798	776	755	736	717	698	681	665	649
	405	*388*	*372*	*357*	*343*	*331*	*319*	*308*	*298*
17	806	785	765	745	727	709	692	676	660
	423	*406*	*389*	*374*	*360*	*347*	*335*	*324*	*314*

CONFIDENCE LIMITS FOR PROPORTIONS (CONFIDENCE COEFFICIENT .95)

x DENOTES THE NUMERATOR AND n THE DENOMINATOR OF THE RELATIVE FREQUENCY

x (Numerator of the Relative Frequency) \ $n-x$ (Denominator minus Numerator)	10	11	12	13	14	15	16	17	18
18	814	793	773	755	736	719	702	686	671
	440	*422*	*406*	*391*	*376*	*363*	*351*	*340*	*329*
19	821	801	782	763	745	728	712	696	681
	456	*439*	*422*	*406*	*392*	*379*	*366*	*355*	*344*
20	827	808	789	771	753	737	720	705	690
	472	*454*	*437*	*421*	*407*	*393*	*381*	*369*	*358*
22	839	820	803	785	768	752	737	722	707
	500	*481*	*465*	*449*	*434*	*421*	*408*	*396*	*385*
24	849	831	814	798	782	766	751	737	723
	525	*507*	*490*	*475*	*460*	*446*	*433*	*421*	*410*
26	858	841	825	809	794	779	764	750	736
	548	*530*	*513*	*497*	*483*	*469*	*456*	*444*	*432*
28	866	850	834	819	804	790	776	762	749
	569	*551*	*535*	*519*	*504*	*491*	*478*	*465*	*453*
30	873	858	843	828	814	800	786	773	760
	588	*571*	*554*	*539*	*524*	*510*	*498*	*485*	*473*
35	888	874	860	847	834	821	809	797	785
	628	*612*	*596*	*581*	*567*	*554*	*541*	*529*	*517*
40	900	887	875	862	850	838	827	815	804
	662	*646*	*631*	*616*	*602*	*590*	*578*	*566*	*555*
45	909	898	886	875	864	853	842	831	821
	690	*675*	*661*	*647*	*633*	*621*	*609*	*598*	*587*
50	917	906	896	885	875	865	854	844	835
	714	*700*	*686*	*673*	*660*	*648*	*636*	*625*	*614*
60	929	920	911	902	893	884	874	866	857
	752	*740*	*727*	*715*	*703*	*692*	*681*	*670*	*660*
80	945	938	931	923	916	909	901	894	887
	804	*793*	*783*	*773*	*763*	*753*	*744*	*734*	*726*
100	955	949	943	937	931	925	919	913	907
	838	*829*	*820*	*811*	*802*	*794*	*786*	*778*	*770*
200	977	974	970	967	964	961	957	954	950
	914	*909*	*903*	*898*	*893*	*888*	*883*	*878*	*873*
500	991	989	988	986	985	984	982	981	979
	964	*962*	*960*	*957*	*955*	*953*	*950*	*948*	*946*
∞	1000	1000	1000	1000	1000	1000	1000	1000	1000
	1000	*1000*	*1000*	*1000*	*1000*	*1000*	*1000*	*1000*	*1000*

CONFIDENCE LIMITS FOR PROPORTIONS (CONFIDENCE COEFFICIENT .95)

x Denotes the Numerator and n the Denominator of the Relative Frequency

Denominator minus Numerator ($n-x$); Numerator of the Relative Frequency (x)

x \ $n-x$	19	20	22	24	26	28	30	35	40
0	176	168	154	142	132	123	116	100	088
	000	*000*	*000*	*000*	*000*	*000*	*000*	*000*	*000*
1	249	238	219	203	190	178	167	145	129
	001	*001*	*001*	*001*	*001*	*001*	*001*	*001*	*001*
2	304	292	270	251	235	221	208	182	162
	012	*011*	*010*	*009*	*009*	*008*	*008*	*007*	*006*
3	349	336	312	292	274	257	243	214	191
	029	*028*	*025*	*024*	*022*	*020*	*019*	*017*	*015*
4	388	374	349	327	307	290	275	242	217
	050	*047*	*044*	*040*	*038*	*035*	*033*	*029*	*025*
5	421	407	381	358	337	319	303	268	241
	071	*068*	*063*	*058*	*055*	*051*	*048*	*042*	*037*
6	451	436	410	386	364	345	328	292	263
	094	*090*	*083*	*077*	*072*	*068*	*064*	*056*	*049*
7	478	463	435	411	389	369	351	314	283
	116	*111*	*103*	*096*	*090*	*084*	*080*	*070*	*062*
8	502	487	459	434	412	391	373	334	302
	138	*132*	*123*	*115*	*107*	*101*	*096*	*084*	*075*
9	524	508	481	455	433	412	393	353	321
	159	*153*	*142*	*133*	*125*	*118*	*111*	*098*	*088*
10	544	528	500	475	452	431	412	372	338
	179	*173*	*161*	*151*	*142*	*134*	*127*	*112*	*100*
11	561	546	519	493	470	449	429	388	354
	199	*192*	*180*	*169*	*159*	*150*	*142*	*126*	*113*
12	578	563	535	510	487	465	446	404	369
	218	*211*	*197*	*186*	*175*	*166*	*157*	*140*	*125*
13	594	579	551	525	503	481	461	419	384
	237	*229*	*215*	*202*	*191*	*181*	*172*	*153*	*138*
14	608	593	566	540	517	496	476	433	398
	255	*247*	*232*	*218*	*206*	*196*	*186*	*166*	*150*
15	621	607	579	554	531	509	490	446	410
	272	*263*	*248*	*234*	*221*	*210*	*200*	*179*	*162*
16	634	619	592	567	544	522	502	459	422
	288	*280*	*263*	*249*	*236*	*224*	*214*	*191*	*173*
17	645	631	604	579	556	535	515	471	434
	304	*295*	*278*	*263*	*250*	*238*	*227*	*203*	*185*

CONFIDENCE LIMITS FOR PROPORTIONS (CONFIDENCE COEFFICIENT .95)

x Denotes the Numerator and n the Denominator of the Relative Frequency

Numerator of the Relative Frequency x \ $n-x$	Denominator minus Numerator 19	20	22	24	26	28	30	35	40
18	656	642	615	590	568	547	527	483	445
	319	*310*	*293*	*277*	*264*	*251*	*240*	*215*	*196*
19	666	652	626	601	578	557	538	494	456
	334	*324*	*307*	*291*	*277*	*264*	*252*	*227*	*207*
20	676	662	636	612	589	568	548	504	467
	348	*338*	*320*	*304*	*289*	*276*	*264*	*238*	*217*
22	693	680	654	631	614	588	568	524	487
	374	*364*	*346*	*329*	*314*	*300*	*287*	*260*	*237*
24	709	696	671	648	626	605	586	543	505
	399	*388*	*369*	*352*	*337*	*322*	*309*	*281*	*257*
26	723	711	686	663	642	622	603	559	522
	422	*411*	*386*	*374*	*358*	*343*	*330*	*300*	*276*
28	736	724	700	678	657	637	618	575	538
	443	*432*	*412*	*395*	*378*	*363*	*349*	*319*	*294*
30	748	736	713	691	670	651	632	590	552
	462	*452*	*432*	*414*	*397*	*382*	*368*	*337*	*311*
35	773	762	740	719	700	681	663	622	586
	506	*496*	*476*	*457*	*441*	*425*	*410*	*378*	*351*
40	793	783	763	743	724	706	689	649	614
	544	*533*	*513*	*495*	*478*	*462*	*448*	*414*	*386*
45	811	801	781	763	745	728	711	673	639
	576	*566*	*546*	*528*	*511*	*495*	*480*	*447*	*419*
50	825	816	797	780	763	746	731	694	660
	604	*594*	*575*	*557*	*540*	*525*	*510*	*476*	*447*
60	848	840	823	807	792	777	763	728	697
	650	*641*	*622*	*605*	*589*	*574*	*559*	*526*	*497*
80	880	874	860	846	833	820	808	778	750
	717	*708*	*692*	*676*	*662*	*647*	*634*	*603*	*575*
100	901	895	883	872	860	847	838	812	787
	762	*755*	*740*	*726*	*713*	*700*	*687*	*658*	*632*
200	947	943	937	930	923	917	910	894	878
	868	*863*	*854*	*845*	*836*	*828*	*819*	*799*	*780*
500	978	976	973	970	967	964	961	954	947
	944	*941*	*937*	*933*	*928*	*924*	*920*	*910*	*901*
∞	1000	1000	1000	1000	1000	1000	1000	1000	1000
	1000	*1000*	*1000*	*1000*	*1000*	*1000*	*1000*	*1000*	*1000*

CONFIDENCE LIMITS FOR PROPORTIONS (CONFIDENCE COEFFICIENT .95)

x Denotes the Numerator and *n* the Denominator of the Relative Frequency

Numerator of the Relative Frequency (x) / Denominator minus Numerator (n − x)

x \ n−x	45	50	60	80	100	200	500	∞
0	079 *000*	071 *000*	060 *000*	045 *000*	036 *000*	018 *000*	007 *000*	000 *000*
1	115 *001*	104 *001*	088 *000*	067 *000*	054 *000*	027 *000*	011 *000*	000 *000*
2	145 *005*	132 *005*	112 *004*	085 *003*	069 *002*	035 *001*	014 *000*	000 *000*
3	172 *013*	157 *012*	133 *010*	102 *008*	083 *006*	043 *003*	017 *001*	000 *000*
4	196 *023*	179 *021*	152 *017*	118 *013*	096 *011*	049 *005*	020 *002*	000 *000*
5	218 *033*	200 *030*	170 *025*	132 *019*	108 *016*	056 *008*	023 *003*	000 *000*
6	239 *044*	219 *040*	187 *034*	145 *026*	119 *021*	062 *011*	026 *004*	000 *000*
7	258 *056*	237 *051*	203 *043*	158 *033*	130 *027*	068 *014*	028 *005*	000 *000*
8	276 *067*	254 *061*	218 *052*	171 *040*	141 *033*	074 *017*	031 *007*	000 *000*
9	293 *079*	270 *072*	233 *061*	184 *047*	151 *038*	080 *020*	033 *008*	000 *000*
10	310 *091*	286 *083*	248 *071*	196 *055*	162 *045*	086 *023*	036 *009*	000 *000*
11	325 *102*	300 *094*	260 *080*	207 *062*	171 *051*	091 *026*	038 *011*	000 *000*
12	339 *114*	314 *104*	273 *089*	217 *069*	180 *057*	097 *030*	040 *012*	000 *000*
13	353 *125*	327 *115*	285 *098*	227 *077*	189 *063*	102 *033*	043 *014*	000 *000*
14	367 *136*	340 *125*	297 *107*	237 *084*	198 *069*	107 *036*	045 *015*	000 *000*
15	379 *147*	352 *135*	308 *116*	247 *091*	206 *075*	112 *039*	047 *016*	000 *000*
16	391 *158*	364 *146*	319 *126*	256 *099*	214 *081*	117 *043*	050 *018*	000 *000*
17	402 *169*	375 *156*	330 *134*	266 *106*	222 *087*	122 *046*	052 *019*	000 *000*

CONFIDENCE LIMITS FOR PROPORTIONS (CONFIDENCE COEFFICIENT .95)

x Denotes the Numerator and n the Denominator of the Relative Frequency

x (Numerator of the Relative Frequency) \ $n-x$ (Denominator minus Numerator)	45	50	60	80	100	200	500	∞
18	413	386	340	274	230	127	054	000
	179	*165*	*143*	*113*	*093*	*050*	*021*	*000*
19	424	396	350	283	238	132	056	000
	189	*175*	*152*	*120*	*099*	*053*	*022*	*000*
20	434	406	359	292	245	137	059	000
	199	*184*	*160*	*126*	*105*	*057*	*024*	*000*
22	454	425	378	308	260	146	063	000
	219	*203*	*177*	*140*	*117*	*063*	*027*	*000*
24	472	443	395	324	274	155	067	000
	237	*220*	*193*	*154*	*128*	*070*	*030*	*000*
26	489	460	411	338	287	164	072	000
	255	*237*	*208*	*167*	*140*	*077*	*033*	*000*
28	505	475	426	353	300	172	076	000
	272	*254*	*223*	*180*	*153*	*083*	*036*	*000*
30	520	490	441	366	313	181	080	000
	289	*269*	*237*	*192*	*162*	*090*	*039*	*000*
35	553	524	474	397	342	201	090	000
	327	*306*	*272*	*222*	*188*	*106*	*046*	*000*
40	581	553	503	425	368	220	099	000
	361	*340*	*303*	*250*	*213*	*122*	*053*	*000*
45	607	579	529	451	392	238	109	000
	393	*370*	*332*	*276*	*236*	*137*	*061*	*000*
50	630	602	552	474	415	255	118	000
	421	*398*	*359*	*301*	*259*	*152*	*068*	*000*
60	668	641	593	515	455	287	136	000
	471	*448*	*407*	*345*	*300*	*181*	*083*	*000*
80	724	699	655	580	520	342	169	000
	549	*526*	*485*	*420*	*370*	*234*	*111*	*000*
100	764	741	700	630	571	395	199	000
	608	*585*	*545*	*480*	*429*	*280*	*138*	*000*
200	863	848	819	766	720	550	319	000
	762	*745*	*713*	*658*	*605*	*450*	*253*	*000*
500	939	932	917	889	862	747	531	000
	891	*882*	*864*	*831*	*801*	*681*	*469*	*000*
∞	1000	1000	1000	1000	1000	1000	1000	—
	1000	*1000*	*1000*	*1000*	*1000*	*1000*	*1000*	—

CONFIDENCE LIMITS FOR PROPORTIONS (CONFIDENCE COEFFICIENT .99)

x Denotes the Numerator and n the Denominator of the Relative Frequency

x (Numerator of the Relative Frequency) \ $n-x$ (Denominator minus Numerator)	1	2	3	4	5	6	7	8	9
0	995 *000*	929 *000*	829 *000*	734 *000*	653 *000*	586 *000*	531 *000*	484 *000*	445 *000*
1	997 *003*	959 *002*	889 *001*	815 *001*	746 *001*	685 *001*	632 *001*	585 *001*	544 *001*
2	998 *041*	971 *029*	917 *023*	856 *019*	797 *016*	742 *014*	693 *012*	648 *011*	608 *010*
3	999 *111*	977 *083*	934 *066*	882 *055*	830 *047*	781 *042*	735 *037*	693 *033*	655 *030*
4	999 *185*	981 *144*	945 *118*	900 *100*	854 *087*	809 *077*	767 *069*	728 *062*	691 *057*
5	999 *254*	984 *203*	953 *170*	913 *146*	872 *128*	831 *114*	791 *103*	755 *094*	720 *087*
6	999 *315*	986 *258*	958 *219*	923 *191*	886 *169*	848 *152*	811 *138*	777 *127*	744 *117*
7	999 *368*	988 *307*	963 *265*	931 *233*	897 *209*	862 *189*	828 *172*	795 *159*	764 *147*
8	999 *415*	989 *352*	967 *307*	938 *272*	906 *245*	873 *223*	841 *205*	811 *189*	781 *176*
9	999 *456*	990 *392*	970 *345*	943 *309*	913 *280*	883 *256*	853 *236*	824 *219*	795 *205*
10	1000 *491*	991 *427*	972 *379*	947 *342*	920 *312*	891 *286*	863 *265*	835 *247*	808 *232*
11	1000 *523*	992 *459*	974 *411*	951 *373*	925 *342*	899 *315*	872 *293*	845 *274*	819 *257*
12	1000 *551*	992 *488*	976 *439*	955 *401*	930 *369*	905 *342*	879 *319*	854 *299*	829 *282*
13	1000 *576*	993 *514*	978 *466*	957 *427*	935 *395*	910 *367*	886 *343*	862 *323*	838 *305*
14	1000 *598*	993 *537*	979 *490*	960 *451*	938 *418*	915 *390*	892 *366*	869 *345*	846 *326*
15	1000 *619*	994 *559*	980 *512*	962 *473*	942 *440*	920 *412*	898 *388*	875 *366*	854 *347*
16	1000 *637*	994 *578*	981 *532*	964 *493*	945 *461*	924 *433*	903 *408*	881 *386*	860 *366*
17	1000 *654*	994 *596*	982 *551*	966 *512*	947 *480*	927 *452*	907 *427*	887 *405*	866 *385*

CONFIDENCE LIMITS FOR PROPORTIONS (CONFIDENCE COEFFICIENT .99)

x Denotes the Numerator and n the Denominator of the Relative Frequency

x (Numerator of the Relative Frequency) \ $n-x$ (Denominator minus Numerator)	1	2	3	4	5	6	7	8	9
18	1000	995	983	968	950	931	911	891	872
	669	*613*	*568*	*530*	*498*	*469*	*445*	*422*	*402*
19	1000	995	984	969	952	934	915	896	877
	683	*628*	*584*	*547*	*515*	*486*	*462*	*439*	*419*
20	1000	995	985	971	954	936	918	900	881
	696	*642*	*599*	*562*	*530*	*502*	*478*	*455*	*435*
22	1000	996	986	973	958	941	924	907	890
	719	*668*	*626*	*590*	*559*	*531*	*507*	*484*	*464*
24	1000	996	987	975	961	946	930	913	897
	738	*690*	*649*	*615*	*584*	*557*	*533*	*511*	*490*
26	1000	996	988	977	963	949	934	919	903
	755	*709*	*670*	*637*	*607*	*580*	*557*	*535*	*515*
28	1000	996	989	978	966	952	938	924	909
	770	*726*	*689*	*656*	*627*	*602*	*578*	*557*	*537*
30	1000	997	989	980	968	955	942	928	914
	784	*741*	*705*	*674*	*646*	*621*	*598*	*577*	*557*
35	1000	997	991	982	972	961	949	937	924
	811	*773*	*740*	*711*	*685*	*661*	*639*	*619*	*600*
40	1000	998	992	984	975	965	955	944	933
	832	*797*	*767*	*740*	*716*	*694*	*673*	*654*	*636*
45	1000	998	993	986	978	969	959	949	939
	849	*817*	*790*	*765*	*742*	*721*	*701*	*683*	*666*
50	1000	998	994	987	980	972	963	954	945
	863	*834*	*808*	*785*	*763*	*743*	*725*	*708*	*691*
60	1000	998	995	989	983	976	969	961	953
	884	*859*	*836*	*816*	*797*	*780*	*763*	*748*	*733*
80	1000	999	996	992	987	982	976	970	964
	912	*892*	*874*	*857*	*842*	*827*	*814*	*801*	*788*
100	1000	999	997	993	990	985	981	976	971
	929	*912*	*897*	*884*	*871*	*858*	*847*	*836*	*825*
200	1000	999	998	997	995	992	990	988	985
	964	*955*	*947*	*939*	*932*	*925*	*919*	*913*	*907*
500	1000	1000	999	999	998	997	996	995	994
	985	*982*	*978*	*975*	*972*	*969*	*967*	*964*	*961*
∞	1000	1000	1000	1000	1000	1000	1000	1000	1000
	1000	*1000*	*1000*	*1000*	*1000*	*1000*	*1000*	*1000*	*1000*

CONFIDENCE LIMITS FOR PROPORTIONS (CONFIDENCE COEFFICIENT .99)

x Denotes the Numerator and n the Denominator of the Relative Frequency

Numerator of the Relative Frequency

x \ $n-x$	Denominator minus Numerator								
	10	11	12	13	14	15	16	17	18
0	411	382	357	335	315	298	282	268	255
	000	*000*	*000*	*000*	*000*	*000*	*000*	*000*	*000*
1	509	477	449	424	402	381	363	346	331
	000	*000*	*000*	*000*	*000*	*000*	*000*	*000*	*000*
2	573	541	512	486	463	441	422	404	387
	009	*008*	*008*	*007*	*007*	*006*	*006*	*006*	*005*
3	621	589	561	534	510	488	468	449	432
	028	*026*	*024*	*022*	*021*	*020*	*019*	*018*	*017*
4	658	627	599	573	549	527	507	488	470
	053	*049*	*045*	*043*	*040*	*038*	*036*	*034*	*032*
5	688	658	631	605	582	560	539	520	502
	080	*075*	*070*	*065*	*062*	*058*	*055*	*053*	*050*
6	714	685	658	633	610	588	567	548	531
	109	*101*	*095*	*090*	*085*	*080*	*076*	*073*	*069*
7	735	707	681	657	634	612	592	573	555
	137	*128*	*121*	*114*	*108*	*102*	*097*	*093*	*089*
8	753	726	701	677	655	634	614	595	578
	165	*155*	*146*	*138*	*131*	*125*	*119*	*113*	*109*
9	768	743	718	695	674	653	634	615	598
	192	*181*	*171*	*162*	*154*	*146*	*140*	*134*	*128*
10	782	758	734	712	690	670	651	633	616
	218	*205*	*195*	*185*	*176*	*168*	*161*	*154*	*148*
11	795	771	748	726	705	686	667	649	632
	242	*229*	*218*	*207*	*197*	*189*	*181*	*173*	*167*
12	805	782	760	739	719	700	682	664	647
	266	*252*	*240*	*228*	*218*	*209*	*200*	*192*	*185*
13	815	793	772	751	731	713	695	678	661
	288	*274*	*261*	*249*	*238*	*228*	*219*	*211*	*203*
14	824	803	782	762	743	724	707	691	674
	310	*295*	*281*	*269*	*257*	*247*	*237*	*228*	*220*
15	832	811	791	772	753	735	718	702	685
	330	*314*	*300*	*287*	*276*	*265*	*255*	*246*	*237*
16	839	819	800	781	763	745	728	712	696
	349	*333*	*318*	*305*	*293*	*282*	*272*	*262*	*253*
17	846	827	808	789	772	754	738	722	706
	367	*351*	*336*	*322*	*309*	*298*	*288*	*278*	*269*

CONFIDENCE LIMITS FOR PROPORTIONS (CONFIDENCE COEFFICIENT .99)

x Denotes the Numerator and n the Denominator of the Relative Frequency

x \ $n-x$ (Numerator of the Relative Frequency)	Denominator minus Numerator 10	11	12	13	14	15	16	17	18
18	852	833	815	797	780	763	747	731	716
	384	*368*	*353*	*339*	*326*	*315*	*304*	*294*	*284*
19	858	840	822	804	787	771	755	740	725
	401	*384*	*369*	*355*	*342*	*330*	*319*	*308*	*299*
20	863	845	828	811	794	778	763	748	733
	417	*400*	*384*	*370*	*357*	*345*	*334*	*323*	*313*
22	873	856	839	823	807	792	777	762	748
	445	*429*	*413*	*398*	*385*	*372*	*361*	*350*	*339*
24	881	865	849	834	819	804	789	775	762
	471	*455*	*439*	*424*	*410*	*398*	*386*	*375*	*364*
26	888	873	858	843	829	814	800	787	774
	496	*479*	*463*	*448*	*434*	*422*	*410*	*398*	*388*
28	894	880	866	852	838	824	811	798	785
	518	*501*	*485*	*471*	*457*	*444*	*432*	*420*	*409*
30	900	886	873	859	846	833	820	807	795
	539	*522*	*506*	*492*	*478*	*464*	*452*	*441*	*430*
35	912	900	887	875	863	851	839	827	816
	582	*566*	*550*	*535*	*522*	*510*	*498*	*486*	*475*
40	921	910	899	888	876	865	854	844	833
	619	*603*	*588*	*574*	*560*	*548*	*536*	*525*	*514*
45	929	919	908	898	888	877	867	857	847
	649	*634*	*620*	*606*	*593*	*582*	*570*	*558*	*547*
50	935	926	916	906	897	888	878	869	859
	676	*661*	*648*	*634*	*621*	*610*	*599*	*588*	*577*
60	945	937	928	920	912	904	895	887	878
	719	*705*	*693*	*680*	*668*	*657*	*646*	*636*	*626*
80	957	951	944	938	931	924	918	911	904
	776	*765*	*754*	*743*	*733*	*724*	*715*	*705*	*696*
100	965	960	955	949	943	938	932	927	921
	815	*805*	*795*	*786*	*777*	*769*	*761*	*753*	*745*
200	982	979	976	973	970	967	964	961	958
	901	*896*	*890*	*884*	*878*	*873*	*868*	*863*	*858*
500	993	992	990	989	988	987	985	984	982
	959	*956*	*953*	*951*	*949*	*946*	*944*	*941*	*939*
∞	1000	1000	1000	1000	1000	1000	1000	1000	1000
	1000	*1000*	*1000*	*1000*	*1000*	*1000*	*1000*	*1000*	*1000*

CONFIDENCE LIMITS FOR PROPORTIONS (CONFIDENCE COEFFICIENT .99)

x Denotes the Numerator and n the Denominator of the Relative Frequency

x (Numerator of the Relative Frequency) \ $n-x$ (Denominator minus Numerator)	19	20	22	24	26	28	30	35	40
0	243 *000*	233 *000*	214 *000*	198 *000*	184 *000*	172 *000*	162 *000*	140 *000*	124 *000*
1	317 *000*	304 *000*	281 *000*	262 *000*	245 *000*	230 *000*	216 *000*	189 *000*	168 *000*
2	372 *005*	358 *005*	332 *004*	310 *004*	291 *004*	274 *004*	259 *003*	227 *003*	203 *002*
3	416 *016*	401 *015*	374 *014*	351 *013*	330 *012*	311 *011*	295 *011*	260 *009*	233 *008*
4	453 *031*	438 *029*	410 *027*	385 *025*	363 *023*	344 *022*	326 *020*	289 *018*	260 *016*
5	485 *048*	470 *046*	441 *042*	416 *039*	393 *037*	373 *034*	354 *032*	315 *028*	284 *025*
6	514 *066*	498 *064*	469 *059*	443 *054*	420 *051*	398 *048*	379 *045*	339 *039*	306 *035*
7	538 *085*	522 *082*	493 *076*	467 *070*	443 *066*	422 *062*	402 *058*	361 *051*	327 *045*
8	561 *104*	545 *100*	516 *093*	489 *087*	465 *081*	443 *076*	423 *072*	381 *063*	346 *056*
9	581 *123*	565 *119*	536 *110*	510 *103*	485 *097*	463 *091*	443 *086*	400 *076*	364 *067*
10	599 *142*	583 *137*	555 *127*	529 *119*	504 *112*	482 *106*	461 *100*	418 *088*	381 *079*
11	616 *160*	600 *155*	571 *144*	545 *135*	521 *127*	499 *120*	478 *114*	434 *100*	397 *090*
12	631 *178*	616 *172*	587 *161*	561 *151*	537 *142*	515 *134*	494 *127*	450 *113*	412 *101*
13	645 *196*	630 *189*	602 *177*	576 *166*	552 *157*	529 *148*	508 *141*	465 *125*	426 *112*
14	658 *213*	643 *206*	615 *193*	590 *181*	566 *171*	543 *162*	522 *154*	478 *137*	440 *124*
15	670 *229*	655 *222*	628 *208*	602 *196*	578 *186*	556 *176*	536 *167*	490 *149*	452 *135*
16	681 *245*	666 *237*	639 *223*	614 *211*	590 *200*	568 *189*	548 *180*	502 *161*	464 *146*
17	692 *260*	677 *252*	650 *238*	625 *225*	602 *213*	580 *202*	559 *193*	514 *173*	475 *156*

CONFIDENCE LIMITS FOR PROPORTIONS (CONFIDENCE COEFFICIENT .99)

x Denotes the Numerator and n the Denominator of the Relative Frequency

Rows: x = Numerator of the Relative Frequency. Columns: $n-x$ = Denominator minus Numerator. Upper values in roman type, lower values in italics.

x \ $n-x$	19	20	22	24	26	28	30	35	40
18	701	687	661	636	612	591	570	525	486
	275	*267*	*252*	*238*	*226*	*215*	*205*	*184*	*167*
19	711	697	670	646	623	601	581	536	497
	289	*281*	*265*	*251*	*239*	*228*	*217*	*195*	*177*
20	719	705	679	655	632	611	591	546	507
	303	*295*	*279*	*264*	*251*	*239*	*229*	*206*	*187*
22	735	721	696	673	650	629	609	565	526
	330	*321*	*304*	*289*	*274*	*263*	*251*	*227*	*207*
24	749	736	711	688	666	646	626	582	543
	354	*345*	*327*	*312*	*298*	*285*	*273*	*247*	*226*
26	761	749	726	702	681	661	642	598	560
	377	*368*	*350*	*334*	*319*	*306*	*293*	*267*	*244*
28	772	761	737	715	694	675	656	613	575
	399	*389*	*371*	*354*	*339*	*325*	*312*	*285*	*262*
30	783	771	749	727	707	688	669	626	589
	419	*409*	*391*	*374*	*358*	*344*	*331*	*303*	*278*
35	805	794	773	753	733	715	697	657	620
	464	*454*	*435*	*418*	*402*	*387*	*374*	*343*	*318*
40	823	813	793	774	756	738	722	682	646
	503	*493*	*474*	*457*	*440*	*425*	*411*	*380*	*354*
45	838	828	810	792	775	758	742	704	670
	537	*527*	*508*	*491*	*474*	*459*	*445*	*413*	*386*
50	850	842	824	807	791	775	759	723	690
	567	*557*	*538*	*521*	*505*	*490*	*475*	*443*	*415*
60	870	863	847	832	817	802	788	755	724
	616	*606*	*589*	*572*	*556*	*541*	*527*	*495*	*466*
80	898	891	878	866	853	841	829	800	773
	687	*679*	*663*	*647*	*632*	*618*	*605*	*574*	*547*
100	916	910	899	888	878	867	857	831	807
	737	*729*	*714*	*700*	*687*	*674*	*661*	*632*	*606*
200	955	952	946	939	933	927	921	905	890
	853	*848*	*838*	*829*	*820*	*811*	*803*	*782*	*763*
500	981	980	977	974	971	969	966	959	952
	937	*934*	*930*	*925*	*921*	*917*	*912*	*902*	*892*
∞	1000	1000	1000	1000	1000	1000	1000	1000	1000
	1000	*1000*	*1000*	*1000*	*1000*	*1000*	*1000*	*1000*	*1000*

CONFIDENCE LIMITS FOR PROPORTIONS (CONFIDENCE COEFFICIENT .99)

x Denotes the Numerator and n the Denominator of the Relative Frequency

x (Numerator of the Relative Frequency) \ $n-x$ (Denominator minus Numerator)	45	50	60	80	100	200	500	∞
0	111	101	085	064	052	026	011	000
	000	*000*	*000*	*000*	*000*	*000*	*000*	*000*
1	151	137	116	088	071	036	015	000
	000	*000*	*000*	*000*	*000*	*000*	*000*	*000*
2	183	166	141	108	088	045	018	000
	002	*002*	*002*	*001*	*001*	*001*	*000*	*000*
3	210	192	164	126	103	053	022	000
	007	*006*	*005*	*004*	*003*	*002*	*001*	*000*
4	235	215	184	143	116	061	025	000
	014	*013*	*011*	*008*	*007*	*003*	*001*	*000*
5	258	237	203	158	129	068	028	000
	022	*020*	*017*	*013*	*010*	*005*	*002*	*000*
6	279	257	220	173	142	075	031	000
	031	*028*	*024*	*018*	*015*	*008*	*003*	*000*
7	299	275	237	186	153	081	033	000
	041	*037*	*031*	*024*	*019*	*010*	*004*	*000*
8	317	292	252	199	164	087	036	000
	051	*046*	*039*	*030*	*024*	*012*	*005*	*000*
9	334	309	267	212	175	093	039	000
	061	*055*	*047*	*036*	*029*	*015*	*006*	*000*
10	351	324	281	224	185	099	041	000
	071	*065*	*055*	*043*	*035*	*018*	*007*	*000*
11	366	339	295	235	195	104	044	000
	081	*074*	*063*	*049*	*040*	*021*	*008*	*000*
12	380	352	307	246	205	110	047	000
	092	*084*	*072*	*056*	*045*	*024*	*010*	*000*
13	394	366	320	257	214	116	049	000
	102	*094*	*080*	*062*	*051*	*027*	*011*	*000*
14	407	379	332	267	223	122	051	000
	112	*103*	*088*	*069*	*057*	*030*	*012*	*000*
15	418	390	343	276	231	127	054	000
	123	*112*	*096*	*076*	*062*	*033*	*013*	*000*
16	430	401	354	285	239	132	056	000
	133	*122*	*105*	*082*	*068*	*036*	*015*	*000*
17	442	412	364	295	247	137	059	000
	143	*131*	*113*	*089*	*073*	*039*	*016*	*000*

CONFIDENCE LIMITS FOR PROPORTIONS (CONFIDENCE COEFFICIENT .99)

x Denotes the Numerator and n the Denominator of the Relative Frequency

x (Numerator of the Relative Frequency) \ $n-x$ (Denominator minus Numerator)	45	50	60	80	100	200	500	∞
18	453	423	374	304	255	142	061	000
	153	*141*	*122*	*096*	*079*	*042*	*018*	*000*
19	463	433	384	313	263	147	063	000
	162	*150*	*130*	*102*	*084*	*045*	*019*	*000*
20	473	443	394	321	271	152	066	000
	172	*158*	*137*	*109*	*090*	*048*	*020*	*000*
22	492	462	411	337	286	162	070	000
	190	*176*	*153*	*122*	*101*	*054*	*023*	*000*
24	509	479	428	353	300	171	075	000
	208	*193*	*168*	*134*	*112*	*061*	*026*	*000*
26	526	495	444	368	313	180	079	000
	225	*209*	*183*	*147*	*122*	*067*	*029*	*000*
28	541	510	459	382	326	189	083	000
	242	*225*	*198*	*159*	*133*	*073*	*031*	*000*
30	555	525	473	395	339	197	088	000
	258	*241*	*212*	*171*	*143*	*079*	*034*	*000*
35	587	557	505	426	368	218	098	000
	296	*277*	*245*	*200*	*169*	*095*	*041*	*000*
40	614	585	534	453	394	237	108	000
	330	*310*	*276*	*227*	*193*	*110*	*048*	*000*
45	638	609	559	478	418	255	118	000
	362	*341*	*305*	*253*	*216*	*125*	*055*	*000*
50	659	631	581	501	440	273	127	000
	391	*369*	*332*	*277*	*238*	*139*	*062*	*000*
60	695	668	620	541	479	305	145	000
	441	*419*	*380*	*321*	*278*	*167*	*076*	*000*
80	747	723	679	604	543	360	179	000
	522	*499*	*459*	*396*	*349*	*219*	*103*	*000*
100	784	762	722	651	593	407	209	000
	582	*560*	*521*	*457*	*407*	*265*	*129*	*000*
200	875	861	833	781	735	565	332	000
	745	*727*	*695*	*640*	*593*	*435*	*243*	*000*
500	945	938	924	897	871	757	541	000
	882	*873*	*855*	*821*	*791*	*668*	*459*	*000*
∞	1000	1000	1000	1000	1000	1000	1000	—
	1000	*1000*	*1000*	*1000*	*1000*	*1000*	*1000*	—

III.4 CONFIDENCE LIMITS FOR THE EXPECTED VALUE OF A POISSON DISTRIBUTION

The general term of a Poisson distributed variable is given by

$$f(x;\lambda) = \frac{e^{-\lambda}\lambda^x}{x!}, \qquad x = 0, 1, 2, \ldots.$$

For any given value x' and $\alpha < 0.5$, lower and upper limits of λ may be determined, say λ_a and λ_b, such that $\lambda_a < \lambda_b$ and

$$\sum_{x=x'}^{\infty} \frac{e^{-\lambda_a}\lambda_a^x}{x!} = \alpha \qquad \text{and} \qquad \sum_{x=0}^{x'} \frac{e^{-\lambda_b}\lambda_b^x}{x!} = \alpha.$$

Within the range of tabulation, λ_a and λ_b may be determined from the cumulative Poisson distribution tables, or from a table of percentage points of the χ^2 distribution, since

$$1 - P(\chi^2;n) = \sum_{x=0}^{x'-1} \frac{e^{-\lambda}\lambda^x}{x!}.$$

This table gives values of λ_a and λ_b for values of x' and for $2\alpha = 0.01$ and 0.05. Beyond $x' = 50$, λ_a and λ_b may be computed from

$$\lambda_b = \tfrac{1}{2}\chi_1^2 \qquad \text{where } 1 - P(\chi^2;n) = \alpha,\ n = 2(x'+1)$$
$$\lambda_a = \tfrac{1}{2}\chi_2^2 \qquad \text{where } P(\chi^2;n) = \alpha,\ n = 2x'\ .$$

CONFIDENCE LIMITS FOR THE EXPECTED VALUE OF A POISSON DISTRIBUTION

Total observed count $x' = \Sigma x_i$	Significance level $2\alpha = 0.01$		$2\alpha = 0.05$		Total observed count $x' = \Sigma x_i$	Significance level $2\alpha = 0.01$		$2\alpha = 0.05$	
	Lower Limit	*Upper Limit*	*Lower Limit*	*Upper Limit*		*Lower Limit*	*Upper Limit*	*Lower Limit*	*Upper Limit*
0	0.0	5.3	0.0	3.7					
1	0.0	7.4	0.1	5.6	26	14.7	42.2	17.0	38.0
2	0.1	9.3	0.2	7.2	27	15.4	43.5	17.8	39.2
3	0.3	11.0	0.6	8.8	28	16.2	44.8	18.6	40.4
4	0.6	12.6	1.0	10.2	29	17.0	46.0	19.4	41.6
5	1.0	14.1	1.6	11.7	30	17.7	47.2	20.2	42.8
6	1.5	15.6	2.2	13.1	31	18.5	48.4	21.0	44.0
7	2.0	17.1	2.8	14.4	32	19.3	49.6	21.8	45.1
8	2.5	18.5	3.4	15.8	33	20.0	50.8	22.7	46.3
9	3.1	20.0	4.0	17.1	34	20.8	52.1	23.5	47.5
10	3.7	21.3	4.7	18.4	35	21.6	53.3	24.3	48.7
11	4.3	22.6	5.4	19.7	36	22.4	54.5	25.1	49.8
12	4.9	24.0	6.2	21.0	37	23.2	55.7	26.0	51.0
13	5.5	25.4	6.9	22.3	38	24.0	56.9	26.8	52.2
14	6.2	26.7	7.7	23.5	39	24.8	58.1	27.7	53.3
15	6.8	28.1	8.4	24.8	40	25.6	59.3	28.6	54.5
16	7.5	29.4	9.4	26.0	41	26.4	60.5	29.4	55.6
17	8.2	30.7	9.9	27.2	42	27.2	61.7	30.3	56.8
18	8.9	32.0	10.7	28.4	43	28.0	62.9	31.1	57.9
19	9.6	33.3	11.5	29.6	44	28.8	64.1	32.0	59.0
20	10.3	34.6	12.2	30.8	45	29.6	65.3	32.8	60.2
21	11.0	35.9	13.0	32.0	46	30.4	66.5	33.6	61.3
22	11.8	37.2	13.8	33.2	47	31.2	67.7	34.5	62.5
23	12.5	38.4	14.6	34.4	48	32.0	68.9	35.3	63.6
24	13.2	39.7	15.4	35.6	49	32.8	70.1	36.1	64.8
25	14.0	41.0	16.2	36.8	50	33.6	71.3	37.0	65.9

III.5 HYPERGEOMETRIC DISTRIBUTION

The hypergeometric probability function is given by

$$f(x;N,n,k) = \frac{\binom{k}{x}\binom{N-k}{n-x}}{\binom{N}{n}} = \frac{\dfrac{k!}{x!(k-x)!}\,\dfrac{(N-k)!}{(n-x)!(N-k-n+x)!}}{\dfrac{N!}{n!(N-n)!}}$$

$$= \frac{k!n!}{x!(k-x)!(n-x)!}\,\frac{(N-k)!(N-n)!}{N!(N-k-n+x)!},$$

where N = number of items in a finite population consisting of A successes and B failures ($A + B = N$)
n = number of items drawn in sample without replacement, from the N items
k = number of failures in finite population $= B$
x = number of failures in sample .

$f(x;N,n,k)$ gives the probability of exactly x failures and $n - x$ successes in the sample of n items.

$$F(x;N,n,k) = \sum_{r=0}^{x} \frac{\binom{k}{r}\binom{N-k}{n-r}}{\binom{N}{n}}.$$

$F(x;N,n,k)$ gives the probability of x or fewer failures in the sample of n items.

HYPERGEOMETRIC PROBABILITY AND DISTRIBUTION FUNCTIONS

$$f(x;N,n,k) = \frac{\binom{k}{x}\binom{N-k}{n-x}}{\binom{N}{n}}, \qquad F(x;N,n,k) = \sum_{r=0}^{x} \frac{\binom{k}{r}\binom{N-k}{n-r}}{\binom{N}{n}}$$

N	n	k	x	$F(x)$	$f(x)$	N	n	k	x	$F(x)$	$f(x)$
2	1	1	0	0.500000	0.500000	6	2	2	2	1.000000	0.066667
2	1	1	1	1.000000	0.500000	6	3	1	0	0.500000	0.500000
3	1	1	0	0.666667	0.666667	6	3	1	1	1.000000	0.500000
3	1	1	1	1.000000	0.333333	6	3	2	0	0.200000	0.200000
3	2	1	0	0.333333	0.333333	6	3	2	1	0.800000	0.600000
3	2	1	1	1.000000	0.666667	6	3	2	2	1.000000	0.200000
3	2	2	1	0.666667	0.666667	6	3	3	0	0.050000	0.050000
3	2	2	2	1.000000	0.333333	6	3	3	1	0.500000	0.450000
4	1	1	0	0.750000	0.750000	6	3	3	2	0.950000	0.450000
4	1	1	1	1.000000	0.250000	6	3	3	3	1.000000	0.050000
4	2	1	0	0.500000	0.500000	6	4	1	0	0.333333	0.333333
4	2	1	1	1.000000	0.500000	6	4	1	1	1.000000	0.666667
4	2	2	0	0.166667	0.166667	6	4	2	0	0.066667	0.066667
4	2	2	1	0.833333	0.666667	6	4	2	1	0.600000	0.533333
4	2	2	2	1.000000	0.166667	6	4	2	2	1.000000	0.400000
4	3	1	0	0.250000	0.250000	6	4	3	1	0.200000	0.200000
4	3	1	1	1.000000	0.750000	6	4	3	2	0.800000	0.600000
4	3	2	1	0.500000	0.500000	6	4	3	3	1.000000	0.200000
4	3	2	2	1.000000	0.500000	6	4	4	2	0.400000	0.400000
4	3	3	2	0.750000	0.750000	6	4	4	3	0.933333	0.533333
4	3	3	3	1.000000	0.250000	6	4	4	4	1.000000	0.066667
5	1	1	0	0.800000	0.800000	6	5	1	0	0.166667	0.166667
5	1	1	1	1.000000	0.200000	6	5	1	1	1.000000	0.833333
5	2	1	0	0.600000	0.600000	6	5	2	1	0.333333	0.333333
5	2	1	1	1.000000	0.400000	6	5	2	2	1.000000	0.666667
5	2	2	0	0.300000	0.300000	6	5	3	2	0.500000	0.500000
5	2	2	1	0.900000	0.600000	6	5	3	3	1.000000	0.500000
5	2	2	2	1.000000	0.100000	6	5	4	3	0.666667	0.666667
5	3	1	0	0.400000	0.400000	6	5	4	4	1.000000	0.333333
5	3	1	1	1.000000	0.600000	6	5	5	4	0.833333	0.833333
5	3	2	0	0.100000	0.100000	6	5	5	5	1.000000	0.166667
5	3	2	1	0.700000	0.600000	7	1	1	0	0.857143	0.857143
5	3	2	2	1.000000	0.300000	7	1	1	1	1.000000	0.142857
5	3	3	1	0.300000	0.300000	7	2	1	0	0.714286	0.714286
5	3	3	2	0.900000	0.600000	7	2	1	1	1.000000	0.285714
5	3	3	3	1.000000	0.100000	7	2	2	0	0.476190	0.476190
5	4	1	0	0.200000	0.200000	7	2	2	1	0.952381	0.476190
5	4	1	1	1.000000	0.800000	7	2	2	2	1.000000	0.047619
5	4	2	1	0.400000	0.400000	7	3	1	0	0.571429	0.571429
5	4	2	2	0.000000	0.600000	7	3	1	1	1.000000	0.428571
5	4	3	2	0.600000	0.600000	7	3	2	0	0.285714	0.285714
5	4	3	3	1.000000	0.400000	7	3	2	1	0.857143	0.571429
5	4	4	3	0.800000	0.800000	7	3	2	2	1.000000	0.142857
5	4	4	4	1.000000	0.200000	7	3	3	0	0.114286	0.114286
6	1	1	0	0.833333	0.833333	7	3	3	1	0.628571	0.514286
6	1	1	1	1.000000	0.166667	7	3	3	2	0.971428	0.342857
6	2	1	0	0.666667	0.666667	7	3	3	3	1.000000	0.028571
6	2	1	1	1.000000	0.333333	7	4	1	0	0.428571	0.428571
6	2	2	0	0.400000	0.400000	7	4	1	1	1.000000	0.571429
6	2	2	1	0.933333	0.533333	7	4	2	0	0.142857	0.142857

HYPERGEOMETRIC PROBABILITY AND DISTRIBUTION FUNCTIONS

N	n	k	x	$F(x)$	$f(x)$	N	n	k	x	$F(x)$	$f(x)$
7	4	2	1	0.714286	0.571429	8	3	3	2	0.982143	0.267857
7	4	2	2	1.000000	0.285714	8	3	3	3	1.000000	0.017857
7	4	3	0	0.028571	0.028571	8	4	1	0	0.500000	0.500000
7	4	3	1	0.371429	0.342857	8	4	1	1	1.000000	0.500000
7	4	3	2	0.885714	0.514286	8	4	2	0	0.214286	0.214286
7	4	3	3	1.000000	0.114286	8	4	2	1	0.785714	0.571429
7	4	4	1	0.114286	0.114286	8	4	2	2	1.000000	0.214286
7	4	4	2	0.628571	0.514286	8	4	3	0	0.071429	0.071429
7	4	4	3	0.971428	0.342857	8	4	3	1	0.500000	0.428571
7	4	4	4	1.000000	0.028571	8	4	3	2	0.928571	0.428571
7	5	1	0	0.285714	0.285714	8	4	3	3	1.000000	0.071429
7	5	1	1	1.000000	0.714286	8	4	4	0	0.014286	0.014286
7	5	2	0	0.047619	0.047619	8	4	4	1	0.242857	0.228571
7	5	2	1	0.523809	0.476190	8	4	4	2	0.757143	0.514286
7	5	2	2	1.000000	0.476190	8	4	4	3	0.985714	0.228571
7	5	3	1	0.142857	0.142857	8	4	4	4	1.000000	0.014286
7	5	3	2	0.714286	0.571429	8	5	1	0	0.375000	0.375000
7	5	3	3	1.000000	0.285714	8	5	1	1	1.000000	0.625000
7	5	4	2	0.285714	0.285714	8	5	2	0	0.107143	0.107143
7	5	4	3	0.857143	0.571429	8	5	2	1	0.642857	0.535714
7	5	4	4	1.000000	0.142857	8	5	2	2	1.000000	0.357143
7	5	5	3	0.476190	0.476190	8	5	3	0	0.017857	0.017857
7	5	5	4	0.952381	0.476190	8	5	3	1	0.285714	0.267857
7	5	5	5	1.000000	0.047619	8	5	3	2	0.821429	0.535714
7	6	1	0	0.142857	0.142857	8	5	3	3	1.000000	0.178571
7	6	1	1	1.000000	0.857143	8	5	4	1	0.071429	0.071429
7	6	2	1	0.285714	0.285714	8	5	4	2	0.500000	0.428571
7	6	2	2	1.000000	0.714286	8	5	4	3	0.928571	0.428571
7	6	3	2	0.428571	0.428571	8	5	4	4	1.000000	0.071429
7	6	3	3	1.000000	0.571429	8	5	5	2	0.178571	0.178571
7	6	4	3	0.571429	0.571429	8	5	5	3	0.714286	0.535714
7	6	4	4	1.000000	0.428571	8	5	5	4	0.982143	0.267857
7	6	5	4	0.714286	0.714286	8	5	5	5	1.000000	0.017857
7	6	5	5	1.000000	0.285714	8	6	1	0	0.250000	0.250000
7	6	6	5	0.857143	0.857143	8	6	1	1	1.000000	0.750000
7	6	6	6	1.000000	0.142857	8	6	2	0	0.035714	0.035714
8	1	1	0	0.875000	0.875000	8	6	2	1	0.464286	0.428571
8	1	1	1	1.000000	0.125000	8	6	2	2	1.000000	0.535714
8	2	1	0	0.750000	0.750000	8	6	3	1	0.107143	0.107143
8	2	1	1	1.000000	0.250000	8	6	3	2	0.642857	0.535714
8	2	2	0	0.535714	0.535714	8	6	3	3	1.000000	0.357143
8	2	2	1	0.964286	0.428571	8	6	4	2	0.214286	0.214286
8	2	2	2	1.000000	0.035714	8	6	4	3	0.785714	0.571429
8	3	1	0	0.625000	0.625000	8	6	4	4	1.000000	0.214286
8	3	1	1	1.000000	0.375000	8	6	5	3	0.357143	0.357143
8	3	2	0	0.357143	0.357143	8	6	5	4	0.892857	0.535714
8	3	2	1	0.892857	0.535714	8	6	5	5	1.000000	0.107143
8	3	2	2	1.000000	0.107143	8	6	6	4	0.535714	0.535714
8	3	3	0	0.178571	0.178571	8	6	6	5	0.964286	0.428571
8	3	3	1	0.714286	0.535714	8	6	6	6	1.000000	0.035714

HYPERGEOMETRIC PROBABILITY AND DISTRIBUTION FUNCTIONS

N	n	k	x	$F(x)$	$f(x)$	N	n	k	x	$F(x)$	$f(x)$
8	7	1	0	0.125000	0.125000	9	5	3	1	0.404762	0.357143
8	7	1	1	1.000000	0.875000	9	5	3	2	0.880952	0.476190
8	7	2	1	0.250000	0.250000	9	5	3	3	1.000000	0.119048
8	7	2	2	1.000000	0.750000	9	5	4	0	0.007936	0.007936
8	7	3	2	0.375000	0.375000	9	5	4	1	0.166667	0.158730
8	7	3	3	1.000000	0.625000	9	5	4	2	0.642857	0.476190
8	7	4	3	0.500000	0.500000	9	5	4	3	0.960317	0.317460
8	7	4	4	1.000000	0.500000	9	5	4	4	1.000000	0.039683
8	7	5	4	0.625000	0.625000	9	5	5	1	0.039683	0.039683
8	7	5	5	1.000000	0.375000	9	5	5	2	0.357143	0.317460
8	7	6	5	0.750000	0.750000	9	5	5	3	0.833333	0.476190
8	7	6	6	1.000000	0.250000	9	5	5	4	0.992063	0.158730
8	7	7	6	0.875000	0.875000	9	5	5	5	1.000000	0.007936
8	7	7	7	1.000000	0.125000	9	6	1	0	0.333333	0.333333
9	1	1	0	0.888889	0.888889	9	6	1	1	1.000000	0.666667
9	1	1	1	1.000000	0.111111	9	6	2	0	0.083333	0.083333
9	2	1	0	0.777778	0.777778	9	6	2	1	0.583333	0.500000
9	2	1	1	1.000000	0.222222	9	6	2	2	1.000000	0.416667
9	2	2	0	0.583333	0.583333	9	6	3	0	0.011905	0.011905
9	2	2	1	0.972222	0.388889	9	6	3	1	0.226190	0.214286
9	2	2	2	1.000000	0.027778	9	6	3	2	0.761905	0.535714
9	3	1	0	0.666667	0.666667	9	6	3	3	1.000000	0.238095
9	3	1	1	1.000000	0.333333	9	6	4	1	0.047619	0.047619
9	3	2	0	0.416667	0.416667	9	6	4	2	0.404762	0.357143
9	3	2	1	0.916667	0.500000	9	6	4	3	0.880952	0.476190
9	3	2	2	1.000000	0.083333	9	6	4	4	1.000000	0.119048
9	3	3	0	0.238095	0.238095	9	6	5	2	0.119048	0.119048
9	3	3	1	0.773809	0.535714	9	6	5	3	0.595238	0.476190
9	3	3	2	0.988095	0.214286	9	6	5	4	0.952381	0.357143
9	3	3	3	1.000000	0.011905	9	6	5	5	1.000000	0.047619
9	4	1	0	0.555556	0.555556	9	6	6	3	0.238095	0.238095
9	4	1	1	1.000000	0.444444	9	6	6	4	0.773809	0.535714
9	4	2	0	0.277778	0.277778	9	6	6	5	0.988095	0.214286
9	4	2	1	0.833333	0.555556	9	6	6	6	1.000000	0.011905
9	4	2	2	1.000000	0.166667	9	7	1	0	0.222222	0.222222
9	4	3	0	0.119048	0.119048	9	7	1	1	1.000000	0.777778
9	4	3	1	0.595238	0.476190	9	7	2	0	0.027778	0.027778
9	4	3	2	0.952381	0.357143	9	7	2	1	0.416667	0.388889
9	4	3	3	1.000000	0.047619	9	7	2	2	1.000000	0.583333
9	4	4	0	0.039683	0.039683	9	7	3	1	0.083333	0.083333
9	4	4	1	0.357143	0.317460	9	7	3	2	0.583333	0.500000
9	4	4	2	0.833333	0.476190	9	7	3	3	1.000000	0.416667
9	4	4	3	0.992063	0.158730	9	7	4	2	0.166667	0.166667
9	4	4	4	1.000000	0.007936	9	7	4	3	0.722222	0.555556
9	5	1	0	0.444444	0.444444	9	7	4	4	1.000000	0.277778
9	5	1	1	1.000000	0.555556	9	7	5	3	0.277778	0.277778
9	5	2	0	0.166667	0.166667	9	7	5	4	0.833333	0.555556
9	5	2	1	0.722222	0.555556	9	7	5	5	1.000000	0.166667
9	5	2	2	1.000000	0.277778	9	7	6	4	0.416667	0.416667
9	5	3	0	0.047619	0.047619	9	7	6	5	0.916667	0.500000

HYPERGEOMETRIC PROBABILITY AND DISTRIBUTION FUNCTIONS

N	n	k	x	F(x)	f(x)	N	n	k	x	F(x)	f(x)
9	7	6	6	1.000000	0.083333	10	5	1	0	0.500000	0.500000
9	7	7	5	0.583333	0.583333	10	5	1	1	1.000000	0.500000
9	7	7	6	0.972222	0.388889	10	5	2	0	0.222222	0.222222
9	7	7	7	1.000000	0.027778	10	5	2	1	0.777778	0.555556
9	8	1	0	0.111111	0.111111	10	5	2	2	1.000000	0.222222
9	8	1	1	1.000000	0.888889	10	5	3	0	0.083333	0.083333
9	8	2	1	0.222222	0.222222	10	5	3	1	0.500000	0.416667
9	8	2	2	1.000000	0.777778	10	5	3	2	0.916667	0.416667
9	8	3	2	0.333333	0.333333	10	5	3	3	1.000000	0.083333
9	8	3	3	1.000000	0.666667	10	5	4	0	0.023810	0.023810
9	8	4	3	0.444444	0.444444	10	5	4	1	0.261905	0.238095
9	8	4	4	1.000000	0.555556	10	5	4	2	0.738095	0.476190
9	8	5	4	0.555556	0.555556	10	5	4	3	0.976190	0.238095
9	8	5	5	1.000000	0.444444	10	5	4	4	1.000000	0.023810
9	8	6	5	0.666667	0.666667	10	5	5	0	0.003968	0.003968
9	8	6	6	1.000000	0.333333	10	5	5	1	0.103175	0.099206
9	8	7	6	0.777778	0.777778	10	5	5	2	0.500000	0.396825
9	8	7	7	1.000000	0.222222	10	5	5	3	0.896825	0.396825
9	8	8	7	0.888889	0.888889	10	5	5	4	0.996032	0.099206
9	8	8	8	1.000000	0.111111	10	5	5	5	1.000000	0.003968
10	1	1	0	0.900000	0.900000	10	6	1	0	0.400000	0.400000
10	1	1	1	1.000000	0.100000	10	6	1	1	1.000000	0.600000
10	2	1	0	0.800000	0.800000	10	6	2	0	0.133333	0.133333
10	2	1	1	1.000000	0.200000	10	6	2	1	0.666667	0.533333
10	2	2	0	0.622222	0.622222	10	6	2	2	1.000000	0.333333
10	2	2	1	0.977778	0.355556	10	6	3	0	0.033333	0.033333
10	2	2	2	1.000000	0.022222	10	6	3	1	0.333333	0.300000
10	3	1	0	0.700000	0.700000	10	6	3	2	0.833333	0.500000
10	3	1	1	1.000000	0.300000	10	6	3	3	1.000000	0.166667
10	3	2	0	0.466667	0.466667	10	6	4	0	0.004762	0.004762
10	3	2	1	0.933333	0.466667	10	6	4	1	0.119048	0.114286
10	3	2	2	1.000000	0.066667	10	6	4	2	0.547619	0.428571
10	3	3	0	0.291667	0.291667	10	6	4	3	0.928571	0.380952
10	3	3	1	0.816667	0.525000	10	6	4	4	1.000000	0.071429
10	3	3	2	0.991667	0.175000	10	6	5	1	0.023810	0.023810
10	3	3	3	1.000000	0.008333	10	6	5	2	0.261905	0.238095
10	4	1	0	0.600000	0.600000	10	6	5	3	0.738095	0.476190
10	4	1	1	1.000000	0.400000	10	6	5	4	0.976190	0.238095
10	4	2	0	0.333333	0.333333	10	6	5	5	1.000000	0.023810
10	4	2	1	0.866667	0.533333	10	6	6	2	0.071429	0.071429
10	4	2	2	1.000000	0.133333	10	6	6	3	0.452381	0.380952
10	4	3	0	0.166667	0.166667	10	6	6	4	0.880952	0.428571
10	4	3	1	0.666667	0.500000	10	6	6	5	0.995238	0.114286
10	4	3	2	0.966667	0.300000	10	6	6	6	1.000000	0.004762
10	4	3	3	1.000000	0.033333	10	7	1	0	0.300000	0.300000
10	4	4	0	0.071429	0.071429	10	7	1	1	1.000000	0.700000
10	4	4	1	0.452381	0.380952	10	7	2	0	0.066667	0.066667
10	4	4	2	0.880952	0.428571	10	7	2	1	0.533333	0.466667
10	4	4	3	0.995238	0.114286	10	7	2	2	1.000000	0.466667
10	4	4	4	1.000000	0.004762	10	7	3	0	0.008333	0.008333

III.6 TESTS OF SIGNIFICANCE IN 2 × 2 CONTINGENCY TABLES

Suppose that N elements are categorized as 1 or 2 and simultaneously as I or II. The 2 × 2 contingency table in standard form is represented by

	I	II	Totals
1	a	$A - a$	A
2	b	$B - b$	B
Totals	r	$N - r$	N

The probability of a given configuration, given fixed marginal totals is

$$f(a|r,A,B) = \frac{A!B!r!(N-r)!}{a!b!(A-a)!(B-b)!N!}.$$

This table is designed to provide a significance test for the discrepancy of observed from expected frequencies. The table shows, in bold type, for given a, A, and B, the highest value of $b(<a)$ which is just significant at the significance levels .05, .025, .01, .005.

Rules to follow in using the table:

(i) Category 1 in the sense of the 2 × 2 table is that for which $A \geq B$.

(ii) $\frac{a}{A} \geq \frac{b}{B}$ (or $aB \geq bA$)

(iii) If b is less than or equal to the integer in bold type, $\frac{a}{A}$ is significantly greater than $\frac{b}{B}$ (single-tail test) at the probability level indicated by the column heading. For a double-tail test, if b is less than or equal to the integer in bold type, $\frac{a}{A}$ is significantly different from $\frac{b}{B}$ at a probability level equal to twice that indicated by the column heading.

(iv) A dash for some combination of A, B, and a indicates that no 2 × 2 table in that class can show a significant effect at that level.

(v) The true probability that, for given r, b will be less than or equal to the integer in bold type, is shown in small type following an entry.

TESTS OF SIGNIFICANCE IN A 2 × 2 CONTINGENCY TABLE

	a	Probability			
		0.05	0.025	0.01	0.005
$A = 3\ B = 3$	3	0.050	—	—	—
$A = 4\ B = 4$	4	0.014	0.014	—	—
3	4	0.029	—	—	—
$A = 5\ B = 5$	5	1.024	1.024	0.004	0.004
	4	0.024	0.024	—	—
4	5	1.048	0.008	0.008	—
	4	0.040	—	—	—
3	5	0.018	0.018	—	—
2	5	0.048	—	—	—
$A = 6\ B = 6$	6	2.030	1.008	1.008	0.001
	5	1.040	0.008	0.008	—
	4	0.030	—	—	—
5	6	1.015+	0.015+	0.002	0.002
	5	0.013	0.013	—	—
	4	0.045+	—	—	—
4	6	1.033	0.005−	0.005−	0.005−
	5	0.024	0.024	—	—
3	6	0.012	0.012	—	—
	5	0.048	—	—	—
2	6	0.036	—	—	—
$A = 7\ B = 7$	7	3.035−	2.010+	1.002	1.002
	6	1.015−	1.015−	0.002	0.002
	5	0.010+	0.010+	—	—
	4	0.035−	—	—	—
6	7	2.021	2.021	1.005−	1.005−
	6	1.025+	0.004	0.004	0.004
	5	0.016	0.016	—	—
	4	0.049	—	—	—
5	7	2.045+	1.010+	0.001	0.001
	6	1.045+	0.008	0.008	—
	5	0.027	—	—	—
4	7	1.024	1.024	0.003	0.003
	6	0.015+	0.015+	—	—
	5	0.045+	—	—	—
3	7	0.008	0.008	0.008	—
	6	0.033	—	—	—
2	7	0.028	—	—	—
$A = 8\ B = 8$	8	4.038	3.013	2.003	2.003
	7	2.020	2.020	1.005+	0.001
	6	1.020	1.020	0.003	0.003
	5	0.013	0.013	—	—
	4	0.038	—	—	—
7	8	3.026	2.007	2.007	1.001
	7	2.035−	1.009	1.009	0.001
	6	1.032	0.006	0.006	—
	5	0.019	0.019	—	—
6	8	2.015−	2.015−	1.003	1.003
	7	1.016	1.016	0.002	0.002
	6	0.009	0.009	0.009	—
	5	0.028	—	—	—
5	8	2.035−	1.007	1.007	0.001
	7	1.032	0.005−	0.005−	0.005−

	a	Probability			
		0.05	0.025	0.01	0.005
$A = 8\ B = 5$	6	0.016	0.016	—	—
	5	0.044	—	—	—
4	8	1.018	1.018	0.002	0.002
	7	0.010+	0.010+	—	—
	6	0.030	—	—	—
3	8	0.006	0.006	0.006	—
	7	0.024	0.024	—	—
2	8	0.022	0.022	—	—
$A = 9\ B = 9$	9	5.041	4.015−	3.005−	3.005−
	8	3.025−	3.025−	2.008	1.002
	7	2.028	1.008	1.008	0.001
	6	1.025−	1.025−	0.005−	0.005−
	5	0.015−	0.015−	—	—
	4	0.041	—	—	—
8	9	4.029	3.009	3.009	2.002
	8	3.043	2.013	1.003	1.003
	7	2.044	1.012	0.002	0.002
	6	1.036	0.007	0.007	—
	5	0.020	0.020	—	—
7	9	3.019	3.019	2.005−	2.005−
	8	2.024	2.024	1.006	0.001
	7	1.020	1.020	0.003	0.003
	6	0.010+	0.010+	—	—
	5	0.029	—	—	—
6	9	3.044	2.011	1.002	1.002
	8	2.047	1.011	0.001	0.001
	7	1.035−	0.006	0.006	—
	6	0.017	0.017	—	—
	5	0.042	—	—	—
5	9	2.027	1.005−	1.005−	1.005−
	8	1.023	1.023	0.003	0.003
	7	0.010+	0.010+	—	—
	6	0.028	—	—	—
4	9	1.014	1.014	0.001	0.001
	8	0.007	0.007	0.007	—
	7	0.021	0.021	—	—
	6	0.049	—	—	—
3	9	1.045+	0.005−	0.005−	0.005−
	8	0.018	0.018	—	—
	7	0.045+	—	—	—
2	9	0.018	0.018	—	—
$A = 10\ B = 10$	10	6.043	5.016	4.005+	3.002
	9	4.029	3.010−	3.010−	2.003
	8	3.035−	2.012	1.003	1.003
	7	2.035−	1.010−	1.010−	0.002
	6	1.029	0.005+	0.005+	—
	5	0.016	0.016	—	—
	4	0.043	—	—	—
9	10	5.033	4.011	3.003	3.003
	9	4.050−	3.017	2.005−	2.005−
	8	2.019	2.019	1.004	1.004
	7	1.015−	1.015−	0.002	0.002
	6	1.040	0.008	0.008	—
	5	0.022	0.022	—	—

TESTS OF SIGNIFICANCE IN A 2 × 2 CONTINGENCY TABLE

	a	Probability 0.05	0.025	0.01	0.005
A = 10 *B* = 8	10	4.023	4.023	3.007	2.002
	9	3.032	2.009	2.009	1.002
	8	2.031	1.008	1.008	0.001
	7	1.023	1.023	0.004	0.004
	6	0.011	0.011	—	—
	5	0.029	—	—	—
7	10	3.015−	3.015−	2.003	2.003
	9	2.018	2.018	1.004	1.004
	8	1.013	1.013	0.002	0.002
	7	1.036	0.006	0.006	—
	6	0.017	0.017	—	—
	5	0.041	—	—	—
6	10	3.036	2.008	2.008	1.001
	9	2.036	1.008	1.008	0.001
	8	1.024	1.024	0.003	0.003
	7	0.010+	0.010+	—	—
	6	0.026	—	—	—
5	10	2.022	2.022	1.004	1.004
	9	1.017	1.017	0.002	0.002
	8	1.047	0.007	0.007	—
	7	0.019	0.019	—	—
	6	0.042	—	—	—
4	10	1.011	1.011	0.001	0.001
	9	1.041	0.005−	0.005−	0.005−
	8	0.015−	0.015−	—	—
	7	0.035−	—	—	—
3	10	1.038	0.003	0.003	0.003
	9	0.014	0.014	—	—
	8	0.035−	—	—	—
2	10	0.015+	0.015+	—	—
	9	0.045+	—	—	—
A = 11 *B* = 11	11	7.045+	6.018	5.006	4.002
	10	5.032	4.012	3.004	3.004
	9	4.040	3.015−	2.004	2.004
	8	3.043	2.015−	1.004	1.004
	7	2.040	1.012	0.002	0.002
	6	1.032	0.006	0.006	—
	5	0.018	0.018	—	—
	4	0.045+	—	—	—
10	11	6.035+	5.012	4.004	4.004
	10	4.021	4.021	3.007	2.002
	9	3.024	3.024	2.007	1.002
	8	2.023	2.023	1.006	0.001
	7	1.017	1.017	0.003	0.003
	6	1.043	0.009	0.009	—
	5	0.023	0.023	—	—
9	11	5.026	4.008	4.008	3.002
	10	4.038	3.012	2.003	2.003
	9	3.040	2.012	1.003	1.003
	8	2.035−	1.009	1.009	0.001
	7	1.025−	1.025−	0.004	0.004
	6	0.012	0.012	—	—
	5	0.030	—	—	—
8	11	4.018	4.018	3.005−	3.005−
	10	3.024	3.024	2.006	1.001
A = 11 *B* = 8	9	2.022	2.022	1.005−	1.005−
	8	1.015−	1.015−	0.002	0.002
	7	1.037	0.007	0.007	—
	6	0.017	0.017	—	—
	5	0.040	—	—	—
7	11	4.043	3.011	2.002	2.002
	10	3.047	2.013	1.002	1.002
	9	2.039	1.009	1.009	0.001
	8	1.025−	1.025−	0.004	0.004
	7	0.010+	0.010+	—	—
	6	0.025−	0.025−	—	—
6	11	3.029	2.006	2.006	1.001
	10	2.028	1.005+	1.005+	0.001
	9	1.018	1.018	0.002	0.002
	8	1.043	0.007	0.007	—
	7	0.017	0.017	—	—
	6	0.037	—	—	—
5	11	2.018	2.018	1.003	1.003
	10	1.013	1.013	0.001	0.001
	9	1.036	0.005−	0.005−	0.005−
	8	0.013	0.013	—	—
	7	0.029	—	—	—
4	11	1.009	1.009	1.009	0.001
	10	1.033	0.004	0.004	0.004
	9	0.011	0.011	—	—
	8	0.026	—	—	—
3	11	1.033	0.003	0.003	0.003
	10	0.011	0.011	—	—
	9	0.027	—	—	—
2	11	0.013	0.013	—	—
	10	0.038	—	—	—
A = 12 *B* = 12	12	8.047	7.019	6.007	5.002
	11	6.034	5.014	4.005−	4.005−
	10	5.045−	4.018	3.006	2.002
	9	4.050−	3.020	2.006	1.001
	8	3.050−	2.018	1.005−	1.005−
	7	2.045−	1.014	0.002	0.002
	6	1.034	0.007	0.007	—
	5	0.019	0.019	—	—
	4	0.047	—	—	—
11	12	7.037	6.014	5.005−	5.005−
	11	5.024	5.024	4.008	3.002
	10	4.029	3.010+	2.003	2.003
	9	3.030	2.009	2.009	1.002
	8	2.026	1.007	1.007	0.001
	7	1.019	1.019	0.003	0.003
	6	1.045−	0.009	0.009	—
	5	0.024	0.024	—	—
10	12	6.029	5.010−	5.010−	4.003
	11	5.043	4.015+	3.005−	3.005−
	10	4.048	3.017	2.005−	2.005−
	9	3.046	2.015−	1.004	1.004
	8	2.038	1.010+	0.002	0.002
	7	1.026	0.005−	0.005−	0.005−
	6	0.012	0.012	—	—

TESTS OF SIGNIFICANCE IN A 2 × 2 CONTINGENCY TABLE

	a	Probability 0.05	0.025	0.01	0.005
A = 12 B = 10	5	0.030	—	—	—
9	12	5.021	5.021	4.006	3.002
	11	4.029	3.009	3.009	2.002
	10	3.029	2.008	2.008	1.002
	9	2.024	2.024	1.006	0.001
	8	1.016	1.016	0.002	0.002
	7	1.037	0.007	0.007	—
	6	0.017	0.017	—	—
	5	0.039	—	—	—
8	12	5.049	4.014	3.004	3.004
	11	3.018	3.018	2.004	2.004
	10	2.015+	2.015+	1.003	1.003
	9	2.040	1.010−	1.010−	0.001
	8	1.025−	1.025−	0.004	0.004
	7	0.010+	0.010+	—	—
	6	0.024	0.024	—	—
7	12	4.036	3.009	3.009	2.002
	11	3.038	2.010−	2.010−	1.002
	10	2.029	1.006	1.006	0.001
	9	1.017	1.017	0.002	0.002
	8	1.040	0.007	0.007	—
	7	0.016	0.016	—	—
	6	0.034	—	—	—
6	12	3.025−	3.025−	2.005−	2.005−
	11	2.022	2.022	1.004	1.004
	10	1.013	1.013	0.002	0.002
	9	1.032	0.005−	0.005−	0.005−
	8	0.011	0.011	—	—
	7	0.025−	0.025−	—	—
	6	0.050−	—	—	—
5	12	2.015−	2.015−	1.002	1.002
	11	1.010−	1.010−	1.010−	0.001
	10	1.028	0.003	0.003	0.003
	9	0.009	0.009	0.009	—
	8	0.020	0.020	—	—
	7	0.041	—	—	—
4	12	2.050	1.007	1.007	0.001
	11	1.027	0.003	0.003	0.003
	10	0.008	0.008	0.008	—
	9	0.019	0.019	—	—
	8	0.038	—	—	—
3	12	1.029	0.002	0.002	0.002
	11	0.009	0.009	0.009	—
	10	0.022	0.022	—	—
	9	0.044	—	—	—
2	12	0.011	0.011	—	—
	11	0.033	—	—	—
A = 13 B = 13	13	9.048	8.020	7.007	6.003
	12	7.037	6.015+	5.006	4.002
	11	6.048	5.021	4.008	3.002
	10	4.024	4.024	3.008	2.002
	9	3.024	3.024	2.008	1.002
	8	2.021	2.021	1.006	0.001
	7	2.048	1.015+	0.003	0.003
	6	1.037	0.007	0.007	—
A = 13 B = 13	5	0.020	0.020	—	—
	4	0.048	—	—	—
12	13	8.039	7.015−	6.005+	5.002
	12	6.027	5.010−	5.010−	4.003
	11	5.033	4.013	3.004	3.004
	10	4.036	3.013	2.004	2.004
	9	3.034	2.011	1.003	1.003
	8	2.029	1.008	1.008	0.001
	7	1.020	1.020	0.004	0.004
	6	1.046	0.010−	0.010−	—
	5	0.024	0.024	—	—
11	13	7.031	6.011	5.003	5.003
	12	6.048	5.018	4.006	3.002
	11	4.021	4.021	3.007	2.002
	10	3.021	3.021	2.006	1.001
	9	3.050−	2.017	1.004	1.004
	8	2.040	1.011	0.002	0.002
	7	1.027	0.005−	0.005−	0.005−
	6	0.013	0.013	—	—
	5	0.030	—	—	—
10	13	6.024	6.024	5.007	4.002
	12	5.035−	4.012	3.003	3.003
	11	4.037	3.012	2.003	2.003
	10	3.033	2.010+	1.002	1.002
	9	2.026	1.006	1.006	0.001
	8	1.017	1.017	0.003	0.003
	7	1.038	0.007	0.007	—
	6	0.017	0.017	—	—
	5	0.038	—	—	—
9	13	5.017	5.017	4.005−	4.005−
	12	4.023	4.023	3.007	2.001
	11	3.022	3.022	2.006	1.001
	10	2.017	2.017	1.004	1.004
	9	2.040	1.010+	0.001	0.001
	8	1.025−	1.025−	0.004	0.004
	7	0.010+	0.010+	—	—
	6	0.023	0.023	—	—
	5	0.049	—	—	—
8	13	5.042	4.012	3.003	3.003
	12	4.047	3.014	2.003	2.003
	11	3.041	2.011	1.002	1.002
	10	2.029	1.007	1.007	0.001
	9	1.017	1.017	0.002	0.002
	8	1.037	0.006	0.006	—
	7	0.015−	0.015−	—	—
	6	0.032	—	—	—
7	13	4.031	3.007	3.007	2.001
	12	3.031	2.007	2.007	1.001
	11	2.022	2.022	1.004	1.004
	10	1.012	1.012	0.002	0.002
	9	1.029	0.004	0.004	0.004
	8	0.010+	0.010+	—	—
	7	0.022	0.022	—	—
	6	0.044	—	—	—
6	13	3.021	3.021	2.004	2.004

TESTS OF SIGNIFICANCE IN A 2 × 2 CONTINGENCY TABLE

	a	Probability 0.05	0.025	0.01	0.005
$A = 13$ $B = 6$	12	2.017	2.017	1.003	1.003
	11	2.046	1.010−	1.010−	0.001
	10	1.024	1.024	0.003	0.003
	9	1.050−	0.008	0.008	—
	8	0.017	0.017	—	—
	7	0.034	—	—	—
5	13	2.012	2.012	1.002	1.002
	12	2.044	1.008	1.008	0.001
	11	1.022	1.022	0.002	0.002
	10	1.047	0.007	0.007	—
	9	0.015−	0.015−	—	—
	8	0.029	—	—	—
4	13	2.044	1.006	1.006	0.000
	12	1.022	1.022	0.002	0.002
	11	0.006	0.006	0.006	—
	10	0.015−	0.015−	—	—
	9	0.029	—	—	—
3	13	1.025	1.025	0.002	0.002
	12	0.007	0.007	0.007	—
	11	0.018	0.018	—	—
	10	0.036	—	—	—
2	13	0.010−	0.010−	0.010−	—
	12	0.029	—	—	—
$A = 14$ $B = 14$	14	10.049	9.020	8.008	7.003
	13	8.038	7.016	6.006	5.002
	12	6.023	6.023	5.009	4.003
	11	5.027	4.011	3.004	3.004
	10	4.028	3.011	2.003	2.003
	9	3.027	2.009	2.009	1.002
	8	2.023	2.023	1.006	0.001
	7	1.016	1.016	0.003	0.003
	6	1.038	0.008	0.008	—
	5	0.020	0.020	—	—
	4	0.049	—	—	—
13	14	9.041	8.016	7.006	6.002
	13	7.029	6.011	5.004	5.004
	12	6.037	5.015+	4.005+	3.002
	11	5.041	4.017	3.006	2.001
	10	4.041	3.016	2.005−	2.005−
	9	3.038	2.013	1.003	1.003
	8	2.031	1.009	1.009	0.001
	7	1.021	1.021	0.004	0.004
	6	1.048	0.010+	—	—
	5	0.025−	0.025−	—	—
12	14	8.033	7.012	6.004	6.004
	13	6.021	6.021	5.007	4.002
	12	5.025+	4.009	4.009	3.003
	11	4.026	3.009	3.009	2.002
	10	3.024	3.024	2.007	1.002
	9	2.019	2.019	1.005−	1.005−
	8	2.042	1.012	0.002	0.002
	7	1.028	0.005+	0.005+	—
	6	0.013	0.013	—	—
	5	0.030	—	—	—
11	14	7.026	6.009	6.009	5.003

	a	Probability 0.05	0.025	0.01	0.005
$A = 14$ $B = 11$	13	6.039	5.014	4.004	4.004
	12	5.043	4.016	3.005−	3.005−
	11	4.042	3.015−	2.004	2.004
	10	3.036	2.011	1.003	1.003
	9	2.027	1.007	1.007	0.001
	8	1.017	1.017	0.003	0.003
	7	1.038	0.007	0.007	—
	6	0.017	0.017	—	—
	5	0.038	—	—	—
10	14	6.020	6.020	5.006	4.002
	13	5.028	4.009	4.009	3.002
	12	4.028	3.009	3.009	2.002
	11	3.024	3.024	2.007	1.001
	10	2.018	2.018	1.004	1.004
	9	2.040	1.011	0.002	0.002
	8	1.024	1.024	0.004	0.004
	7	0.010−	0.010−	0.010−	—
	6	0.022	0.022	—	—
	5	0.047	—	—	—
9	14	6.047	5.014	4.004	4.004
	13	4.018	4.018	3.005−	3.005−
	12	3.017	3.017	2.004	2.004
	11	3.042	2.012	1.002	1.002
	10	2.029	1.007	1.007	0.001
	9	1.017	1.017	0.002	0.002
	8	1.036	0.006	0.006	—
	7	0.014	0.014	—	—
	6	0.030	—	—	—
8	14	5.036	4.010−	4.010−	3.002
	13	4.039	3.011	2.002	2.002
	12	3.032	2.008	2.008	1.001
	11	2.022	2.022	1.005−	1.005−
	10	2.048	1.012	0.002	0.002
	9	1.026	0.004	0.004	0.004
	8	0.009	0.009	0.009	—
	7	0.020	0.020	—	—
	6	0.040	—	—	—
7	14	4.026	3.006	3.006	2.001
	13	3.025	2.006	2.006	1.001
	12	2.017	2.017	1.003	1.003
	11	2.041	1.009	1.009	0.001
	10	1.021	1.021	0.003	0.003
	9	1.043	0.007	0.007	—
	8	0.015−	0.015−	—	—
	7	0.030	—	—	—
6	14	3.018	3.018	2.003	2.003
	13	2.014	2.014	1.002	1.002
	12	2.037	1.007	1.007	0.001
	11	1.018	1.018	0.002	0.002
	10	1.038	0.005+	0.005+	—
	9	0.012	0.012	—	—
	8	0.024	0.024	—	—
	7	0.044	—	—	—
5	14	2.010+	2.010+	1.001	1.001
	13	2.037	1.006	1.006	0.001

TESTS OF SIGNIFICANCE IN A 2 × 2 CONTINGENCY TABLE

	a	Probability			
		0.05	0.025	0.01	0.005
A = 14 B = 5	12	1.017	1.017	0.002	0.002
	11	1.038	0.005−	0.005−	0.005−
	10	0.011	0.011	—	—
	9	0.022	0.022	—	—
	8	0.040	—	—	—
4	14	2.039	1.005−	1.005−	1.005−
	13	1.019	1.019	0.002	0.002
	12	1.044	0.005−	0.005−	0.005−
	11	0.011	0.011	—	—
	10	0.023	0.023	—	—
	9	0.041	—	—	—
3	14	1.022	1.022	0.001	0.001
	13	0.006	0.006	0.006	—
	12	0.015−	0.015−	—	—
	11	0.029	—	—	—
2	14	0.008	0.008	0.008	—
	13	0.025	0.025	—	—
	12	0.050	—	—	—
A = 15 B = 15	15	11.050−	10.021	9.008	8.003
	14	9.040	8.018	7.007	6.003
	13	7.025+	6.010+	5.004	5.004
	12	6.030	5.013	4.005−	4.005−
	11	5.033	4.013	3.005−	3.005−
	10	4.033	3.013	2.004	2.004
	9	3.030	2.010+	1.003	1.003
	8	2.025+	1.007	1.007	0.001
	7	1.018	1.018	0.003	0.003
	6	1.040	0.008	0.008	—
	5	0.021	0.021	—	—
	4	0.050−	—	—	—
14	15	10.042	9.017	8.006	7.002
	14	8.031	7.013	6.005−	6.005−
	13	7.041	6.017	5.007	4.002
	12	6.046	5.020	4.007	3.002
	11	5.048	4.020	3.007	2.002
	10	4.046	3.018	2.006	1.001
	9	3.041	2.014	1.004	1.004
	8	2.033	1.009	1.009	0.001
	7	1.022	1.022	0.004	0.004
	6	1.049	0.011	—	—
	5	0.025+	—	—	—
13	15	9.035−	8.013	7.005−	7.005−
	14	7.023	7.023	6.009	5.003
	13	6.029	5.011	4.004	4.004
	12	5.031	4.012	3.004	3.004
	11	4.030	3.011	2.003	2.003
	10	3.026	2.008	2.008	1.002
	9	2.020	2.020	1.005+	0.001
	8	2.043	1.013	0.002	0.002
	7	1.029	0.005+	0.005+	—
	6	0.013	0.013	—	—
	5	0.031	—	—	—
12	15	8.028	7.010−	7.010−	6.003
	14	7.043	6.016	5.006	4.002
	13	6.049	5.019	4.007	3.002

	a	Probability			
		0.05	0.025	0.01	0.005
A = 15 B = 12	12	5.049	4.019	3.006	2.002
	11	4.045+	3.017	2.005−	2.005−
	10	3.038	2.012	1.003	1.003
	9	2.028	1.007	1.007	0.001
	8	1.018	1.018	0.003	0.003
	7	1.038	0.007	0.007	—
	6	0.017	0.017	—	—
	5	0.037	—	—	—
11	15	7.022	7.022	6.007	5.002
	14	6.032	5.011	4.003	4.003
	13	5.034	4.012	3.003	3.003
	12	4.032	3.010+	2.003	2.003
	11	3.026	2.008	2.008	1.002
	10	2.019	2.019	1.004	1.004
	9	2.040	1.011	0.002	0.002
	8	1.024	1.024	0.004	0.004
	7	1.049	0.010−	0.010−	—
	6	0.022	0.022	—	—
	5	0.046	—	—	—
10	15	6.017	6.017	5.005−	5.005−
	14	5.023	5.023	4.007	3.002
	13	4.022	4.022	3.007	2.001
	12	3.018	3.018	2.005−	2.005−
	11	3.042	2.013	1.003	1.003
	10	2.029	1.007	1.007	0.001
	9	1.016	1.016	0.002	0.002
	8	1.034	0.006	0.006	—
	7	0.013	0.013	—	—
	6	0.028	—	—	—
9	15	6.042	5.012	4.003	4.003
	14	5.047	4.015−	3.004	3.004
	13	4.042	3.013	2.003	2.003
	12	3.032	2.009	2.009	1.002
	11	2.021	2.021	1.005−	1.005−
	10	2.045−	1.011	0.002	0.002
	9	1.024	1.024	0.004	0.004
	8	1.048	0.009	0.009	—
	7	0.019	0.019	—	—
	6	0.037	—	—	—
8	15	5.032	4.008	4.008	3.002
	14	4.033	3.009	3.009	2.002
	13	3.026	2.006	2.006	1.001
	12	2.017	2.017	1.003	1.003
	11	2.037	1.008	1.008	0.001
	10	1.019	1.019	0.003	0.003
	9	1.038	0.006	0.006	—
	8	0.013	0.013	—	—
	7	0.026	—	—	—
	6	0.050−	—	—	—
7	15	4.023	4.023	3.005−	3.005−
	14	3.021	3.021	2.004	2.004
	13	2.014	2.014	1.002	1.002
	12	2.032	1.007	1.007	0.001
	11	1.015+	1.015+	0.002	0.002
	10	1.032	0.005−	0.005−	0.005−

TESTS OF SIGNIFICANCE IN A 2 × 2 CONTINGENCY TABLE

	a	Probability 0.05	0.025	0.01	0.005
$A = 15$ $B = 7$	9	0.010+	0.010+	—	—
	8	0.020	0.020	—	—
	7	0.038	—	—	—
6	15	3.015+	3.015+	2.003	2.003
	14	2.011	2.011	1.002	1.002
	13	2.031	1.006	1.006	0.001
	12	1.014	1.014	0.002	0.002
	11	1.029	0.004	0.004	0.004
	10	0.009	0.009	0.009	—
	9	0.017	0.017	—	—
	8	0.032	—	—	—
5	15	2.009	2.009	2.009	1.001
	14	2.032	1.005−	1.005−	1.005−
	13	1.014	1.014	0.001	0.001
	12	1.031	0.004	0.004	0.004
	11	0.008	0.008	0.008	—
	10	0.016	0.016	—	—
	9	0.030	—	—	—
4	15	2.035+	1.004	1.004	1.004
	14	1.016	1.016	0.001	0.001
	13	1.037	0.004	0.004	0.004
	12	0.009	0.009	0.009	—
	11	0.018	0.018	—	—
	10	0.033	—	—	—
3	15	1.020	1.020	0.001	0.001
	14	0.005−	0.005−	0.005−	0.005−
	13	0.012	0.012	—	—
	12	0.025−	0.025−	—	—
	11	0.043	—	—	—
2	15	0.007	0.007	0.007	—
	14	0.022	0.022	—	—
	13	10.044	—	—	—
$A = 16$ $B = 16$	16	11.022	11.022	10.009	9.003
	15	10.041	9.019	8.008	7.003
	14	8.027	7.012	6.005−	6.005−
	13	7.033	6.015−	5.006	4.002
	12	6.037	5.016	4.006	3.002
	11	5.038	4.016	3.006	2.002
	10	4.037	3.015−	2.005−	2.005−
	9	3.033	2.012	1.003	1.003
	8	2.027	1.008	1.008	0.001
	7	1.019	1.019	0.003	0.003
	6	1.041	0.009	0.009	—
	5	0.022	0.022	—	—
15	16	11.043	10.018	9.007	8.002
	15	9.033	8.014	7.005+	6.002
	14	8.044	7.019	6.008	5.003
	13	6.023	6.023	5.009	4.003
	12	5.024	5.024	4.009	3.003
	11	4.023	4.023	3.008	2.002
	10	4.049	3.020	2.006	1.001
	9	3.043	2.016	1.004	1.004
	8	2.035−	1.010+	0.002	0.002
	7	1.023	1.023	0.004	0.004
	6	0.011	0.011	—	—
$A = 16$ $B = 15$	5	0.026	—	—	—
14	16	10.037	9.014	8.005+	7.002
	15	8.025+	7.010−	7.010−	6.003
	14	7.032	6.013	5.005−	5.005−
	13	6.035+	5.014	4.005+	3.001
	12	5.035+	4.014	3.005−	3.005−
	11	4.033	3.012	2.004	2.004
	10	3.028	2.009	2.009	1.002
	9	2.021	2.021	1.006	0.001
	8	2.015−	1.013	0.002	0.002
	7	1.030	0.006	0.006	—
	6	0.013	0.013	—	—
	5	0.031	—	—	—
13	16	9.030	8.011	7.004	7.004
	15	8.037	7.019	6.007	5.002
	14	6.023	6.023	5.008	4.003
	13	5.023	5.023	4.008	3.003
	12	4.022	4.022	3.007	2.002
	11	4.078	3.018	2.005+	1.001
	10	3.039	2.013	1.003	1.003
	9	2.029	1.008	1.008	0.001
	8	1.018	1.018	0.003	0.003
	7	1.038	0.007	0.007	—
	6	0.017	0.017	—	—
	5	0.033	—	—	—
12	16	8.024	8.024	7.008	6.002
	15	7.036	6.013	5.004	5.004
	14	6.040	5.015−	4.005−	4.005−
	13	5.039	4.014	3.004	3.004
	12	4.034	3.012	2.003	2.003
	11	3.027	2.008	2.008	1.002
	10	2.019	2.019	1.005−	1.005−
	9	2.040	1.011	0.002	0.002
	8	1.024	1.024	0.004	0.004
	7	1.048	0.010−	0.010−	—
	6	0.021	0.021	—	—
	5	0.044	—	—	—
11	16	7.019	7.019	6.005	5.002
	15	6.027	5.009	5.009	4.002
	14	5.027	4.009	4.009	3.002
	13	4.024	4.024	3.008	2.002
	12	3.019	3.019	2.005+	1.001
	11	3.041	2.013	1.003	1.003
	10	2.028	1.007	1.007	0.001
	9	1.016	1.016	0.002	0.002
	8	1.033	0.006	0.066	—
	7	0.013	0.013	—	—
	6	0.027	—	—	—
10	16	7.046	6.014	5.004	5.004
	15	5.018	5.018	4.005+	3.001
	14	4.017	4.017	3.005−	3.005−
	13	4.042	3.014	2.003	2.003
	12	3.032	2.009	2.009	1.002
	11	2.021	2.021	1.005−	1.005−
	10	2.042	1.011	0.002	0.002

TESTS OF SIGNIFICANCE IN A 2 × 2 CONTINGENCY TABLE

	a	Probability 0.05	0.025	0.01	0.005
$A = 16$ $B = 10$	9	1.023	1.023	0.004	0.004
	8	1.045−	0.008	0.008	—
	7	0.017	0.017	—	—
	6	0.035−	—	—	—
9	16	6.037	5.010−	5.010−	4.002
	15	5.040	4.012	3.003	3.003
	14	4.034	3.010−	3.010−	2.002
	13	3.025+	2.007	2.007	1.001
	12	2.016	2.016	1.003	1.003
	11	2.033	1.008	1.008	0.001
	10	1.017	1.017	0.002	0.002
	9	1.034	0.006	0.006	—
	8	0.012	0.012	—	—
	7	0.024	0.024	—	—
	6	0.045+	—	—	—
8	16	5.028	4.007	4.007	3.001
	15	4.028	3.007	3.007	2.001
	14	3.021	3.021	2.005−	2.005−
	13	3.047	2.013	1.002	1.002
	12	2.028	1.006	1.006	0.001
	11	1.014	1.014	0.002	0.002
	10	1.027	0.004	0.004	0.004
	9	0.009	0.009	0.009	—
	8	0.017	0.017	—	—
	7	0.033	—	—	—
7	16	4.020	4.020	3.004	3.004
	15	3.017	3.017	2.003	2.003
	14	3.045+	2.011	1.002	1.002
	13	2.026	1.005−	1.005−	1.005−
	12	1.012	1.012	0.001	0.001
	11	1.024	1.024	0.003	0.003
	10	1.045−	0.007	0.007	—
	9	0.014	0.014	—	—
	8	0.026	—	—	—
	7	0.047	—	—	—
6	16	3.013	3.013	2.002	2.002
	15	3.046	2.009	2.009	1.001
	14	2.025+	1.004	1.004	1.004
	13	1.011	1.011	0.001	0.001
	12	1.023	1.023	0.003	0.003
	11	1.043	0.006	0.006	—
	10	0.012	0.012	—	—
	9	0.023	0.023	—	—
	8	0.040	—	—	—
5	16	3.048	2.008	2.008	1.001
	15	2.028	1.004	1.004	1.004
	14	1.011	1.011	0.001	0.001
	13	1.025+	0.003	0.003	0.003
	12	1.047	0.006	0.006	—
	11	0.012	0.012	—	—
	10	0.023	0.023	—	—
	9	0.039	—	—	—
4	16	2.032	1.004	1.004	1.004
	15	1.013	1.013	0.001	0.001
	14	1.032	0.003	0.003	0.003
$A = 16$ $B = 4$	13	0.007	0.007	0.007	—
	12	0.014	0.014	—	—
	11	0.026	—	—	—
	10	0.043	—	—	—
3	16	1.018	1.018	0.001	0.001
	15	0.004	0.004	0.004	0.004
	14	0.010+	0.010+	—	—
	13	0.021	0.021	—	—
	12	0.036	—	—	—
2	16	0.007	0.007	0.007	—
	15	0.020	0.020	—	—
	14	0.039	—	—	—
$A = 17$ $B = 17$	17	12.022	12.022	11.009	10.004
	16	11.043	10.020	9.008	8.003
	15	9.029	8.013	7.005+	6.002
	14	8.035+	7.016	6.007	5.002
	13	7.040	6.018	5.007	4.003
	12	6.042	5.019	4.007	3.002
	11	5.042	4.018	3.007	2.002
	10	4.040	3.016	2.005+	1.001
	9	3.035+	2.013	1.003	1.003
	8	2.029	1.008	1.008	0.001
	7	1.020	1.020	0.004	0.004
	6	1.043	0.009	0.009	—
	5	0.022	0.022	—	—
16	17	12.044	11.018	10.007	9.003
	16	10.035−	9.015−	8.006	7.002
	15	9.046	8.021	7.009	6.003
	14	7.025+	6.011	5.004	5.004
	13	6.027	5.011	4.004	4.004
	12	5.027	4.011	3.004	3.004
	11	4.025+	3.009	3.009	2.003
	10	3.022	3.022	2.007	1.002
	9	3.046	2.017	1.004	1.004
	8	2.036	1.011	0.002	0.002
	7	1.024	1.024	0.005−	0.005−
	6	0.011	0.011	—	—
	5	0.026	—	—	—
15	17	11.038	10.015−	9.006	8.002
	16	9.027	8.011	7.004	7.004
	15	8.035+	7.015−	6.006	5.002
	14	7.040	6.017	5.006	4.002
	13	6.041	5.017	4.006	3.002
	12	5.039	4.016	3.005+	2.001
	11	4.035+	3.013	2.004	2.004
	10	3.029	2.010−	2.010−	1.002
	9	2.022	2.022	1.006	0.001
	8	2.046	1.014	0.002	0.002
	7	1.030	0.006	0.006	—
	6	0.014	0.014	—	—
	5	0.031	—	—	—
14	17	10.032	9.012	8.004	8.004
	16	8.021	8.021	7.008	6.003
	15	7.026	6.010−	6.010−	5.003
	14	6.028	5.011	4.004	4.004

TESTS OF SIGNIFICANCE IN A 2 × 2 CONTINGENCY TABLE

	a	Probability					a	Probability			
		0.05	0.025	0.01	0.005			0.05	0.025	0.01	0.005
$A = 17$ $B = 14$	13	5.027	4.010−	4.010−	3.003	$A = 17$ $B = 10$	8	0.011	0.011	—	—
	12	4.024	4.024	3.008	2.002		7	0.022	0.022	—	—
	11	4.049	3.019	2.006	1.001		6	0.042	—	—	—
	10	3.040	2.014	1.003	1.003	9	17	6.032	5.008	5.008	4.002
	9	2.029	1.008	1.008	0.001		16	5.034	4.010−	4.010−	3.002
	8	1.018	1.018	0.003	0.003		15	4.028	3.008	3.008	2.002
	7	1.038	0.007	0.007	—		14	3.020	3.020	2.005−	2.005−
	6	0.017	0.017	—	—		13	3.042	2.012	1.002	1.002
	5	0.036	—	—	—		12	2.025+	1.006	1.006	0.001
13	17	9.026	8.009	8.009	7.003		11	2.048	1.012	0.002	0.002
	16	8.040	7.015+	6.005+	5.002		10	1.024	1.024	0.004	0.004
	15	7.045+	6.018	5.006	4.002		9	1.045−	0.008	0.008	—
	14	6.045+	5.018	4.006	3.002		8	0.016	0.016	—	—
	13	5.042	4.016	3.005+	2.001		7	0.030	—	—	—
	12	4.035+	3.013	2.004	2.004	8	17	5.024	5.024	4.006	3.001
	11	3.028	2.009	2.009	1.002		16	4.023	4.023	3.006	2.001
	10	2.019	2.019	1.005−	1.005−		15	3.017	3.017	2.004	2.004
	9	2.040	1.011	0.002	0.002		14	3.039	2.010−	2.010−	1.002
	8	1.024	1.024	0.004	0.004		13	2.022	2.022	1.004	1.004
	7	1.047	0.010−	0.010−	—		12	2.043	1.010−	1.010−	0.001
	6	0.021	0.021	—	—		11	1.020	1.020	0.003	0.003
	5	0.043	—	—	—		10	1.038	0.006	0.006	—
12	17	8.021	8.021	7.007	6.002		9	0.012	0.012	—	—
	16	7.030	6.011	5.003	5.003		8	0.022	0.022	—	—
	15	6.033	5.012	4.004	4.004		7	0.040	—	—	—
	14	5.030	4.011	3.003	3.003	7	17	4.017	4.017	3.003	3.003
	13	4.026	3.008	3.008	2.002		16	3.014	3.014	2.003	2.003
	12	3.020	3.020	2.006	1.001		15	3.038	2.009	2.009	1.001
	11	3.041	2.013	1.003	1.003		14	2.021	2.021	1.004	1.004
	10	2.028	1.007	1.007	0.001		13	2.042	1.009	1.009	0.001
	9	1.016	1.016	0.002	0.002		12	1.018	1.018	0.002	0.002
	8	1.032	0.006	0.006	—		11	1.034	0.005−	0.005−	0.005−
	7	0.012	0.012	—	—		10	0.010−	0.010−	0.010−	—
	6	0.026	—	—	—		9	0.019	0.019	—	—
11	17	7.016	7.016	6.005−	6.005−		8	0.033	—	—	—
	16	6.022	6.022	5.007	4.002	6	17	3.011	3.011	2.002	2.002
	15	5.022	5.022	4.007	3.002		16	3.040	2.008	2.008	1.001
	14	4.019	4.019	3.006	2.001		15	2.021	2.021	1.003	1.003
	13	4.042	3.014	2.004	2.004		14	2.045+	1.009	1.009	0.001
	12	3.031	2.009	2.009	1.002		13	1.018	1.018	0.002	0.002
	11	2.020	2.020	1.005−	1.005−		12	1.035−	0.005−	0.005−	0.005−
	10	2.040	1.011	0.001	0.001		11	0.009	0.009	0.009	—
	9	1.022	1.022	0.004	0.004		10	0.017	0.017	—	—
	8	1.042	0.008	0.008	—		9	0.030	—	—	—
	7	0.016	0.016	—	—		8	0.050−	—	—	—
	6	0.033	—	—	—	5	17	3.043	2.006	2.006	1.001
10	17	7.041	6.012	5.003	5.003		16	2.024	2.024	1.003	1.003
	16	6.047	5.015+	4.004	4.004		15	1.009	1.009	1.009	0.001
	15	5.043	4.014	3.004	3.004		14	1.021	1.021	0.002	0.002
	14	4.034	3.010+	2.002	2.002		13	1.039	0.005−	0.005−	0.005−
	13	3.024	3.024	2.007	1.001		12	0.010−	0.010−	0.010−	—
	12	3.049	2.015+	1.003	1.003		11	0.018	0.018	—	—
	11	2.031	1.007	1.007	0.001		10	0.030	—	—	—
	10	1.016	1.016	0.002	0.002		9	0.049	—	—	—
	9	1.031	0.005+	0.005+	—	4	17	2.029	1.003	1.003	1.003

TESTS OF SIGNIFICANCE IN A 2 × 2 CONTINGENCY TABLE

	a	Probability 0.05	0.025	0.01	0.005
$A = 17$ $B = 4$	16	1.012	1.012	0.001	0.001
	15	1.028	0.003	0.003	0.003
	14	0.006	0.006	0.006	—
	13	0.012	0.012	—	—
	12	0.021	0.021	—	—
	11	0.035+	—	—	—
3	17	1.016	1.016	0.001	0.001
	16	1.046	0.004	0.004	0.004
	15	0.009	0.009	0.009	—
	14	0.018	0.018	—	—
	13	0.031	—	—	—
	12	0.049	—	—	—
2	17	0.006	0.006	0.006	—
	16	0.018	0.018	—	—
	15	0.035+	—	—	—
$A = 18$ $B = 18$	18	13.023	13.023	12.010−	11.004
	17	12.044	11.020	10.009	9.004
	16	10.030	9.014	8.006	7.002
	15	9.038	8.018	7.008	6.003
	14	8.043	7.020	6.009	5.003
	13	7.046	6.022	5.009	4.003
	12	6.047	5.022	4.009	3.003
	11	5.046	4.020	3.008	2.002
	10	4.043	3.018	2.006	1.001
	9	3.038	2.014	1.004	1.004
	8	2.030	1.009	1.009	0.001
	7	1.020	1.020	0.004	0.004
	6	1.044	0.010−	0.010−	—
	5	0.023	0.023	—	—
17	18	13.045+	12.019	11.008	10.003
	17	11.036	10.016	9.007	8.002
	16	10.049	9.023	8.010−	7.004
	15	8.028	7.012	6.005−	6.005−
	14	7.030	6.013	5.005+	4.002
	13	6.031	5.013	4.005−	4.005−
	12	5.030	4.012	3.004	3.004
	11	4.028	3.010+	2.003	2.003
	10	3.023	3.023	2.008	1.002
	9	3.047	2.018	1.005−	1.005−
	8	2.037	1.011	0.002	0.002
	7	1.025−	1.025−	0.005−	0.005−
	6	0.011	0.011	—	—
	5	0.026	—	—	—
16	18	12.039	11.016	10.006	9.002
	17	10.029	9.012	8.005−	8.005−
	16	9.038	8.017	7.007	6.002
	15	8.043	7.019	6.008	5.003
	14	7.046	6.020	5.008	4.003
	13	6.045+	5.020	4.007	3.002
	12	5.042	4.018	3.006	2.002
	11	4.037	3.015−	2.004	2.004
	10	3.031	2.011	1.003	1.003
	9	2.023	2.023	1.006	0.001
	8	2.046	1.014	0.002	0.002
	7	1.030	0.006	0.006	—
$A = 18$ $B = 16$	6	0.014	0.014	—	—
	5	0.031	—	—	—
15	18	11.033	10.013	9.005−	9.005−
	17	9.023	9.023	8.009	7.003
	16	8.029	7.012	6.004	6.004
	15	7.031	6.013	5.005−	5.005−
	14	6.031	5.013	4.004	4.004
	13	5.029	4.011	3.004	3.004
	12	4.025+	3.009	3.009	2.003
	11	3.020	3.020	2.006	1.001
	10	3.041	2.014	1.004	1.004
	9	2.030	1.008	1.008	0.001
	8	1.018	1.018	0.003	0.003
	7	1.038	0.007	0.007	—
	6	0.017	0.017	—	—
	5	0.036	—	—	—
14	18	10.028	9.010−	9.010−	8.003
	17	9.043	8.017	7.006	6.002
	16	8.050−	7.021	6.008	5.003
	15	6.022	6.022	5.008	4.003
	14	6.049	5.020	4.007	3.002
	13	5.044	4.017	3.006	2.001
	12	4.037	3.013	2.004	2.004
	11	3.028	2.009	2.009	1.002
	10	2.020	2.020	1.005−	1.005−
	9	2.039	1.011	0.002	0.002
	8	1.024	1.024	0.004	0.004
	7	1.047	0.009	0.009	—
	6	0.020	0.020	—	—
	5	0.043	—	—	—
13	18	9.023	9.023	8.008	7.002
	17	8.034	7.012	6.004	6.004
	16	7.037	6.014	5.005−	5.005−
	15	6.036	5.014	4.004	4.004
	14	5.032	4.012	3.004	3.004
	13	4.027	3.009	3.009	2.002
	12	3.020	3.020	2.006	1.001
	11	3.040	2.013	1.003	1.003
	10	2.027	1.007	1.007	0.001
	9	1.015+	1.015+	0.002	0.002
	8	1.031	0.006	0.006	—
	7	0.012	0.012	—	—
	6	0.025+	—	—	—
12	18	8.018	8.018	7.006	6.002
	17	7.026	6.009	6.009	5.003
	16	6.027	5.009	5.009	4.003
	15	5.024	5.024	4.008	3.002
	14	4.020	4.020	3.006	2.001
	13	4.042	3.014	2.004	2.004
	12	3.030	2.009	2.009	1.002
	11	2.019	2.019	1.005−	1.005−
	10	2.038	1.010+	0.001	0.001
	9	1.021	1.021	0.003	0.003
	8	1.040	0.007	0.007	—
	7	0.016	0.016	—	—

TESTS OF SIGNIFICANCE IN A 2 × 2 CONTINGENCY TABLE

	a	Probability 0.05	0.025	0.01	0.005
$A = 18$ $B = 12$	6	0.031	—	—	—
11	18	8.045+	7.014	6.004	6.004
	17	6.018	6.018	5.006	4.001
	16	5.018	5.018	4.005+	3.001
	15	5.043	4.015−	3.004	3.004
	14	4.033	3.011	2.003	2.003
	13	3.023	3.023	2.007	1.001
	12	3.046	2.014	1.003	1.003
	11	2.029	1.007	1.007	0.001
	10	1.015−	1.015−	0.002	0.002
	9	1.029	0.005−	0.005−	0.005−
	8	0.010+	0.010+	—	—
	7	0.020	0.020	—	—
	6	0.039	—	—	—
10	18	7.037	6.010+	5.003	5.003
	17	6.041	5.013	4.003	4.003
	16	5.036	4.011	3.003	3.003
	15	4.028	3.008	3.008	2.002
	14	3.019	3.019	2.005−	2.005−
	13	3.039	2.011	1.002	1.002
	12	2.023	2.023	1.005+	0.001
	11	2.043	1.011	0.001	0.001
	10	1.022	1.022	0.003	0.003
	9	1.040	0.007	0.007	—
	8	0.014	0.014	—	—
	7	0.027	—	—	—
	6	0.049	—	—	—
9	18	6.029	5.007	5.007	4.002
	17	5.030	4.008	4.008	3.002
	16	4.023	4.023	3.006	2.001
	15	3.016	3.016	2.004	2.004
	14	3.034	2.009	2.009	1.002
	13	2.019	2.019	1.004	1.004
	12	2.037	1.009	1.009	0.001
	11	1.018	1.018	0.002	0.002
	10	1.033	0.005+	0.005+	—
	9	0.010+	0.010+	—	—
	8	0.020	0.020	—	—
	7	0.036	—	—	—
8	18	5.022	5.022	4.005−	4.005−
	17	4.020	4.020	3.004	3.004
	16	3.014	3.014	2.003	2.003
	15	3.032	2.008	2.008	1.001
	14	2.017	2.017	1.003	1.003
	13	2.034	1.007	1.007	0.001
	12	1.015+	1.015+	0.002	0.002
	11	1.023	0.004	0.004	0.004
	10	1.049	0.008	0.008	—
	9	0.016	0.016	—	—
	8	0.028	—	—	—
	7	0.048	—	—	—
7	18	4.015+	4.015+	3.003	3.003
	17	3.012	3.012	2.002	2.002
	16	3.032	2.007	2.007	1.001
	15	2.017	2.017	1.003	1.003
$A = 18$ $B = 7$	14	2.034	1.007	1.007	0.001
	13	1.014	1.014	0.002	0.002
	12	1.027	0.004	0.004	0.004
	11	1.046	0.007	0.007	—
	10	0.013	0.013	—	—
	9	0.024	0.024	—	—
	8	0.040	—	—	—
6	18	3.010−	3.010−	3.010−	2.001
	17	3.035+	2.006	2.006	1.001
	16	2.018	2.018	1.003	1.003
	15	2.038	1.007	1.007	0.001
	14	1.015−	1.015−	0.002	0.002
	13	1.028	0.003	0.003	0.003
	12	1.048	0.007	0.007	—
	11	0.013	0.013	—	—
	10	0.022	0.022	—	—
	9	0.037	—	—	—
5	18	3.040	2.006	2.006	1.001
	17	2.021	2.021	1.003	1.003
	16	2.048	1.008	1.008	0.001
	15	1.017	1.017	0.002	0.002
	14	1.033	0.004	0.004	0.004
	13	0.007	0.007	0.007	—
	12	0.014	0.014	—	—
	11	0.024	0.024	—	—
	10	0.038	—	—	—
4	18	2.026	1.003	1.003	1.033
	17	1.010−	1.010−	1.010−	0.001
	16	1.024	1.024	0.002	0.002
	15	1.046	0.005−	0.005−	0.005−
	14	0.010−	0.010−	0.010−	—
	13	0.017	0.017	—	—
	12	0.029	—	—	—
	11	0.045+	—	—	—
3	18	1.014	1.014	0.001	0.001
	17	1.041	0.003	0.003	0.003
	16	0.008	0.008	0.008	—
	15	0.015+	0.015+	—	—
	14	0.026	—	—	—
	13	0.042	—	—	—
2	18	0.005+	0.005+	0.005+	—
	17	0.016	0.016	—	—
	16	0.032	—	—	—
$A = 19$ $B = 19$	19	14.023	14.023	13.010−	12.004
	18	13.045−	12.021	11.009	10.004
	17	11.031	10.015−	9.006	8.003
	16	10.039	9.019	8.009	7.003
	15	9.046	8.022	6.004	6.004
	14	8.050−	7.024	5.004	5.004
	13	6.025+	5.011	4.004	4.004
	12	5.024	5.024	3.003	3.003
	11	5.050−	4.022	3.009	2.003
	10	4.046	3.019	2.006	1.002
	9	3.039	2.015−	1.004	1.004
	8	2.031	1.009	1.009	0.002

TESTS OF SIGNIFICANCE IN A 2 × 2 CONTINGENCY TABLE

	a	Probability 0.05	0.025	0.01	0.005
$A = 19$ $B = 19$	7	1.021	1.021	0.004	0.004
	6	1.045−	0.010−	0.010−	—
	5	0.023	0.023	—	—
18	19	14.046	13.020	12.008	11.003
	18	12.037	11.017	10.007	9.003
	17	10.024	10.024	8.004	8.004
	16	9.030	8.014	7.006	6.002
	15	8.033	7.015+	6.006	5.002
	14	7.035+	6.016	5.006	4.002
	13	6.035−	5.015+	4.006	3.002
	12	5.033	4.014	3.005−	3.005−
	11	4.030	3.011	2.004	2.004
	10	3.025−	3.025−	2.008	1.002
	9	3.049	2.019	1.005+	0.001
	8	2.038	1.012	0.002	0.002
	7	1.025+	0.005−	0.005−	0.005−
	7	0.012	0.012	—	—
	5	0.027	—	—	—
17	19	13.040	12.016	11.006	10.002
	18	11.030	10.013	9.005+	8.002
	17	10.040	9.018	8.008	7.003
	16	9.047	8.022	7.009	6.003
	15	8.050−	7.023	6.010−	5.004
	14	6.023	6.023	5.010−	4.003
	13	6.049	5.022	4.008	3.003
	12	5.045−	4.019	3.007	2.002
	11	4.039	3.015+	2.005−	2.005−
	10	3.032	2.011	1.003	1.003
	9	2.024	2.024	1.007	0.001
	8	2.047	1.015−	0.002	0.002
	7	1.031	0.006	0.006	—
	6	0.014	0.014	—	—
	5	0.031	—	—	—
16	19	12.035−	11.013	10.005−	10.005−
	18	10.024	10.024	9.010−	8.004
	17	9.031	8.013	7.005+	6.002
	16	8.035−	7.015+	6.006	5.002
	15	7.036	6.015+	5.006	4.002
	14	6.034	5.014	4.005+	3.002
	13	5.031	4.012	3.004	3.004
	12	4.027	3.010−	3.010−	2.003
	11	3.021	3.021	2.007	1.002
	10	3.042	2.015−	1.004	1.004
	9	2.030	1.009	1.009	0.001
	8	1.018	1.018	0.003	0.003
	7	1.037	0.007	0.007	—
	6	0.017	0.017	—	—
	5	0.036	—	—	—
15	19	11.029	10.011	9.004	9.004
	18	10.046	9.019	8.007	7.002
	17	8.023	8.023	7.009	6.003
	16	7.025−	7.025−	6.010−	5.003
	15	6.024	6.024	5.009	4.003
	14	5.022	5.022	4.008	3.002
	13	5.045+	4.018	3.006	2.002

	a	Probability 0.05	0.025	0.01	0.005
$A = 19$ $B = 15$	12	4.037	3.014	2.004	2.004
	11	3.029	2.009	2.009	1.002
	10	2.020	2.020	1.005+	0.001
	9	2.039	1.011	0.002	0.002
	8	1.023	1.023	0.004	0.004
	7	1.046	0.009	0.009	—
	6	0.020	0.020	—	—
	5	0.042	—	—	—
14	19	10.024	10.024	9.008	8.003
	18	9.037	8.014	7.005−	7.005−
	17	8.042	7.017	6.006	5.002
	16	7.042	6.017	5.006	4.002
	15	6.039	5.015+	4.005+	3.001
	14	5.034	4.013	3.004	3.004
	13	4.027	3.009	3.009	2.003
	12	3.020	3.020	2.006	1.001
	11	3.040	2.013	1.003	1.003
	10	2.027	1.007	1.007	0.001
	9	1.015−	1.015−	0.002	0.002
	8	1.030	0.005+	0.005+	—
	7	0.012	0.012	—	—
	6	0.024	0.024	—	—
	5	0.049	—	—	—
13	19	9.020	9.020	8.006	7.002
	18	8.029	7.010+	6.003	6.003
	17	7.031	6.011	5.004	5.004
	16	6.029	5.011	4.003	4.003
	15	5.025+	4.009	4.009	3.003
	14	4.020	4.020	3.006	2.002
	13	4.041	3.015−	2.004	2.004
	12	3.029	2.009	2.009	1.002
	11	2.019	2.019	1.005−	1.005−
	10	2.036	1.010−	1.010−	0.001
	9	1.020	1.020	0.003	0.003
	8	1.038	0.007	0.007	—
	7	0.015−	0.015−	—	—
	6	0.030	—	—	—
12	19	9.049	8.016	7.005−	7.005−
	18	7.022	7.022	6.007	5.002
	17	6.022	6.022	5.007	4.002
	16	5.019	5.019	4.006	3.002
	15	5.042	4.015+	3.004	3.004
	14	4.032	3.011	2.003	2.003
	13	3.023	3.023	2.006	1.001
	12	3.043	2.014	1.003	1.003
	11	2.027	1.007	1.007	0.001
	10	2.050−	1.014	0.002	0.002
	9	1.027	0.005−	0.005−	0.005−
	8	1.050−	0.010−	0.010−	—
	7	0.019	0.019	—	—
	6	0.037	—	—	—
11	19	8.041	7.012	6.003	6.003
	18	7.047	6.016	5.004	5.004
	17	6.043	5.015−	4.004	4.004
	16	5.035+	4.012	3.003	3.003

TESTS OF SIGNIFICANCE IN A 2 × 2 CONTINGENCY TABLE

	a	Probability 0.05	0.025	0.01	0.005
$A = 19\ B = 11$	15	4.027	3.008	3.008	2.002
	14	3.018	3.018	2.005−	2.005−
	13	3.035+	2.010+	1.002	1.002
	12	2.021	2.021	1.005−	1.005−
	11	2.040	1.010+	0.001	0.001
	10	1.020	1.020	0.003	0.003
	9	1.037	0.006	0.006	—
	8	0.013	0.013	—	—
	7	0.025−	0.025−	—	—
	6	0.046	—	—	—
10	19	7.033	6.009	6.009	5.002
	18	6.036	5.011	4.003	4.003
	17	5.030	4.009	4.009	3.002
	16	4.022	4.022	3.006	2.001
	15	4.047	3.015−	2.004	2.004
	14	3.030	2.008	2.008	1.002
	13	2.017	2.017	1.004	1.004
	12	2.033	1.008	1.008	0.001
	11	1.016	1.016	0.002	0.002
	10	1.029	0.005−	0.005−	0.005−
	9	0.009	0.009	0.009	—
	8	0.018	0.018	—	—
	7	0.032	—	—	—
9	19	6.026	5.006	5.006	4.001
	18	5.026	4.007	4.007	3.001
	17	4.020	4.020	3.005−	3.005−
	16	4.044	3.013	2.003	2.003
	15	3.028	2.007	2.007	1.001
	14	2.015−	2.015−	1.003	1.003
	13	2.029	1.006	1.006	0.001
	12	1.013	1.013	0.002	0.002
	11	1.024	1.024	0.004	0.004
	10	1.042	0.007	0.007	—
	9	0.013	0.013	—	—
	8	0.024	0.024	—	—
	7	0.043	—	—	—
8	19	5.019	5.019	4.004	4.004
	18	4.017	4.017	3.004	3.004
	17	4.044	3.011	2.002	2.002
	16	3.027	2.006	2.006	1.001
	15	2.014	2.014	1.002	1.002
	14	2.027	1.006	1.006	0.001
	13	2.049	1.011	0.001	0.001
	12	1.021	1.021	0.003	0.003
	11	1.038	0.006	0.006	—
	10	0.011	0.011	—	—
	9	0.020	0.020	—	—
	8	0.034	—	—	—
7	19	4.013	4.013	3.002	3.002
	18	4.047	3.010+	2.002	2.002
	17	3.028	2.006	2.006	1.001
	16	2.014	2.014	1.002	1.002
	15	2.028	1.005+	1.005+	0.001
	14	1.011	1.011	0.001	0.001
	13	1.021	1.021	0.003	0.003
$A = 19\ B = 7$	12	1.037	0.005+	0.005+	—
	11	0.010−	0.010−	0.010−	—
	10	0.017	0.017	—	—
	9	0.030	—	—	—
	8	0.048	—	—	—
6	19	4.050	3.009	3.009	2.001
	18	3.031	2.005+	2.005+	1.001
	17	2.015+	2.015+	1.002	1.002
	16	2.032	1.006	1.006	0.000
	15	1.012	1.012	0.001	0.001
	14	1.023	1.023	0.003	0.003
	13	1.039	0.005+	0.005+	—
	12	0.010−	0.010−	0.010−	—
	11	0.017	0.017	—	—
	10	0.028	—	—	—
	9	0.045+	—	—	—
5	19	3.036	2.005−	2.005−	2.005−
	18	2.018	2.018	1.002	1.002
	17	2.042	1.006	1.006	0.000
	16	1.014	1.014	0.001	0.001
	15	1.028	0.003	0.003	0.003
	14	1.047	0.006	0.006	—
	13	0.011	0.011	—	—
	12	0.019	0.019	—	—
	11	0.030	—	—	—
	10	0.047	—	—	—
4	19	2.024	2.024	1.002	1.002
	18	1.009	1.009	1.009	0.001
	17	1.021	1.021	0.002	0.002
	16	1.040	0.004	0.004	0.004
	15	0.008	0.008	0.008	—
	14	0.014	0.014	—	—
	13	0.024	0.024	—	—
	12	0.037	—	—	—
3	19	1.013	1.013	0.001	0.001
	19	1.038	0.003	0.003	0.003
	17	0.006	0.006	0.006	—
	16	0.013	0.013	—	—
	15	0.023	0.023	—	—
	14	0.036	—	—	—
2	19	0.005−	0.005−	0.005−	0.005−
	18	0.014	0.014	—	—
	17	0.029	—	—	—
	16	0.048	—	—	—
$A = 20\ B = 20$	20	15.024	15.024	13.004	13.004
	19	14.046	13.022	12.010−	11.004
	18	12.032	11.015+	10.007	9.003
	17	11.041	10.020	9.009	8.004
	16	10.048	9.024	7.005−	7.005−
	15	8.027	7.012	6.005+	5.002
	14	7.028	6.013	5.005+	4.002
	13	6.028	5.012	4.005−	4.005−
	12	5.027	4.011	3.004	3.004
	11	4.024	4.024	3.009	2.003
	10	4.048	3.020	2.007	1.002

TESTS OF SIGNIFICANCE IN A 2 × 2 CONTINGENCY TABLE

	a	Probability 0.05	0.025	0.01	0.005
$A = 20$ $B = 20$	9	3.041	2.015+	1.004	1.004
	8	2.032	1.010−	1.010−	0.002
	7	1.022	1.022	0.004	0.004
	6	1.046	0.010+	—	—
	5	0.024	0.024	—	—
19	20	15.047	14.020	13.008	12.003
	19	13.039	12.018	11.008	10.003
	18	11.026	10.012	9.005−	9.005−
	17	10.032	9.015−	8.006	7.002
	16	9.036	8.017	7.007	6.003
	15	8.038	7.018	6.008	5.003
	14	7.039	6.018	5.007	4.003
	13	6.038	5.017	4.007	3.002
	12	5.035+	4.015+	3.005+	2.002
	11	4.031	3.012	2.004	2.004
	10	3.026	2.009	2.009	1.002
	9	2.019	2.019	1.005+	0.001
	8	2.039	1.012	0.002	0.002
	7	1.026	0.005+	0.005+	—
	6	0.012	0.012	—	—
	5	0.027	—	—	—
18	20	14.041	13.017	12.007	11.003
	19	12.032	11.014	10.006	9.002
	18	11.043	10.020	9.008	8.003
	17	10.050−	9.024	7.004	7.004
	16	8.026	7.011	6.005−	6.005−
	15	7.027	6.012	5.004	5.004
	14	6.026	5.011	4.004	4.004
	13	5.024	5.024	4.009	3.003
	12	5.047	4.020	3.007	2.002
	11	4.041	3.016	2.005+	1.001
	10	3.033	2.012	1.003	1.003
	9	2.024	2.024	1.007	0.001
	8	2.048	1.015−	0.003	0.003
	7	1.031	0.006	0.006	—
	6	0.014	0.014	—	—
	5	0.031	—	—	—
17	20	13.036	12.014	11.005+	10.002
	19	11.026	10.011	9.004	9.004
	18	10.034	9.015−	8.006	7.002
	17	9.038	8.017	7.007	6.003
	16	8.040	7.018	6.007	5.003
	15	7.039	6.017	5.007	4.002
	14	6.037	5.016	4.006	3.002
	13	5.033	4.013	3.005−	3.005−
	12	4.028	3.010+	2.003	2.003
	11	3.022	3.022	2.007	1.002
	10	3.042	2.015+	1.004	1.004
	9	2.031	1.009	1.009	0.001
	8	1.019	1.019	0.003	0.003
	7	1.037	0.008	0.008	—
	6	0.017	0.017	—	—
	5	0.036	—	—	—
16	20	12.031	11.012	10.004	10.004
	19	11.049	10.021	9.008	8.003
$A = 20$ $B = 16$	18	9.026	8.011	7.004	7.004
	17	8.028	7.012	6.004	6.004
	16	7.028	6.012	5.004	5.004
	15	6.026	5.011	4.004	4.004
	14	5.023	5.023	4.009	3.003
	13	5.046	4.019	3.007	2.002
	12	4.038	3.014	2.004	2.004
	11	3.029	2.010−	2.010−	1.002
	10	2.020	2.020	1.005+	0.001
	9	2.039	1.011	0.002	0.002
	8	1.023	1.023	0.004	0.004
	7	1.045+	0.009	0.009	—
	6	0.020	0.020	—	—
	5	0.041	—	—	—
15	20	11.026	10.009	10.009	9.003
	19	10.040	9.016	8.006	7.002
	18	9.046	8.019	7.007	6.002
	17	8.047	7.020	6.008	5.003
	16	7.045−	6.019	5.007	4.002
	15	6.040	5.017	4.006	3.002
	14	5.034	4.013	3.004	3.004
	13	4.028	3.010−	3.010−	2.003
	12	3.020	3.020	2.006	1.001
	11	3.039	2.013	1.003	1.003
	10	2.026	1.007	1.007	0.001
	9	2.049	1.015−	0.002	0.002
	8	1.029	0.005+	0.005+	—
	7	0.012	0.012	—	—
	6	0.024	0.024	—	—
	5	0.048	—	—	—
14	20	10.022	10.022	9.007	8.002
	19	9.032	8.012	7.004	7.004
	18	8.035+	7.014	6.005−	6.005−
	17	7.035−	6.013	5.005−	5.005−
	16	6.031	5.012	4.004	4.004
	15	5.026	4.009	4.009	3.003
	14	4.020	4.020	3.007	2.002
	13	4.040	3.015−	2.004	2.004
	12	3.029	2.009	2.009	1.002
	11	2.018	2.018	1.005−	1.005−
	10	2.035+	1.010−	1.010−	0.001
	9	1.019	1.019	0.003	0.003
	8	1.037	0.007	0.007	—
	7	0.014	0.014	—	—
	6	0.029	—	—	—
13	20	9.017	9.017	8.005	7.002
	19	8.025−	8.025−	7.008	6.003
	18	7.026	6.009	6.009	5.003
	17	6.024	6.024	5.008	4.002
	16	5.020	5.020	4.007	3.002
	15	5.041	4.015+	3.005	3.005
	14	4.031	3.011	2.003	2.003
	13	3.022	3.022	2.006	1.001
	12	3.041	2.013	1.003	1.003
	11	2.026	1.007	1.007	0.001

TESTS OF SIGNIFICANCE IN A 2 × 2 CONTINGENCY TABLE

	a	Probability 0.05	0.025	0.01	0.005
A = 20 *B* = 13	10	2.047	1.013	0.002	0.002
	9	1.026	0.004	0.004	0.004
	8	1.047	0.009	0.009	—
	7	0.018	0.018	—	—
	6	0.035−	—	—	—
12	20	9.044	8.014	7.004	7.004
	19	7.018	7.018	6.006	5.002
	18	6.018	6.018	5.006	4.002
	17	6.043	5.016	4.005−	4.005−
	16	5.034	4.012	3.003	3.003
	15	4.025+	3.008	3.008	2.002
	14	4.049	3.017	2.005−	2.005−
	13	3.033	2.010−	2.010−	1.002
	12	2.020	2.020	1.005−	1.005−
	11	2.036	1.009	1.009	0.001
	10	1.018	1.018	0.003	0.003
	9	1.034	0.006	0.006	—
	8	0.012	0.012	—	—
	7	0.023	0.023	—	—
	6	0.043	—	—	—
11	20	8.037	7.010+	6.003	6.003
	19	7.042	6.013	5.004	5.004
	18	6.037	5.012	4.003	4.003
	17	5.029	4.009	4.009	3.002
	16	4.021	4.021	3.006	2.001
	15	4.042	3.003	2.003	2.003
	14	3.028	2.008	2.008	1.001
	13	2.016	2.016	1.003	1.003
	12	2.029	1.007	1.007	0.001
	11	1.014	1.014	0.002	0.002
	10	1.026	0.004	0.004	0.004
	9	1.046	0.008	0.008	—
	8	0.016	0.016	—	—
	7	0.029	—	—	—
10	20	7.030	6.008	6.008	5.002
	19	6.031	5.009	5.009	4.002
	18	5.026	4.007	4.007	3.002
	17	4.018	4.018	3.005−	3.005−
	16	4.039	3.012	2.003	2.003
	15	3.024	3.024	2.006	1.001
	14	3.045+	2.013	1.003	1.003
	13	2.025+	1.006	1.006	0.001
	12	2.045−	1.011	0.001	0.001
	11	1.021	1.021	0.003	0.003
	10	1.037	0.006	0.006	—
	9	0.012	0.012	—	—
	8	0.022	0.022	—	—
	7	0.038	—	—	—
9	20	6.023	6.023	5.005+	4.001
	19	5.022	5.022	4.005+	3.001
	18	4.016	4.016	3.004	3.004
	17	4.037	3.010+	2.002	2.002
	16	3.022	3.022	2.005+	1.001
	15	3.043	2.012	1.002	1.002
	14	2.023	2.023	1.005−	1.005−
A = 20 *B* = 9	13	2.041	1.009	1.009	0.001
	12	1.018	1.018	0.002	0.002
	11	1.032	0.005−	0.005−	0.005−
	10	0.009	0.009	0.009	—
	9	0.017	0.017	—	—
	8	0.029	—	—	—
	7	0.050−	—	—	—
8	20	5.017	5.017	4.003	4.003
	19	4.015−	4.015−	3.003	3.003
	18	4.038	3.009	3.009	2.002
	17	3.022	3.022	2.005−	2.005−
	16	3.044	2.011	1.002	1.002
	15	0.022	2.022	1.004	1.004
	14	2.040	1.009	1.009	0.001
	13	1.016	1.016	0.002	0.002
	12	1.029	0.004	0.004	0.004
	11	1.048	0.008	0.008	—
	10	0.014	0.014	—	—
	9	0.024	0.024	—	—
	8	0.041	—	—	—
7	20	4.012	4.012	3.002	3.002
	19	4.042	3.009	3.009	2.001
	18	3.024	3.024	2.005−	2.005−
	17	3.050−	2.011	1.002	1.002
	16	2.023	2.023	1.004	1.004
	15	2.043	1.009	1.009	0.001
	14	1.016	1.016	0.002	0.002
	13	1.029	0.004	0.004	0.004
	12	1.048	0.007	0.007	—
	11	0.013	0.013	—	—
	10	0.022	0.022	—	—
	9	0.036	—	—	—
6	20	4.046	3.008	3.008	2.001
	19	3.028	2.005−	2.005−	2.005−
	18	2.013	2.013	1.002	1.002
	17	2.028	1.004	1.004	1.004
	16	1.010−	1.010−	1.010−	0.001
	15	1.018	1.018	0.002	0.002
	14	1.032	0.004	0.004	0.004
	13	0.007	0.007	0.007	—
	12	0.013	0.013	—	—
	11	0.022	0.022	—	—
	10	0.035−	—	—	—
5	20	3.033	2.004	2.004	2.004
	19	2.016	2.016	1.002	1.002
	18	2.038	1.005+	1.005+	0.000
	17	1.012	1.012	0.001	0.001
	16	1.023	1.023	0.002	0.002
	15	1.040	0.005−	0.005−	0.005−
	14	0.009	0.009	0.009	—
	13	0.015−	0.015−	—	—
	12	0.024	0.024	—	—
	11	0.038	—	—	—
4	20	2.022	2.022	1.002	1.002
	19	1.008	1.008	1.008	0.000

TESTS OF SIGNIFICANCE IN A 2 × 2 CONTINGENCY TABLE

	a	Probability					a	Probability			
		0.05	0.025	0.01	0.005			0.05	0.025	0.01	0.005
$A = 20\ B = 4$	18	1.018	1.018	0.001	0.001	$A = 20\ B = 3$	17	0.011	0.011	—	—
	17	1.035+	0.003	0.003	0.003		16	0.020	0.020	—	—
	16	0.007	0.007	0.007	—		15	0.032	—	—	—
	15	0.012	0.012	—	—		14	0.047	—	—	—
	14	0.020	0.020	—	—	2	20	0.004	0.004	0.004	0.004
	13	0.031	—	—	—		19	0.013	0.013	—	—
	12	0.047	—	—	—		18	0.026	—	—	—
3	20	1.012	1.012	0.001	0.001		17	0.043	—	—	—
	19	1.034	0.002	0.002	0.002	1	20	0.048	—	—	—
	18	0.006	0.006	0.006	—						

IV. STUDENT'S *t*-DISTRIBUTION

IV.1 PERCENTAGE POINTS, STUDENT'S *t*-DISTRIBUTION

This table gives values of t such that

$$F(t) = \int_{-\infty}^{t} \frac{\Gamma\left(\frac{n+1}{2}\right)}{\sqrt{n\pi}\,\Gamma\left(\frac{n}{2}\right)} \left(1 + \frac{x^2}{n}\right)^{-\frac{n+1}{2}} dx$$

for n, the number of degrees of freedom, equal to 1, 2, . . ., 30, 40, 60, 120, ∞; and for $F(t) = 0.60, 0.75, 0.90, 0.95, 0.975, 0.99, 0.995$, and 0.9995. The *t*-distribution is symmetrical, so that $F(-t) = 1 - F(t)$

n \ F	.60	.75	.90	.95	.975	.99	.995	.9995
1	.325	1.000	3.078	6.314	12.706	31.821	63.657	636.619
2	.289	.816	1.886	2.920	4.303	6.965	9.925	31.598
3	.277	.765	1.638	2.353	3.182	4.541	5.841	12.924
4	.271	.741	1.533	2.132	2.776	3.747	4.604	8.610
5	.267	.727	1.476	2.015	2.571	3.365	4.032	6.869
6	.265	.718	1.440	1.943	2.447	3.143	3.707	5.959
7	.263	.711	1.415	1.895	2.365	2.998	3.499	5.408
8	.262	.706	1.397	1.860	2.306	2.896	3.355	5.041
9	.261	.703	1.383	1.833	2.262	2.821	3.250	4.781
10	.260	.700	1.372	1.812	2.228	2.764	3.169	4.587
11	.260	.697	1.363	1.796	2.201	2.718	3.106	4.437
12	.259	.695	1.356	1.782	2.179	2.681	3.055	4.318
13	.259	.694	1.350	1.771	2.160	2.650	3.012	4.221
14	.258	.692	1.345	1.761	2.145	2.624	2.977	4.140
15	.258	.691	1.341	1.753	2.131	2.602	2.947	4.073
16	.258	.690	1.337	1.746	2.120	2.583	2.921	4.015
17	.257	.689	1.333	1.740	2.110	2.567	2.898	3.965
18	.257	.688	1.330	1.734	2.101	2.552	2.878	3.922
19	.257	.688	1.328	1.729	2.093	2.539	2.861	3.883
20	.257	.687	1.325	1.725	2.086	2.528	2.845	3.850
21	.257	.686	1.323	1.721	2.080	2.518	2.831	3.819
22	.256	.686	1.321	1.717	2.074	2.508	2.819	3.792
23	.256	.685	1.319	1.714	2.069	2.500	2.807	3.767
24	.256	.685	1.318	1.711	2.064	2.492	2.797	3.745
25	.256	.684	1.316	1.708	2.060	2.485	2.787	3.725
26	.256	.684	1.315	1.706	2.056	2.479	2.779	3.707
27	.256	.684	1.314	1.703	2.052	2.473	2.771	3.690
28	.256	.683	1.313	1.701	2.048	2.467	2.763	3.674
29	.256	.683	1.311	1.699	2.045	2.462	2.756	3.659
30	.256	.683	1.310	1.697	2.042	2.457	2.750	3.646
40	.255	.681	1.303	1.684	2.021	2.423	2.704	3.551
60	.254	.679	1.296	1.671	2.000	2.390	2.660	3.460
120	.254	.677	1.289	1.658	1.980	2.358	2.617	3.373
∞	.253	.674	1.282	1.645	1.960	2.326	2.576	3.291

* This table is abridged from the "Statistical Tables" of R. A. Fisher and Frank Yates published by Oliver & Boyd. Ltd., Edinburgh and London, 1938. It is here published with the kind permission of the authors and their publishers.

IV.2 NOMOGRAPH FOR STUDENT'S *t*-DISTRIBUTION

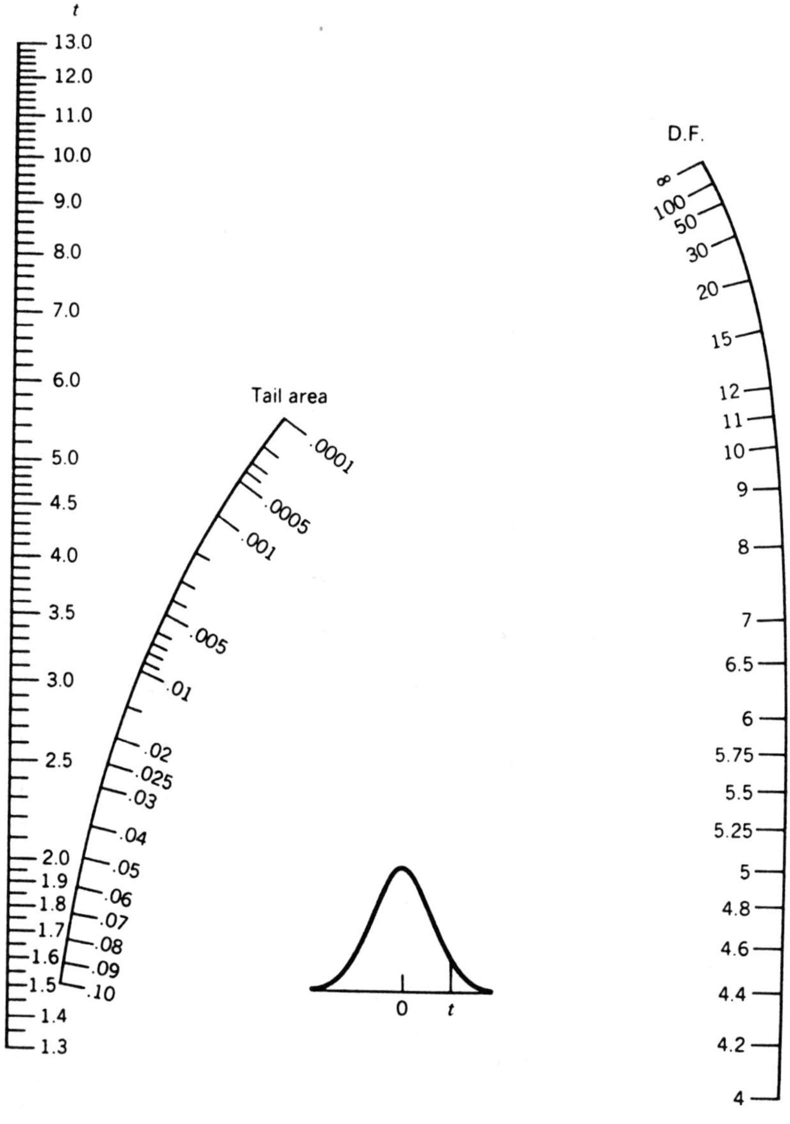

IV.3 POWER FUNCTION OF THE *t*-TEST

Any statistic of the form

$$t' = \frac{z + \delta}{s_z} = \frac{z'}{s_z},$$

where z is normally distributed with expectation zero and standard deviation σ_z, s_z^2 is an independent estimate of σ_z^2 based on ν degrees of freedom, and δ is the noncentrality parameter, is distributed as the non-central t-distribution, denoted by $f(t')$.

The power function of the t-test is the value of the following integrals considered as a function of $\frac{\delta}{\sigma_z}$

(a) $$\int_{-\infty}^{-t_{\alpha/2}} f(t')\,dt' + \int_{t_{\alpha/2}}^{\infty} f(t')\,dt' \quad \text{for the double-tail } t\text{-test}$$

(b) $$\int_{t_\alpha}^{\infty} f(t')\,dt' \quad \text{for the single-tail } t\text{-test } (\delta \geq 0)\ ,$$

where t_α denotes the α-level significance point for t.

The graph in this table shows the integral (*a*) for $\alpha = 0.05$ and 0.01, and for various values of ν, the degrees of freedom associated with s_z. The horizontal scale is in terms of $\phi = \frac{\delta}{\sigma_z \sqrt{2}}$. The graph can also be used to give the integral (*b*) for significance levels $\alpha = 0.025$ and 0.005.

POWER FUNCTION OF THE *t*-TEST

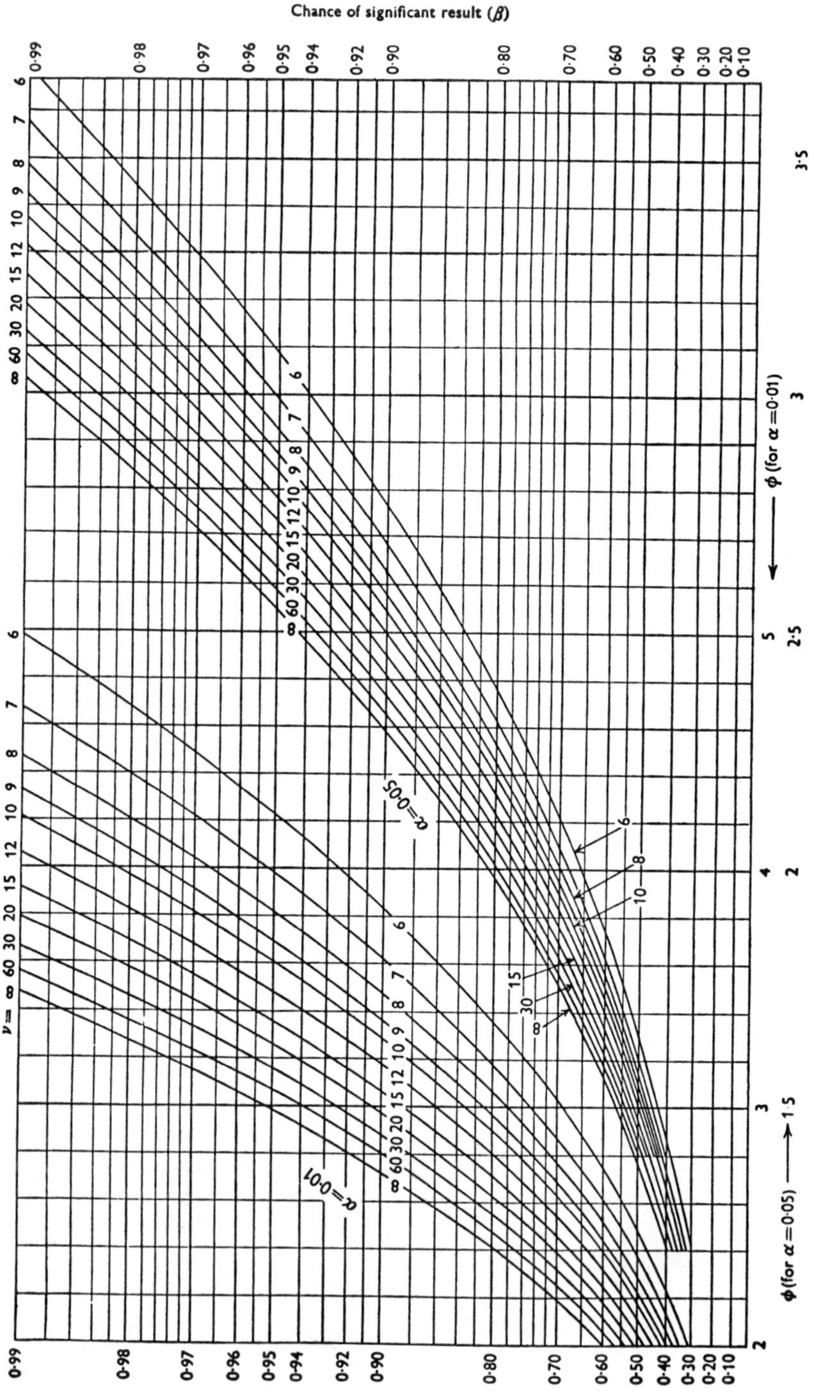

IV.4 NUMBER OF OBSERVATIONS FOR *t*-TEST OF MEAN

This table gives the sample size needed for given values of $\alpha = P$ (Type I error) and $\beta = P$ (Type II error) for a test on a single mean with unknown standard deviation.

To test the hypothesis H_0: $\mu = \mu_0$ against the alternative H_a: $\mu < \mu_0$, the statistic $t = \dfrac{(\bar{x} - \mu_0)\sqrt{n}}{s}$ is used. The distribution of t when H_0 is true is the t-distribution with $n - 1$ degrees of freedom and the critical region $t > t_{n-1,1-\alpha}$ would have a significance level α. The distribution of $t(\delta) = \dfrac{\sqrt{n}(\bar{x} - \mu) + \delta\sigma}{s}$ is noncentral t with $n - 1$ degrees of freedom and noncentrality parameter δ. Here $\delta = \dfrac{(\mu - \mu_0)\sqrt{n}}{\sigma}$. This table is used to obtain sample sizes needed to control the values of α and β for various values of $\Delta = \dfrac{\mu - \mu_0}{\sigma}$ for both one-sided tests and two-sided tests.

NUMBER OF OBSERVATIONS FOR *t*-TEST OF MEAN

	Level of *t*-test																				
Single-sided test	$\alpha = 0.005$					$\alpha = 0.01$					$\alpha = 0.025$					$\alpha = 0.05$					
Double-sided test	$\alpha = 0.01$					$\alpha = 0.02$					$\alpha = 0.05$					$\alpha = 0.1$					
$\beta =$	0.01	0.05	0.1	0.2	0.5	0.01	0.05	0.1	0.2	0.5	0.01	0.05	0.1	0.2	0.5	0.01	0.05	0.1	0.2	0.5	
0.05																					0.05
0.10																					0.10
0.15																				122	0.15
0.20										139					99					70	0.20
0.25					110					90				128	64			139	101	45	0.25
0.30				134	78				115	63			119	90	45		122	97	71	32	0.30
0.35			125	99	58			109	85	47		109	88	67	34		90	72	52	24	0.35
0.40		115	97	77	45		101	85	66	37	117	84	68	51	26	101	70	55	40	19	0.40
0.45		92	77	62	37	110	81	68	53	30	93	67	54	41	21	80	55	44	33	15	0.45
0.50	100	75	63	51	30	90	66	55	43	25	76	54	44	34	18	65	45	36	27	13	0.50
0.55	83	63	53	42	26	75	55	46	36	21	63	45	37	28	15	54	38	30	22	11	0.55
0.60	71	53	45	36	22	63	47	39	31	18	53	38	32	24	13	46	32	26	19	9	0.60
0.65	61	46	39	31	20	55	41	34	27	16	46	33	27	21	12	39	28	22	17	8	0.65
0.70	53	40	34	28	17	47	35	30	24	14	40	29	24	19	10	34	24	19	15	8	0.70
0.75	47	36	30	25	16	42	31	27	21	13	35	26	21	16	9	30	21	17	13	7	0.75
0.80	41	32	27	22	14	37	28	24	19	12	31	22	19	15	9	27	19	15	12	6	0.80
0.85	37	29	24	20	13	33	25	21	17	11	28	21	17	13	8	24	17	14	11	6	0.85
0.90	34	26	22	18	12	29	23	19	16	10	25	19	16	12	7	21	15	13	10	5	0.90
Value of 0.95	31	24	20	17	11	27	21	18	14	9	23	17	14	11	7	19	14	11	9	5	0.95
$\Delta = \frac{\mu - \mu_0}{\sigma}$ 1.00	28	22	19	16	10	25	19	16	13	9	21	16	13	10	6	18	13	11	8	5	1.00
1.1	24	19	16	14	9	21	16	14	12	8	18	13	11	9	6	15	11	9	7		1.1
1.2	21	16	14	12	8	18	14	12	10	7	15	12	10	8	5	13	10	8	6		1.2
1.3	18	15	13	11	8	16	13	11	9	6	14	10	9	7		11	8	7	6		1.3
1.4	16	13	12	10	7	14	11	10	9	6	12	9	8	7		10	8	7	5		1.4
1.5	15	12	11	9	7	13	10	9	8	6	11	8	7	6		9	7	6			1.5
1.6	13	11	10	8	6	12	10	9	7	5	10	8	7	6		8	6	6			1.6
1.7	12	10	9	8	6	11	9	8	7		9	7	6	5		8	6	5			1.7
1.8	12	10	9	8	6	10	8	7	7		8	7	6			7	6				1.8
1.9	11	9	8	7	6	10	8	7	6		8	6	6			7	5				1.9
2.0	10	8	8	7	5	9	7	7	6		7	6	5			6					2.0
2.1	10	8	7	7		8	7	6	6		7	6				6					2.1
2.2	9	8	7	6		8	7	6	5		7	6				6					2.2
2.3	9	7	7	6		8	6	6			6	5				5					2.3
2.4	8	7	7	6		7	6	6			6										2.4
2.5	8	7	6	6		7	6	6			6										2.5
3.0	7	6	6	5		6	5	5			5										3.0
3.5	6	5	5			5															3.5
4.0	6																				4.0

IV.5 NUMBER OF OBSERVATIONS FOR *t*-TEST OF DIFFERENCE BETWEEN TWO MEANS

This table gives the sample size needed for given values of $\alpha = P$ (Type I error) and $\beta = P$ (Type II error) for a test of the hypothesis of the equality of two means H_0: $\mu_x = \mu_y$, where there is a common but unknown variance. The statistic used is

$$t = \frac{\bar{x} - \bar{y}}{s\sqrt{\frac{1}{n_x} + \frac{1}{n_y}}}$$

which is distributed as Students t-distribution with $n_x + n_y - 2$ degrees of freedom. Here

$$s = \left[\frac{(n_x - 1)s_x^2 + (n_y - 1)s_y^2}{n_x + n_y - 2}\right]^{\frac{1}{2}}.$$

The noncentrality parameter in this case is

$$\sigma = \frac{\mu_x - \mu_y}{\sigma\sqrt{\frac{1}{n_x} + \frac{1}{n_y}}}.$$

This table is used to obtain sample sizes needed to control the values of α and β for various values of $\Delta = \frac{\mu_x - \mu_y}{\sigma}$ for both one-sided and two-sided tests, where it is assumed $n_x = n_y = n$.

NUMBER OF OBSERVATIONS FOR *t*-TEST OF DIFFERENCE BETWEEN TWO MEANS

	Level of *t*-test																				
Single-sided test	$\alpha = 0.005$					$\alpha = 0.01$					$\alpha = 0.025$					$\alpha = 0.05$					
Double-sided test	$\alpha = 0.01$					$\alpha = 0.02$					$\alpha = 0.05$					$\alpha = 0.1$					
$\beta =$	0.01	0.05	0.1	0.2	0.5	0.01	0.05	0.1	0.2	0.5	0.01	0.05	0.1	0.2	0.5	0.01	0.05	0.1	0.2	0.5	
Value of $\Delta = \frac{\mu_x - \mu}{\sigma}$																					
0.05																					0.05
0.10																					0.10
0.15																					0.15
0.20																				137	0.20
0.25															124					88	0.25
0.30										123					87					61	0.30
0.35					110					90					64				102	45	0.35
0.40					85					70				100	50			108	78	35	0.40
0.45				118	68				101	55			105	79	39		108	86	62	28	0.45
0.50				96	55			106	82	45		106	86	64	32		88	70	51	23	0.50
0.55			101	79	46		106	88	68	38		87	71	53	27	112	73	58	42	19	0.55
0.60		101	85	67	39		90	74	58	32	104	74	60	45	23	89	61	49	36	16	0.60
0.65		87	73	57	34	104	77	64	49	27	88	63	51	39	20	76	52	42	30	14	0.65
0.70	100	75	63	50	29	90	66	55	43	24	76	55	44	34	17	66	45	36	26	12	0.70
0.75	88	66	55	44	26	79	58	48	38	21	67	48	39	29	15	57	40	32	23	11	0.75
0.80	77	58	49	39	23	70	51	43	33	19	59	42	34	26	14	50	35	28	21	10	0.80
0.85	69	51	43	35	21	62	46	38	30	17	52	37	31	23	12	45	31	25	18	9	0.85
0.90	62	46	39	31	19	55	41	34	27	15	47	34	27	21	11	40	28	22	16	8	0.90
0.95	55	42	35	28	17	50	37	31	24	14	42	30	25	19	10	36	25	20	15	7	0.95
1.00	50	38	32	26	15	45	33	28	22	13	38	27	23	17	9	33	23	18	14	7	1.00
1.1	42	32	27	22	13	38	28	23	19	11	32	23	19	14	8	27	19	15	12	6	1.1
1.2	36	27	23	18	11	32	24	20	16	9	27	20	16	12	7	23	16	13	10	5	1.2
1.3	31	23	20	16	10	28	21	17	14	8	23	17	14	11	6	20	14	11	9	5	1.3
1.4	27	20	17	14	9	24	18	15	12	8	20	15	12	10	6	17	12	10	8	4	1.4
1.5	24	18	15	13	8	21	16	14	11	7	18	13	11	9	5	15	11	9	7	4	1.5
1.6	21	16	14	11	7	19	14	12	10	6	16	12	10	8	5	14	10	8	6	4	1.6
1.7	19	15	13	10	7	17	13	11	9	6	14	11	9	7	4	12	9	7	6	3	1.7
1.8	17	13	11	10	6	15	12	10	8	5	13	10	8	6	4	11	8	7	5		1.8
1.9	16	12	11	9	6	14	11	9	8	5	12	9	7	6	4	10	7	6	5		1.9
2.0	14	11	10	8	6	13	10	9	7	5	11	8	7	6	4	9	7	6	4		2.0
2.1	13	10	9	8	5	12	9	8	7	5	10	8	6	5	3	8	6	5	4		2.1
2.2	12	10	8	7	5	11	9	7	6	4	9	7	6	5		8	6	5	4		2.2
2.3	11	9	8	7	5	10	8	7	6	4	9	7	6	5		7	5	5	4		2.3
2.4	11	9	8	6	5	10	8	7	6	4	8	6	5	4		7	5	4	4		2.4
2.5	10	8	7	6	4	9	7	6	5	4	8	6	5	4		6	5	4	3		2.5
3.0	8	6	6	5	4	7	6	5	4	3	6	5	4	4		5	4	3			3.0
3.5	6	5	5	4	3	6	5	4	4		5	4	4	3		4	3				3.5
4.0	6	5	4	4		5	4	4	3		4	4	3			4					4.0

IV.6 OPERATING CHARACTERISTIC (OC) CURVES FOR A TEST ON THE MEAN OF A NORMAL DISTRIBUTION WITH UNKNOWN STANDARD DEVIATION

The OC curves give the sample sizes needed for given values of $\alpha = P$ (Type I error) and $\beta = P$ (Type II error) for a test of the hypothesis H_0: $\mu = \mu_0$, where the standard deviation is unknown. The statistic used is $t = \dfrac{(\bar{x} - \mu_0)\sqrt{n}}{s}$ which is distributed as Student's t-distribution with $n - 1$ degrees of freedom. The required sample size is obtained by entering the appropriate set of curves for given α and β for various values of $\Delta = \dfrac{|\mu_1 - \mu_0|}{\sigma}$ for both one-sided and two-sided tests.

The OC curves can also be used to give the sample sizes for a test of the hypothesis Ho: $\mu_x = \mu_y$ where the standard deviations σ_x and σ_y are unknown. If $\sigma_x = \sigma_y = \sigma$, then the statistic used is

$$t = \frac{\bar{x} - \bar{y}}{\sqrt{\dfrac{(n_x - 1)s_x^2 + (n_y - 1)s_y^2}{n_x + n_y - 2}}\sqrt{\dfrac{1}{n_x} + \dfrac{1}{n_y}}}$$

which is distributed as Student's t-distribution with $(n_x + n_y - 2)$ degrees of freedom. The required sample size is obtained by entering the appropriate set of curves for given α and β for various values of $\Delta = \dfrac{|\mu_x - \mu_y|}{2\sigma}$ for both one-sided and two-sided tests, where it is assumed that $n_x = n_y = n$. If the value read from the OC curve is denoted by n', the required sample size is given by $n = \dfrac{n' + 1}{2}$.

OC CURVES FOR A TEST ON THE MEAN OF A NORMAL DISTRIBUTION WITH UNKNOWN STANDARD DEVIATION

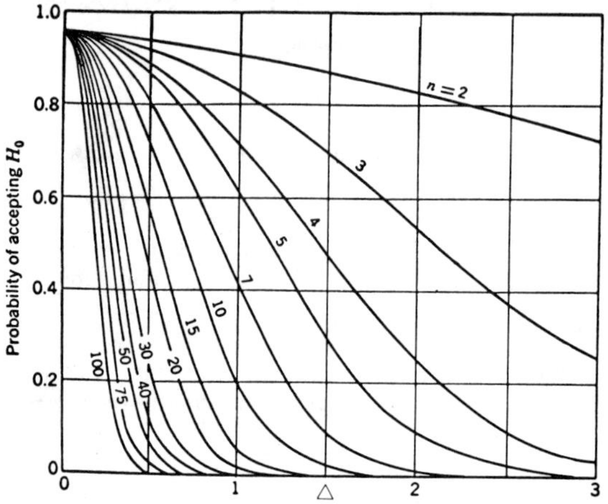

a) OC curves for different values of n for the two-sided t test for a level of significance $\alpha = 0.05$.

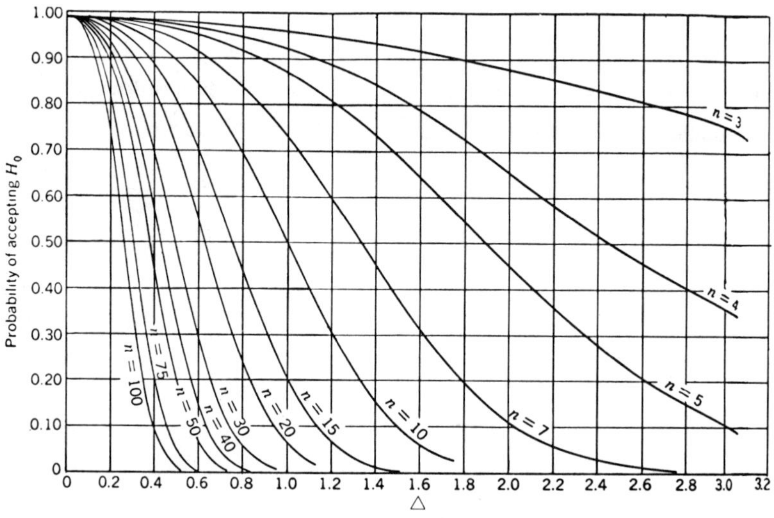

b) OC curves for different values of n for the two-sided t test for a level of significance $\alpha = 0.01$.

OC CURVES FOR A TEST ON THE MEAN OF A NORMAL DISTRIBUTION WITH UNKNOWN STANDARD DEVIATION

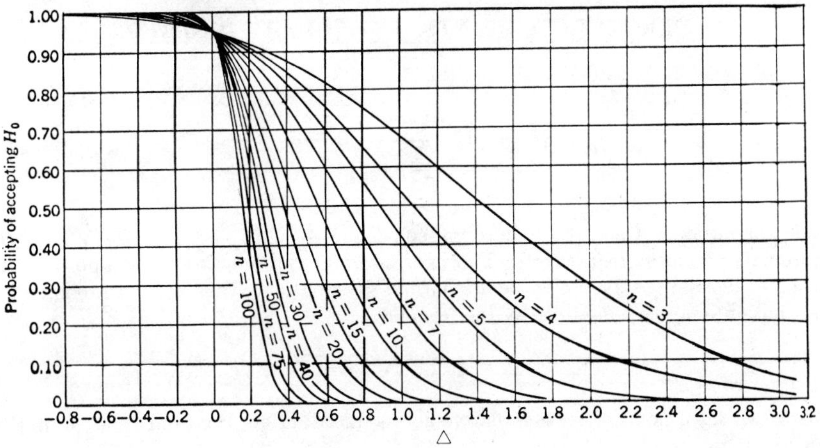

c) OC curves for different values of n for the one-sided t test for a level of significance $\alpha = 0.05$.

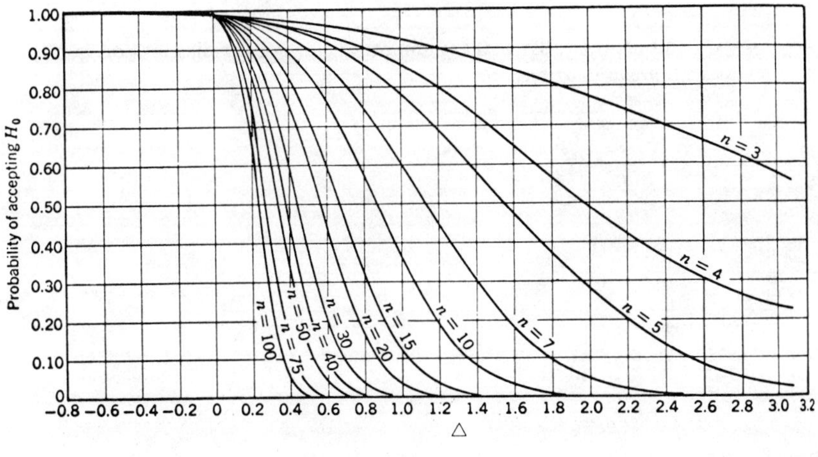

d) OC curves for different values of n for the one-sided t test for a level of significance $\alpha = 0.01$.

V. CHI-SQUARE DISTRIBUTION

V.1 PERCENTAGE POINTS, CHI-SQUARE DISTRIBUTION

This table gives values of χ^2 such that

$$F(\chi^2) = \int_0^{\chi^2} \frac{1}{2^{\frac{n}{2}}\,\Gamma\left(\frac{n}{2}\right)} x^{\frac{n-2}{2}} e^{-\frac{x}{2}}\,dx$$

for n, the number of degrees of freedom, equal to 1, 2, . . . , 30. For $n > 30$, a normal approximation is quite accurate. The expression $\sqrt{2\chi^2} - \sqrt{2n-1}$ is approximately normally distributed as the standard normal distribution. Thus χ^2_α, the α-point of the distribution, may be computed by the formula

$$\chi^2_\alpha = \tfrac{1}{2}[x_\alpha + \sqrt{2n-1}]^2,$$

where x_α is the α-point of the cumulative normal distribution. For even values of n, $F(\chi^2)$ can be written as

$$1 - F(\chi^2) = \sum_{x=0}^{x'-1} \frac{e^{-\lambda}\lambda^x}{x!}$$

with $\lambda = \frac{1}{2}\chi^2$ and $x' = \frac{1}{2}n$. Thus the cumulative Chi-Square distribution is related to the cumulative Poisson distribution.

PERCENTAGE POINTS, CHI-SQUARE DISTRIBUTION

$$F(\chi^2) = \int_0^{\chi^2} \frac{1}{2^{\frac{n}{2}}\Gamma\left(\frac{n}{2}\right)} x^{\frac{n-2}{2}} e^{-\frac{x}{2}} dx$$

n \ F	.005	.010	.025	.050	.100	.250	.500	.750	.900	.950	.975	.990	.995
1	.0000393	.000157	.000982	.00393	.0158	.102	.455	1.32	2.71	3.84	5.02	6.63	7.88
2	.0100	.0201	.0506	.103	.211	.575	1.39	2.77	4.61	5.99	7.38	9.21	10.6
3	.0717	.115	.216	.352	.584	1.21	2.37	4.11	6.25	7.81	9.35	11.3	12.8
4	.207	.297	.484	.711	1.06	1.92	3.36	5.39	7.78	9.49	11.1	13.3	14.9
5	.412	.554	.831	1.15	1.61	2.67	4.35	6.63	9.24	11.1	12.8	15.1	16.7
6	.676	.872	1.24	1.64	2.20	3.45	5.35	7.84	10.6	12.6	14.4	16.8	18.5
7	.989	1.24	1.69	2.17	2.83	4.25	6.35	9.04	12.0	14.1	16.0	18.5	20.3
8	1.34	1.65	2.18	2.73	3.49	5.07	7.34	10.2	13.4	15.5	17.5	20.1	22.0
9	1.73	2.09	2.70	3.33	4.17	5.90	8.34	11.4	14.7	16.9	19.0	21.7	23.6
10	2.16	2.56	3.25	3.94	4.87	6.74	9.34	12.5	16.0	18.3	20.5	23.2	25.2
11	2.60	3.05	3.82	4.57	5.58	7.58	10.3	13.7	17.3	19.7	21.9	24.7	26.8
12	3.07	3.57	4.40	5.23	6.30	8.44	11.3	14.8	18.5	21.0	23.3	26.2	28.3
13	3.57	4.11	5.01	5.89	7.04	9.30	12.3	16.0	19.8	22.4	24.7	27.7	29.8
14	4.07	4.66	5.63	6.57	7.79	10.2	13.3	17.1	21.1	23.7	26.1	29.1	31.3
15	4.60	5.23	6.26	7.26	8.55	11.0	.4.3	18.2	22.3	25.0	27.5	30.6	32.8
16	5.14	5.81	6.91	7.96	9.31	11.9	15.3	19.4	23.5	26.3	28.8	32.0	34.3
17	5.70	6.41	7.56	8.67	10.1	12.8	16.3	20.5	24.8	27.6	30.2	33.4	35.7
18	6.26	7.01	8.23	9.39	10.9	13.7	17.3	21.6	26.0	28.9	31.5	34.8	37.2
19	6.84	7.63	8.91	10.1	11.7	14.6	18.3	22.7	27.2	30.1	32.9	36.2	38.6
20	7.43	8.26	9.59	10.9	12.4	15.5	19.3	23.8	28.4	31.4	34.2	37.6	40.0
21	8.03	8.90	10.3	11.6	13.2	16.3	20.3	24.9	29.6	32.7	35.5	38.9	41.4
22	8.64	9.54	11.0	12.3	14.0	17.2	21.3	26.0	30.8	33.9	36.8	40.3	42.8
23	9.26	10.2	11.7	13.1	14.8	18.1	22.3	27.1	32.0	35.2	38.1	41.6	44.2
24	9.89	10.9	12.4	13.8	15.7	19.0	23.3	28.2	33.2	36.4	39.4	43.0	45.6
25	10.5	11.5	13.1	14.6	16.5	19.9	24.3	29.3	34.4	37.7	40.6	44.3	46.9
26	11.2	12.2	13.8	15.4	17.3	20.8	25.3	30.4	35.6	38.9	41.9	45.6	48.3
27	11.8	12.9	14.6	16.2	18.1	21.7	26.3	31.5	36.7	40.1	43.2	47.0	49.6
28	12.5	13.6	15.3	16.9	18.9	22.7	27.3	32.6	37.9	41.3	44.5	48.3	51.0
29	13.1	14.3	16.0	17.7	19.8	23.6	28.3	33.7	39.1	42.6	45.7	49.6	52.3
30	13.8	15.0	16.8	18.5	20.6	24.5	29.3	34.8	40.3	43.8	47.0	50.9	53.7

V.2 PERCENTAGE POINTS, CHI-SQUARE OVER DEGREES OF FREEDOM DISTRIBUTION

This table gives the percentage points of the sampling distribution of $\frac{s^2}{\sigma^2}$, referred to as the percentage points of the $\frac{\chi^2}{\text{d.f.}}$ distribution (read "chi-square over degrees of freedom"). The percentage points are different for different sample sizes.

PERCENTAGE POINTS, CHI-SQUARE OVER DEGREES OF FREEDOM DISTRIBUTION

F / n	Probability in per cent						Probability in per cent					
	0.05	0.1	0.5	1.0	2.5	5.0	95.0	97.5	99.0	99.5	99.9	99.95
1	.0000	.0000	.0000	.0002	.0010	.0039	3.8410	5.0240	6.6350	7.8790	10.8280	12.1160
2	.0005	.0010	.0050	.0100	.0253	.0515	2.9955	3.6890	4.6050	5.2985	6.9080	7.6010
3	.0051	.0081	.0239	.0383	.0720	.1173	2.6050	3.1160	3.7817	4.2793	5.4220	5.9100
4	.0160	.0227	.0518	.0742	.1210	.1778	2.3720	2.7858	3.3192	3.7150	4.6168	4.9995
5	.0316	.0420	.0824	.1108	.1662	.2290	2.2140	2.5664	3.0172	3.3500	4.1030	4.4210
6	.0499	.0635	.1127	.1453	.2062	.2725	2.0987	2.4082	2.8020	3.0913	3.7430	4.0172
7	.0693	.0854	.1413	.1770	.2414	.3096	2.0096	2.2876	2.6393	2.8969	3.4746	3.7169
8	.0888	.1071	.1680	.2058	.2725	.3416	1.9384	2.1919	2.5112	2.7444	3.2656	3.4835
9	.1080	.1281	.1928	.2320	.3000	.3694	1.8799	2.1137	2.4073	2.6210	3.0974	3.2962
10	.1265	.1479	.2156	.2558	.3247	.3940	1.8307	2.0483	2.3209	2.5188	2.9588	3.1419
11	.1443	.1667	.2366	.2775	.3469	.4159	1.7886	1.9927	2.2477	2.4325	2.8422	3.0124
12	.1612	.1845	.2562	.2976	.3670	.4355	1.7522	1.9447	2.1848	2.3583	2.7424	2.9018
13	.1773	.2013	.2742	.3159	.3853	.4532	1.7202	1.9028	2.1298	2.2938	2.6560	2.8060
14	.1926	.2172	.2911	.3329	.4021	.4694	1.6918	1.8656	2.0815	2.2371	2.5802	2.7221
15	.2072	.2322	.3067	.3486	.4175	.4841	1.6664	1.8325	2.0385	2.1867	2.5131	2.6479
16	.2210	.2464	.3214	.3632	.4318	.4976	1.6435	1.8028	2.0000	2.1417	2.4532	2.5818
17	.2341	.2598	.3351	.3769	.4449	.5101	1.6228	1.7759	1.9652	2.1011	2.3994	2.5223
18	.2466	.2725	.3481	.3897	.4573	.5217	1.6038	1.7514	1.9336	2.0642	2.3507	2.4686
19	.2585	.2846	.3602	.4017	.4688	.5325	1.5865	1.7291	1.9048	2.0306	2.3063	2.4196
20	.2699	.2961	.3717	.4130	.4796	.5426	1.5705	1.7085	1.8783	1.9998	2.2658	2.3749
21	.2808	.3070	.3826	.4237	.4897	.5520	1.5558	1.6895	1.8539	1.9715	2.2284	2.3338
22	.2911	.3174	.3929	.4337	.4992	.5608	1.5420	1.6719	1.8313	1.9453	2.1940	2.2960
23	.3010	.3273	.4026	.4433	.5082	.5692	1.5292	1.6555	1.8103	1.9209	2.1621	2.2609
24	.3105	.3369	.4119	.4523	.5167	.5770	1.5173	1.6402	1.7908	1.8982	2.1325	2.2283
25	.3196	.3460	.4208	.4610	.5248	.5844	1.5061	1.6258	1.7726	1.8771	2.1048	2.1979
26	.3284	.3547	.4292	.4692	.5325	.5915	1.4956	1.6124	1.7555	1.8573	2.0789	2.1695
27	.3368	.3631	.4373	.4770	.5397	.5982	1.4857	1.5998	1.7394	1.8387	2.0547	2.1429
28	.3449	.3711	.4450	.4845	.5467	.6046	1.4763	1.5879	1.7242	1.8212	2.0319	2.1179
29	.3527	.3788	.4524	.4916	.5533	.6106	1.4675	1.5766	1.7099	1.8047	2.0104	2.0943
30	.3601	.3863	.4596	.4984	.5597	.6164	1.4591	1.5660	1.6964	1.7891	1.9901	2.0720
31	.3674	.3934	.4664	.5050	.5658	.6220	1.4511	1.5559	1.6836	1.7743	1.9709	2.0510
32	.3743	.4003	.4729	.5113	.5716	.6272	1.4436	1.5462	1.6714	1.7602	1.9527	2.0311
33	.3811	.4070	.4792	.5174	.5772	.6323	1.4364	1.5371	1.6599	1.7469	1.9355	2.0122
34	.3876	.4134	.4853	.5232	.5825	.6372	1.4295	1.5284	1.6489	1.7342	1.9190	1.9942
35	.3939	.4197	.4912	.5288	.5877	.6419	1.4229	1.5201	1.6383	1.7221	1.9034	1.9771
36	.4000	.4257	.4969	.5342	.5927	.6464	1.4166	1.5121	1.6283	1.7106	1.8885	1.9608
37	.4059	.4315	.5023	.5395	.5975	.6507	1.4106	1.5045	1.6187	1.6995	1.8742	1.9452
38	.4117	.4371	.5076	.5445	.6021	.6548	1.4048	1.4972	1.6095	1.6890	1.8606	1.9303
39	.4173	.4426	.5127	.5494	.6065	.6588	1.3993	1.4903	1.6007	1.6789	1.8476	1.9160
40	.4226	.4479	.5177	.5541	.6108	.6627	1.3940	1.4836	1.5923	1.6692	1.8350	1.9024
41	.4279	.4530	.5225	.5587	.6150	.6665	1.3888	1.4771	1.5841	1.6598	1.8230	1.8892
42	.4330	.4580	.5271	.5631	.6190	.6701	1.3839	1.4709	1.5763	1.6509	1.8115	1.8767
43	.4380	.4629	.5316	.5674	.6229	.6736	1.3792	1.4649	1.5688	1.6422	1.8004	1.8646
44	.4428	.4676	.5360	.5715	.6267	.6770	1.3746	1.4591	1.5616	1.6339	1.7898	1.8529
45	.4475	.4722	.5402	.5756	.6304	.6803	1.3701	1.4536	1.5546	1.6259	1.7795	1.8417
46	.4520	.4767	.5444	.5795	.6339	.6835	1.3659	1.4482	1.5478	1.6182	1.7696	1.8309
47	.4565	.4811	.5484	.5833	.6374	.6866	1.3617	1.4430	1.5413	1.6107	1.7600	1.8204
48	.4609	.4853	.5523	.5870	.6407	.6895	1.3577	1.4380	1.5351	1.6035	1.7508	1.8104
49	.4651	.4894	.5561	.5906	.6440	.6924	1.3539	1.4331	1.5290	1.5966	1.7418	1.8006
50	.4692	.4935	.5598	.5941	.6471	.6953	1.3501	1.4284	1.5231	1.5898	1.7332	1.7912

PERCENTAGE POINTS, CHI-SQUARE OVER DEGREES OF FREEDOM DISTRIBUTION

F / n	Probability in per cent						Probability in per cent					
	0.05	0.1	0.5	1.0	2.5	5.0	95.0	97.5	99.0	99.5	99.9	99.95
51	.4733	.4974	.5634	.5975	.6502	.6980	1.3465	1.4238	1.5174	1.5833	1.7249	1.7821
52	.4772	.5012	.5669	.6009	.6532	.7007	1.3429	1.4194	1.5118	1.5769	1.7168	1.7733
53	.4810	.5050	.5704	.6041	.6562	.7033	1.3395	1.4151	1.5065	1.5708	1.7089	1.7648
54	.4848	.5087	.5737	.6073	.6590	.7059	1.3362	1.4110	1.5013	1.5649	1.7013	1.7565
55	.4885	.5122	.5770	.6104	.6618	.7083	1.3329	1.4069	1.4962	1.5591	1.6939	1.7484
56	.4921	.5157	.5802	.6134	.6645	.7107	1.3298	1.4030	1.4913	1.5535	1.6868	1.7406
57	.4956	.5191	.5833	.6163	.6671	.7131	1.3267	1.3992	1.4865	1.5480	1.6798	1.7331
58	.4990	.5225	.5863	.6192	.6697	.7154	1.3238	1.3954	1.4819	1.5427	1.6731	1.7257
59	.5024	.5258	.5893	.6220	.6722	.7176	1.3209	1.3918	1.4774	1.5375	1.6665	1.7185
60	.5057	.5290	.5922	.6248	.6747	.7198	1.3180	1.3883	1.4730	1.5325	1.6601	1.7116
61	.5089	.5321	.5951	.6274	.6771	.7219	1.3153	1.3849	1.4687	1.5276	1.6539	1.7048
62	.5121	.5352	.5979	.6300	.6795	.7240	1.3126	1.3815	1.4645	1.5229	1.6478	1.6982
63	.5152	.5382	.6006	.6326	.6817	.7260	1.3100	1.3783	1.4605	1.5182	1.6419	1.6918
64	.5182	.5411	.6033	.6351	.6840	.7280	1.3074	1.3751	1.4565	1.5137	1.6362	1.6855
65	.5212	.5440	.6059	.6376	.6862	.7300	1.3049	1.3720	1.4526	1.5093	1.6306	1.6794
66	.5241	.5469	.6085	.6400	.6883	.7319	1.3025	1.3689	1.4489	1.5050	1.6251	1.6735
67	.5270	.5496	.6110	.6424	.6905	.7338	1.3001	1.3660	1.4452	1.5008	1.6198	1.6677
68	.5298	.5524	.6134	.6447	.6925	.7356	1.2978	1.3631	1.4416	1.4967	1.6146	1.6620
69	.5325	.5550	.6159	.6469	.6946	.7374	1.2955	1.3602	1.4381	1.4927	1.6095	1.6565
70	.5352	.5577	.6182	.6492	.6965	.7391	1.2933	1.3575	1.4346	1.4888	1.6045	1.6511
71	.5379	.5602	.6205	.6514	.6985	.7408	1.2911	1.3548	1.4313	1.4850	1.5997	1.6458
72	.5405	.5628	.6228	.6535	.7004	.7425	1.2890	1.3521	1.4280	1.4812	1.5949	1.6407
73	.5431	.5653	.6251	.6556	.7023	.7442	1.2869	1.3495	1.4248	1.4776	1.5903	1.6356
74	.5456	.5677	.6273	.6576	.7041	.7458	1.2849	1.3470	1.4216	1.4740	1.5858	1.6307
75	.5481	.5701	.6294	.6597	.7059	.7474	1.2829	1.3445	1.4186	1.4705	1.5813	1.6259
76	.5505	.5724	.6316	.6617	.7077	.7489	1.2809	1.3421	1.4156	1.4670	1.5770	1.6212
77	.5529	.5748	.6336	.6636	.7094	.7505	1.2790	1.3397	1.4126	1.4637	1.5727	1.6166
78	.5553	.5771	.6357	.6655	.7111	.7520	1.2771	1.3374	1.4097	1.4604	1.5686	1.6120
79	.5576	.5793	.6377	.6674	.7128	.7534	1.2753	1.3351	1.4069	1.4572	1.5645	1.6076
80	.5599	.5815	.6396	.6692	.7144	.7549	1.2735	1.3329	1.4041	1.4540	1.5605	1.6033
81	.5621	.5837	.6416	.6711	.7160	.7563	1.2717	1.3307	1.4014	1.4509	1.5566	1.5990
82	.5643	.5858	.6435	.6729	.7176	.7577	1.2700	1.3285	1.3987	1.4479	1.5527	1.5948
83	.5665	.5879	.6454	.6746	.7192	.7591	1.2683	1.3264	1.3961	1.4449	1.5490	1.5908
84	.5687	.5900	.6472	.6763	.7207	.7604	1.2666	1.3243	1.3935	1.4420	1.5453	1.5868
85	.5708	.5920	.6491	.6780	.7222	.7618	1.2650	1.3223	1.3910	1.4391	1.5417	1.5828
86	.5728	.5940	.6508	.6797	.7237	.7631	1.2633	1.3203	1.3885	1.4363	1.5381	1.5790
87	.5749	.5960	.6526	.6814	.7252	.7643	1.2618	1.3183	1.3861	1.4335	1.5346	1.5752
88	.5769	.5979	.6543	.6830	.7266	.7656	1.2602	1.3164	1.3837	1.4308	1.5312	1.5715
89	.5789	.5998	.6561	.6846	.7280	.7668	1.2587	1.3145	1.3814	1.4282	1.5278	1.5678
90	.5808	.6017	.6577	.6862	.7294	.7681	1.2572	1.3126	1.3791	1.4255	1.5245	1.5643
91	.5828	.6036	.6594	.6877	.7308	.7693	1.2557	1.3108	1.3768	1.4230	1.5213	1.5607
92	.5847	.6054	.6610	.6892	.7321	.7705	1.2542	1.3090	1.3746	1.4204	1.5181	1.5573
93	.5865	.6072	.6626	.6907	.7335	.7716	1.2528	1.3072	1.3724	1.4180	1.5150	1.5539
94	.5884	.6090	.6642	.6922	.7348	.7728	1.2514	1.3055	1.3702	1.4155	1.5119	1.5505
95	.5902	.6108	.6658	.6937	.7361	.7739	1.2500	1.3038	1.3681	1.4131	1.5089	1.5473
96	.5920	.6125	.6673	.6951	.7373	.7750	1.2487	1.3021	1.3661	1.4108	1.5059	1.5440
97	.5938	.6142	.6688	.6965	.7386	.7761	1.2473	1.3004	1.3640	1.4084	1.5030	1.5409
98	.5955	.6159	.6703	.6979	.7398	.7772	1.2460	1.2988	1.3620	1.4062	1.5001	1.5377
99	.5973	.6175	.6718	.6993	.7410	.7782	1.2447	1.2972	1.3600	1.4039	1.4973	1.5347
100	.5990	.6192	.6733	.7007	.7422	.7793	1.2434	1.2956	1.3581	1.4017	1.4945	1.5317

PERCENTAGE POINTS, CHI-SQUARE OVER DEGREES OF FREEDOM DISTRIBUTION

F / n	Probability in per cent						Probability in per cent					
	0.05	0.1	0.5	1.0	2.5	5.0	95.0	97.5	99.0	99.5	99.9	99.95
100	.5990	.6192	.6733	.7007	.7422	.7793	1.2434	1.2956	1.3581	1.4017	1.4945	1.5317
105	.6072	.6271	.6802	.7071	.7480	.7843	1.2373	1.2881	1.3488	1.3911	1.4812	1.5173
110	.6148	.6344	.6868	.7132	.7534	.7890	1.2316	1.2811	1.3401	1.3813	1.4689	1.5040
115	.6221	.6414	.6930	.7190	.7584	.7934	1.2263	1.2746	1.3321	1.3722	1.4575	1.4916
120	.6289	.6480	.6988	.7243	.7632	.7975	1.2214	1.2685	1.3246	1.3637	1.4468	1.4801
125	.6353	.6542	.7042	.7294	.7676	.8014	1.2167	1.2627	1.3175	1.3557	1.4368	1.4692
130	.6414	.6600	.7094	.7342	.7718	.8051	1.2124	1.2574	1.3109	1.3484	1.4275	1.4592
135	.6473	.6656	.7143	.7388	.7757	.8085	1.2083	1.2523	1.3047	1.3413	1.4187	1.4496
140	.6528	.6709	.7190	.7431	.7795	.8119	1.2043	1.2475	1.2988	1.3346	1.4104	1.4406
145	.6581	.6760	.7234	.7472	.7831	.8150	1.2007	1.2430	1.2933	1.3284	1.4026	1.4321
150	.6631	.6808	.7276	.7511	.7865	.8180	1.1972	1.2387	1.2880	1.3224	1.3951	1.4241
155	.6679	.6854	.7316	.7549	.7898	.8208	1.1939	1.2346	1.2830	1.3168	1.3881	1.4166
160	.6725	.6898	.7355	.7584	.7930	.8235	1.1907	1.2308	1.2783	1.3114	1.3813	1.4093
165	.6769	.6939	.7392	.7618	.7959	.8260	1.1877	1.2270	1.2737	1.3063	1.3751	1.4024
170	.6811	.6980	.7427	.7651	.7987	.8285	1.1848	1.2235	1.2694	1.3014	1.3690	1.3958
175	.6852	.7019	.7461	.7682	.8015	.8309	1.1821	1.2201	1.2653	1.2968	1.3632	1.3896
180	.6891	.7056	.7494	.7712	.8041	.8332	1.1795	1.2170	1.2614	1.2924	1.3577	1.3836
185	.6929	.7092	.7525	.7741	.8066	.8353	1.1769	1.2138	1.2576	1.2881	1.3523	1.3779
190	.6964	.7127	.7555	.7768	.8090	.8374	1.1745	1.2109	1.2541	1.2840	1.3472	1.3725
195	.6999	.7160	.7584	.7795	.8114	.8394	1.1722	1.2081	1.2506	1.2801	1.3424	1.3672
200	.7033	.7192	.7612	.7821	.8136	.8414	1.1700	1.2053	1.2473	1.2763	1.3377	1.3622
210	.7097	.7254	.7665	.7870	.8179	.8451	1.1657	1.2001	1.2409	1.2692	1.3288	1.3526
220	.7157	.7311	.7715	.7916	.8219	.8485	1.1618	1.1953	1.2351	1.2626	1.3207	1.3438
230	.7213	.7365	.7762	.7959	.8256	.8517	1.1582	1.1908	1.2297	1.2564	1.3131	1.3356
240	.7266	.7415	.7805	.7999	.8291	.8547	1.1547	1.1867	1.2246	1.2507	1.3060	1.3279
250	.7317	.7463	.7847	.8037	.8324	.8576	1.1515	1.1828	1.2198	1.2453	1.2994	1.3207
260	.7364	.7507	.7886	.8073	.8355	.8602	1.1485	1.1791	1.2153	1.2403	1.2931	1.3140
270	.7408	.7550	.7923	.8107	.8384	.8628	1.1457	1.1756	1.2111	1.2356	1.2872	1.3077
280	.7450	.7590	.7958	.8139	.8412	.8652	1.1430	1.1723	1.2071	1.2312	1.2817	1.3017
290	.7491	.7629	.7991	.8170	.8438	.8674	1.1404	1.1692	1.2033	1.2269	1.2764	1.2961
300	.7529	.7665	.8023	.8199	.8463	.8696	1.1380	1.1663	1.1997	1.2229	1.2714	1.2907
350	.7698	.7826	.8160	.8326	.8573	.8790	1.1275	1.1535	1.1843	1.2055	1.2500	1.2676
400	.7836	.7957	.8272	.8429	.8662	.8866	1.1191	1.1433	1.1718	1.1915	1.2378	1.2491
450	.7951	.8066	.8366	.8515	.8736	.8929	1.1121	1.1349	1.1616	1.1801	1.2187	1.2340
500	.8050	.8160	.8446	.8588	.8799	.8983	1.1063	1.1277	1.1530	1.1704	1.2070	1.2214
550	.8135	.8239	.8515	.8651	.8853	.9029	1.1012	1.1216	1.1456	1.1622	1.1968	1.2105
600	.8208	.8310	.8575	.8706	.8900	.9070	1.0968	1.1163	1.1392	1.1550	1.1880	1.2010
650	.8275	.8373	.8629	.8755	.8942	.9106	1.0929	1.1116	1.1335	1.1487	1.1803	1.1927
700	.8334	.8429	.8677	.8799	.8980	.9137	1.0895	1.1074	1.1285	1.1430	1.1734	1.1853
750	.8387	.8480	.8720	.8838	.9013	.9166	1.0864	1.1037	1.1240	1.1380	1.1672	1.1787
800	.8436	.8526	.8759	.8874	.9044	.9192	1.0836	1.1004	1.1200	1.1335	1.1617	1.1728
850	.8480	.8568	.8795	.8906	.9072	.9216	1.0811	1.0973	1.1163	1.1294	1.1567	1.1674
900	.8521	.8606	.8827	.8936	.9097	.9237	1.0788	1.0945	1.1129	1.1256	1.1520	1.1624
950	.8559	.8642	.8858	.8964	.9121	.9257	1.0767	1.0919	1.1098	1.1221	1.1478	1.1579
1000	.8594	.8675	.8886	.8989	.9143	.9276	1.0747	1.0895	1.1070	1.1190	1.1440	1.1538
2000	.8992	.9051	.9204	.9279	.9390	.9486	1.0526	1.0629	1.0750	1.0833	1.1006	1.1074
3000	.9172	.9221	.9348	.9409	.9500	.9579	1.0429	1.0513	1.0611	1.0678	1.0817	1.0872
4000	.9280	.9323	.9433	.9487	.9566	.9635	1.0370	1.0443	1.0527	1.0585	1.0705	1.0752
5000	.9355	.9393	.9493	.9541	.9612	.9673	1.0331	1.0396	1.0471	1.0523	1.0630	1.0671
10000	.9541	.9569	.9640	.9674	.9725	.9769	1.0234	1.0279	1.0332	1.0368	1.0443	1.0472

V.3 NUMBER OF OBSERVATIONS REQUIRED FOR THE COMPARISON OF A POPULATION VARIANCE WITH A STANDARD VALUE USING THE CHI-SQUARE TEST

The tabular entries show the value of the ratio R of the population variance σ_1^2 to a standard variance σ_0^2 which is undetected with probability β in a χ^2 test at significance level α of an estimate s_1^2 of σ_1^2 based on n degrees of freedom.

NUMBER OF OBSERVATIONS REQUIRED FOR THE COMPARISON OF A POPULATION VARIANCE WITH A STANDARD VALUE USING THE CHI-SQUARE TEST

n	$\alpha = 0.01$				$\alpha = 0.05$			
	$\beta = 0.01$	$\beta = 0.05$	$\beta = 0.1$	$\beta = 0.5$	$\beta = 0.01$	$\beta = 0.05$	$\beta = 0.1$	$\beta = 0.5$
1	42,240	1,687	420.2	14.58	25,450	977.0	243.3	8.444
2	458.2	89.78	43.71	6.644	298.1	58.40	28.43	4.322
3	98.79	32.24	19.41	4.795	68.05	22.21	13.37	3.303
4	44.69	18.68	12.48	3.955	31.93	13.35	8.920	2.826
5	27.22	13.17	9.369	3.467	19.97	9.665	6.875	2.544
6	19.28	10.28	7.628	3.144	14.44	7.699	5.713	2.354
7	14.91	8.524	6.521	2.911	11.35	6.491	4.965	2.217
8	12.20	7.352	5.757	2.736	9.418	5.675	4.444	2.112
9	10.38	6.516	5.198	2.597	8.103	5.088	4.059	2.028
10	9.072	5.890	4.770	2.484	7.156	4.646	3.763	1.960
12	7.343	5.017	4.159	2.312	5.889	4.023	3.335	1.854
15	5.847	4.211	3.578	2.132	4.780	3.442	2.925	1.743
20	4.548	3.462	3.019	1.943	3.802	2.895	2.524	1.624
24	3.959	3.104	2.745	1.842	3.354	2.630	2.326	1.560
30	3.403	2.752	2.471	1.735	2.927	2.367	2.125	1.492
40	2.874	2.403	2.192	1.619	2.516	2.103	1.919	1.418
60	2.358	2.046	1.902	1.490	2.110	1.831	1.702	1.333
120	1.829	1.661	1.580	1.332	1.686	1.532	1.457	1.228
∞	1.000	1.000	1.000	1.000	1.000	1.000	1.000	1.000

Examples

Testing for an increase in variance. Let $\alpha = 0.05$, $\beta = 0.01$, and $R = 4$. Entering the table with these values it is found that the value 4 occurs between the rows corresponding to $n = 15$ and $n = 20$. Using rough interpolation it is indicated that the estimate of variance should be based on 19 degrees of freedom.

Testing for a decrease in variance. Let $\alpha = 0.05$, $\beta = 0.01$, and $R = 0.33$. The table is entered with $\alpha' = \beta = 0.01$, $\beta' = \alpha = 0.05$, and $R' = 1/R = 3$. It is found that the value 3 occurs between the rows corresponding to $n = 24$ and $n = 30$. Using rough interpolation it is indicated that the estimate of variance should be based on 26 degrees of freedom.

V.4 OPERATING CHARACTERISTIC (OC) CURVES FOR A TEST ON THE STANDARD DEVIATION OF A NORMAL DISTRIBUTION

The OC curves give the sample sizes needed for given values of $\alpha = P$ (Type I error) and $\beta = P$ (Type II error) for a test of the hypothesis H_0: $\sigma = \sigma_0$. The statistic used is $\chi^2 = \dfrac{(n-1)s^2}{\sigma_0{}^2}$, which is distributed as the Chi-square distribution with $n - 1$ degrees of freedom. The required sample size is obtained by entering the appropriate set of curves for given α and β for various values of $\lambda = \dfrac{\sigma_1}{\sigma_0}$ for both one-sided and two-sided tests.

OC CURVES FOR A TEST ON THE STANDARD DEVIATION OF A NORMAL DISTRIBUTION

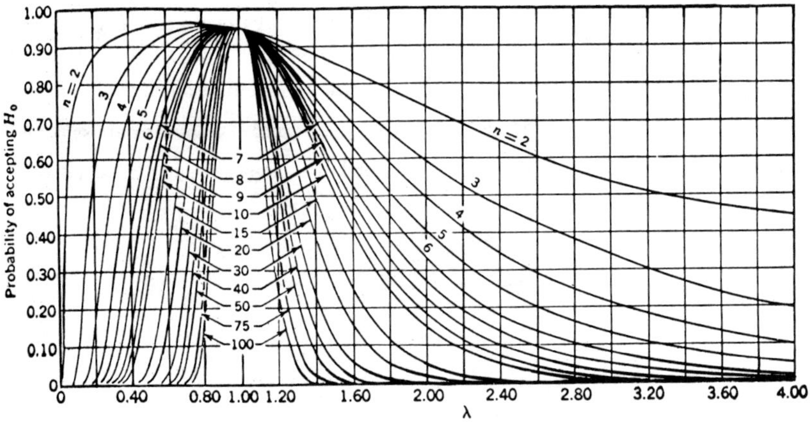

a) OC curves for different values of *n* for the two-sided chi-square test for a level of significance $\alpha = 0.05$.

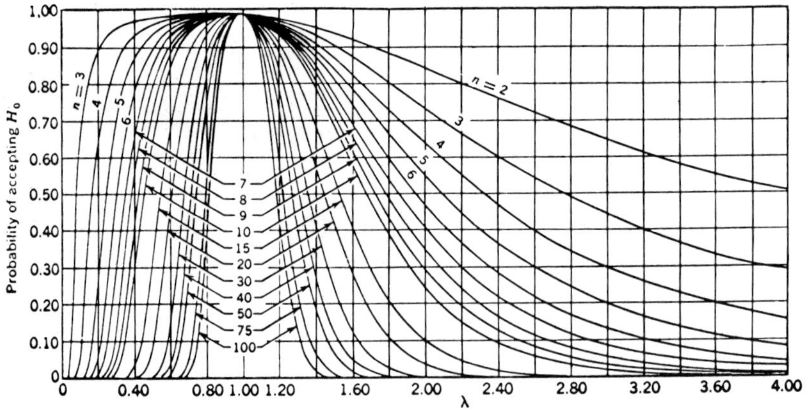

b) OC curves for different values of *n* for the two-sided chi-square test for a level of significance $\alpha = 0.01$.

OC CURVES FOR A TEST ON THE STANDARD DEVIATION OF A NORMAL DISTRIBUTION

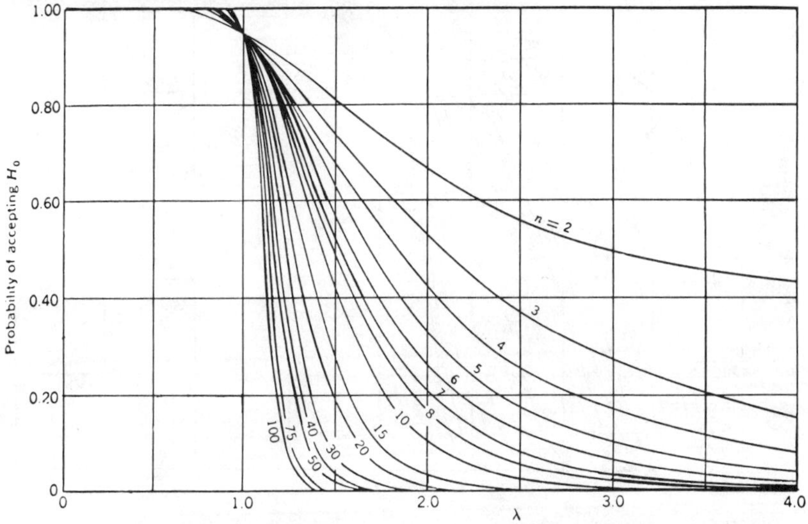

c) OC curves for different values of n for the one-sided (upper tail) chi-square test for a level of significance $\alpha = 0.05$.

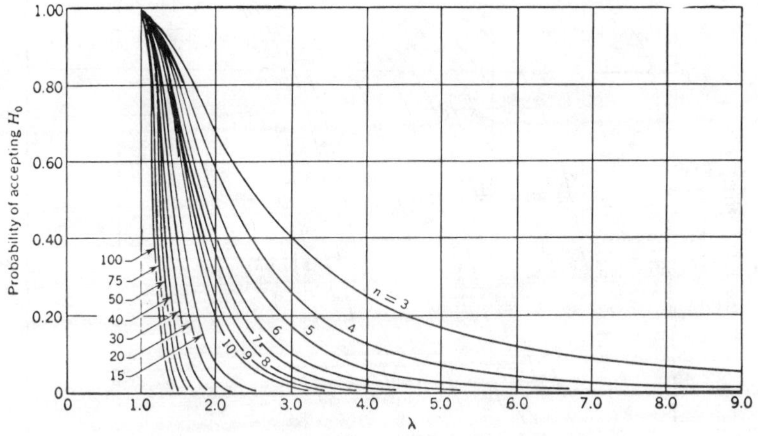

d) OC curves for different values of n for the one-sided (upper tail) chi-square test for a level of significance $\alpha = 0.01$.

OC CURVES FOR A TEST ON THE STANDARD DEVIATION OF A NORMAL DISTRIBUTION

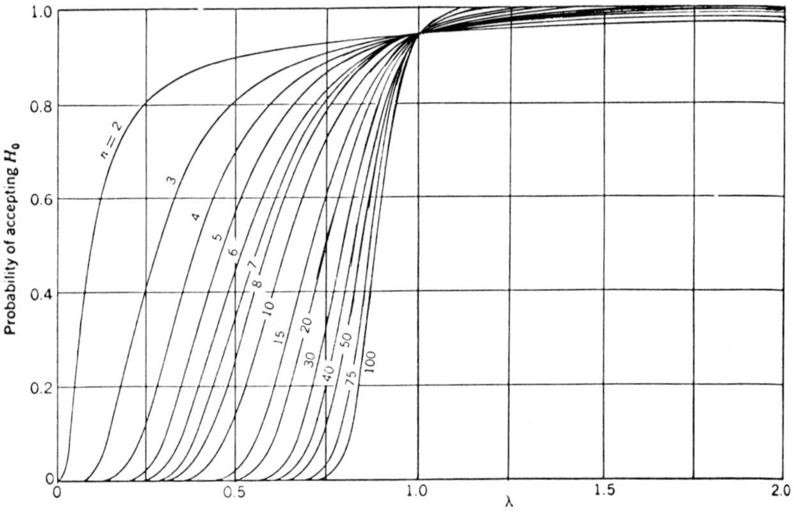

e) OC curves for different values of n for the one-sided (lower tail) chi-square test for a level of significance $\alpha = 0.05$.

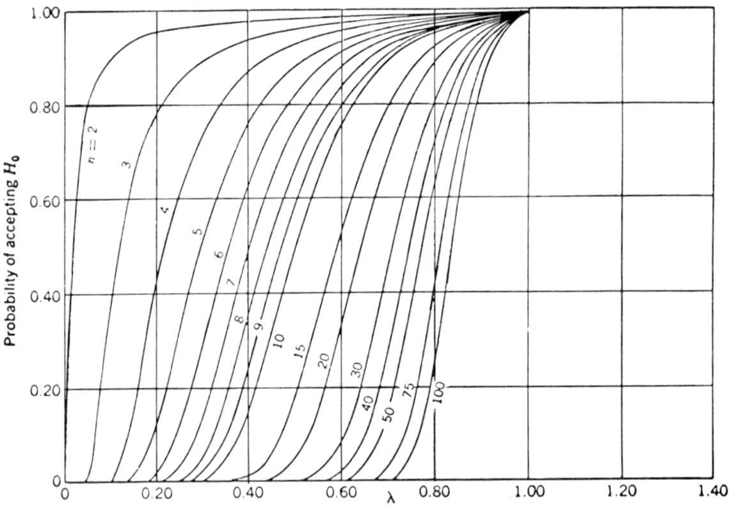

f) OC curves for different values of n for the one-sided (lower tail) chi-square test for a level of significance $\alpha = 0.01$.

VI. *F*-DISTRIBUTION

VI.1 PERCENTAGE POINTS, *F*-DISTRIBUTION

This table gives values of F such that

$$F(F) = \int_0^F \frac{\Gamma\left(\frac{m+n}{2}\right)}{\Gamma\left(\frac{m}{2}\right)\Gamma\left(\frac{n}{2}\right)} m^{\frac{m}{2}} n^{\frac{n}{2}} x^{\frac{m-2}{2}} (n+mx)^{-\frac{m+n}{2}} dx$$

for selected values of m, the number of degrees of freedom of the numerator of F; and for selected values of n, the number of degrees of freedom of the denominator of F. The table also provides values corresponding to $F(F) = .10, .05, .025, .01, .005, .001$ since $F_{1-\alpha}$ for m and n degrees of freedom is the reciprocal of F_{α} for n and m degrees of freedom. Thus

$$F_{.05}(4, 7) = \frac{1}{F_{.95}(7, 4)} = \frac{1}{6.09} = .164 \ .$$

PERCENTAGE POINTS, *F*-DISTRIBUTION

$$F(F) = \int_0^F \frac{\Gamma\left(\frac{m+n}{2}\right)}{\Gamma\left(\frac{m}{2}\right)\Gamma\left(\frac{n}{2}\right)} m^{\frac{m}{2}} n^{\frac{n}{2}} x^{\frac{m}{2}-1} (n+mx)^{-\frac{m+n}{2}}\, dx = .90$$

n \ m	1	2	3	4	5	6	7	8	9	10	12	15	20	24	30	40	60	120	∞
1	39.86	49.50	53.59	55.83	57.24	58.20	58.91	59.44	59.86	60.19	60.71	61.22	61.74	62.00	62.26	62.53	62.79	63.06	63.33
2	8.53	9.00	9.16	9.24	9.29	9.33	9.35	9.37	9.38	9.39	9.41	9.42	9.44	9.45	9.46	9.47	9.47	9.48	9.49
3	5.54	5,46	5.39	5.34	5.31	5.28	5.27	5.25	5.24	5.23	5.22	5.20	5.18	5.18	5.17	5.16	5.15	5.14	5.13
4	4.54	4.32	4.19	4.11	4.05	4.01	3.98	3.95	3.94	3.92	3.90	3.87	3.84	3.83	3.82	3.80	3.79	3.78	3.76
5	4.06	3.78	3.62	3.52	3.45	3.40	3.37	3.34	3.32	3.30	3.27	3.24	3.21	3.19	3.17	3.16	3.14	3.12	3.10
6	3.78	3.46	3.29	3.18	3.11	3.05	3.01	2.98	2.96	2.94	2.90	2.87	2.84	2.82	2.80	2.78	2.76	2.74	2.72
7	3.59	3.26	3.07	2.96	2.88	2.83	2.78	2.75	2.72	2.70	2.67	2.63	2.59	2.58	2.56	2.54	2.51	2.49	2.47
8	3.46	3.11	2.92	2.81	2.73	2.67	2.62	2.59	2.56	2.54	2.50	2.46	2.42	2.40	2.38	2.36	2.34	2.32	2.29
9	3.36	3.01	2.81	2.69	2.61	2.55	2.51	2.47	2.44	2.42	2.38	2.34	2.30	2.28	2.25	2.23	2.21	2.18	2.16
10	3.29	2.92	2.73	2.61	2.52	2.46	2.41	2.38	2.35	2.32	2.28	2.24	2.20	2.18	2.16	2.13	2.11	2.08	2.06
11	3.23	2.86	2.66	2.54	2.45	2.39	2.34	2.30	2.27	2.25	2.21	2.17	2.12	2.10	2.08	2.05	2.03	2.00	1.97
12	3.18	2.81	2.61	2.48	2.39	2.33	2.28	2.24	2.21	2.19	2.15	2.10	2.06	2.04	2.01	1.99	1.96	1.93	1.90
13	3.14	2.76	2.56	2.43	2.35	2.28	2.23	2.20	2.16	2.14	2.10	2.05	2.01	1.98	1.96	1.93	1.90	1.88	1.85
14	3.10	2.73	2.52	2.39	2.31	2.24	2.19	2.15	2.12	2.10	2.05	2.01	1.96	1.94	1.91	1.89	1.86	1.83	1.80
15	3.07	2.70	2.49	2.36	2.27	2.21	2.16	2.12	2.09	2.06	2.02	1.97	1.92	1.90	1.87	1.85	1.82	1.79	1.76
16	3.05	2.67	2.46	2.33	2.24	2.18	2.13	2.09	2.06	2.03	1.99	1.94	1.89	1.87	1.84	1.81	1.78	1.75	1.72
17	3.03	2.64	2.44	2.31	2.22	2.15	2.10	2.06	2.03	2.00	1.96	1.91	1.86	1.84	1.81	1.78	1.75	1.72	1.69
18	3.01	2.62	2.42	2.29	2.20	2.13	2.08	2.04	2.00	1.98	1.93	1.89	1.84	1.81	1.78	1.75	1.72	1.69	1.66
19	2.99	2.61	2.40	2.27	2.18	2.11	2.06	2.02	1.98	1.96	1.91	1.86	1.81	1.79	1.76	1.73	1.70	1.67	1.63
20	2.97	2.59	2.38	2.25	2.16	2.09	2.04	2.00	1.96	1.94	1.89	1.84	1.79	1.77	1.74	1.71	1.68	1.64	1.61
21	2.96	2.57	2.36	2.23	2.14	2.08	2.02	1.98	1.95	1.92	1.87	1.83	1.78	1.75	1.72	1.69	1.66	1.62	1.59
22	2.95	2.56	2.35	2.22	2.13	2.06	2.01	1.97	1.93	1.90	1.86	1.81	1.76	1.73	1.70	1.67	1.64	1.60	1.57
23	2.94	2.55	2.34	2.21	2.11	2.05	1.99	1.95	1.92	1.89	1.84	1.80	1.74	1.72	1.69	1.66	1.62	1.59	1.55
24	2.93	2.54	2.33	2.19	2.10	2.04	1.98	1.94	1.91	1.88	1.83	1.78	1.73	1.70	1.67	1.64	1.61	1.57	1.53
25	2.92	2.53	2.32	2.18	2.09	2.02	1.97	1.93	1.89	1.87	1.82	1.77	1.72	1.69	1.66	1.63	1.59	1.56	1.52
26	2.91	2.52	2.31	2.17	2.08	2.01	1.96	1.92	1.88	1.86	1.81	1.76	1.71	1.68	1.65	1.61	1.58	1.54	1.50
27	2.90	2.51	2.30	2.17	2.07	2.00	1.95	1.91	1.87	1.85	1.80	1.75	1.70	1.67	1.64	1.60	1.57	1.53	1.49
28	2.89	2.50	2.29	2.16	2.06	2.00	1.94	1.90	1.87	1.84	1.79	1.74	1.69	1.66	1.63	1.59	1.56	1.52	1.48
29	2.89	2.50	2.28	2.15	2.06	1.99	1.93	1.89	1.86	1.83	1.78	1.73	1.68	1.65	1.62	1.58	1.55	1.51	1.47
30	2.88	2.49	2.28	2.14	2.05	1.98	1.93	1.88	1.85	1.82	1.77	1.72	1.67	1.64	1.61	1.57	1.54	1.50	1.46
40	2.84	2.44	2.23	2.09	2.00	1.93	1.87	1.83	1.79	1.76	1.71	1.66	1.61	1.57	1.54	1.51	1.47	1.42	1.38
60	2.79	2.39	2.18	2.04	1.95	1.87	1.82	1.77	1.74	1.71	1.66	1.60	1.54	1.51	1.48	1.44	1.40	1.35	1.29
120	2.75	2.35	2.13	1.99	1.90	1.82	1.77	1.72	1.68	1.65	1.60	1.55	1.48	1.45	1.41	1.37	1.32	1.26	1.19
∞	2.71	2.30	2.08	1.94	1.85	1.77	1.72	1.67	1.63	1.60	1.55	1.49	1.42	1.38	1.34	1.30	1.24	1.17	1.00

$F = \frac{s_1^2}{s_2^2} = \frac{S_1}{m} \Big/ \frac{S_2}{n}$, where $s_1^2 = S_1/m$ and $s_2^2 = S_2/n$ are independent mean squares estimating a common variance σ^2 and based on m and n degrees of freedom, respectively.

PERCENTAGE POINTS, F-DISTRIBUTION

$$F(F) = \int_0^F \frac{\Gamma\left(\frac{m+n}{2}\right)}{\Gamma\left(\frac{m}{2}\right)\Gamma\left(\frac{n}{2}\right)} m^{\frac{m}{2}} n^{\frac{n}{2}} x^{\frac{m}{2}-1} (n+mx)^{-\frac{m+n}{2}} dx = .95$$

n \ m	1	2	3	4	5	6	7	8	9	10	12	15	20	24	30	40	60	120	∞
1	161.4	199.5	215.7	224.6	230.2	234.0	236.8	238.9	240.5	241.9	243.9	245.9	248.0	249.1	250.1	251.1	252.2	253.3	254.3
2	18.51	19.00	19.16	19.25	19.30	19.33	19.35	19.37	19.38	19.40	19.41	19.43	19.45	19.45	19.46	19.47	19.48	19.49	19.50
3	10.13	9.55	9.28	9.12	9.01	8.94	8.89	8.85	8.81	8.79	8.74	8.70	8.66	8.64	8.62	8.59	8.57	8.55	8.53
4	7.71	6.94	6.59	6.39	6.26	6.16	6.09	6.04	6.00	5.96	5.91	5.86	5.80	5.77	5.75	5.72	5.69	5.66	5.63
5	6.61	5.79	5.41	5.19	5.05	4.95	4.88	4.82	4.77	4.74	4.68	4.62	4.56	4.53	4.50	4.46	4.43	4.40	4.36
6	5.99	5.14	4.76	4.53	4.39	4.28	4.21	4.15	4.10	4.06	4.00	3.94	3.87	3.84	3.81	3.77	3.74	3.70	3.67
7	5.59	4.74	4.35	4.12	3.97	3.87	3.79	3.73	3.68	3.64	3.57	3.51	3.44	3.41	3.38	3.34	3.30	3.27	3.23
8	5.32	4.46	4.07	3.84	3.69	3.58	3.50	3.44	3.39	3.35	3.28	3.22	3.15	3.12	3.08	3.04	3.01	2.97	2.93
9	5.12	4.26	3.86	3.63	3.48	3.37	3.29	3.23	3.18	3.14	3.07	3.01	2.94	2.90	2.86	2.83	2.79	2.75	2.71
10	4.96	4.10	3.71	3.48	3.33	3.22	3.14	3.07	3.02	2.98	2.91	2.85	2.77	2.74	2.70	2.66	2.62	2.58	2.54
11	4.84	3.98	3.59	3.36	3.20	3.09	3.01	2.95	2.90	2.85	2.79	2.72	2.65	2.61	2.57	2.53	2.49	2.45	2.40
12	4.75	3.89	3.49	3.26	3.11	3.00	2.91	2.85	2.80	2.75	2.69	2.62	2.54	2.51	2.47	2.43	2.38	2.34	2.30
13	4.67	3.81	3.41	3.18	3.03	2.92	2.83	2.77	2.71	2.67	2.60	2.53	2.46	2.42	2.38	2.34	2.30	2.25	2.21
14	4.60	3.74	3.34	3.11	2.96	2.85	2.76	2.70	2.65	2.60	2.53	2.46	2.39	2.35	2.31	2.27	2.22	2.18	2.13
15	4.54	3.68	3.29	3.06	2.90	2.79	2.71	2.64	2.59	2.54	2.48	2.40	2.33	2.29	2.25	2.20	2.16	2.11	2.07
16	4.49	3.63	3.24	3.01	2.85	2.74	2.66	2.59	2.54	2.49	2.42	2.35	2.28	2.24	2.19	2.15	2.11	2.06	2.01
17	4.45	3.59	3.20	2.96	2.81	2.70	2.61	2.55	2.49	2.45	2.38	2.31	2.23	2.19	2.15	2.10	2.06	2.01	1.96
18	4.41	3.55	3.16	2.93	2.77	2.66	2.58	2.51	2.46	2.41	2.34	2.27	2.19	2.15	2.11	2.06	2.02	1.97	1.92
19	4.38	3.52	3.13	2.90	2.74	2.63	2.54	2.48	2.42	2.38	2.31	2.23	2.16	2.11	2.07	2.03	1.98	1.93	1.88
20	4.35	3.49	3.10	2.87	2.71	2.60	2.51	2.45	2.39	2.35	2.28	2.20	2.12	2.08	2.04	1.99	1.95	1.90	1.84
21	4.32	3.47	3.07	2.84	2.68	2.57	2.49	2.42	2.37	2.32	2.25	2.18	2.10	2.05	2.01	1.96	1.92	1.87	1.81
22	4.30	3.44	3.05	2.82	2.66	2.55	2.46	2.40	2.34	2.30	2.23	2.15	2.07	2.03	1.98	1.94	1.89	1.84	1.78
23	4.28	3.42	3.03	2.80	2.64	2.53	2.44	2.37	2.32	2.27	2.20	2.13	2.05	2.01	1.96	1.91	1.86	1.81	1.76
24	4.26	3.40	3.01	2.78	2.62	2.51	2.42	2.36	2.30	2.25	2.18	2.11	2.03	1.98	1.94	1.89	1.84	1.79	1.73
25	4.24	3.39	2.99	2.76	2.60	2.49	2.40	2.34	2.28	2.24	2.16	2.09	2.01	1.96	1.92	1.87	1.82	1.77	1.71
26	4.23	3.37	2.98	2.74	2.59	2.47	2.39	2.32	2.27	2.22	2.15	2.07	1.99	1.95	1.90	1.85	1.80	1.75	1.69
27	4.21	3.35	2.96	2.73	2.57	2.46	2.37	2.31	2.25	2.20	2.13	2.06	1.97	1.93	1.88	1.84	1.79	1.73	1.67
28	4.20	3.34	2.95	2.71	2.56	2.45	2.36	2.29	2.24	2.19	2.12	2.04	1.96	1.91	1.87	1.82	1.77	1.71	1.65
29	4.18	3.33	2.93	2.70	2.55	2.43	2.35	2.28	2.22	2.18	2.10	2.03	1.94	1.90	1.85	1.81	1.75	1.70	1.64
30	4.17	3.32	2.92	2.69	2.53	2.42	2.33	2.27	2.21	2.16	2.09	2.01	1.93	1.89	1.84	1.79	1.74	1.68	1.62
40	4.08	3.23	2.84	2.61	2.45	2.34	2.25	2.18	2.12	2.08	2.00	1.92	1.84	1.79	1.74	1.69	1.64	1.58	1.51
60	4.00	3.15	2.76	2.53	2.37	2.25	2.17	2.10	2.04	1.99	1.92	1.84	1.75	1.70	1.65	1.59	1.53	1.47	1.39
120	3.92	3.07	2.68	2.45	2.29	2.17	2.09	2.02	1.96	1.91	1.83	1.75	1.66	1.61	1.55	1.50	1.43	1.35	1.25
∞	3.84	3.00	2.60	2.37	2.21	2.10	2.01	1.94	1.88	1.83	1.75	1.67	1.57	1.52	1.46	1.39	1.32	1.22	1.00

$F = \frac{s_1^2}{s_2^2} = \frac{S_1}{m} \Big/ \frac{S_2}{n}$, where $s_1^2 = S_1/m$ and $s_2^2 = S_2/n$ are independent mean squares estimating a common variance σ^2 and based on m and n degrees of freedom, respectively.

PERCENTAGE POINTS, *F*-DISTRIBUTION

$$F(F) = \int_0^F \frac{\Gamma\left(\frac{m+n}{2}\right)}{\Gamma\left(\frac{m}{2}\right)\Gamma\left(\frac{n}{2}\right)} m^{\frac{m}{2}} n^{\frac{n}{2}} x^{\frac{m}{2}-1} (n+mx)^{-\frac{m+n}{2}} dx = .975$$

n \ m	1	2	3	4	5	6	7	8	9	10	12	15	20	24	30	40	60	120	∞
1	647.8	799.5	864.2	899.6	921.8	937.1	948.2	956.7	963.3	968.6	976.7	984.9	993.1	997.2	1001	1006	1010	1014	1018
2	38.51	39.00	39.17	39.25	39.30	39.33	39.36	39.37	39.39	39.40	39.41	39.43	39.45	39.46	39.46	39.47	39.48	39.49	39.50
3	17.44	16.04	15.44	15.10	14.88	14.73	14.62	14.54	14.47	14.42	14.34	14.25	14.17	14.12	14.08	14.04	13.99	13.95	13.90
4	12.22	10.65	9.98	9.60	9.36	9.20	9.07	8.98	8.90	8.84	8.75	8.66	8.56	8.51	8.46	8.41	8.36	8.31	8.26
5	10.01	8.43	7.76	7.39	7.15	6.98	6.85	6.76	6.68	6.62	6.52	6.43	6.33	6.28	6.23	6.18	6.12	6.07	6.02
6	8.81	7.26	6.60	6.23	5.99	5.82	5.70	5.60	5.52	5.46	5.37	5.27	5.17	5.12	5.07	5.01	4.96	4.90	4.85
7	8.07	6.54	5.89	5.52	5.29	5.12	4.99	4.90	4.82	4.76	4.67	4.57	4.47	4.42	4.36	4.31	4.25	4.20	4.14
8	7.57	6.06	5.42	5.05	4.82	4.65	4.53	4.43	4.36	4.30	4.20	4.10	4.00	3.95	3.89	3.84	3.78	3.73	3.67
9	7.21	5.71	5.08	4.72	4.48	4.32	4.20	4.10	4.03	3.96	3.87	3.77	3.67	3.61	3.56	3.51	3.45	3.39	3.33
10	6.94	5.46	4.83	4.47	4.24	4.07	3.95	3.85	3.78	3.72	3.62	3.52	3.42	3.37	3.31	3.26	3.20	3.14	3.08
11	6.72	5.26	4.63	4.28	4.04	3.88	3.76	3.66	3.59	3.53	3.43	3.33	3.23	3.17	3.12	3.06	3.00	2.94	2.88
12	6.55	5.10	4.47	4.12	3.89	3.73	3.61	3.51	3.44	3.37	3.28	3.18	3.07	3.02	2.96	2.91	2.85	2.79	2.72
13	6.41	4.97	4.35	4.00	3.77	3.60	3.48	3.39	3.31	3.25	3.15	3.05	2.95	2.89	2.84	2.78	2.72	2.66	2.60
14	6.30	4.86	4.24	3.89	3.66	3.50	3.38	3.29	3.21	3.15	3.05	2.95	2.84	2.79	2.73	2.67	2.61	2.55	2.49
15	6.20	4.77	4.15	3.80	3.58	3.41	3.29	3.20	3.12	3.06	2.96	2.86	2.76	2.70	2.64	2.59	2.52	2.46	2.40
16	6.12	4.69	4.08	3.73	3.50	3.34	3.22	3.12	3.05	2.99	2.89	2.79	2.68	2.63	2.57	2.51	2.45	2.38	2.32
17	6.04	4.62	4.01	3.66	3.44	3.28	3.16	3.06	2.98	2.92	2.82	2.72	2.62	2.56	2.50	2.44	2.38	2.32	2.25
18	5.98	4.56	3.95	3.61	3.38	3.22	3.10	3.01	2.93	2.87	2.77	2.67	2.56	2.50	2.44	2.38	2.32	2.26	2.19
19	5.92	4.51	3.90	3.56	3.33	3.17	3.05	2.96	2.88	2.82	2.72	2.62	2.51	2.45	2.39	2.33	2.27	2.20	2.13
20	5.87	4.46	3.86	3.51	3.29	3.13	3.01	2.91	2.84	2.77	2.68	2.57	2.46	2.41	2.35	2.29	2.22	2.16	2.09
21	5.83	4.42	3.82	3.48	3.25	3.09	2.97	2.87	2.80	2.73	2.64	2.53	2.42	2.37	2.31	2.25	2.18	2.11	2.04
22	5.79	4.38	3.78	3.44	3.22	3.05	2.93	2.84	2.76	2.70	2.60	2.50	2.39	2.33	2.27	2.21	2.14	2.08	2.00
23	5.75	4.35	3.75	3.41	3.18	3.02	2.90	2.81	2.73	2.67	2.57	2.47	2.36	2.30	2.24	2.18	2.11	2.04	1.97
24	5.72	4.32	3.72	3.38	3.15	2.99	2.87	2.78	2.70	2.64	2.54	2.44	2.33	2.27	2.21	2.15	2.08	2.01	1.94
25	5.69	4.29	3.69	3.35	3.13	2.97	2.85	2.75	2.68	2.61	2.51	2.41	2.30	2.24	2.18	2.12	2.05	1.98	1.91
26	5.66	4.27	3.67	3.33	3.10	2.94	2.82	2.73	2.65	2.59	2.49	2.39	2.28	2.22	2.16	2.09	2.03	1.95	1.88
27	5.63	4.24	3.65	3.31	3.08	2.92	2.80	2.71	2.63	2.57	2.47	2.36	2.25	2.19	2.13	2.07	2.00	1.93	1.85
28	5.61	4.22	3.63	3.29	3.06	2.90	2.78	2.69	2.61	2.55	2.45	2.34	2.23	2.17	2.11	2.05	1.98	1.91	1.83
29	5.59	4.20	3.61	3.27	3.04	2.88	2.76	2.67	2.59	2.53	2.43	2.32	2.21	2.15	2.09	2.03	1.96	1.89	1.81
30	5.57	4.18	3.59	3.25	3.03	2.87	2.75	2.65	2.57	2.51	2.41	2.31	2.20	2.14	2.07	2.01	1.94	1.87	1.79
40	5.42	4.05	3.46	3.13	2.90	2.74	2.62	2.53	2.45	2.39	2.29	2.18	2.07	2.01	1.94	1.88	1.80	1.72	1.64
60	5.29	3.93	3.34	3.01	2.79	2.63	2.51	2.41	2.33	2.27	2.17	2.06	1.94	1.88	1.82	1.74	1.67	1.58	1.48
120	5.15	3.80	3.23	2.89	2.67	2.52	2.39	2.30	2.22	2.16	2.05	1.94	1.82	1.76	1.69	1.61	1.53	1.43	1.31
∞	5.02	3.69	3.12	2.79	2.57	2.41	2.29	2.19	2.11	2.05	1.94	1.83	1.71	1.64	1.57	1.48	1.39	1.27	1.00

$F = \frac{s_1^2}{s_2^2} = \frac{S_1}{m} \Big/ \frac{S_2}{n}$, where $s_1^2 = S_1/m$ and $s_2^2 = S_2/n$ are independent mean squares estimating a common variance σ^2 and based on m and n degrees of freedom, respectively.

PERCENTAGE POINTS, *F*-DISTRIBUTION

$$F(F) = \int_0^F \frac{\Gamma\left(\frac{m+n}{2}\right)}{\Gamma\left(\frac{m}{2}\right)\Gamma\left(\frac{n}{2}\right)} m^{\frac{m}{2}} n^{\frac{n}{2}} x^{\frac{m}{2}-1} (n+mx)^{-\frac{m+n}{2}}\, dx = .99$$

n \ m	1	2	3	4	5	6	7	8	9	10	12	15	20	24	30	40	60	120	∞
1	4052	4999.5	5403	5625	5764	5859	5928	5982	6022	6056	6106	6157	6209	6235	6261	6287	6313	6339	6366
2	98.50	99.00	99.17	99.25	99.30	99.33	99.36	99.37	99.39	99.40	99.42	99.43	99.45	99.46	99.47	99.47	99.48	99.49	99.50
3	34.12	30.82	29.46	28.71	28.24	27.91	27.67	27.49	27.35	27.23	27.05	26.87	26.69	26.60	26.50	26.41	26.32	26.22	26.13
4	21.20	18.00	16.69	15.98	15.52	15.21	14.98	14.80	14.66	14.55	14.37	14.20	14.02	13.93	13.84	13.75	13.65	13.56	13.46
5	16.26	13.27	12.06	11.39	10.97	10.67	10.46	10.29	10.16	10.05	9.89	9.72	9.55	9.47	9.38	9.29	9.20	9.11	9.02
6	13.75	10.92	9.78	9.15	8.75	8.47	8.26	8.10	7.98	7.87	7.72	7.56	7.40	7.31	7.23	7.14	7.06	6.97	6.88
7	12.25	9.55	8.45	7.85	7.46	7.19	6.99	6.84	6.72	6.62	6.47	6.31	6.16	6.07	5.99	5.91	5.82	5.74	5.65
8	11.26	8.65	7.59	7.01	6.63	6.37	6.18	6.03	5.91	5.81	5.67	5.52	5.36	5.28	5.20	5.12	5.03	4.95	4.86
9	10.56	8.02	6.99	6.42	6.06	5.80	5.61	5.47	5.35	5.26	5.11	4.96	4.81	4.73	4.65	4.57	4.48	4.40	4.31
10	10.04	7.56	6.55	5.99	5.64	5.39	5.20	5.06	4.94	4.85	4.71	4.56	4.41	4.33	4.25	4.17	4.08	4.00	3.91
11	9.65	7.21	6.22	5.67	5.32	5.07	4.89	4.74	4.63	4.54	4.40	4.25	4.10	4.02	3.94	3.86	3.78	3.69	3.60
12	9.33	6.93	5.95	5.41	5.06	4.82	4.64	4.50	4.39	4.30	4.16	4.01	3.86	3.78	3.70	3.62	3.54	3.45	3.36
13	9.07	6.70	5.74	5.21	4.86	4.62	4.44	4.30	4.19	4.10	3.96	3.82	3.66	3.59	3.51	3.43	3.34	3.25	3.17
14	8.86	6.51	5.56	5.04	4.69	4.46	4.28	4.14	4.03	3.94	3.80	3.66	3.51	3.43	3.35	3.27	3.18	3.09	3.00
15	8.68	6.36	5.42	4.89	4.56	4.32	4.14	4.00	3.89	3.80	3.67	3.52	3.37	3.29	3.21	3.13	3.05	2.96	2.87
16	8.53	6.23	5.29	4.77	4.44	4.20	4.03	3.89	3.78	3.69	3.55	3.41	3.26	3.18	3.10	3.02	2.93	2.84	2.75
17	8.40	6.11	5.18	4.67	4.34	4.10	3.93	3.79	3.68	3.59	3.46	3.31	3.16	3.08	3.00	2.92	2.83	2.75	2.65
18	8.29	6.01	5.09	4.58	4.25	4.01	3.84	3.71	3.60	3.51	3.37	3.23	3.08	3.00	2.92	2.84	2.75	2.66	2.57
19	8.18	5.93	5.01	4.50	4.17	3.94	3.77	3.63	3.52	3.43	3.30	3.15	3.00	2.92	2.84	2.76	2.67	2.58	2.49
20	8.10	5.85	4.94	4.43	4.10	3.87	3.70	3.56	3.46	3.37	3.23	3.09	2.94	2.86	2.78	2.69	2.61	2.52	2.42
21	8.02	5.78	4.87	4.37	4.04	3.81	3.64	3.51	3.40	3.31	3.17	3.03	2.88	2.80	2.72	2.64	2.55	2.46	2.36
22	7.95	5.72	4.82	4.31	3.99	3.76	3.59	3.45	3.35	3.26	3.12	2.98	2.83	2.75	2.67	2.58	2.50	2.40	2.31
23	7.88	5.66	4.76	4.26	3.94	3.71	3.54	3.41	3.30	3.21	3.07	2.93	2.78	2.70	2.62	2.54	2.45	2.35	2.26
24	7.82	5.61	4.72	4.22	3.90	3.67	3.50	3.36	3.26	3.17	3.03	2.89	2.74	2.66	2.58	2.49	2.40	2.31	2.21
25	7.77	5.57	4.68	4.18	3.85	3.63	3.46	3.32	3.22	3.13	2.99	2.85	2.70	2.62	2.54	2.45	2.36	2.27	2.17
26	7.72	5.53	4.64	4.14	3.82	3.59	3.42	3.29	3.18	3.09	2.96	2.81	2.66	2.58	2.50	2.42	2.33	2.23	2.13
27	7.68	5.49	4.60	4.11	3.78	3.56	3.39	3.26	3.15	3.06	2.93	2.78	2.63	2.55	2.47	2.38	2.29	2.20	2.10
28	7.64	5.45	4.57	4.07	3.75	3.53	3.36	3.23	3.12	3.03	2.90	2.75	2.60	2.52	2.44	2.35	2.26	2.17	2.06
29	7.60	5.42	4.54	4.04	3.73	3.50	3.33	3.20	3.09	3.00	2.87	2.73	2.57	2.49	2.41	2.33	2.23	2.14	2.03
30	7.56	5.39	4.51	4.02	3.70	3.47	3.30	3.17	3.07	2.98	2.84	2.70	2.55	2.47	2.39	2.30	2.21	2.11	2.01
40	7.31	5.18	4.31	3.83	3.51	3.29	3.12	2.99	2.89	2.80	2.66	2.52	2.37	2.29	2.20	2.11	2.02	1.92	1.80
60	7.08	4.98	4.13	3.65	3.34	3.12	2.95	2.82	2.72	2.63	2.50	2.35	2.20	2.12	2.03	1.94	1.84	1.73	1.60
120	6.85	4.79	3.95	3.48	3.17	2.96	2.79	2.66	2.56	2.47	2.34	2.19	2.03	1.95	1.86	1.76	1.66	1.53	1.38
∞	6.63	4.61	3.78	3.32	3.02	2.80	2.64	2.51	2.41	2.32	2.18	2.04	1.88	1.79	1.70	1.59	1.47	1.32	1.00

$F = \frac{s_1^2}{s_2^2} = \frac{S_1}{m} \Big/ \frac{S_2}{n}$, where $s_1^2 = S_1/m$ and $s_2^2 = S_2/n$ are independent mean squares estimating a common variance σ^2 and based on m and n degrees of freedom, respectively.

PERCENTAGE POINTS, F-DISTRIBUTION

$$F(F) = \int_0^F \frac{\Gamma\left(\frac{m+n}{2}\right)}{\Gamma\left(\frac{m}{2}\right)\Gamma\left(\frac{n}{2}\right)} m^{\frac{m}{2}} n^{\frac{n}{2}} x^{\frac{m}{2}-1} (n+mx)^{-\frac{m+n}{2}}\, dx = .995$$

n \ m	1	2	3	4	5	6	7	8	9	10	12	15	20	24	30	40	60	120	∞
1	16211	20000	21615	22500	23056	23437	23715	23925	24091	24224	24426	24630	24836	24940	25044	25148	25253	25359	25465
2	198.5	199.0	199.2	199.2	199.3	199.3	199.4	199.4	199.4	199.4	199.4	199.4	199.4	199.5	199.5	199.5	199.5	199.5	199.5
3	55.55	49.80	47.47	46.19	45.39	44.84	44.43	44.13	43.88	43.69	43.39	43.08	42.78	42.62	42.47	42.31	42.15	41.99	41.83
4	31.33	26.28	24.26	23.15	22.46	21.97	21.62	21.35	21.14	20.97	20.70	20.44	20.17	20.03	19.89	19.75	19.61	19.47	19.32
5	22.78	18.31	16.53	15.56	14.94	14.51	14.20	13.96	13.77	13.62	13.38	13.15	12.90	12.78	12.66	12.53	12.40	12.27	12.14
6	18.63	14.54	12.92	12.03	11.46	11.07	10.79	10.57	10.39	10.25	10.03	9.81	9.59	9.47	9.36	9.24	9.12	9.00	8.88
7	16.24	12.40	10.88	10.05	9.52	9.16	8.89	8.68	8.51	8.38	8.18	7.97	7.75	7.65	7.53	7.42	7.31	7.19	7.08
8	14.69	11.04	9.60	8.81	8.30	7.95	7.69	7.50	7.34	7.21	7.01	6.81	6.61	6.50	6.40	6.29	6.18	6.06	5.95
9	13.61	10.11	8.72	7.96	7.47	7.13	6.88	6.69	6.54	6.42	6.23	6.03	5.83	5.73	5.62	5.52	5.41	5.30	5.19
10	12.83	9.43	8.08	7.34	6.87	6.54	6.30	6.12	5.97	5.85	5.66	5.47	5.27	5.17	5.07	4.97	4.86	4.75	4.64
11	12.23	8.91	7.60	6.88	6.42	6.10	5.86	5.68	5.54	5.42	5.24	5.05	4.86	4.76	4.65	4.55	4.44	4.34	4.23
12	11.75	8.51	7.23	6.52	6.07	5.76	5.52	5.35	5.20	5.09	4.91	4.72	4.53	4.43	4.33	4.23	4.12	4.01	3.90
13	11.37	8.19	6.93	6.23	5.79	5.48	5.25	5.08	4.94	4.82	4.64	4.46	4.27	4.17	4.07	3.97	3.87	3.76	3.65
14	11.06	7.92	6.68	6.00	5.56	5.26	5.03	4.86	4.72	4.60	4.43	4.25	4.06	3.96	3.86	3.76	3.66	3.55	3.44
15	10.80	7.70	6.48	5.80	5.37	5.07	4.85	4.67	4.54	4.42	4.25	4.07	3.88	3.79	3.69	3.58	3.48	3.37	3.26
16	10.58	7.51	6.30	5.64	5.21	4.91	4.69	4.52	4.38	4.27	4.10	3.92	3.73	3.64	3.54	3.44	3.33	3.22	3.11
17	10.38	7.35	6.16	5.50	5.07	4.78	4.56	4.39	4.25	4.14	3.97	3.79	3.61	3.51	3.41	3.31	3.21	3.10	2.98
18	10.22	7.21	6.03	5.37	4.96	4.66	4.44	4.28	4.14	4.03	3.86	3.68	3.50	3.40	3.30	3.20	3.10	2.99	2.87
19	10.07	7.09	5.92	5.27	4.85	4.56	4.34	4.18	4.04	3.93	3.76	3.59	3.40	3.31	3.21	3.11	3.00	2.89	2.78
20	9.94	6.99	5.82	5.17	4.76	4.47	4.26	4.09	3.96	3.85	3.68	3.50	3.32	3.22	3.12	3.02	2.92	2.81	2.69
21	9.83	6.89	5.73	5.09	4.68	4.39	4.18	4.01	3.88	3.77	3.60	3.43	3.24	3.15	3.05	2.95	2.84	2.73	2.61
22	9.73	6.81	5.65	5.02	4.61	4.32	4.11	3.94	3.81	3.70	3.54	3.36	3.18	3.08	2.98	2.88	2.77	2.66	2.55
23	9.63	6.73	5.58	4.95	4.54	4.26	4.05	3.88	3.75	3.64	3.47	3.30	3.12	3.02	2.92	2.82	2.71	2.60	2.48
24	9.55	6.66	5.52	4.89	4.49	4.20	3.99	3.83	3.69	3.59	3.42	3.25	3.06	2.97	2.87	2.77	2.66	2.55	2.43
25	9.48	6.60	5.46	4.84	4.43	4.15	3.94	3.78	3.64	3.54	3.37	3.20	3.01	2.92	2.82	2.72	2.61	2.50	2.38
26	9.41	6.54	5.41	4.79	4.38	4.10	3.89	3.73	3.60	3.49	3.33	3.15	2.97	2.87	2.77	2.67	2.56	2.45	2.33
27	9.34	6.49	5.36	4.74	4.34	4.06	3.85	3.69	3.56	3.45	3.28	3.11	2.93	2.83	2.73	2.63	2.52	2.41	2.25
28	9.28	6.44	5.32	4.70	4.30	4.02	3.81	3.65	3.52	3.41	3.25	3.07	2.89	2.79	2.69	2.59	2.48	2.37	2.29
29	9.23	6.40	5.28	4.66	4.26	3.98	3.77	3.61	3.48	3.38	3.21	3.04	2.86	2.76	2.66	2.56	2.45	2.33	2.24
30	9.18	6.35	5.24	4.62	4.23	3.95	3.74	3.58	3.45	3.34	3.18	3.01	2.82	2.73	2.63	2.52	2.42	2.30	2.18
40	8.83	6.07	4.98	4.37	3.99	3.71	3.51	3.35	3.22	3.12	2.95	2.78	2.60	2.50	2.40	2.30	2.18	2.06	1.93
60	8.49	5.79	4.73	4.14	3.76	3.49	3.29	3.13	3.01	2.90	2.74	2.57	2.39	2.29	2.19	2.08	1.96	1.83	1.69
120	8.18	5.54	4.50	3.92	3.55	3.28	3.09	2.93	2.81	2.71	2.54	2.37	2.19	2.09	1.98	1.87	1.75	1.61	1.43
∞	7.88	5.30	4.28	3.72	3.35	3.09	2.90	2.74	2.62	2.52	2.36	2.19	2.00	1.90	1.79	1.67	1.53	1.36	1.00

$F = \frac{s_1^2}{s_2^2} = \frac{S_1}{m} \Big/ \frac{S_2}{n}$, where $s_1^2 = S_1/m$ and $s_2^2 = S_2/n$ are independent mean squares estimating a common variance σ^2 and based on m and n degrees of freedom, respectively.

PERCENTAGE POINTS, *F*-DISTRIBUTION

$$F(F) = \int_0^F \frac{\Gamma\left(\frac{m+n}{2}\right)}{\Gamma\left(\frac{m}{2}\right)\Gamma\left(\frac{n}{2}\right)} m^{\frac{m}{2}} n^{\frac{n}{2}} x^{\frac{m}{2}-1} (n+mx)^{-\frac{m+n}{2}} \, dx = .999$$

n \ m	1	2	3	4	5	6	7	8	9	10	12	15	20	24	30	40	60	120	∞
1	4053*	5000*	5404*	5625*	5764*	5859*	5929*	5981*	6023*	6056*	6107*	6158*	6209*	6235*	6261*	6287*	6313*	6340*	6366*
2	998.5	999.0	999.2	999.2	999.3	999.3	999.4	999.4	999.4	999.4	999.4	999.4	999.4	999.5	999.5	999.5	999.5	999.5	999.5
3	167.0	148.5	141.1	137.1	134.6	132.8	131.6	130.6	129.9	129.2	128.3	127.4	126.4	125.9	125.4	125.0	124.5	124.0	123.5
4	74.14	61.25	56.18	53.44	51.71	50.53	49.66	49.00	48.47	48.05	47.41	46.76	46.10	45.77	45.43	45.09	44.75	44.40	44.05
5	47.18	37.12	33.20	31.09	29.75	28.84	28.16	27.64	27.24	26.92	26.42	25.91	25.39	25.14	24.87	24.60	24.33	24.06	23.79
6	35.51	27.00	23.70	21.92	20.81	20.03	19.46	19.03	18.69	18.41	17.99	17.56	17.12	16.89	16.67	16.44	16.21	15.99	15.75
7	29.25	21.69	18.77	17.19	16.21	15.52	15.02	14.63	14.33	14.08	13.71	13.32	12.93	12.73	12.53	12.33	12.12	11.91	11.70
8	25.42	18.49	15.83	14.39	13.49	12.86	12.40	12.04	11.77	11.54	11.19	10.84	10.48	10.30	10.11	9.92	9.73	9.53	9.33
9	22.86	16.39	13.90	12.56	11.71	11.13	10.70	10.37	10.11	9.89	9.57	9.24	8.90	8.72	8.55	8.37	8.19	8.00	7.81
10	21.04	14.91	12.55	11.28	10.48	9.92	9.52	9.20	8.96	8.75	8.45	8.13	7.80	7.64	7.47	7.30	7.12	6.94	6.76
11	19.69	13.81	11.56	10.35	9.58	9.05	8.66	8.35	8.12	7.92	7.63	7.32	7.01	6.85	6.68	6.52	6.35	6.17	6.00
12	18.64	12.97	10.80	9.63	8.89	8.38	8.00	7.71	7.48	7.29	7.00	6.71	6.40	6.25	6.09	5.93	5.76	5.59	5.42
13	17.81	12.31	10.21	9.07	8.35	7.86	7.49	7.21	6.98	6.80	6.52	6.23	5.93	5.78	5.63	5.47	5.30	5.14	4.97
14	17.14	11.78	9.73	8.62	7.92	7.43	7.08	6.80	6.58	6.40	6.13	5.85	5.56	5.41	5.25	5.10	4.94	4.77	4.60
15	16.59	11.34	9.34	8.25	7.57	7.09	6.74	6.47	6.26	6.08	5.81	5.54	5.25	5.10	4.95	4.80	4.64	4.47	4.31
16	16.12	10.97	9.00	7.94	7.27	6.81	6.46	6.19	5.98	5.81	5.55	5.27	4.99	4.85	4.70	4.54	4.39	4.23	4.06
17	15.72	10.66	8.73	7.68	7.02	6.56	6.22	5.96	5.75	5.58	5.32	5.05	4.78	4.63	4.48	4.33	4.18	4.02	3.85
18	15.38	10.39	8.49	7.46	6.81	6.35	6.02	5.76	5.56	5.39	5.13	4.87	4.59	4.45	4.30	4.15	4.00	3.84	3.67
19	15.08	10.16	8.28	7.26	6.62	6.18	5.85	5.59	5.39	5.22	4.97	4.70	4.43	4.29	4.14	3.99	3.84	3.68	3.51
20	14.82	9.95	8.10	7.10	6.46	6.02	5.69	5.44	5.24	5.08	4.82	4.56	4.29	4.15	4.00	3.86	3.70	3.54	3.38
21	14.59	9.77	7.94	6.95	6.32	5.88	5.56	5.31	5.11	4.95	4.70	4.44	4.17	4.03	3.88	3.74	3.58	3.42	3.26
22	14.38	9.61	7.80	6.81	6.19	5.76	5.44	5.19	4.99	4.83	4.58	4.33	4.06	3.92	3.78	3.63	3.48	3.32	3.15
23	14.19	9.47	7.67	6.69	6.08	5.65	5.33	5.09	4.89	4.73	4.48	4.23	3.96	3.82	3.68	3.53	3.38	3.22	3.05
24	14.03	9.34	7.55	6.59	5.98	5.55	5.23	4.99	4.80	4.64	4.39	4.14	3.87	3.74	3.59	3.45	3.29	3.14	2.97
25	13.88	9.22	7.45	6.49	5.88	5.46	5.15	4.91	4.71	4.56	4.31	4.06	3.79	3.66	3.52	3.37	3.22	3.06	2.89
26	13.74	9.12	7.36	6.41	5.80	5.38	5.07	4.83	4.64	4.48	4.24	3.99	3.72	3.59	3.44	3.30	3.15	2.99	2.82
27	13.61	9.02	7.27	6.33	5.73	5.31	5.00	4.76	4.57	4.41	4.17	3.92	3.66	3.52	3.38	3.23	3.08	2.92	2.75
28	13.50	8.93	7.19	6.25	5.66	5.24	4.93	4.69	4.50	4.35	4.11	3.86	3.60	3.46	3.32	3.18	3.02	2.86	2.69
29	13.39	8.85	7.12	6.19	5.59	5.18	4.87	4.64	4.45	4.29	4.05	3.80	3.54	3.41	3.27	3.12	2.97	2.81	2.64
30	13.29	8.77	7.05	6.12	5.53	5.12	4.82	4.58	4.39	4.24	4.00	3.75	3.49	3.36	3.22	3.07	2.92	2.76	2.59
40	12.61	8.25	6.60	5.70	5.13	4.73	4.44	4.21	4.02	3.87	3.64	3.40	3.15	3.01	2.87	2.73	2.57	2.41	2.23
60	11.97	7.76	6.17	5.31	4.76	4.37	4.09	3.87	3.69	3.54	3.31	3.08	2.83	2.69	2.55	2.41	2.25	2.08	1.89
120	11.38	7.32	5.79	4.95	4.42	4.04	3.77	3.55	3.38	3.24	3.02	2.78	2.53	2.40	2.26	2.11	1.95	1.76	1.54
∞	10.83	6.91	5.42	4.62	4.10	3.74	3.47	3.27	3.10	2.96	2.74	2.51	2.27	2.13	1.99	1.84	1.66	1.45	1.00

* Multiply these entries by 100.

VI.2 POWER FUNCTIONS OF THE ANALYSIS-OF-VARIANCE TESTS

The noncentral F-distribution, $f(F')$, arises in the ratio of a non-central chi-square with m degrees of freedom and noncentrality parameter λ to an independent chi-square with n degrees of freedom.

P. C. Tang has compiled tables of

$$\int_0^{F_\alpha} f(F')\,dF'$$

for certain values of F_α. These tables are given in terms of E^2, where

$$E^2 = \frac{mF'}{mF' + n} \cdot$$

If the frequency function of E^2 is denoted by $g(E^2;m,n,\lambda)$, $g(E^2)$ is a beta distribution if $\lambda = 0$ and a noncentral beta distribution if $\lambda \neq 0$.

The integral

$$\int_0^{E_\alpha^2} g(E^2;m,n,\lambda)\,dE^2$$

equals $1 - \beta(\lambda)$, or unity minus the power of the test, which is the probability of a type II error. Here E_α^2 is obtained from the integral

$$\int_{E_\alpha^2}^1 g(E^2;m,n,\ \lambda = 0)\,dE^2 = \lambda.$$

P. C. Tang evaluated the integral

$$P(\mathrm{II}) = 1 - \beta(\phi) = \int_0^{E_\alpha^2} g(E^2;f_1,f_2,\phi)\,dE^2$$

for various values of f_1, f_2, ϕ, and E_α^2 for $\alpha = 0.05$ and 0.01, where

$$\phi = \sqrt{\frac{2\lambda}{f_1 + 1}}$$

and where f_1 is the degrees of freedom in the numerator of the F statistic.

In this table, graphs are shown with $1 - \beta$ on the vertical scale corresponding to ϕ on the horizontal. The graphs are for two levels of significance, $\alpha = 0.01$ and 0.05, for eight values of ν_1, the number of degrees of freedom for the numerator, and several values of ν_2, the number of degrees of freedom for the denominator of the F ratio. There is a different curve for each set of values α, ν_1, and ν_2.

POWER OF THE ANALYSIS-OF-VARIANCE TEST

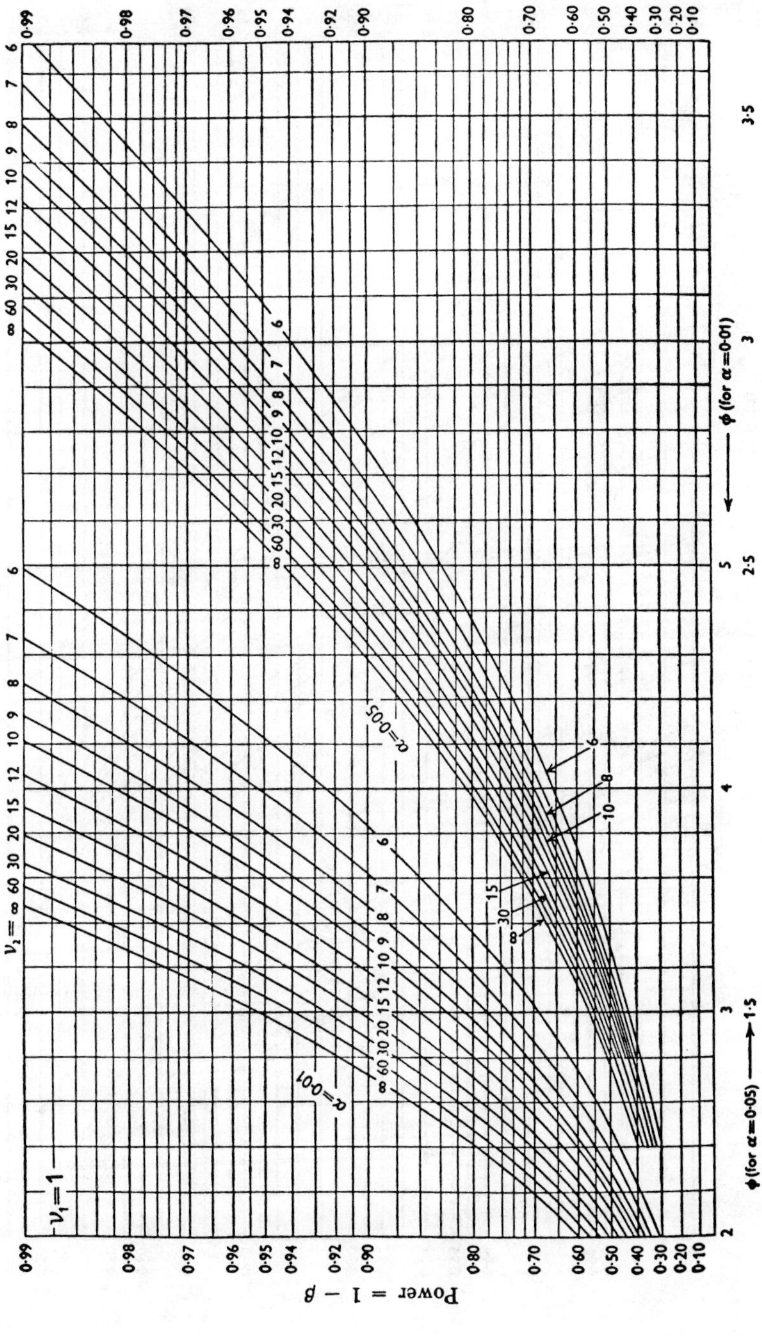

POWER OF THE ANALYSIS-OF-VARIANCE TEST

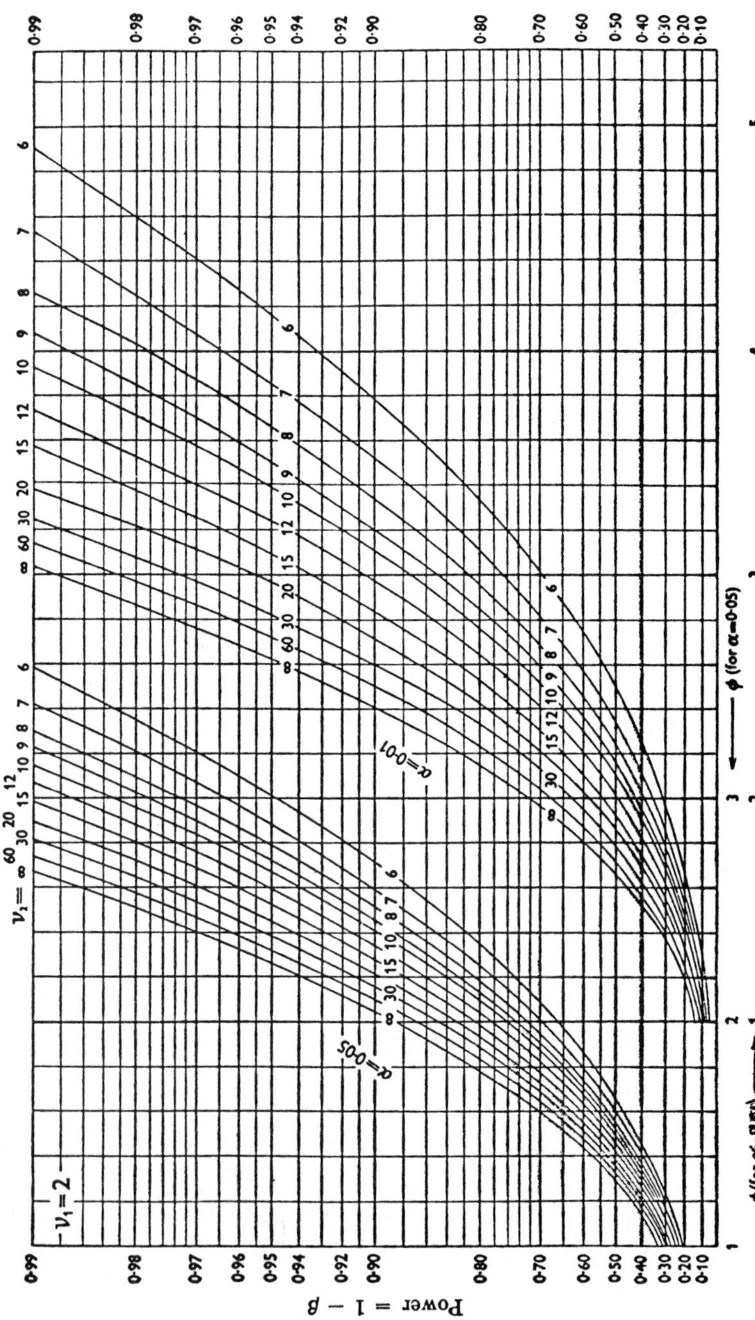

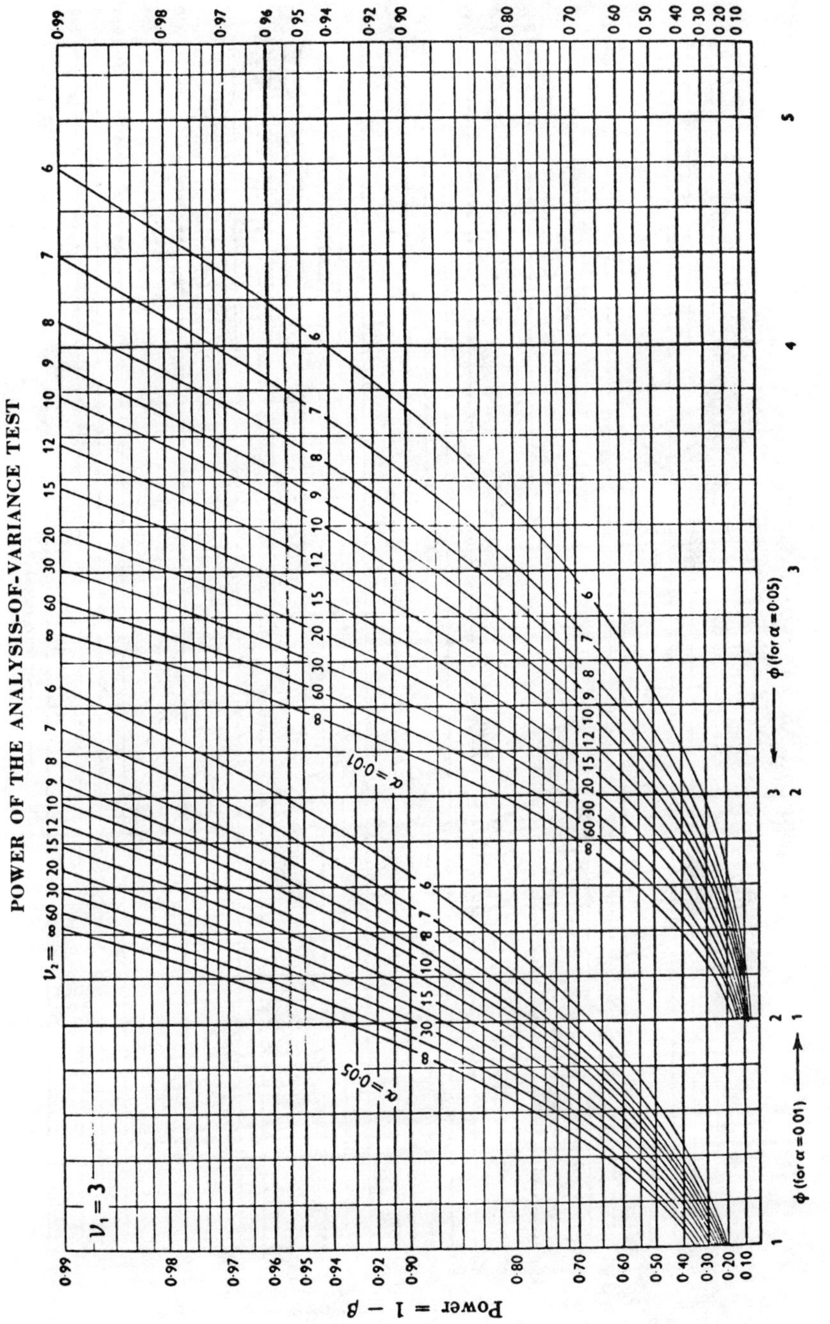
POWER OF THE ANALYSIS-OF-VARIANCE TEST
ν₁ = 3
ν₂ = ∞ 60 30 20 15 12 10 9 8 7 6
α = 0·05
α = 0·01
Power = 1 − β
φ (for α = 0·01) ⟶
⟵ φ (for α = 0·05)

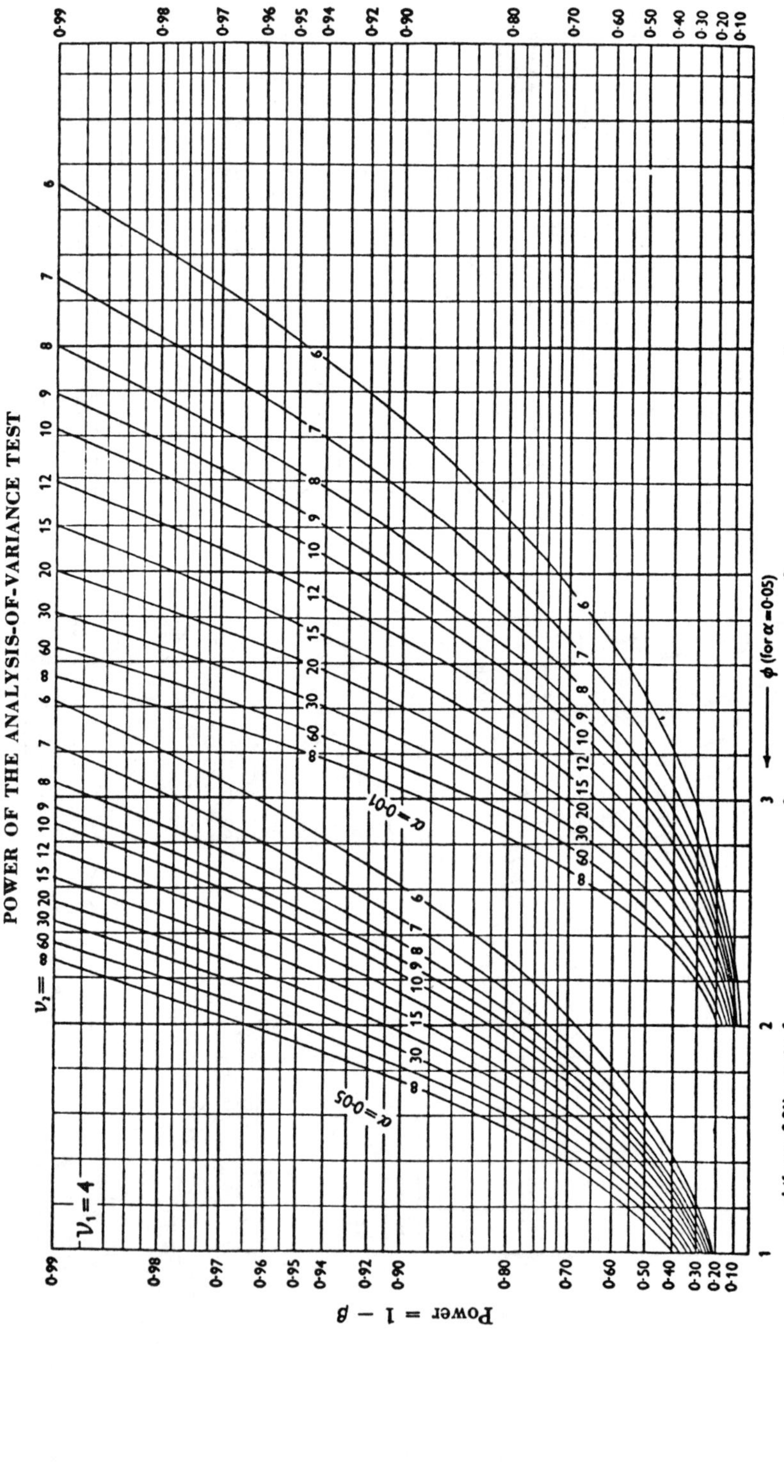
POWER OF THE ANALYSIS-OF-VARIANCE TEST
$\nu_1 = 4$
$\nu_2 = \infty$ 60 30 20 15 12 10 9 8 7 6 ∞ 60 30 20 15 12 10 9 8 7 6
$\alpha = 0{\cdot}05$
$\alpha = 0{\cdot}01$
Power = 1 − β
φ (for α=0·01) ⟶
φ (for α=0·05)

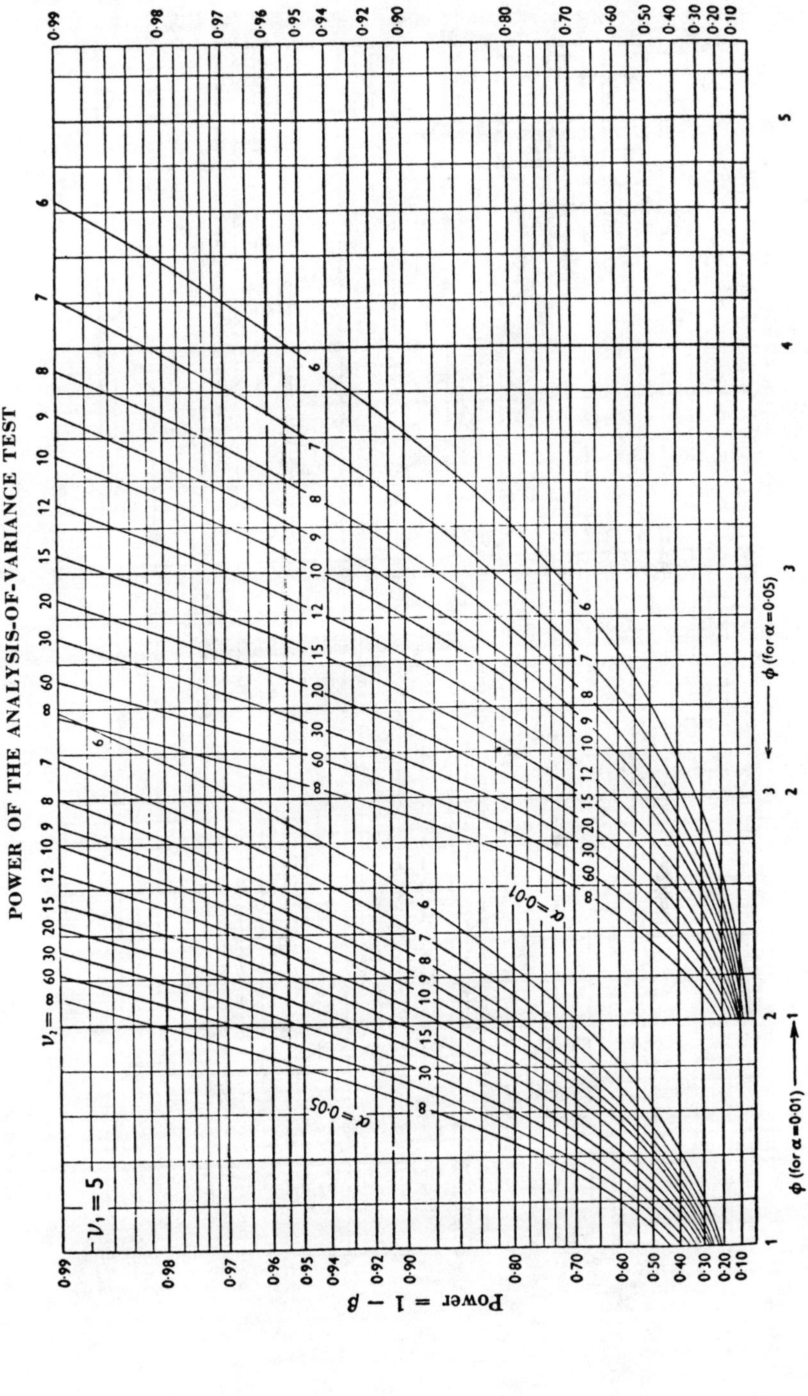
POWER OF THE ANALYSIS-OF-VARIANCE TEST
ν₁ = 5
ν₂ = ∞ 60 30 20 15 12 10 9 8 7 6
∞ 60 30 20 15 12 10 9 8 7 6
α = 0·05
α = 0·01
Power = 1 − β
0·99 0·98 0·97 0·96 0·95 0·94 0·92 0·90 0·80 0·70 0·60 0·50 0·40 0·30 0·20 0·10
φ (for α = 0·01) ⟶ 1 2 3
φ (for α = 0·05) ⟵ 1 2 3 4 5

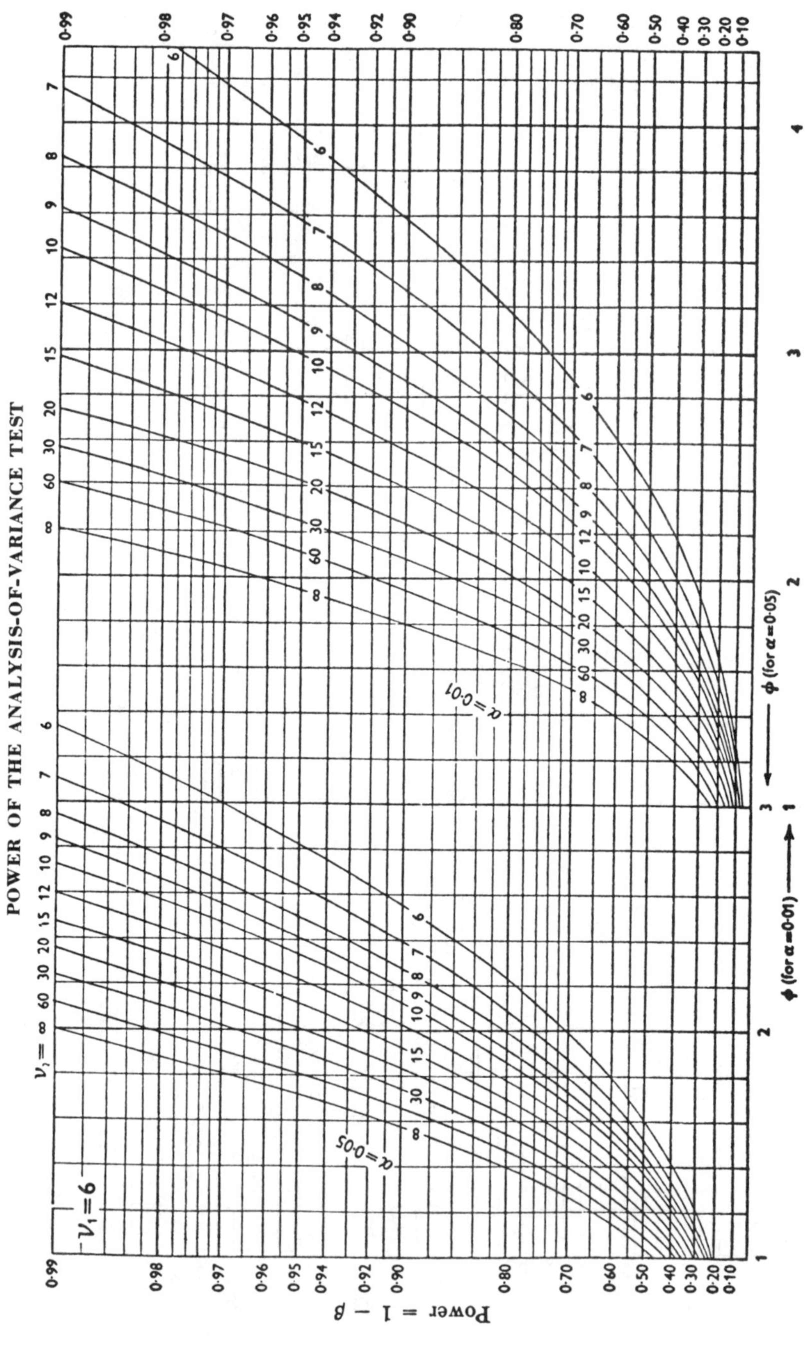
POWER OF THE ANALYSIS-OF-VARIANCE TEST
$\nu_1 = 6$
$\nu_2 = \infty$ 60 30 20 15 12 10 9 8 7 6
$\alpha = 0{\cdot}05$
$\alpha = 0{\cdot}01$
Power = 1 − β
ϕ (for $\alpha = 0{\cdot}01$)
ϕ (for $\alpha = 0{\cdot}05$)
0·99
0·98
0·97
0·96
0·95
0·94
0·92
0·90
0·80
0·70
0·60
0·50
0·40
0·30
0·20
0·10

POWER OF THE ANALYSIS-OF-VARIANCE TEST

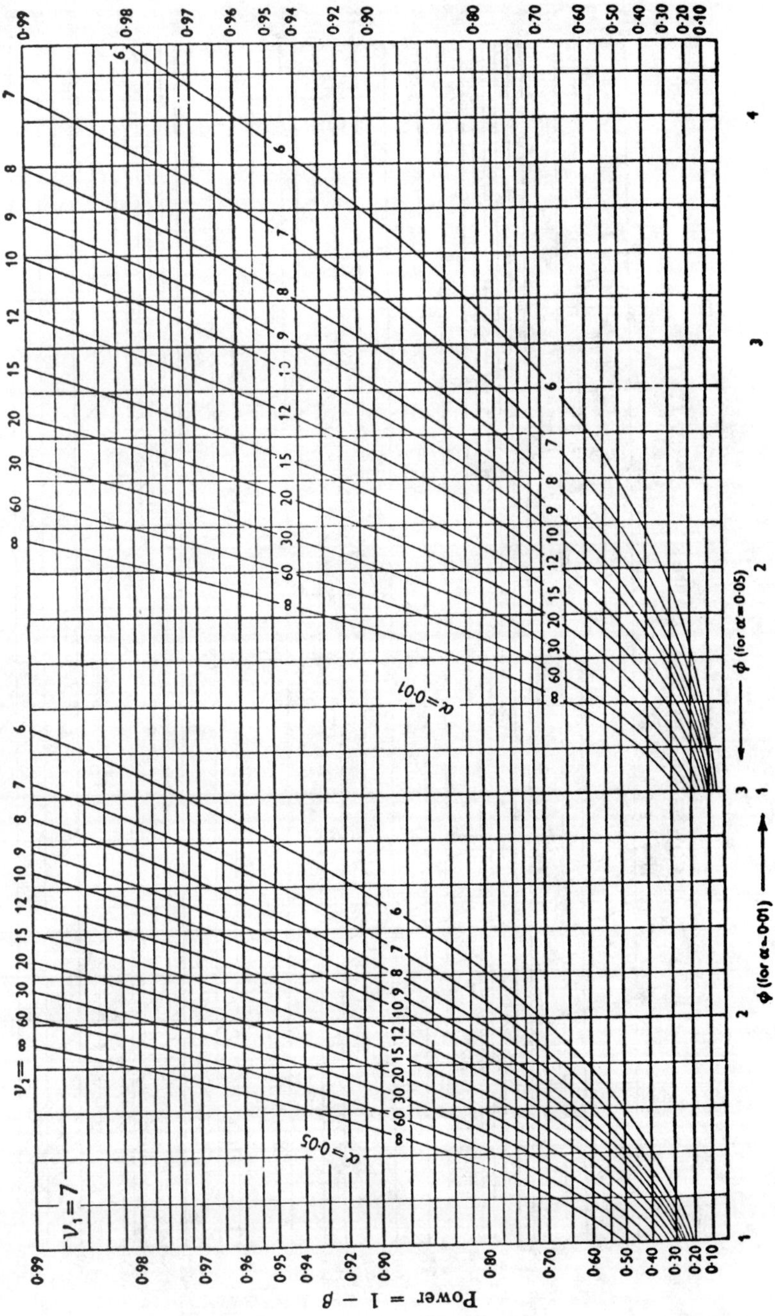

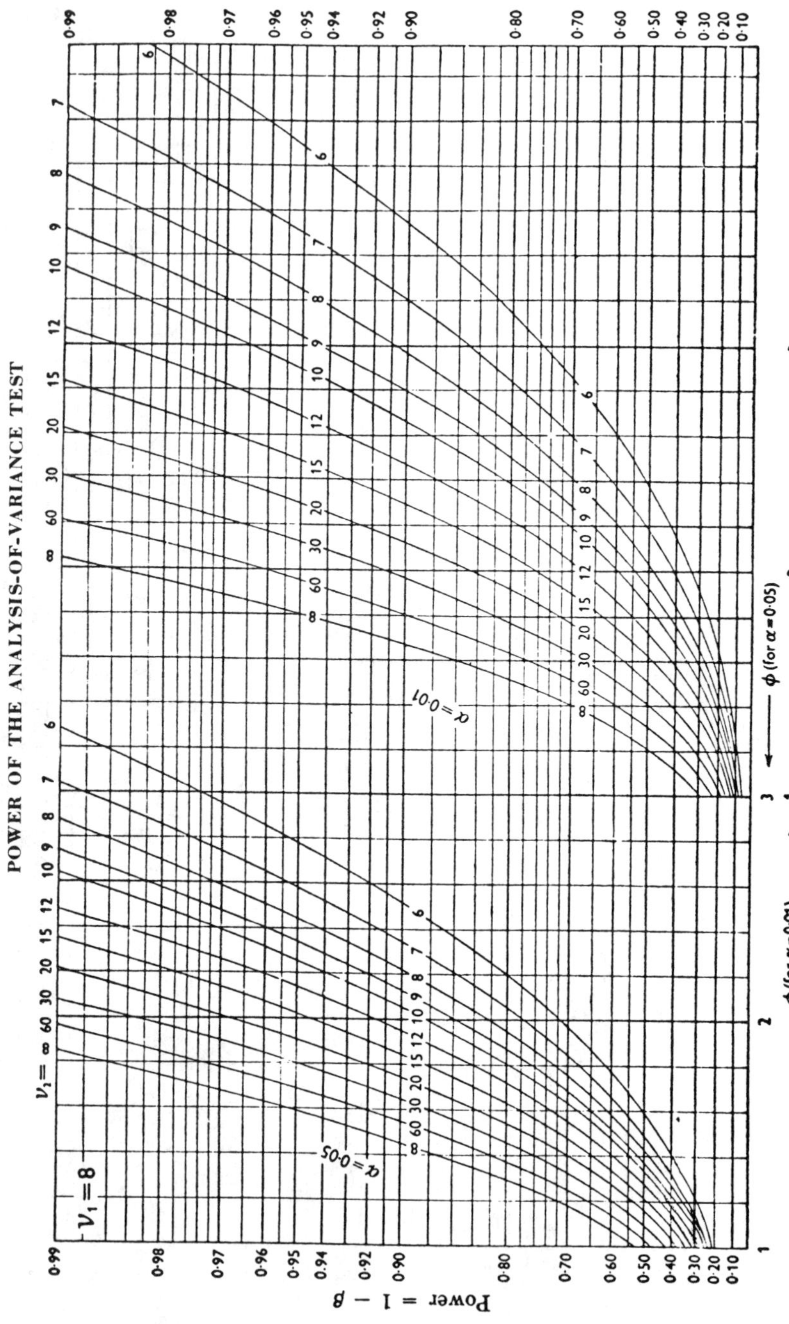
POWER OF THE ANALYSIS-OF-VARIANCE TEST
$\nu_1 = 8$
$\nu_2 = \infty$ 60 30 20 15 12 10 9 8 7 6
$\alpha = 0{\cdot}05$
$\alpha = 0{\cdot}01$
Power = 1 − β
ϕ (for α = 0·01)
ϕ (for α = 0·05)

VI.3 NUMBER OF OBSERVATIONS REQUIRED FOR THE COMPARISON OF TWO POPULATION VARIANCES USING THE *F*-TEST

The tabular entries show the value of the ratio R of two population variances $\frac{\sigma_2^2}{\sigma_1^2}$, which remains undetected with probability β in a variance ratio test at significance level α of the ratio $\frac{s_2^2}{s_1^2}$ of estimates of the two variances, each being based on n degrees of freedom.

NUMBER OF OBSERVATIONS REQUIRED FOR THE COMPARISON OF TWO POPULATION VARIANCES USING THE F-TEST

η	$\alpha = 0.01$				$\alpha = 0.05$				$\alpha = 0.5$			
	$\beta = 0.01$	$\beta = 0.05$	$\beta = 0.1$	$\beta = 0.5$	$\beta = 0.01$	$\beta = 0.05$	$\beta = 0.1$	$\beta = 0.5$	$\beta = 0.01$	$\beta = 0.05$	$\beta = 0.1$	$\beta = 0.5$
1	16,420,000	654,200	161,500	4052	654,200	26,070	6,436	161.5	4,052	161.5	39.85	1.000
2	9,000	1,881	891.0	99.00	1,881	361.0	171.0	19.00	99.00	19.00	9.000	1.000
3	867.7	273.3	158.8	29.46	273.3	86.06	50.01	9.277	29.46	9.277	5.391	1.000
4	255.3	102.1	65.62	15.98	102.1	40.81	26.24	6.388	15.98	6.388	4.108	1.000
5	120.3	55.39	37.87	10.97	55.39	25.51	17.44	5.050	10.97	5.050	3.453	1.000
6	71.67	36.27	25.86	8.466	36.27	18.35	13.09	4.284	8.466	4.284	3.056	1.000
7	48.90	26.48	19.47	6.993	26.48	14.34	10.55	3.787	6.993	3.787	2.786	1.000
8	36.35	20.73	15.61	6.029	20.73	11.82	8.902	3.438	6.029	3.438	2.589	1.000
9	28.63	17.01	13.06	5.351	17.01	10.11	7.757	3.179	5.351	3.179	2.440	1.000
10	23.51	14.44	11.26	4.849	14.44	8.870	6.917	2.978	4.849	2.978	2.323	1.000
12	17.27	11.16	8.923	4.155	11.16	7.218	5.769	2.687	4.155	2.687	2.147	1.000
15	12.41	8.466	6.946	3.522	8.466	5.777	4.740	2.404	3.522	2.404	1.972	1.000
20	8.630	6.240	5.270	2.938	6.240	4.512	3.810	2.124	2.938	2.124	1.794	1.000
24	7.071	5.275	4.526	2.659	5.275	3.935	3.376	1.984	2.659	1.984	1.702	1.000
30	5.693	4.392	3.833	2.386	4.392	3.389	2.957	1.841	2.386	1.841	1.606	1.000
40	4.470	3.579	3.183	2.114	3.579	2.866	2.549	1.693	2.114	1.693	1.506	1.000
60	3.372	2.817	2.562	1.836	2.817	2.354	2.141	1.534	1.836	1.534	1.396	1.000
120	2.350	2.072	1.939	1.533	2.072	1.828	1.710	1.352	1.533	1.352	1.265	1.000
∞	1.000	1.000	1.000	1.000	1.000	1.000	1.000	1.000	1.000	1.000	1.000	1.000

VI.4 OPERATING CHARACTERISTIC (OC) CURVES FOR A TEST ON THE STANDARD DEVIATIONS OF TWO NORMAL DISTRIBUTIONS

The OC curves give the sample sizes needed for given values of $\alpha = P$ (Type I error) and $\beta = P$ (Type II error) for a test of the hypothesis H_0: $\sigma_x = \sigma_y$. The test statistic used is $F = \frac{s_x^2}{s_y^2}$ which is distributed as the F-distribution with $n_x - 1$ and $n_y - 1$ degrees of freedom. The required sample size is obtained by entering the appropriate set of curves for given α and β and for various values of $\lambda = \frac{\sigma_x}{\sigma_y}$ for both one-sided and two-sided tests for the case $n_x = n_y = n$.

OC CURVES FOR A TEST ON THE STANDARD DEVIATIONS OF TWO NORMAL DISTRIBUTIONS

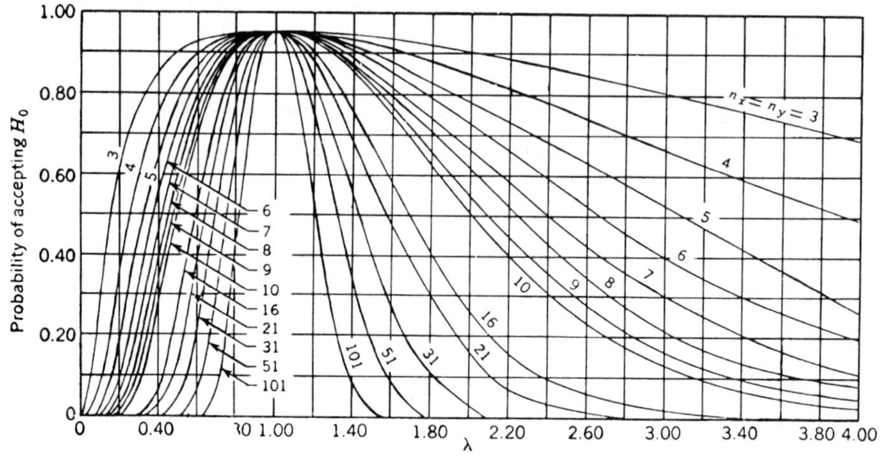

a) OC curves for different values of n for the two-sided F test for a level of significance $\alpha = 0.05$.

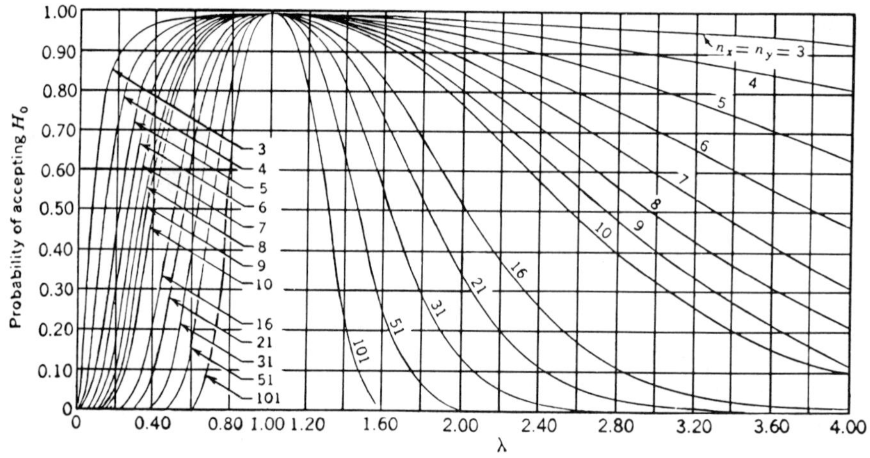

b) OC curves for different values of n for the two-sided F test for a level of significance $\alpha = 0.01$.

OC CURVES FOR A TEST ON THE STANDARD DEVIATIONS OF TWO NORMAL DISTRIBUTIONS

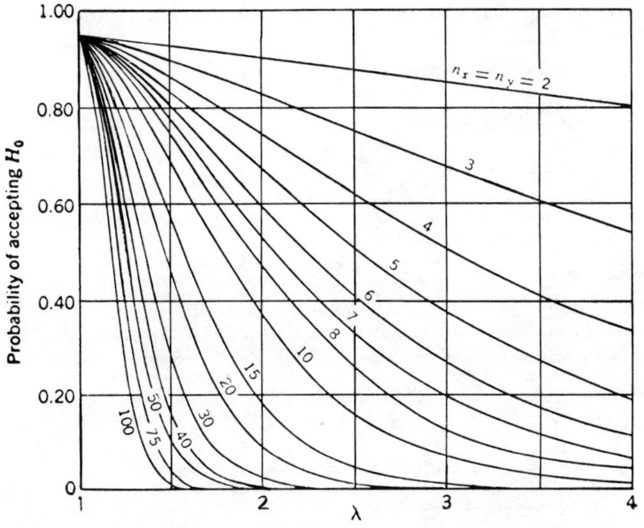

c) OC curves for different values of *n* for the one-sided *F* test for a level of significance $\alpha = 0.05$.

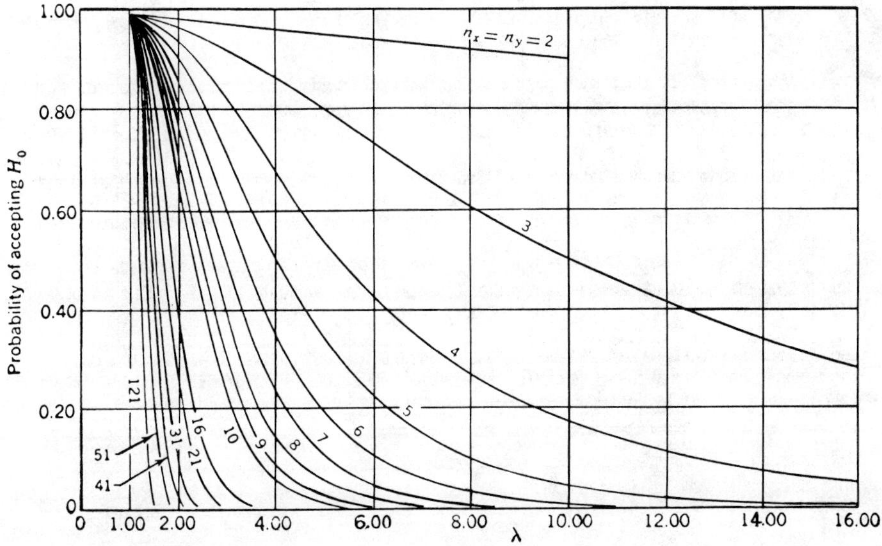

d) OC curves for different values of *n* for the one sided *F* test for a level of significance $\alpha = 0.01$.

VI.5 COCHRAN'S TEST FOR THE HOMOGENEITY OF VARIANCES

Let s_i^2, $i = 1, 2, \ldots, k$ denote a set of mean squares which are independent estimates of σ_i^2, respectively, each based upon n independent normally distributed random variables. Let

$$g = \frac{\max s_i^2}{\sum_{i=1}^{k} s_i^2}$$

be the ratio of the largest s^2 to their total. The hypothesis that $\sigma_1^2 = \sigma_2^2 = \cdots = \sigma_k^2$ is accepted if

$$g \leq g_\alpha$$

where g_α is given in the table for levels of significance α, equal to 0.05 and 0.01. The table is entered with n, the number of observations within each group, and k, the number of variances being considered.

UPPER 5 PERCENTAGE POINTS OF THE RATIO OF THE LARGEST TO THE SUM OF k INDEPENDENT ESTIMATES OF VARIANCE, EACH OF WHICH IS BASED ON n OBSERVATIONS

k \ n	2	3	4	5	6	7	8	9	10	11	17	37	145	∞
2	0.9985	0.9750	0.9392	0.9057	0.8772	0.8534	0.8332	0.8159	0.8010	0.7880	0.7341	0.6602	0.5813	0.5000
3	0.9669	0.8709	0.7977	0.7457	0.7071	0.6771	0.6530	0.6333	0.6167	0.6025	0.5466	0.4748	0.4031	0.3333
4	0.9065	0.7679	0.6841	0.6287	0.5895	0.5598	0.5365	0.5175	0.5017	0.4884	0.4366	0.3720	0.3093	0.2500
5	0.8412	0.6838	0.5981	0.5441	0.5065	0.4783	0.4564	0.4387	0.4241	0.4118	0.3645	0.3066	0.2513	0.2000
6	0.7808	0.6161	0.5321	0.4803	0.4447	0.4184	0.3980	0.3817	0.3682	0.3568	0.3135	0.2612	0.2119	0.1667
7	0.7271	0.5612	0.4800	0.4307	0.3974	0.3726	0.3535	0.3384	0.3259	0.3154	0.2756	0.2278	0.1833	0.1429
8	0.6798	0.5157	0.4377	0.3910	0.3595	0.3362	0.3185	0.3043	0.2926	0.2829	0.2462	0.2022	0.1616	0.1250
9	0.6385	0.4775	0.4027	0.3584	0.3286	0.3067	0.2901	0.2768	0.2659	0.2568	0.2226	0.1820	0.1446	0.1111
10	0.6020	0.4450	0.3733	0.3311	0.3029	0.2823	0.2666	0.2541	0.2439	0.2353	0.2032	0.1655	0.1308	0.1000
12	0.5410	0.3924	0.3264	0.2880	0.2624	0.2439	0.2299	0.2187	0.2098	0.2020	0.1737	0.1403	0.1100	0.0833
15	0.4709	0.3346	0.2758	0.2419	0.2195	0.2034	0.1911	0.1815	0.1736	0.1671	0.1429	0.1144	0.0889	0.0667
20	0.3894	0.2705	0.2205	0.1921	0.1735	0.1602	0.1501	0.1422	0.1357	0.1303	0.1108	0.0879	0.0675	0.0500
24	0.3434	0.2354	0.1907	0.1656	0.1493	0.1374	0.1286	0.1216	0.1160	0.1113	0.0942	0.0743	0.0567	0.0417
30	0.2929	0.1980	0.1593	0.1377	0.1237	0.1137	0.1061	0.1002	0.0958	0.0921	0.0771	0.0604	0.0457	0.0333
40	0.2370	0.1576	0.1259	0.1082	0.0968	0.0887	0.0827	0.0780	0.0745	0.0713	0.0595	0.0462	0.0347	0.0250
60	0.1737	0.1131	0.0895	0.0765	0.0682	0.0623	0.0583	0.0552	0.0520	0.0497	0.0411	0.0316	0.0234	0.0167
120	0.0998	0.0632	0.0495	0.0419	0.0371	0.0337	0.0312	0.0292	0.0279	0.0266	0.0218	0.0165	0.0120	0.0083
∞	0	0	0	0	0	0	0	0	0	0	0	0	0	0

ERRATA

The following table should replace the table found on page 237.

UPPER 1 PERCENTAGE POINTS OF THE RATIO OF THE LARGEST TO THE SUM OF k INDEPENDENT ESTIMATES OF VARIANCE, EACH OF WHICH IS BASED ON n OBSERVATIONS

k \ n	2	3	4	5	6	7	8	9	10	11	17	37	145	∞
2	0.9999	0.9950	0.9794	0.9586	0.9373	0.9172	0.8988	0.8823	0.8674	0.8539	0.7949	0.7067	0.6062	0.5000
3	0.9933	0.9423	0.8831	0.8335	0.7933	0.7606	0.7335	0.7107	0.6912	0.6743	0.6059	0.5153	0.4230	0.3333
4	0.9676	0.8643	0.7814	0.7212	0.6761	0.6410	0.6129	0.5897	0.5702	0.5536	0.4884	0.4057	0.3251	0.2500
5	0.9279	0.7885	0.6957	0.6329	0.5875	0.5531	0.5259	0.5037	0.4854	0.4697	0.4094	0.3351	0.2644	0.2000
6	0.8828	0.7218	0.6258	0.5635	0.5195	0.4866	0.4608	0.4401	0.4229	0.4084	0.3529	0.2858	0.2229	0.1667
7	0.8376	0.6644	0.5685	0.5080	0.4659	0.4347	0.4105	0.3911	0.3751	0.3616	0.3105	0.2494	0.1929	0.1429
8	0.7945	0.6152	0.5209	0.4627	0.4226	0.3932	0.3704	0.3522	0.3373	0.3248	0.2779	0.2214	0.1700	0.1250
9	0.7544	0.5727	0.4810	0.4251	0.3870	0.3592	0.3378	0.3207	0.3067	0.2950	0.2514	0.1992	0.1521	0.1111
10	0.7175	0.5358	0.4469	0.3934	0.3572	0.3308	0.3106	0.2945	0.2813	0.2704	0.2297	0.1811	0.1376	0.1000
12	0.6528	0.4751	0.3919	0.3428	0.3099	0.2861	0.2680	0.2535	0.2419	0.2320	0.1961	0.1535	0.1157	0.0833
15	0.5747	0.4069	0.3317	0.2882	0.2593	0.2386	0.2228	0.2104	0.2002	0.1918	0.1612	0.1251	0.0934	0.0667
20	0.4799	0.3297	0.2654	0.2288	0.2048	0.1877	0.1748	0.1646	0.1567	0.1501	0.1248	0.0960	0.0709	0.0500
24	0.4247	0.2871	0.2295	0.1970	0.1759	0.1608	0.1495	0.1406	0.1338	0.1283	0.1060	0.0810	0.0595	0.0417
30	0.3632	0.2412	0.1913	0.1635	0.1454	0.1327	0.1232	0.1157	0.1100	0.1054	0.0867	0.0658	0.0480	0.0333
40	0.2940	0.1915	0.1508	0.1281	0.1135	0.1033	0.0957	0.0898	0.0853	0.0816	0.0668	0.0503	0.0363	0.0250
60	0.2151	0.1371	0.1069	0.0902	0.0796	0.0722	0.0668	0.0625	0.0594	0.0567	0.0461	0.0344	0.0245	0.0167
120	0.1225	0.0759	0.0585	0.0489	0.0429	0.0387	0.0357	0.0334	0.0316	0.0302	0.0242	0.0178	0.0125	0.0083
∞	0	0	0	0	0	0	0	0	0	0	0	0	0	0

UPPER 5 PERCENTAGE POINTS OF THE RATIO OF THE LARGEST TO THE SUM OF k INDEPENDENT ESTIMATES OF VARIANCE, EACH OF WHICH IS BASED ON n OBSERVATIONS

k \ n	2	3	4	5	6	7	8	9	10	11	17	37	145	∞
2	0.9985	0.9750	0.9392	0.9057	0.8772	0.8534	0.8332	0.8159	0.8010	0.7880	0.7341	0.6602	0.5813	0.5000
3	0.9669	0.8709	0.7977	0.7457	0.7071	0.6771	0.6530	0.6333	0.6167	0.6025	0.5466	0.4748	0.4031	0.3333
4	0.9065	0.7679	0.6841	0.6287	0.5895	0.5598	0.5365	0.5175	0.5017	0.4884	0.4366	0.3720	0.3093	0.2500
5	0.8412	0.6838	0.5981	0.5441	0.5065	0.4783	0.4564	0.4387	0.4241	0.4118	0.3645	0.3066	0.2513	0.2000
6	0.7808	0.6161	0.5321	0.4803	0.4447	0.4184	0.3980	0.3817	0.3682	0.3568	0.3135	0.2612	0.2119	0.1667
7	0.7271	0.5612	0.4800	0.4307	0.3974	0.3726	0.3535	0.3384	0.3259	0.3154	0.2756	0.2278	0.1833	0.1429
8	0.6798	0.5157	0.4377	0.3910	0.3595	0.3362	0.3185	0.3043	0.2926	0.2829	0.2462	0.2022	0.1616	0.1250
9	0.6385	0.4775	0.4027	0.3584	0.3286	0.3067	0.2901	0.2768	0.2659	0.2568	0.2226	0.1820	0.1446	0.1111
10	0.6020	0.4450	0.3733	0.3311	0.3029	0.2823	0.2666	0.2541	0.2439	0.2353	0.2032	0.1655	0.1308	0.1000
12	0.5410	0.3924	0.3264	0.2880	0.2624	0.2439	0.2299	0.2187	0.2098	0.2020	0.1737	0.1403	0.1100	0.0833
15	0.4709	0.3346	0.2758	0.2419	0.2195	0.2034	0.1911	0.1815	0.1736	0.1671	0.1429	0.1144	0.0889	0.0667
20	0.3894	0.2705	0.2205	0.1921	0.1735	0.1602	0.1501	0.1422	0.1357	0.1303	0.1108	0.0879	0.0675	0.0500
24	0.3434	0.2354	0.1907	0.1656	0.1493	0.1374	0.1286	0.1216	0.1160	0.1113	0.0942	0.0743	0.0567	0.0417
30	0.2929	0.1980	0.1593	0.1377	0.1237	0.1137	0.1061	0.1002	0.0958	0.0921	0.0771	0.0604	0.0457	0.0333
40	0.2370	0.1576	0.1259	0.1082	0.0968	0.0887	0.0827	0.0780	0.0745	0.0713	0.0595	0.0462	0.0347	0.0250
60	0.1737	0.1131	0.0895	0.0765	0.0682	0.0623	0.0583	0.0552	0.0520	0.0497	0.0411	0.0316	0.0234	0.0167
120	0.0998	0.0632	0.0495	0.0419	0.0371	0.0337	0.0312	0.0292	0.0279	0.0266	0.0218	0.0165	0.0120	0.0083
∞	0	0	0	0	0	0	0	0	0	0	0	0	0	0

← See inserted sheet

VI.6 PERCENTAGE POINTS OF THE MAXIMUM *F*-RATIO

The maximum *F*-ratio $s^2_{\text{max}}/s^2_{\text{min}}$ can be used as a short-cut test for the heterogeneity of variance. Let s_i^2, $i = 1, 2, \ldots, k$ denote a set of mean squares, each based on ν degrees of freedom and arranged in ascending order of magnitude. Then

$$\begin{aligned} \log_e (s^2_{\text{max}}/s^2_{\text{min}}) &= \log_e (s^2_{\text{max}}) - \log_e (s^2_{\text{min}}) \\ &= \text{range} (\log_e s_i^2). \end{aligned}$$

Since $(\log_e s_i^2)$ are approximately normally distributed with mean $\log_e \sigma^2$ and variance $\frac{2}{\nu - 1}$, approximate percentage points of $s^2_{\text{max}}/s^2_{\text{min}}$ can be computed from percentage points of the range in normal samples. This table gives 5% and 1% points of the maximum F-ratio.

PERCENTAGE POINTS OF THE MAXIMUM *F*-RATIO

Upper 5% points

ν \ k	2	3	4	5	6	7	8	9	10	11	12
2	39.0	87.5	142	202	266	333	403	475	550	626	704
3	15.4	27.8	39.2	50.7	62.0	72.9	83.5	93.9	104	114	124
4	9.60	15.5	20.6	25.2	29.5	33.6	37.5	41.1	44.6	48.0	51.4
5	7.15	10.8	13.7	16.3	18.7	20.8	22.9	24.7	26.5	28.2	29.9
6	5.82	8.38	10.4	12.1	13.7	15.0	16.3	17.5	18.6	19.7	20.7
7	4.99	6.94	8.44	9.70	10.8	11.8	12.7	13.5	14.3	15.1	15.8
8	4.43	6.00	7.18	8.12	9.03	9.78	10.5	11.1	11.7	12.2	12.7
9	4.03	5.34	6.31	7.11	7.80	8.41	8.95	9.45	9.91	10.3	10.7
10	3.72	4.85	5.67	6.34	6.92	7.42	7.87	8.28	8.66	9.01	9.34
12	3.28	4.16	4.79	5.30	5.72	6.09	6.42	6.72	7.00	7.25	7.48
15	2.86	3.54	4.01	4.37	4.68	4.95	5.19	5.40	5.59	5.77	5.93
20	2.46	2.95	3.29	3.54	3.76	3.94	4.10	4.24	4.37	4.49	4.59
30	2.07	2.40	2.61	2.78	2.91	3.02	3.12	3.21	3.29	3.36	3.39
60	1.67	1.85	1.96	2.04	2.11	2.17	2.22	2.26	2.30	2.33	2.36
∞	1.00	1.00	1.00	1.00	1.00	1.00	1.00	1.00	1.00	1.00	1.00

Upper 1% points

ν \ k	2	3	4	5	6	7	8	9	10	11	12
2	199	448	729	1036	1362	1705	2063	2432	2813	3204	3605
3	47.5	85	120	151	184	21(6)	24(9)	28(1)	31(0)	33(7)	36(1)
4	23.2	37	49	59	69	79	89	97	106	113	120
5	14.9	22	28	33	38	42	46	50	54	57	60
6	11.1	15.5	19.1	22	25	27	30	32	34	36	37
7	8.89	12.1	14.5	16.5	18.4	20	22	23	24	26	27
8	7.50	9.9	11.7	13.2	14.5	15.8	16.9	17.9	18.9	19.8	21
9	6.54	8.5	9.9	11.1	12.1	13.1	13.9	14.7	15.3	16.0	16.6
10	5.85	7.4	8.6	9.6	10.4	11.1	11.8	12.4	12.9	13.4	13.9
12	4.91	6.1	6.9	7.6	8.2	8.7	9.1	9.5	9.9	10.2	10.6
15	4.07	4.9	5.5	6.0	6.4	6.7	7.1	7.3	7.5	7.8	8.0
20	3.32	3.8	4.3	4.6	4.9	5.1	5.3	5.5	5.6	5.8	5.9
30	2.63	3.0	3.3	3.4	3.6	3.7	3.8	3.9	4.0	4.1	4.2
60	1.96	2.2	2.3	2.4	2.4	2.5	2.5	2.6	2.6	2.7	2.7
∞	1.00	1.0	1.0	1.0	1.0	1.0	1.0	1.0	1.0	1.0	1.0

s^2_{max} is the largest and s^2_{min} the smallest in a set of k independent mean squares, each based on ν degrees of freedom.

Values in the column $k = 2$ and in the rows $\nu = 2$ and ∞ are exact. Elsewhere the third digit may be in error by a few units for the 5% points and several units for the 1% points. The third digit figures in brackets for $\nu = 3$ are the most uncertain.

VII. ORDER STATISTICS

VII.1 EXPECTED VALUES OF ORDER STATISTICS FROM A STANDARD NORMAL POPULATION

If a sample of n observations $x_1, x_2, \ldots, x_n$ is drawn from a standard normal distribution, and the observations are arranged in ascending order of magnitude $x_{(1)}, \ldots, x_{(n)}$, the ith value of the set $\{x_{(i)}\}$ is called the ith normal order statistic and its expectation is given by

$$E[x_{(i)}] = \frac{n!}{(i-1)!(n-i)!} \int_{-\infty}^{\infty} x f(x) F^{i-1}(x)[1 - F(x)]^{n-i}\, dx ,$$

where $f(x) = \dfrac{1}{\sqrt{2\pi}} e^{-\frac{1}{2}x^2}$,

$$F(x) = \int_{-\infty}^{x} \frac{1}{\sqrt{2\pi}} e^{-t^2/2}\, dt.$$

This table gives value of $E[x_{(i)}]$ for various values of n. Missing values may be obtained by noting that

$$E[x_{(i)}] = -E[x_{(n-i+1)}].$$

Tabular values are the expected values of the ith largest normal order statistic from a sample of size n from $N(0,1)$; or when preceded by a minus sign, they are the expected values of the ith smallest normal order statistic.

EXPECTED VALUES OF NORMAL ORDER STATISTICS

i \ n	2	3	4	5	6	7	8	9
1	0.56419	0.84628	1.02938	1.16296	1.26721	1.35218	1.42360	1.48501
2	—	.00000	0.29701	0.49502	0.64176	0.75737	0.85222	0.93230
3	—	—	—	.00000	.20155	.35271	.47282	.57197
4	—	—	—	—	—	.00000	.15251	.27453
5	—	—	—	—	—	—	—	.00000

i \ n	10	11	12	13	14	15	16	17	18	19
1	1.53875	1.58644	1.62923	1.66799	1.70338	1.73591	1.76599	1.79394	1.82003	1.84448
2	1.00136	1.06192	1.11573	1.16408	1.20790	1.24794	1.28474	1.31878	1.35041	1.37994
3	0.65606	0.72884	0.79284	0.84983	0.90113	0.94769	0.99027	1.02946	1.06573	1.09945
4	.37576	.46198	.53684	.60285	.66176	.71488	.76317	0.80738	0.84812	0.88586
5	.12267	.22489	.31225	.38833	.45557	.51570	.57001	.61946	.66479	.70661
6	—	0.00000	0.10259	0.19052	0.26730	0.33530	0.39622	0.45133	0.50158	0.54771
7	—	—	—	.00000	0.08816	.16530	.23375	.29519	.35084	.40164
8	—	—	—	—	—	.00000	.07729	.14599	.20774	.26374
9	—	—	—	—	—	—	—	.00000	.06880	.13072
10	—	—	—	—	—	—	—	—	—	.00000

i \ n	20	21	22	23	24	25	26	27	28	29
1	1.86748	1.88917	1.90969	1.92916	1.94767	1.96531	1.98216	1.99827	2.01371	2.02852
2	1.40760	1.43362	1.45816	1.48137	1.50338	1.52430	1.54423	1.56326	1.58145	1.59888
3	1.13095	1.16047	1.18824	1.21445	1.23924	1.26275	1.28511	1.30641	1.32674	1.34619
4	0.92098	0.95380	0.98459	1.01356	1.04091	1.06679	1.09135	1.11471	1.13697	1.15822
5	.74538	.78150	.81527	0.84697	0.87682	0.90501	0.93171	0.95705	0.98115	1.00414
6	0.59030	0.62982	0.66667	0.70115	0.73354	0.76405	0.79289	0.82021	0.84615	0.87084
7	.44833	.49148	.53157	.56896	.60399	.63690	.66794	.69727	.72508	.75150
8	.31493	.36203	.40559	.44609	.48391	.51935	.55267	.58411	.61385	.64205
9	.18696	.23841	.28579	.32965	.37047	.40860	.44436	.47801	.50977	.53982
10	.06200	.11836	.16997	.21755	.26163	.30268	.34105	.37706	.41096	.44298
11	—	0.00000	0.05642	0.10813	0.15583	0.20006	0.24128	0.27983	0.31603	0.35013
12	—	—	—	.00000	.05176	.09953	.14387	.18520	.22389	.26023
13	—	—	—	—	—	.00000	.04781	.09220	.13361	.17240
14	—	—	—	—	—	—	—	.00000	.04442	.08588
15	—	—	—	—	—	—	—	—	—	.00000

i \ n	30	31	32	33	34	35	36	37	38	39
1	2.04276	2.05646	2.06967	2.08241	2.09471	2.10661	2.11812	2.12928	2.14009	2.15059
2	1.61560	1.63166	1.64712	1.66200	1.67636	1.69023	1.70362	1.71659	1.72914	1.74131
3	1.36481	1.38268	1.39985	1.41637	1.43228	1.44762	1.46244	1.47676	1.49061	1.50402
4	1.17855	1.19803	1.21672	1.23468	1.25196	1.26860	1.28466	1.30016	1.31514	1.32964
5	1.02609	1.04709	1.06721	1.08652	1.10509	1.12295	1.14016	1.15677	1.17280	1.18830
6	0.89439	0.91688	0.93841	0.95905	0.97886	0.99790	1.01624	1.03390	1.05095	1.06741
7	.77666	.80066	.82359	.84555	.86660	.88681	0.90625	0.92496	0.94300	0.96041
8	.66885	.69438	.71875	.74204	.76435	.78574	.80629	.82605	.84508	.86343
9	.56834	.59545	.62129	.64596	.66954	.69214	.71382	.73465	.75468	.77398
10	.47329	.50206	.52943	.55552	.58043	.60427	.62710	.64902	.67009	.69035
11	0.38235	0.41287	0.44185	0.46942	0.49572	0.52084	0.54488	0.56793	0.59005	0.61131
12	.29449	.32686	.35755	.38669	.41444	.44091	.46620	.49042	.51363	.53592
13	.20885	.24322	.27573	.30654	.33582	.36371	.39032	.41576	.44012	.46348
14	.12473	.16126	.19572	.22832	.25924	.28863	.31663	.34336	.36892	.39340
15	.04148	.08037	.11695	.15147	.18415	.21515	.24463	.27272	.29954	.32520
16	—	0.00000	0.03890	0.07552	0.11009	0.14282	0.17388	0.20342	0.23159	0.25849
17	—	—	—	.00000	.03663	.07123	.10399	.13509	.16469	.19292
18	—	—	—	—	—	.00000	.03461	.06739	.09853	.12817
19	—	—	—	—	—	—	—	.00000	.03280	.06395
20	—	—	—	—	—	—	—	—	—	.00000

VII.2 VARIANCES AND COVARIANCES OF ORDER STATISTICS

If a sample of n observations $x_1, x_2, \ldots, x_n$ is drawn from a standard normal distribution, and the observations are arranged in ascending order of magnitude $x_{(1)}, x_{(2)}, \ldots, x_{(n)}$, then the variances and covariances of these order statistics may be obtained from the following expressions for expected values and product moments:

$$E[x_{(i)}] = \frac{n!}{(i-1)!(n-i)!} \int_{-\infty}^{\infty} x f(x)[F(x)]^{i-1}[1 - F(x)]^{n-i}\, dx,$$

$$E[x_{(i)}^2] = \frac{n!}{(i-1)!(n-i)!} \int_{-\infty}^{\infty} x^2 f(x)[F(x)]^{i-1}[1 - F(x)]^{n-i}\, dx,$$

$$E[x_{(i)}x_{(j)}] = \frac{n!}{(i-1)!(j-i-1)!(n-j)!} \int_{-\infty}^{\infty} \int_{-\infty}^{y} xyf(x)f(y)[F(x)]^{i-1}[1 - F(y)]^{n-j}[F(y) - F(x)]^{j-i-1}\, dx\, dy\ ,$$

where $f(x) = \frac{1}{\sqrt{2\pi}} e^{-\frac{1}{2}x^2}$,

$$F(x) = \int_{-\infty}^{x} \frac{1}{\sqrt{2\pi}} e^{-\frac{1}{2}t^2}\, dt.$$

This table gives the variances and covariances of order statistics in samples of sizes up to 20 from a standard normal distribution. Missing values may be supplied from $E[x_{(i)}] = -E[x_{(n-i+1)}]$; $E[x_{(i)}x_{(j)}] = E[x_{(j)}x_{(i)}] = E[x_{(n-i+1)}x_{(n-j+1)}]$.

VARIANCES AND COVARIANCES OF ORDER STATISTICS

n	i	j	Value	n	i	j	Value	n	i	j	Value
2	1	1	.6816901139	8				10	3		
		2	.3183098861		2	2	.2394010458			5	.1077445336
	2	2	.6816901139			3	.1631958727			6	.0892254012
3	1	1	.5594672038			4	.1232633317			7	.0749183943
		2	.2756644477			5	.0975647193			8	.0630332449
		3	.1648683485			6	.0787224662		4	4	.1579389144
	2	2	.4486711046			7	.0632466118			5	.1275089295
4	1	1	.4917152369		3	3	.2007687900			6	.1057858169
		2	.2455926930			4	.1523584312			7	.0889462026
		3	.1580080701			5	.1209637555		5	5	.1510539039
		4	.1046840000			6	.0978171355			6	.1255989678
	2	2	.3604553434		4	4	.1871862195	11	1	1	.3332474428
		3	.2359438935			5	.1491754908			2	.1653647712
5	1	1	.4475340691	9	1	1	.3573533264			3	.1123584351
		2	.2243309596			2	.1781434240			4	.0855170596
		3	.1481477252			3	.1207454442			5	.0688483064
		4	.1057719776			4	.0913071400			6	.0572007586
		5	.0742152685			5	.0727422354			7	.0483754063
	2	2	.3115189521			6	.0594831125			8	.0412423472
		3	.2084354440			7	.0490764061			9	.0351103357
		4	.1499426668			8	.0400936927			10	.0294198503
	3	3	.2868336616			9	.0310552188			11	.0233152868
6	1	1	.4159271090		2	2	.2256968778		2	2	.2051975798
		2	.2085030023			3	.1541163526			3	.1403096511
		3	.1394352565			4	.1170056918			4	.1071492595
		4	.1024293940			5	.0934477394			5	.0864430257
		5	.0773637839			6	.0765461431			6	.0719305024
		6	.0563414544			7	.0632354695			7	.0608869662
	2	2	.2795777392			8	.0517146091			8	.0519504506
		3	.1889859560		3	3	.1863826133			9	.0442549455
		4	.1396640604			4	.1420779776			10	.0371029977
		5	.1059054582			5	.1137680176		3	3	.1657242880
	3	3	.2462125354			6	.0933625386			4	.1269672925
		4	.1832727978			7	.0772351806			5	.1026407291
7	1	1	.3919177761		4	4	.1705588454			6	.0855178832
		2	.1961990246			5	.1369913669			7	.0724741050
		3	.1321155811			6	.1126671842			8	.0618873278
		4	.0984868607		5	5	.1661012814			9	.0527550069
		5	.0765598346	10	1	1	.3443438233		4	4	.1479546565
		6	.0599187124			2	.1712629030			5	.1198752861
		7	.0448022105			3	.1162590989			6	.1000346585
	2	2	.2567328862			4	.0882494247			7	.0848765182
		3	.1744833274			5	.0707413677			8	.0725451434
		4	.1307298656			6	.0583987134		5	5	.1396410804
		5	.1019550089			7	.0489206279			6	.1167449805
		6	.0799811748			8	.0410844589			7	.0991935960
	3	3	.2197215626			9	.0340406470		6	6	.1371624335
		4	.1655598429			10	.0266989351	12	1	1	.3236363870
		5	.1296048425		2	2	.2145241430			2	.1602373762
	4	4	.2104468615			3	.1466226180			3	.1089309641
8	1	1	.3728971434			4	.1117015961			4	.0830686767
		2	.1863073997			5	.0897428245			5	.0670884464
		3	.1259660300			6	.0741995414			6	.0559933694
		4	.0947230277			7	.0622278486			7	.0476620974
		5	.0747650242			8	.0523067222			8	.0410208554
		6	.0602075169			9	.0433711561			9	.0354439060
		7	.0482985508		3	3	.1750032834			10	.0305012591
		8	.0368353073			4	.1338022448			11	.0257945392

VARIANCES AND COVARIANCES OF ORDER STATISTICS

n	i	j	Value	n	i	j	Value	n	i	j	Value
12	1			13	3			14	3		
		12	.0206221233			5	.0944566603			11	.0392352316
	2	2	.1972646039			6	.0792922993			12	.0343322071
		3	.1349020328			7	.0679282354		4	4	.1272273070
		4	.1031959206			8	.0589221432			5	.1036931108
		5	.0835045822			9	.0514460445			6	.0873562483
		6	.0697859658			10	.0449637542			7	.0751519909
		7	.0594590652			11	.0390643799			8	.0655310936
		8	.0512113198		4	4	.1330111820			9	.0576120957
		9	.0442747124			5	.1082512667			10	.0508402240
		10	.0381191478			6	.0909855605			11	.0448243469
		11	.0322507340			7	.0780173339		5	5	.1171012461
	3	3	.1579786877			8	.0677217143			6	.0987747550
		4	.1212063211			9	.0591628729			7	.0850536546
		5	.0982605602			10	.0517328050			8	.0742181416
		6	.0822228461		5	5	.1232503256			9	.0652867776
		7	.0701213964			6	.1037367701			10	.0576401464
		8	.0604384621			7	.0890434754		6	6	.1115324579
		9	.0522825611			8	.0773552864			7	.0961405595
		10	.0450357615			9	.0676230994			8	.0839617110
	4	4	.1398109405		6	6	.1183175325			9	.0739069221
		5	.1135687821			7	.1016824204		7	7	.1090269480
		6	.0951645279			8	.0884194610			8	.0953087256
		7	.0812419810		7	7	.1167989950	15	1	1	.3010415703
		8	.0700795832	14	1	1	.3077301026			2	.1481297708
		9	.0606620874			2	.1517203662			3	.1007223449
	5	5	.1306137359			3	.1031719531			4	.0770594060
		6	.1096212247			4	.0788715916			5	.0625845851
		7	.0936951520			5	.0639657428			6	.0526530129
		8	.0808972960			6	.0537064714			7	.0453078886
	6	6	.1266377911			7	.0460899189			8	.0395736673
		7	.1083945831			8	.0401141688			9	.0349035905
13	1	1	.3152053842			9	.0352141760			10	.0309614122
		2	.1557272904			10	.0310371163			11	.0275211039
		3	.1058908842			11	.0273362865			12	.0244126313
		4	.0808649736			12	.0239061001			13	.0214819828
		5	.0654634499			13	.0205080257			14	.0185333263
		6	.0548221797			14	.0166279801			15	.0151137071
		7	.0468833088		2	2	.1844200252		2	2	.1791215291
		8	.0406132548			3	.1260791989			3	.1224176953
		9	.0354226462			4	.0966524633			4	.0939067144
		10	.0309322744			5	.0785202981			5	.0763912337
		11	.0268537250			6	.0660028340			6	.0643390895
		12	.0228858068			7	.0566896715			7	.0554074400
		13	.0184348220			8	.0493708148			8	.0484238833
	2	2	.1904130721			9	.0433617156			9	.0427294113
		3	.1302055829			10	.0382337404			10	.0379177516
		4	.0997262696			11	.0336863221			11	.0337151721
		5	.0808785938			12	.0294681314			12	.0299152347
		6	.0678145832			13	.0252863928			13	.0263303885
		7	.0580457285		3	3	.1457045665			14	.0227213594
		8	.0503167946			4	.1119816877		3	3	.1407322502
		9	.0439095087			5	.0911181271			4	.1082138452
		10	.0383601798			6	.0766754957			5	.0881605755
		11	.0333147765			7	.0659084825			6	.0743268436
		12	.0284018130			8	.0574341188			7	.0640558183
	3	3	.1513917013			9	.0504677802			8	.0560136122
		4	.1162698131			10	.0445169192			9	.0494485109

VARIANCES AND COVARIANCES OF ORDER STATISTICS

n	*i*	*j*	Value	*n*	*i*	*j*	Value	*n*	*i*	*j*	Value
15	3			16	2			17	1		
		10	.0438960670			14	.0237301562			14	.0199690651
		11	.0390426915			15	.0205785433			15	.0177476891
		12	.0346513382		3	3	.1363385612			16	.0154552071
		13	.0305060359			4	.1048706756			17	.0127264751
	4	4	.1222328270			5	.0855189036		2	2	.1701426762
		5	.0997323941			6	.0722075087			3	.1161866734
		6	.0841705696			7	.0623568515			4	.0891982557
		7	.0725946869			8	.0546749107			5	.0726970385
		8	.0635175907			9	.0484366096			6	.0613998459
		9	.0560990511			10	.0431979377			7	.0530761573
		10	.0498187836			11	.0386652995			8	.0466140918
		11	.0443247452			12	.0346277256			9	.0413928192
		12	.0393501820			13	.0309149135			10	.0370349110
	5	5	.1118698986			14	.0273595378			11	.0332940892
		6	.0945206004		4	4	.1178657554			12	.0299982825
		7	.0815891122			5	.0962513413			13	.0270170379
		8	.0714331681			6	.0813480448			14	.0242386812
		9	.0631224388			7	.0703000911			15	.0215459396
		10	.0560795065			8	.0616728990			16	.0187658306
		11	.0499127743			9	.0546595026		3	3	.1324207975
	6	6	.1058666366			10	.0487647746			4	.1018792434
		7	.0914683204			11	.0436607328			5	.0831421716
		8	.0801407559			12	.0391112669			6	.0702850403
		9	.0708582099			13	.0349253749			7	.0607964413
		10	.0629824402		5	5	.1073517089			8	.0534208202
	7	7	.1026916923			6	.0908232622			9	.0474555487
		8	.0900499964			7	.0785480532			10	.0424726884
		9	.0796738323			8	.0689488802			11	.0381925587
	8	8	.1016946521			9	.0611364182			12	.0344194567
16	1	1	.2950098090			10	.0545638941			13	.0310047771
		2	.1448881689			11	.0488684327			14	.0278210708
		3	.0985009764			12	.0437882959			15	.0247342095
		4	.0754040023		6	6	.1010461906		4	4	.1140068197
		5	.0613086724			7	.0874627156			5	.0931620339
		6	.0516624963			8	.0768239668			6	.0788266621
		7	.0445503705			9	.0681545540			7	.0682298909
		8	.0390194716			10	.0608534805			8	.0599826092
		9	.0345378158			11	.0545210724			9	.0533057575
		10	.0307810093		7	7	.0974026613			10	.0477239973
		11	.0275353612			8	.0856181916			11	.0429261816
		12	.0246479007			9	.0760015577			12	.0386942630
		13	.0219956755			10	.0678931922			13	.0348624030
		14	.0194585037		8	8	.0957213007			14	.0312881041
		15	.0168710289			9	.0850291218		5	5	.1034004377
		16	.0138287378	17	1	1	.2895330037			6	.0875729930
	2	2	.1743940788			2	.1419424629			7	.0758534534
		3	.1191409287			3	.0964748737			8	.0667204245
		4	.0914359918			4	.0738849615			9	.0593187706
		5	.0744591145			5	.0601272302			10	.0531257771
		6	.0628093909			6	.0507326948			11	.0477987292
		7	.0542033941			7	.0438236491			12	.0430970793
		8	.0475009769			8	.0384672834			13	.0388375657
		9	.0420638230			9	.0341441055		6	6	.0968824669
		10	.0375018250			10	.0305389548			7	.0839811738
		11	.0335574912			11	.0274465527			8	.0739130260
		12	.0300461298			12	.0247237144			9	.0657442736
		13	.0268189579			13	.0222620771			10	.0589030403

VARIANCES AND COVARIANCES OF ORDER STATISTICS

n	*i*	*j*	Value	*n*	*i*	*j*	Value	*n*	*i*	*j*	Value
17	6			18	3			19	1		
		11	.0530137275			15	.0252244786			14	.0204007370
		12	.0478122599			16	.0225161109			15	.0185431530
	7	7	.0929031780		4	4	.1105660331			16	.0167731147
		8	.0818194607			5	.0903973787			17	.0150223067
		9	.0728154074			6	.0765579277			18	.0131789994
		10	.0652667274			7	.0663522086			19	.0109382527
		11	.0587626219			8	.0584310521		2	2	.1627856651
	8	8	.0907361650			9	.0520394281			3	.1110590145
		9	.0808000267			10	.0467183404			4	.0852931053
		10	.0724599963			11	.0421694861			5	.0695970759
	9	9	.0900465814			12	.0381869632			6	.0588910196
18	1	1	.2845301297			13	.0346192645			7	.0510351093
		2	.1392501620			14	.0313452497			8	.0449652247
		3	.0946172637			15	.0282548286			9	.0400891754
		4	.0724851730		5	5	.0999084321			10	.0360490040
		5	.0590304274			6	.0846879168			11	.0326137544
		6	.0498600635			7	.0734460811			12	.0296258236
		7	.0431302310			8	.0647101858			13	.0269716592
		8	.0379260195			9	.0576543520			14	.0245641909
		9	.0337388141			10	.0517756675			15	.0223306885
		10	.0302610667			11	.0467468133			16	.0202017247
		11	.0272938041			12	.0423415563			17	.0180952193
		12	.0247002471			13	.0383932046			18	.0158767294
		13	.0223801573			14	.0347682770		3	3	.1257138904
		14	.0202537421		6	6	.0932407331			4	.0967367097
		15	.0182488619			7	.0809202644			5	.0790298792
		16	.0162850441			8	.0713338046			6	.0669273696
		17	.0142368875			9	.0635829688			7	.0580336124
		18	.0117719054			10	.0571197288			8	.0511541418
	2	2	.1662929294			11	.0515868552			9	.0456228816
		3	.1135058132			12	.0467370896			10	.0410365629
		4	.0871597604			13	.0423879846			11	.0371346427
		5	.0710825990		7	7	.0890167025			12	.0337391171
		6	.0600975754			8	.0785179677			13	.0307215918
		7	.0520217423			9	.0700199026			14	.0279835020
		8	.0457683625			10	.0629269074			15	.0254424108
		9	.0407317967			11	.0568501034			16	.0230195063
		10	.0365451034			12	.0515199092			17	.0206214645
		11	.0329704894		8	8	.0864960639		4	4	.1074740839
		12	.0298442464			9	.0771762286			5	.0879051965
		13	.0270462261			10	.0693891332			6	.0745033878
		14	.0244806359			11	.0627116906			7	.0646406188
		15	.0220607111		9	9	.0853127880			8	.0570032284
		16	.0196894667			10	.0767442321			9	.0508572608
		17	.0172154925	19	1	1	.2799358050			10	.0457576598
	3	3	.1288998943			2	.1367768168			11	.0414165091
		4	.0991828539			3	.0929061763			12	.0376368753
		5	.0809899792			4	.0711902425			13	.0342765540
		6	.0685324700			5	.0580094835			14	.0312262549
		7	.0593598602			6	.0490405678			15	.0283944527
		8	.0522488413			7	.0424705246			16	.0256935148
		9	.0465162123			8	.0374006329		5	5	.0967944745
		10	.0417473296			9	.0333319395			6	.0821055695
		11	.0376730987			10	.0299634144			7	.0712796742
		12	.0341080171			11	.0271011338			8	.0628870095
		13	.0309157650			12	.0246129452			9	.0561272025
		14	.0279875014			13	.0224037540			10	.0505141639

VARIANCES AND COVARIANCES OF ORDER STATISTICS

n	i	j	Value	n	i	j	Value	n	i	j	Value
19	5			20	1			20	4		
		11	.0457330144			18	.0139227072			14	.0310045146
		12	.0415681234			19	.0122530117			15	.0283650517
		13	.0378636088			20	.0102047204			16	.0253897454
		14	.0344995261		2	2	.1595731636			17	.0235070343
		15	.0313752928			3	.1088143707		5	5	.0939960007
	6	6	.0900218693			4	.0835758044			6	.0797773755
		7	.0782029063			5	.0682247554			7	.0693175756
		8	.0690294360			6	.0577699656			8	.0612251429
		9	.0616336896			7	.0501109523			9	.0547222526
		10	.0554877905			8	.0442041191			10	.0493374275
		11	.0502493169			9	.0394693443			11	.0447662310
		12	.0456834841			10	.0355565554			12	.0408014074
		13	.0416203596			11	.0322405467			13	.0372948400
		14	.0379290224			12	.0293684960			14	.0341351571
	7	7	.0856172981			13	.0268315105			15	.0312332040
		8	.0756153413			14	.0245479493			16	.0285109200
		9	.0675433161			15	.0224526609		6	6	.0871511254
		10	.0608297030			16	.0204888032			7	.0757703360
		11	.0551032224			17	.0185994024			8	.0669555789
		12	.0501089625			18	.0167136502			9	.0598659769
		13	.0456621835			19	.0147107671			10	.0539910639
	8	8	.0828339961		3	3	.1228134687			11	.0490008080
		9	.0740273546			4	.0945049010			12	.0446702771
		10	.0666958229			5	.0772355098			13	.0408385549
		11	.0604372723			6	.0654510179			14	.0373845194
		12	.0549752083			7	.0568056677			15	.0342111024
	9	9	.0812876330			8	.0501310269		7	7	.0826123955
		10	.0732703911			9	.0447763202			8	.0730383676
		11	.0664202898			10	.0403482354			9	.0653307665
	10	10	.0807909751			11	.0365934287			10	.0589387428
20	1	1	.2756966156			12	.0333397949			11	.0535056766
		2	.1344941714			13	.0304645792			12	.0487882257
		3	.0913234064			14	.0278756579			13	.0446121090
		4	.0699879991			15	.0254994381			14	.0408459989
		5	.0570566384			16	.0232716371		8	8	.0796309757
		6	.0482701093			17	.0211277373			9	.0712591607
		7	.0418437826			18	.0189874448			10	.0643103375
		8	.0368937058		4	4	.1046766243			11	.0583997310
		9	.0329296302			5	.0856442356			12	.0532644495
		10	.0296562523			6	.0726321560			13	.0487159834
		11	.0268838308			7	.0630731775		9	9	.0778118317
		12	.0244839567			8	.0556855081			10	.0702526464
		13	.0223649803			9	.0497539273			11	.0638176734
		14	.0204584277			10	.0448455403			12	.0582229133
		15	.0187096782			11	.0406811669		10	10	.0769474356
		16	.0170711408			12	.0370709493			11	.0699266198
		17	.0154951854			13	.0338793392				

VII.3 CONFIDENCE INTERVALS FOR MEDIANS

If the observations $x_1, x_2, \ldots, x_n$ are arranged in ascending order $x_{(1)}, x_{(2)}, \ldots, x_{(n)}$, a $100(1-\alpha)\%$ confidence interval on the median of the population can be found. This table gives values of k and α such that one can be $100(1-\alpha)\%$ confident that the population median is between $x_{(k)}$ and $x_{(n-k+1)}$.

CONFIDENCE INTERVALS FOR THE MEDIAN

n	Largest k	Actual $\alpha \le 0.05$	Largest k	Actual $\alpha \le 0.01$	N	Largest k	Actual $\alpha \le 0.05$	Largest k	Actual $\alpha \le 0.01$
6	1	0.031			36	12	0.029	10	0.004
7	1	0.016			37	13	0.047	11	0.008
8	1	0.008	1	0.008	38	13	0.034	11	0.005
9	2	0.039	1	0.004	39	13	0.024	12	0.009
10	2	0.021	1	0.002	40	14	0.038	12	0.006
11	2	0.012	1	0.001	41	14	0.028	12	0.004
12	3	0.039	2	0.006	42	15	0.044	13	0.008
13	3	0.022	2	0.003	43	15	0.032	13	0.005
14	3	0.013	2	0.002	44	16	0.049	14	0.010
15	4	0.035	3	0.007	45	16	0.036	14	0.007
16	4	0.021	3	0.004	46	16	0.026	14	0.005
17	5	0.049	3	0.002	47	17	0.040	15	0.008
18	5	0.031	4	0.008	48	17	0.029	15	0.006
19	5	0.019	4	0.004	49	18	0.044	16	0.009
20	6	0.041	4	0.003	50	18	0.033	16	0.007
21	6	0.027	5	0.007	51	19	0.049	16	0.005
22	6	0.017	5	0.004	52	19	0.036	17	0.008
23	7	0.035	5	0.003	53	19	0.027	17	0.005
24	7	0.023	6	0.007	54	20	0.040	18	0.009
25	8	0.043	6	0.004	55	20	0.030	18	0.006
26	8	0.029	7	0.009	56	21	0.044	18	0.005
27	8	0.019	7	0.006	57	21	0.033	19	0.008
28	9	0.036	7	0.004	58	22	0.048	19	0.005
29	9	0.024	8	0.008	59	22	0.036	20	0.009
30	10	0.043	8	0.005	60	22	0.027	20	0.006
31	10	0.029	8	0.003	61	23	0.040	21	0.010
32	10	0.020	9	0.007	62	23	0.030	21	0.007
33	11	0.035	9	0.005	63	24	0.043	21	0.005
34	11	0.024	10	0.009	64	24	0.033	22	0.008
35	12	0.041	10	0.006	65	25	0.046	22	0.006

VII.4 CRITICAL VALUES FOR TESTING OUTLIERS

Tests for outliers may be based on the largest deviation $\max_{i=1,2,\ldots,n} (x_i - \bar{x})$ of the observations from their mean or on the range w, where these statistics have to be divided by the standard deviation σ or by an estimate of σ, depending on whether σ is known or not. An alternate set of statistics is considered in this table.

The following ratios are suitable for detection of outliers.

a) For single outlier $x_{(1)}$:

$$r_{10} = \frac{x_{(2)} - x_{(1)}}{x_{(n)} - x_{(1)}}$$

$$\left(\text{or for } x_{(n)}\text{: } r_{10} = \frac{x_{(n)} - x_{(n-1)}}{x_{(n)} - x_{(1)}}\right)$$

b) For single outlier $x_{(1)}$ avoiding $x_{(n)}$:

$$r_{11} = \frac{x_{(2)} - x_{(1)}}{x_{(n-1)} - x_{(1)}}$$

$$\left(\text{or for } x_{(n)} \text{ avoiding } x_{(1)}\text{: } r_{11} = \frac{x_{(n)} - x_{(n-1)}}{x_{(n)} - x_{(2)}}\right)$$

c) For single outlier $x_{(1)}$, avoiding $x_{(n)}$, $x_{(n-1)}$:

$$r_{12} = \frac{x_{(2)} - x_{(1)}}{x_{(n-2)} - x_{(1)}}$$

$$\left(\text{or for } x_{(n)} \text{ avoiding } x_{(1)}, x_{(2)}\text{: } r_{12} = \frac{x_{(n)} - x_{(n-1)}}{x_{(n)} - x_{(3)}}\right)$$

d) For outlier $x_{(1)}$ avoiding $x_{(2)}$:

$$r_{20} = \frac{x_{(3)} - x_{(1)}}{x_{(n)} - x_{(1)}}$$

$$\left(\text{or for } x_{(n)} \text{ avoiding } x_{(n-1)}\text{: } r_{20} = \frac{x_{(n)} - x_{(n-2)}}{x_{(n)} - x_{(1)}}\right)$$

e) For outlier $x_{(1)}$ avoiding $x_{(2)}$ and $x_{(n)}$:

$$r_{21} = \frac{x_{(3)} - x_{(1)}}{x_{(n-1)} - x_{(1)}}$$

$$\left(\text{or for } x_{(n)} \text{ avoiding } x_{(n-1)}, x_{(1)}\text{: } r_{21} = \frac{x_{(n)} - x_{(n-2)}}{x_{(n)} - x_{(2)}}\right)$$

f) For outlier $x_{(1)}$ avoiding $x_{(2)}$ and $x_{(n)}$, $x_{(n-1)}$:

$$r_{22} = \frac{x_{(3)} - x_{(1)}}{x_{(n-2)} - x_{(1)}}$$

$$\left(\text{or for } x_{(n)} \text{ avoiding } x_{(n-1)}, x_{(1)}, x_{(2)}\text{: } r_{22} = \frac{x_{(n)} - x_{(n-2)}}{x_{(n)} - x_{(3)}}\right)$$

PERCENTAGE VALUES FOR r_{10}

$[\Pr(r_{10} > R) = \alpha]$

n \ α	.005	.01	.02	.05	.10	.20	.30	.40	.50	.60	.70	.80	.90	.95	α / n
3	.994	.988	.976	.941	.886	.781	.684	.591	.500	.409	.316	.219	.114	.059	3
4	.926	.889	.846	.765	.679	.560	.471	.394	.324	.257	.193	.130	.065	.033	4
5	.821	.780	.729	.642	.557	.451	.373	.308	.250	.196	.146	.097	.048	.023	5
6	.740	.698	.644	.560	.482	.386	.318	.261	.210	.164	.121	.079	.038	.018	6
7	.680	.637	.586	.507	.434	.344	.281	.230	.184	.143	.105	.068	.032	.016	7
8	.634	.590	.543	.468	.399	.314	.255	.208	.166	.128	.094	.060	.029	.014	8
9	.598	.555	.510	.437	.370	.290	.234	.191	.152	.118	.086	.055	.026	.013	9
10	.568	.527	.483	.412	.349	.273	.219	.178	.142	.110	.080	.051	.025	.012	10
11	.542	.502	.460	.392	.332	.259	.208	.168	.133	.103	.074	.048	.023	.011	11
12	.522	.482	.441	.376	.318	.247	.197	.160	.126	.097	.070	.045	.022	.011	12
13	.503	.465	.425	.361	.305	.237	.188	.153	.120	.092	.067	.043	.021	.010	13
14	.488	.450	.411	.349	.294	.228	.181	.147	.115	.088	.064	.041	.020	.010	14
15	.475	.438	.399	.338	.285	.220	.175	.141	.111	.085	.062	.040	.019	.010	15
16	.463	.426	.388	.329	.277	.213	.169	.136	.107	.082	.060	.039	.019	.009	16
17	.452	.416	.379	.320	.269	.207	.165	.132	.104	.080	.058	.038	.018	.009	17
18	.442	.407	.370	.313	.263	.202	.160	.128	.101	.078	.056	.036	.018	.009	18
19	.433	.398	.363	.306	.258	.197	.157	.125	.098	.076	.055	.036	.017	.008	19
20	.425	.391	.356	.300	.252	.193	.153	.122	.096	.074	.053	.035	.017	.008	20
21	.418	.384	.350	.295	.247	.189	.150	.119	.094	.072	.052	.034	.016	.008	21
22	.411	.378	.344	.290	.242	.185	.147	.117	.092	.071	.051	.033	.016	.008	22
23	.404	.372	.338	.285	.238	.182	.144	.115	.090	.069	.050	.033	.016	.008	23
24	.399	.367	.333	.281	.234	.179	.142	.113	.089	.068	.049	.032	.016	.008	24
25	.393	.362	.329	.277	.230	.176	.139	.111	.088	.067	.048	.032	.015	.008	25
26	.388	.357	.324	.273	.227	.173	.137	.109	.086	.066	.047	.031	.015	.007	26
27	.384	.353	.320	.269	.224	.171	.135	.108	.085	.065	.047	.031	.015	.007	27
28	.380	.349	.316	.266	.220	.168	.133	.106	.084	.064	.046	.030	.015	.007	28
29	.376	.345	.312	.263	.218	.166	.131	.105	.083	.063	.046	.030	.014	.007	29
30	.372	.341	.309	.260	.215	.164	.130	.103	.082	.062	.045	.029	.014	.007	30

PERCENTAGE VALUES FOR r_{11}

$[\Pr(r_{11} > R) = \alpha]$

n \ α	.005	.01	.02	.05	.10	.20	.30	.40	.50	.60	.70	.80	.90	.95	α / n
4	.995	.991	.981	.955	.910	.822	.737	.648	.554	.459	.362	.250	.131	.069	4
5	.937	.916	.876	.807	.728	.615	.524	.444	.369	.296	.224	.151	.078	.039	5
6	.839	.805	.763	.689	.609	.502	.420	.350	.288	.227	.169	.113	.056	.028	6
7	.782	.740	.689	.610	.530	.432	.359	.298	.241	.189	.140	.093	.045	.022	7
8	.725	.683	.631	.554	.479	.385	.318	.260	.210	.164	.121	.079	.037	.019	8
9	.677	.635	.587	.512	.441	.352	.288	.236	.189	.148	.107	.070	.033	.016	9
10	.639	.597	.551	.477	.409	.325	.265	.216	.173	.134	.098	.063	.030	.014	10
11	.606	.566	.521	.450	.385	.305	.248	.202	.161	.124	.090	.058	.028	.013	11
12	.580	.541	.498	.428	.367	.289	.234	.190	.150	.116	.084	.055	.026	.012	12
13	.558	.520	.477	.410	.350	.275	.222	.180	.142	.109	.079	.052	.025	.012	13
14	.539	.502	.460	.395	.336	.264	.212	.171	.135	.104	.075	.049	.024	.011	14
15	.522	.486	.445	.381	.323	.253	.203	.164	.129	.099	.072	.047	.023	.011	15
16	.508	.472	.432	.369	.313	.244	.196	.158	.124	.095	.069	.045	.022	.011	16
17	.495	.460	.420	.359	.303	.236	.190	.152	.119	.092	.067	.044	.021	.010	17
18	.484	.449	.410	.349	.295	.229	.184	.148	.116	.089	.065	.042	.020	.010	18
19	.473	.439	.400	.341	.288	.223	.179	.143	.112	.087	.063	.041	.020	.010	19
20	.464	.430	.392	.334	.282	.218	.174	.139	.110	.084	.061	.040	.019	.010	20
21	.455	.421	.384	.327	.276	.213	.170	.136	.107	.082	.059	.039	.019	.009	21
22	.446	.414	.377	.320	.270	.208	.166	.132	.104	.081	.058	.038	.018	.009	22
23	.439	.407	.371	.314	.265	.204	.163	.130	.102	.079	.056	.037	.018	.009	23
24	.432	.400	.365	.309	.260	.200	.160	.127	.100	.077	.055	.036	.018	.009	24
25	.426	.394	.359	.304	.255	.197	.156	.124	.098	.076	.054	.036	.017	.009	25
26	.420	.389	.354	.299	.250	.193	.154	.122	.096	.074	.053	.035	.017	.008	26
27	.414	.383	.349	.295	.246	.190	.151	.120	.095	.073	.052	.034	.017	.008	27
28	.409	.378	.344	.291	.243	.188	.149	.118	.093	.072	.051	.034	.016	.008	28
29	.404	.374	.340	.287	.239	.185	.146	.116	.092	.070	.051	.033	.016	.008	29
30	.399	.369	.336	.283	.236	.182	.144	.115	.090	.069	.050	.032	.016	.008	30

PERCENTAGE VALUES FOR r_{12}

$[\Pr(r_{12} > R) = \alpha]$

n \ α	.005	.01	.02	.05	.10	.20	.30	.40	.50	.60	.70	.80	.90	.95	α / n
5	.996	.992	.984	.960	.919	.838	.755	.669	.579	.483	.381	.268	.143	.074	5
6	.951	.925	.891	.824	.745	.635	.545	.465	.390	.316	.240	.165	.088	.049	6
7	.875	.836	.791	.712	.636	.528	.445	.374	.307	.245	.183	.123	.064	.031	7
8	.797	.760	.708	.632	.557	.456	.382	.317	.258	.203	.152	.101	.056	.025	8
9	.739	.701	.656	.580	.504	.409	.339	.270	.227	.177	.130	.086	.044	.021	9
10	.694	.655	.610	.537	.454	.373	.308	.258	.204	.158	.116	.075	.038	.019	10
11	.658	.619	.575	.502	.431	.345	.283	.232	.187	.145	.106	.069	.035	.017	11
12	.629	.590	.546	.473	.406	.324	.265	.217	.174	.135	.098	.063	.032	.016	12
13	.612	.554	.521	.451	.387	.307	.250	.204	.163	.126	.092	.059	.030	.015	13
14	.580	.542	.501	.432	.369	.292	.237	.193	.153	.118	.086	.055	.028	.014	14
15	.560	.523	.482	.416	.354	.280	.226	.184	.146	.112	.082	.053	.026	.013	15
16	.544	.508	.467	.401	.341	.269	.217	.177	.139	.107	.078	.050	.025	.013	16
17	.529	.493	.453	.388	.330	.259	.209	.170	.134	.103	.075	.048	.024	.012	17
18	.516	.480	.440	.377	.320	.251	.202	.163	.129	.099	.072	.047	.023	.012	18
19	.504	.469	.429	.367	.311	.243	.196	.157	.125	.096	.069	.045	.022	.011	19
20	.493	.458	.419	.358	.303	.237	.191	.153	.121	.093	.067	.044	.022	.011	20
21	.483	.449	.410	.349	.296	.231	.186	.148	.118	.090	.065	.042	.021	.010	21
22	.474	.440	.402	.342	.290	.225	.181	.145	.114	.088	.063	.041	.020	.010	22
23	.465	.432	.394	.336	.284	.220	.176	.141	.112	.086	.062	.040	.020	.010	23
24	.457	.423	.387	.330	.278	.216	.173	.138	.109	.084	.060	.039	.019	.010	24
25	.450	.417	.381	.324	.273	.212	.169	.135	.107	.082	.059	.038	.019	.009	25
26	.443	.411	.375	.319	.268	.208	.166	.132	.105	.080	.058	.037	.019	.009	26
27	.437	.405	.370	.314	.263	.204	.163	.130	.103	.079	.057	.037	.018	.009	27
28	.431	.399	.365	.309	.259	.201	.160	.128	.101	.077	.056	.036	.018	.009	28
29	.426	.394	.360	.305	.255	.197	.157	.126	.099	.076	.055	.035	.017	.009	29
30	.420	.389	.355	.301	.251	.194	.154	.124	.098	.075	.054	.035	.017	.009	30

PERCENTAGE VALUES FOR r_{20}

$[\Pr(r_{20} > R) = \alpha]$

n \ α	.005	.01	.02	.05	.10	.20	.30	.40	.50	.60	.70	.80	.90	.95	α / n
4	.996	.992	.987	.967	.935	.871	.807	.743	.676	.606	.529	.440	.321	.235	4
5	.950	.929	.901	.845	.782	.694	.623	.560	.500	.440	.377	.306	.218	.155	5
6	.865	.836	.800	.736	.670	.585	.520	.463	.411	.358	.305	.245	.172	.126	6
7	.814	.778	.732	.661	.596	.516	.454	.402	.355	.306	.261	.208	.144	.099	7
8	.746	.710	.670	.607	.545	.468	.410	.361	.317	.274	.230	.184	.125	.085	8
9	.700	.667	.627	.565	.505	.432	.378	.331	.288	.250	.208	.166	.114	.077	9
10	.664	.632	.592	.531	.474	.404	.354	.307	.268	.231	.192	.153	.104	.070	10
11	.627	.603	.564	.504	.449	.381	.334	.290	.253	.217	.181	.143	.097	.065	11
12	.612	.579	.540	.481	.429	.362	.316	.274	.239	.205	.172	.136	.091	.060	12
13	.590	.557	.520	.461	.411	.345	.301	.261	.227	.195	.164	.129	.086	.057	13
14	.571	.538	.502	.445	.395	.332	.288	.250	.217	.187	.157	.123	.082	.054	14
15	.554	.522	.486	.430	.382	.320	.277	.241	.209	.179	.150	.118	.079	.052	15
16	.539	.508	.472	.418	.370	.310	.268	.233	.202	.173	.144	.113	.076	.050	16
17	.526	.495	.460	.406	.359	.301	.260	.226	.195	.167	.139	.109	.074	.049	17
18	.514	.484	.449	.397	.350	.293	.252	.219	.189	.162	.134	.105	.071	.048	18
19	.503	.473	.439	.379	.341	.286	.246	.213	.184	.157	.130	.101	.069	.047	19
20	.494	.464	.430	.372	.333	.279	.240	.208	.179	.152	.126	.098	.067	.046	20
21	.485	.455	.422	.365	.326	.273	.235	.203	.175	.148	.123	.096	.065	.045	21
22	.477	.447	.414	.358	.320	.267	.230	.199	.171	.145	.120	.094	.064	.044	22
23	.469	.440	.407	.352	.314	.262	.225	.195	.167	.142	.117	.092	.062	.043	23
24	.462	.434	.401	.347	.309	.258	.221	.192	.164	.139	.114	.090	.061	.042	24
25	.456	.428	.395	.343	.304	.254	.217	.189	.161	.136	.112	.089	.060	.041	25
26	.450	.422	.390	.338	.300	.250	.214	.186	.158	.134	.110	.087	.059	.041	26
27	.444	.417	.385	.334	.296	.246	.211	.183	.156	.132	.109	.086	.058	.040	27
28	.439	.412	.381	.330	.292	.243	.208	.180	.154	.130	.107	.085	.058	.040	28
29	.434	.407	.376	.326	.288	.239	.205	.177	.151	.128	.106	.083	.057	.039	29
30	.428	.402	.372	.322	.285	.236	.202	.175	.149	.126	.104	.082	.056	.039	30

PERCENTAGE VALUES FOR r_{21}

$[\Pr(r_{21} > R) = \alpha]$

n \ α	.005	.01	.02	.05	.10	.20	.30	.40	.50	.60	.70	.80	.90	.95	α / n
5	.998	.995	.990	.976	.952	.902	.850	.795	.735	.669	.594	.501	.374	.273	5
6	.970	.951	.924	.872	.821	.745	.680	.621	.563	.504	.439	.364	.268	.195	6
7	.919	.885	.842	.780	.725	.637	.575	.517	.462	.408	.350	.285	.198	.138	7
8	.868	.829	.780	.710	.650	.570	.509	.454	.402	.352	.298	.240	.166	.117	8
9	.816	.776	.725	.657	.594	.516	.458	.407	.360	.313	.265	.212	.146	.103	9
10	.760	.726	.678	.612	.551	.474	.420	.374	.329	.286	.240	.189	.130	.089	10
11	.713	.679	.638	.576	.517	.442	.391	.348	.305	.265	.221	.173	.118	.080	11
12	.675	.642	.605	.546	.490	.419	.370	.326	.285	.247	.206	.161	.110	.074	12
13	.649	.615	.578	.521	.467	.399	.351	.308	.269	.232	.194	.152	.104	.070	13
14	.627	.593	.556	.501	.448	.381	.334	.293	.256	.219	.184	.144	.099	.066	14
15	.607	.574	.537	.483	.431	.366	.319	.280	.245	.208	.175	.138	.094	.062	15
16	.589	.557	.521	.467	.416	.353	.307	.269	.235	.199	.167	.132	.090	.059	16
17	.573	.542	.507	.453	.403	.341	.296	.259	.225	.192	.161	.127	.086	.057	17
18	.559	.529	.494	.440	.391	.331	.287	.250	.218	.186	.155	.122	.082	.054	18
19	.547	.517	.482	.428	.380	.322	.279	.243	.211	.180	.150	.117	.078	.052	19
20	.536	.506	.472	.419	.371	.314	.271	.236	.205	.174	.145	.113	.075	.050	20
21	.526	.496	.462	.410	.363	.306	.264	.229	.199	.170	.141	.110	.073	.049	21
22	.517	.487	.453	.402	.356	.299	.258	.223	.194	.165	.137	.107	.071	.048	22
23	.509	.479	.445	.395	.349	.293	.252	.218	.189	.161	.133	.105	.069	.046	23
24	.501	.471	.438	.388	.343	.287	.247	.214	.185	.158	.130	.103	.068	.045	24
25	.493	.464	.431	.382	.337	.282	.242	.210	.181	.154	.127	.100	.067	.043	25
26	.486	.457	.424	.376	.331	.277	.238	.206	.178	.151	.125	.098	.066	.042	26
27	.479	.450	.418	.370	.325	.273	.234	.203	.175	.149	.123	.096	.064	.041	27
28	.472	.444	.412	.365	.320	.269	.230	.200	.172	.146	.121	.094	.063	.041	28
29	.466	.438	.406	.360	.316	.265	.227	.197	.170	.144	.119	.092	.062	.040	29
30	.460	.433	.401	.355	.312	.261	.224	.194	.167	.142	.117	.091	.061	.040	30

PERCENTAGE VALUES FOR r_{22}

$[\Pr(r_{22} > R) = \alpha]$

n \ α	.005	.01	.02	.05	.10	.20	.30	.40	.50	.60	.70	.80	.90	.95	α / n
6	.998	.995	.992	.983	.965	.930	.880	.830	.780	.720	.640	.540	.410	.300	6
7	.970	.945	.919	.881	.850	.780	.730	.670	.610	.540	.470	.390	.270	.200	7
8	.922	.890	.857	.803	.745	.664	.602	.546	.490	.434	.375	.309	.218	.156	8
9	.873	.840	.800	.737	.676	.592	.530	.478	.425	.373	.320	.261	.186	.128	9
10	.826	.791	.749	.682	.620	.543	.483	.433	.384	.335	.285	.231	.150	.111	10
11	.781	.745	.703	.637	.578	.503	.446	.397	.351	.305	.258	.208	.142	.099	11
12	.740	.704	.661	.600	.543	.470	.416	.370	.325	.282	.238	.190	.130	.090	12
13	.705	.670	.628	.570	.515	.443	.391	.347	.304	.263	.222	.177	.122	.084	13
14	.674	.641	.602	.546	.492	.421	.370	.328	.287	.247	.208	.166	.115	.079	14
15	.647	.616	.579	.525	.472	.402	.353	.312	.273	.234	.196	.156	.109	.075	15
16	.624	.595	.559	.507	.454	.386	.338	.298	.261	.223	.186	.148	.104	.071	16
17	.605	.577	.542	.490	.438	.373	.325	.286	.250	.214	.178	.142	.099	.067	17
18	.589	.561	.527	.475	.424	.361	.314	.276	.241	.206	.171	.135	.094	.063	18
19	.575	.547	.514	.462	.412	.350	.304	.268	.233	.199	.165	.130	.090	.060	19
20	.562	.535	.502	.450	.401	.340	.295	.260	.226	.193	.160	.125	.086	.057	20
21	.551	.524	.491	.440	.391	.331	.287	.252	.220	.187	.155	.120	.082	.054	21
22	.541	.514	.481	.430	.382	.323	.280	.245	.213	.182	.150	.116	.078	.051	22
23	.532	.505	.472	.421	.374	.316	.274	.239	.207	.177	.146	.113	.075	.049	23
24	.524	.497	.484	.413	.367	.310	.268	.232	.201	.172	.142	.111	.074	.047	24
25	.516	.489	.457	.406	.360	.304	.262	.227	.196	.168	.138	.108	.073	.045	25
26	.508	.486	.450	.399	.354	.298	.257	.222	.192	.164	.135	.106	.072	.044	26
27	.501	.475	.443	.393	.348	.292	.252	.218	.189	.161	.132	.104	.071	.043	27
28	.495	.469	.437	.387	.342	.287	.247	.215	.186	.158	.130	.102	.069	.042	28
29	.489	.463	.431	.381	.337	.282	.243	.211	.183	.155	.128	.100	.068	.041	29
30	.483	.457	.425	.376	.332	.278	.239	.208	.180	.153	.126	.098	.067	.041	30

VII.5 PERCENTILE ESTIMATES IN LARGE SAMPLES

A. Estimates of Population Mean

In sampling from a normal population with variance σ^2, the sampling distribution of the median has variance $\frac{1.57\sigma^2}{n}$ for large sample size n. For estimating the mean μ the efficiency of the median P_{50} is .637, i.e.

$$E_{P_{50}} = \frac{\sigma^2/n}{1.57\sigma^2/n} = .637 \ .$$

Higher efficiencies can be obtained from the mean of several percentile values. The efficiencies in this table are for the percentile estimates obtained from the mean of the indicated percentile.

B. Estimates of the Population Standard Deviation

This table gives the efficiencies for estimating the population standard deviation obtained from percentile estimates.

C. Estimates of Mean and Standard Deviation

This table gives percentile values for estimating both the mean and standard deviation and the efficiencies for the estimation of each. The values of K are the multipliers for the estimate of σ.

PERCENTILE ESTIMATES IN LARGE SAMPLES

A. Mean.

	Percentile estimate	Eff.
1	P_{50}	.64
2	$.5(P_{25} + P_{75})$	.81
3	$.3333(P_{17} + P_{50} + P_{83})$	.88
4	$.25(P_{12.5} + P_{37.5} + P_{62.5} + P_{87.5})$	.91
5	$.20(P_{10} + P_{30} + P_{50} + P_{70} + P_{90})$	.93
...	....	...
10	$.10(P_{05} + P_{15} + P_{25} + P_{35} + P_{45} + P_{55} + P_{65} + P_{75} + P_{85} + P_{95})$	.97

B. Standard deviation.

	Percentile estimate	Eff.
2	$.3388(P_{93} - P_{07})$	.65
4	$.1714(P_{97} + P_{85} - P_{15} - P_{03})$	.80
6	$.1180(P_{98} + P_{91} + P_{80} - P_{20} - P_{09} - P_{02})$	.87
8	$.0935(P_{98} + P_{93} + P_{86} + P_{77} - P_{23} - P_{14} - P_{07} - P_{02})$	.90
10	$.0739(P_{98.5} + P_{95} + P_{90} + P_{84} + P_{75} - P_{25} - P_{16} - P_{10} - P_{05} - P_{01.5})$	.92

C. Mean and standard deviation.

	Percentile	Efficiency		K
		Mean	Standard deviation	
2	15, 85	.73	.56	.4824
4	05, 30, 70, 95	.80	.74	.2305
6	05, 15, 40, 60, 85, 95	.89	.80	.1704
8	03, 10, 25, 45, 55, 75, 90, 97	.90	.86	.1262
10	03, 10, 20, 30, 50, 50, 70, 80, 90, 97	.94	.87	.1104

VII.6 SIMPLE ESTIMATES IN SMALL SAMPLES

The observations $x_1, x_2, \ldots, x_n$ are arranged in ascending order $x_{(1)}, x_{(2)}, \ldots, x_{(n)}$.

A. Estimates of the Population Mean

This tables gives variance and efficiency for several alternate estimates of the population mean. The midrange is defined as $(x_{(1)} + x_{(n)})/2$.

B. Estimates of the Population Standard Deviation

(i) The range is a biased estimate of σ. By multiplying the range by a factor, an unbiased estimate is obtained. This table gives values of this factor, along with variance and efficiency of the range.

(ii) The mean deviation can also be used to estimate σ. The mean deviation is given by

$$\text{M.D.} = \frac{1}{n}\sum_{i=1}^{n} |x_i - \bar{x}| \ .$$

It is easy to compute for small samples if the deviations are taken from the median. This table indicates the computation of the sum of these deviations. The multiplier to convert this sum to an unbiased estimate of σ and the efficiencies of this estimate are also included.

(iii) The efficiencies of the range and mean deviation are less than for estimates which are easier to compute than the mean deviation. This table indicates the values to use in computing an estimate of σ which will give the highest efficiency for an estimate of this type. The coefficient is such that this statistic will give an unbiased estimate of σ.

(iv) This table indicates the values to use in computing the best linear estimate of σ. The efficiency of each of these estimates is also given.

SIMPLE ESTIMATES IN SMALL SAMPLES

A. Several estimates of the mean. (Variance to be multiplied by σ^2.)

n	Median		Midrange		Av. of best two			$(x_2 + x_3 + \cdots + x_{n-1})/(n-2)$	
	Var.	Eff.	Var.	Eff.	Statistic	Var.	Eff.	Var.	Eff.
2	.500	1.000	.500	1.000	$\frac{1}{2}(x_1 + x_2)$	.500	1.000		
3	.449	.743	.362	.920	$\frac{1}{2}(x_1 + x_3)$	.362	.920	.449	.743
4	.298	.838	.298	.838	$\frac{1}{2}(x_2 + x_3)$	.298	.838	.298	.838
5	.287	.697	.261	.767	$\frac{1}{2}(x_2 + x_4)$	.231	.867	.227	.881
6	.215	.776	.236	.706	$\frac{1}{2}(x_2 + x_5)$	.193	.865	.184	.906
7	.210	.679	.218	.654	$\frac{1}{2}(x_2 + x_6)$	.168	.849	.155	.922
8	.168	.743	.205	.610	$\frac{1}{2}(x_3 + x_6)$	.149	.837	.134	.934
9	.166	.669	.194	.572	$\frac{1}{2}(x_3 + x_7)$	.132	.843	.118	.942
10	.138	.723	.186	.539	$\frac{1}{2}(x_3 + x_8)$	.119	.840	.105	.949
11	.137	.663	.178	.510	$\frac{1}{2}(x_3 + x_9)$	.109	.832	.0952	.955
12	.118	.709	.172	.484	$\frac{1}{2}(x_4 + x_9)$	.100	.831	.0869	.959
13	.117	.659	.167	.461	$\frac{1}{2}(x_4 + x_{10})$	.0924	.833	.0799	.963
14	.102	.699	.162	.440	$\frac{1}{2}(x_4 + x_{11})$	.0860	.830	.0739	.966
15	.102	.656	.158	.422	$\frac{1}{2}(x_4 + x_{12})$	.0808	.825	.0688	.969
16	.0904	.692	.154	.392	$\frac{1}{2}(x_5 + x_{12})$	.0756	.827	.0644	.971
17	.0901	.653	.151	.389	$\frac{1}{2}(x_5 + x_{13})$	.0711	.827	.0605	.973
18	.0810	.686	.148	.375	$\frac{1}{2}(x_5 + x_{14})$	.0673	.825	.0570	.975
19	.0808	.651	.145	.362	$\frac{1}{2}(x_6 + x_{14})$	.0640	.823	.0539	.976
20	.0734	.681	.143	.350	$\frac{1}{2}(x_6 + x_{15})$	.0607	.824	.0511	.978
∞	$\frac{1.57}{n}$	.637		.000	$\frac{1}{2}(P_{25} + P_{75})$	$\frac{1.24}{n}$	.808		1.000

B. Estimates of mean and dispersion in small samples.
(i) Unbiased estimate of σ using w. (Variance to be multiplied by σ^2.)

Sample size	Estimate	Variance	Eff.	Sample size	Estimate	Variance	Eff.
2	$.886w$	.571	1.000	11	$.315w$	.0616	.831
3	$.591w$	.275	.992	12	$.307w$	.0571	.814
4	$.486w$	.183	.975	13	$.300w$	.0533	.797
5	$.430w$	.138	.955	14	$.294w$	.0502	.781
6	$.395w$	.112	.933	15	$.288w$	.0474	.766
7	$.370w$	.0949	.911	16	$.283w$	.0451	.751
8	$.351w$	.0829	.890	17	$.279w$	.0430	.738
9	$.337w$	.0740	.869	18	$.275w$	.0412	.725
10	$.325w$	.0671	.850	19	$.271w$	.0395	.712
				20	$.268w$	.0381	.700

(ii) Mean deviation estimate of σ.

Sample size	Estimate	Eff.
2	$.8862(x_2 - x_1)$	1.00
3	$.5908(x_3 - x_1)$	.99
4	$.3770(x_4 + x_3 - x_2 - x_1)$	.91
5	$.3016(x_5 + x_4 - x_2 - x_1)$	.94
6	$.2369(x_6 + x_5 + x_4 - x_3 - x_2 - x_1)$	.90
7	$.2031(x_7 + x_6 + x_5 - x_3 - x_2 - x_1)$	.92
8	$.1723(x_8 + x_7 + x_6 + x_5 - x_4 - x_3 - x_2 - x_1)$	.90
9	$.1532(x_9 + x_8 + x_7 + x_6 - x_4 - x_3 - x_2 - x_1)$	.91
10	$.1353(x_{10} + x_9 + x_8 + x_7 + x_6 - x_5 - x_4 - x_3 - x_2 - x_1)$	.89

(iii) Modified linear estimate of σ. (Variance to be multiplied by σ^2.)

Sample size	Estimate	Variance	Eff.
2	$.8862(x_2 - x_1)$	.571	1.000
3	$.5908(x_3 - x_1)$	.275	.992
4	$.4857(x_4 - x_1)$	.183	.975
5	$.4299(x_5 - x_1)$	.138	.955
6	$.2619(x_6 + x_5 - x_2 - x_1)$	.109	.957
7	$.2370(x_7 + x_6 - x_2 - x_1)$	.0895	.967
8	$.2197(x_8 + x_7 - x_2 - x_1)$	.0761	.970
9	$.2068(x_9 + x_8 - x_2 - x_1)$	.0664	.968
10	$.1968(x_{10} + x_9 - x_2 - x_1)$	.0591	.964
11	$.1608(x_{11} + x_{10} + x_8 - x_4 - x_2 - x_1)$	.0529	.967
12	$.1524(x_{12} + x_{11} + x_9 - x_4 - x_2 - x_1)$	.0478	.972
13	$.1456(x_{13} + x_{12} + x_{10} - x_4 - x_2 - x_1)$	.0436	.975
14	$.1399(x_{14} + x_{13} + x_{11} - x_4 - x_2 - x_1)$	.0401	.977
15	$.1352(x_{15} + x_{14} + x_{12} - x_4 - x_2 - x_1)$	.0372	.977
16	$.1311(x_{16} + x_{15} + x_{13} - x_4 - x_2 - x_1)$	.0347	.975
17	$.1050(x_{17} + x_{16} + x_{15} + x_{13} - x_5 - x_3 - x_2 - x_1)$	.0325	.978
18	$.1020(x_{18} + x_{17} + x_{16} + x_{14} - x_5 - x_3 - x_2 - x_1)$	.0305	.978
19	$.09939(x_{19} + x_{18} + x_{17} + x_{15} - x_5 - x_3 - x_2 - x_1)$	.0288	.979
20	$.09706(x_{20} + x_{19} + x_{18} + x_{16} - x_5 - x_3 - x_2 - x_1)$	.0272	.978

(iv) Best linear estimate of σ.

Sample size	Estimate	Eff.
2	$.8862(x_2 - x_1)$	1.000
3	$.5908(x_3 - x_1)$	.992
4	$.4539(x_4 - x_1) + .1102(x_3 - x_2)$	.989
5	$.3724(x_5 - x_1) + .1352(x_4 - x_2)$	.988
6	$.3175(x_6 - x_1) + .1386(x_5 - x_2) + .0432(x_4 - x_3)$	.988
7	$.2778(x_7 - x_1) + .1351(x_6 - x_2) + .0625(x_5 - x_3)$	.989
8	$.2476(x_8 - x_1) + .1294(x_7 - x_2) + .0713(x_6 - x_3) + .0230(x_5 - x_4)$	.989
9	$.2237(x_9 - x_1) + .1233(x_8 - x_2) + .0751(x_7 - x_3) + .0360(x_6 - x_4)$	.989
10	$.2044(x_{10} - x_1) + .1172(x_9 - x_2) + .0763(x_8 - x_3) + .0436(x_7 - x_4) + .0142(x_6 - x_5)$	.990

VIII. RANGE AND STUDENTIZED RANGE

VIII.1 PROBABILITY INTEGRAL OF THE RANGE

Let $x_1, x_2, \ldots, x_n$ denote a random sample of size n from a population with density function $f(x)$ and distribution function $F(x)$.

Let $x_{(1)}, x_{(2)}, \ldots, x_{(n)}$ denote the same values in ascending order of magnitude. Then the sample range w is defined by

$$w = x_{(n)} - x_{(1)} .$$

In standardized form

$$W = \frac{x_{(n)} - x_{(1)}}{\sigma} = X_{(n)} - X_{(1)} .$$

The probability integral for W for a sample of size n is given by

$$P(W;n) = n \int_{-\infty}^{\infty} [F(X + w) - F(X)]^{n-1} f(X)\, dX .$$

This table gives values of $P(W;n)$ for the normal density function $f(x) = \frac{1}{\sqrt{2\pi}} e^{-\frac{1}{2}x^2}$ and for various values of n and W.

PROBABILITY INTEGRAL OF THE RANGE

W \ n	2	3	4	5	6	7	8	9	10
0.00	0.0000	0.0000							
0.05	.0282	.0007	0.0000						
0.10	.0564	.0028	.0001						
0.15	.0845	.0062	.0004	0.0000					
0.20	.1125	.0110	.0010	.0001					
0.25	0.1403	0.0171	0.0020	0.0002					
0.30	.1680	.0245	.0034	.0004	0.0001				
0.35	.1955	.0332	.0053	.0008	.0001				
0.40	.2227	.0431	.0079	.0014	.0002	0.0000			
0.45	.2497	.0543	.0111	.0022	.0004	.0001			
0.50	0.2763	0.0666	0.0152	0.0033	0.0007	0.0002	0.0000		
0.55	.3027	.0800	.0200	.0048	.0011	.0003	.0001		
0.60	.3286	.0944	.0257	.0068	.0017	.0004	.0001	0.0000	
0.65	.3542	.1099	.0322	.0092	.0026	.0007	.0002	.0001	
0.70	.3794	.1263	.0398	.0121	.0036	.0011	.0003	.0001	
0.75	0.4041	0.1436	0.0483	0.0157	0.0050	0.0016	0.0005	0.0002	0.0000
0.80	.4284	.1616	.0578	.0200	.0068	.0023	.0008	.0002	.0001
0.85	.4522	.1805	.0682	.0250	.0090	.0032	.0011	.0004	.0001
0.90	.4755	.2000	.0797	.0308	.0117	.0044	.0016	.0006	.0002
0.95	.4983	.2201	.0922	.0375	.0150	.0059	.0023	.0009	.0003
1.00	0.5205	0.2407	0.1057	0.0450	0.0188	0.0078	0.0032	0.0013	0.0005
1.05	.5422	.2618	.1201	.0535	.0234	.0101	.0043	.0018	.0008
1.10	.5633	.2833	.1355	.0629	.0287	.0129	.0058	.0025	.0011
1.15	.5839	.3052	.1517	.0733	.0348	.0163	.0075	.0035	.0016
1.20	.6039	.3272	.1688	.0847	.0417	.0203	.0098	.0047	.0022
1.25	0.6232	0.3495	0.1867	0.0970	0.0495	0.0250	0.0125	0.0062	0.0030
1.30	.6420	.3719	.2054	.1104	.0583	.0304	.0157	.0080	.0041
1.35	.6602	.3943	.2248	.1247	.0680	.0366	.0195	.0103	.0054
1.40	.6778	.4168	.2448	.1400	.0787	.0437	.0240	.0131	.0071
1.45	.6948	.4392	.2654	.1562	.0904	0.516	.0292	.0164	.0092
1.50	0.7112	0.4614	0.2865	0.1733	0.1031	0.0606	0.0353	0.0204	0.0117
1.55	.7269	.4835	.3080	.1913	.1168	.0705	.0421	.0250	.0148
1.60	.7421	.5053	.3299	.2101	.1315	.0814	.0499	.0304	.0184
1.65	.7567	.5269	.3521	.2296	.1473	.0934	.0587	.0366	.0227
1.70	.7707	.5481	.3745	.2498	.1639	.1064	.0684	.0437	.0278
1.75	0.7841	0.5690	0.3970	0.2706	0.1815	0.1204	0.0792	0.0517	0.0336
1.80	.7969	.5894	.4197	.2920	.2000	.1355	.0910	.0607	.0403
1.85	.8092	.6094	.4423	.3138	.2193	.1516	.1039	.0707	.0479
1.90	.8209	.6290	.4649	.3361	.2394	.1686	.1178	.0818	.0565
1.95	.8321	.6480	.4874	.3587	.2602	.1867	.1329	.0939	.0661
2.00	0.8427	0.6665	0.5096	0.3816	0.2816	0.2056	0.1489	0.1072	0.0768
2.05	.8528	.6845	.5317	.4046	.3035	.2254	.1661	.1216	.0886
2.10	.8624	.7019	.5534	.4277	.3260	.2460	.1842	.1371	.1015
2.15	.8716	.7187	.5748	.4508	.3489	.2673	.2032	.1536	.1155
2.20	.8802	.7349	.5957	.4739	.3720	.2893	.2232	.1712	.1307
2.25	0.8884	0.7505	0.6163	0.4969	0.3955	0.3118	0.2440	0.1899	0.1470

PROBABILITY INTEGRAL OF THE RANGE

W \ n	11	12	13	14	15	16	17	18	19	20
0.85	0.0000									
0.90	.0001									
0.95	.0001	0.0000								
1.00	0.0002	0.0001	0.0000							
1.05	.0003	.0001	.0001	0.0000						
1.10	.0005	.0002	.0001	0.0001						
1.15	.0007	.0003	.0001	.0001	0.0000					
1.20	.0010	.0005	.0002	.0001	0.0001					
1.25	0.0015	0.0007	0.0004	0.0002	0.0001	0.0000				
1.30	.0021	.0010	.0005	.0003	.0001	.0001	0.0000	0.0000		
1.35	.0028	.0015	.0008	.0004	.0002	.0001	.0001	0.0001		
1.40	.0038	.0021	.0011	.0006	.0003	.0002	.0001	.0001		
1.45	.0051	.0028	.0016	.0009	.0005	.0003	.0001	.0001	0.0000	
1.50	0.0067	0.0038	0.0022	0.0012	0.0007	0.0004	0.0002	0.0001	0.0001	0.0000
1.55	.0087	.0051	.0030	.0017	.0010	.0006	.0003	.0002	.0001	.0001
1.60	.0111	.0067	.0040	.0024	.0014	.0008	.0005	.0003	.0002	.0001
1.65	.0140	.0086	.0053	.0032	.0020	.0012	.0007	.0004	.0003	.0002
1.70	.0176	.0111	.0070	.0044	.0027	.0017	.0011	.0007	.0004	.0003
1.75	0.0217	0.0140	0.0090	0.0058	0.0037	0.0023	0.0015	0.0010	0.0006	0.0004
1.80	.0266	.0175	.0115	.0075	.0049	.0032	.0021	.0014	.0009	.0006
1.85	.0323	.0217	.0145	.0097	.0065	.0043	.0029	.0019	.0013	.0008
1.90	.0388	.0266	.0182	.0124	.0084	.0057	.0039	.0026	.0018	.0012
1.95	.0463	.0323	.0070	.0044	.0108	.0075	.0052	.0036	.0024	.0017
2.00	0.0548	0.0389	0.0276	0.0195	0.0137	0.0097	0.0068	0.0048	0.0033	0.0023
2.05	.0643	.0465	.0335	.0241	.0173	.0124	.0088	.0063	.0045	.0032
2.10	.0748	.0550	.0403	.0295	.0215	.0156	.0114	.0082	.0060	.0043
2.15	.0866	.0646	.0481	.0357	.0265	.0196	.0144	.0106	.0078	.0058
2.20	.0994	.0753	.0569	.0429	.0323	.0242	.0182	.0136	.0102	.0076
2.25	0.1134	0.0872	0.0669	0.0511	0.0390	0.0297	0.0226	0.0172	0.0130	0.0099

PROBABILITY INTEGRAL OF THE RANGE

W \ n	2	3	4	5	6	7	8	9	10
2.25	0.8884	0.7505	0.6163	0.4969	0.3955	0.3118	0.2440	0.1899	0.1470
2.30	.8961	.7655	.6363	.5196	.4190	.3348	.2656	.2095	.1645
2.35	.9034	.7799	.6559	.5421	.4427	.3582	.2878	.2300	.1829
2.40	.9103	.7937	.6748	.5643	.4663	.3820	.3107	.2514	.2025
2.45	.9168	.8069	.6932	.5861	.4899	.4059	.3341	.2735	.2229
2.50	0.9229	0.8195	0.7110	0.6075	0.5132	0.4300	0.3579	0.2963	0.2443
2.55	.9286	.8315	.7282	.6283	.5364	.4541	.3820	.3198	.2665
2.60	.9340	.8429	.7448	.6487	.5592	.4782	.4064	.3437	.2894
2.65	.9390	.8537	.7607	.6685	.5816	.5022	.4310	.3680	.3130
2.70	.9438	.8640	.7759	.6877	.6036	.5259	.4555	.3927	.3372
2.75	0.9482	0.8737	0.7905	0.7063	0.6252	0.5494	0.4801	0.4175	0.3617
2.80	.9523	.8828	.8045	.7242	.6461	.5725	.5045	.4425	.3867
2.85	.9561	.8915	.8177	.7415	.6665	.5952	.5286	.4675	.4119
2.90	.9597	.8996	.8304	.7581	.6863	.6174	.5525	.4923	.4372
2.95	.9630	.9073	.8424	.7739	.7055	.6391	.5760	.5171	.4625
3.00	0.9661	0.9145	0.8537	0.7891	0.7239	0.6601	0.5991	0.5415	0.4878
3.05	.9690	.9212	.8645	.8036	.7416	.6806	.6216	.5656	.5129
3.10	.9716	.9275	.8746	.8174	.7587	.7003	.6436	.5892	.5378
3.15	.9741	.9334	.8842	.8305	.7750	.7194	.6649	.6124	.5623
3.20	.9763	.9388	.8931	.8429	.7905	.7377	.6856	.6350	.5864
3.25	0.9784	0.9439	0.9016	0.8546	0.8053	0.7553	0.7055	0.6569	0.6099
3.30	.9804	.9487	.9095	.8657	.8194	.7721	.7248	.6782	.6329
3.35	.9822	.9531	.9168	.8761	.8327	.7881	.7432	.6988	.6553
3.40	.9838	.9572	.9237	.8859	.8454	.8034	.7609	.7186	.6769
3.45	.9853	.9610	.9302	.8951	.8573	.8179	.7778	.7376	.6978
3.50	0.9867	0.9644	0.9361	0.9037	0.8685	0.8316	0.7938	0.7558	0.7180
3.55	.9879	.9677	.9417	.9117	.8790	.8446	.8091	.7732	.7373
3.60	.9891	.9706	.9468	.9192	.8889	.8568	.8236	.7898	.7558
3.65	.9901	.9734	.9516	.9261	.8981	.8683	.8372	.8055	.7735
3.70	.9911	.9759	.9560	.9326	.9067	.8790	.8501	.8204	.7903
3.75	0.9920	0.9782	0.9600	0.9386	0.9147	0.8891	0.8622	0.8345	0.8062
3.80	.9928	.9803	.9637	.9441	.9222	.8985	.8736	.8477	.8212
3.85	.9935	.9822	.9672	.9493	.9291	.9073	.8842	.8602	.8355
3.90	.9942	.9840	.9703	.9540	.9355	.9155	.8941	.8718	.8488
3.95	.9948	.9856	.9732	.9583	.9415	.9230	.9034	.8827	.8614
4.00	0.9953	0.9870	0.9758	0.9623	0.9469	0.9300	0.9120	0.8929	0.8731
4.05	.9958	.9883	.9782	.9660	.9520	.9365	.9199	.9024	.8841
4.10	.9963	.9895	.9804	.9693	.9566	.9425	.9273	.9112	.8943
4.15	.9967	.9906	.9824	.9724	.9608	.9480	.9341	.9193	.9038
4.20	.9970	.9916	.9842	.9752	.9647	.9530	.9404	.9268	.9126
4.25	0.9973	0.9925	0.9859	0.9777	0.9682	0.9576	0.9461	0.9338	0.9208
4.30	.9976	.9933	.9874	.9800	.9715	.9520	.9514	.9402	.9283
4.35	.9979	.9941	.9887	.9821	.9744	.9657	.9562	.9460	.9352
4.40	.9981	.9947	.9899	.9840	.9771	.9692	.9607	.9514	.9416
4.45	.9983	.9953	.9910	.9857	.9795	.9724	.9647	.9563	.9474
4.50	0.9985	0.9958	0.9920	0.9873	0.9817	0.9754	0.9684	0.9608	0.9527

PROBABILITY INTEGRAL OF THE RANGE

W \ n	11	12	13	14	15	16	17	18	19	20
2.25	0.1134	0.0872	0.0669	0.0511	0.0390	0.0297	0.0226	0.0172	0.0130	0.0099
2.30	.1286	.1003	.0779	.0604	.0468	.0361	.0279	.0214	.0165	.0127
2.35	.1450	.1145	.0902	.0709	.0556	.0435	.0340	.0265	.0207	.0161
2.40	.1624	.1299	.1036	.0825	.0655	.0519	.0411	.0325	.0256	.0202
2.45	.1810	.1466	.1183	.0953	.0766	.0615	.0493	.0394	.0315	.0251
2.50	0.2007	0.1643	0.1342	0.1094	0.0890	0.0722	0.0585	0.0474	0.0383	0.0309
2.55	.2213	.1833	.1513	.1247	.1025	.0842	.0690	.0565	.0462	.0377
2.60	.2429	.2032	.1696	.1413	.1174	.0974	.0807	.0668	.0552	.0455
2.65	.2653	.2243	.1891	.1590	.1335	.1119	.0937	.0783	.0654	.0545
2.70	.2885	.2462	.2096	.1780	.1509	.1278	.1080	.0911	.0768	.0647
2.75	0.3124	0.2690	0.2311	0.1981	0.1696	0.1449	0.1236	0.1053	0.0896	0.0761
2.80	.3368	.2926	.2536	.2194	.1894	.1632	.1405	.1208	.1037	.0889
2.85	.3618	.3169	.2770	.2416	.2103	.1828	.1587	.1376	.1191	.1031
2.90	.3870	.3417	.3011	.2647	.2323	.2036	.1782	.1557	.1360	.1186
2.95	.4125	.3670	.3258	.2887	.2553	.2255	.1989	.1752	.1541	.1355
3.00	0.4382	0.3927	0.3511	0.3134	0.2792	0.2484	0.2207	0.1959	0.1736	0.1537
3.05	.4639	.4186	.3769	.3387	.3039	.2723	.2436	.2177	.1944	.1733
3.10	.4895	.4446	.4029	.3645	.3292	.2969	.2675	.2407	.2163	.1942
3.15	.5150	.4706	.4291	.3907	.3551	.3223	.2922	.2646	.2394	.2163
3.20	.5401	.4965	.4554	.4171	.3814	.3483	.3177	.2894	.2634	.2395
3.25	0.5649	0.5222	0.4817	0.4437	0.4080	0.3748	0.3438	0.3151	0.2884	0.2638
3.30	.5893	.5475	.5078	.4703	.4348	.4016	.3704	.3413	.3142	.2890
3.35	.6131	.5725	.5337	.4967	.4617	.4286	.3974	.3681	.3407	.3150
3.40	.6363	.5970	.5592	.5230	.4885	.4557	.4246	.3953	.3676	.3416
3.45	.6589	.6209	.5842	.5489	.5150	.4827	.4519	.4227	.3950	.3688
3.50	0.6807	0.6442	0.6087	0.5744	0.5413	0.5096	0.4792	0.4502	0.4226	0.3964
3.55	.7017	.6668	.6326	.5994	.5672	.5362	.5063	.4777	.4504	.4242
3.60	.7220	.6886	.6558	.6237	.5926	.5624	.5332	.5051	.4781	.4522
3.65	.7414	.7096	.6782	.6474	.6173	.5881	.5597	.5322	.5056	.4801
3.70	.7600	.7298	.6999	.6704	.6414	.6132	.5856	.5588	.5329	.5078
3.75	0.7776	0.7491	0.7206	0.6925	0.6648	0.6376	0.6110	0.5850	0.5598	0.5352
3.80	.7944	.7675	.7406	.7138	.6874	.6613	.6357	.6106	.5861	.5622
3.85	.8103	.7850	.7596	.7342	.7090	.6842	.6596	.6355	.6118	.5887
3.90	.8254	.8016	.7777	.7537	.7298	.7062	.6827	.6596	.6369	.6145
3.95	.8395	.8173	.7948	.7723	.7497	.7273	.7050	.6829	.6611	.6397
4.00	0.8528	0.8321	0.8111	0.7899	0.7686	0.7474	0.7263	0.7053	0.6845	0.6640
4.05	.8653	.8460	.8264	.8066	.7866	.7666	.7466	.7268	.7070	.6874
4.10	.8769	.8590	.8408	.8223	.8036	.7848	.7660	.7472	.7285	.7099
4.15	.8878	.8712	.8543	.8371	.8196	.8021	.7844	.7667	.7491	.7315
4.20	.8978	.8826	.8669	.8509	.8347	.8183	.8018	.7852	.7686	.7520
4.25	0.9072	0.8931	0.8787	0.8639	0.8488	0.8336	0.8182	0.8027	0.7871	0.7715
4.30	.9158	.9029	.8896	.8760	.8620	.8479	.8336	.8191	.8046	.7899
4.35	.9238	.9120	.8998	.8872	.8744	.8613	.8480	.8346	.8210	.8074
4.40	.9312	.9204	.9092	.8976	.8858	.8737	.8615	.8490	.8364	.8237
4.45	.9379	.9281	.9178	.9073	.8964	.8853	.8740	.8625	.8508	.8391
4.50	0.9441	0.9352	0.9258	0.9162	0.9062	0.8960	0.8856	0.8750	0.8643	0.8534

PROBABILITY INTEGRAL OF THE RANGE

W \ n	2	3	4	5	6	7	8	9	10
4.50	0.9985	0.9958	0.9920	0.9873	0.9817	0.9754	0.9684	0.9608	0.9527
4.55	.9987	.9963	.9929	.9887	.9837	.9780	.9717	.9649	.9576
4.60	.9989	.9967	.9937	.9899	.9855	.9804	.9747	.9686	.9620
4.65	.9990	.9971	.9944	.9911	.9871	.9825	.9775	.9719	.9660
4.70	.9991	.9974	.9951	.9921	.9885	.9845	.9799	.9750	.9696
4.75	0.9992	0.9977	0.9956	0.9930	0.9898	0.9862	0.9822	0.9777	0.9729
4.80	.9993	.9980	.9962	.9938	.9910	.9878	.9842	.9802	.9759
4.85	.9994	.9982	.9966	.9945	.9920	.9892	.9860	.9824	.9786
4.90	.9995	.9985	.9970	.9952	.9930	.9904	.9876	.9844	.9810
4.95	.9995	.9986	.9974	.9958	.9938	.9916	.9890	.9862	.9832
5.00	0.9996	0.9988	0.9977	0.9963	0.9945	0.9926	0.9903	0.9878	0.9851
5.05	.9996	.9990	.9980	.9967	.9952	.9935	.9915	.9893	.9869
5.10	.9997	.9991	.9982	.9971	.9958	.9942	.9925	.9906	.9884
5.15	.9997	.9992	.9985	.9975	.9963	.9950	.9934	.9917	.9898
5.20	.9998	.9993	.9987	.9978	.9968	.9956	.9942	.9927	.9911
5.25	0.9998	0.9994	0.9988	0.9981	0.9972	0.9961	0.9949	0.9936	0.9922
5.30	.9998	.9995	.9990	.9983	.9975	.9966	.9956	.9944	.9931
5.35	.9998	.9995	.9991	.9985	.9979	.9971	.9961	.9951	.9940
5.40	.9999	.9996	.9992	.9987	.9981	.9974	.9966	.9957	.9948
5.45	.9999	.9997	.9993	.9989	.9984	.9978	.9971	.9963	.9954
5.50	0.9999	0.9997	0.9994	0.9990	0.9986	0.9981	0.9974	0.9968	0.9960
5.55	.9999	.9997	.9995	.9992	.9988	.9983	.9978	.9972	.9965
5.60	.9999	.9998	.9996	.9993	.9989	.9985	.9981	.9976	.9970
5.65	.9999	.9998	.9996	.9994	.9991	.9987	.9983	.9979	.9974
5.70	0.9999	.9998	.9997	.9995	.9992	.9989	.9986	.9982	.9977
5.75	1.0000	0.9999	0.9997	0.9995	0.9993	0.9991	0.9988	0.9984	0.9980
5.80		.9999	.9998	.9996	.9994	.9992	.9989	.9986	.9983
5.85		.9999	.9998	.9997	.9995	.9993	.9991	.9988	.9985
5.90		.9999	.9998	.9997	.9996	.9994	.9992	.9990	.9988
5.95		.9999	.9998	.9997	.9996	.9995	.9993	.9991	.9989
6.00		0.9999	0.9999	0.9998	0.9997	0.9996	0.9994	0.9993	0.9991

PROBABILITY INTEGRAL OF THE RANGE

W \ n	11	12	13	14	15	16	17	18	19	20
4.50	0.9441	0.9352	0.9258	0.9162	0.9062	0.8960	0.8856	0.8750	0.8643	0.8534
4.55	.9498	.9417	.9332	.9244	.9153	.9060	.8964	.8867	.8768	.8667
4.60	.9550	.9476	.9399	.9319	.9236	.9151	.9064	.8975	.8884	.8791
4.65	.9597	.9530	.9460	.9388	.9313	.9235	.9155	.9074	.8991	.8906
4.70	.9639	.9579	.9516	.9451	.9382	.9312	.9240	.9165	.9089	.9012
4.75	0.9678	0.9624	0.9567	0.9508	0.9446	0.9383	0.9317	0.9249	0.9180	0.9110
4.80	.9713	.9665	.9614	.9560	.9505	.9447	.9387	.9326	.9263	.9199
4.85	.9745	.9702	.9656	.9608	.9557	.9505	.9452	.9396	.9339	.9281
4.90	.9774	.9735	.9694	.9650	.9605	.9559	.9510	.9460	.9409	.9356
4.95	.9799	.9765	.9728	.9689	.9649	.9607	.9563	.9518	.9472	.9424
5.00	0.9822	0.9791	0.9759	0.9724	0.9688	0.9650	0.9611	0.9571	0.9529	0.9486
5.05	.9843	.9816	.9786	.9756	.9723	.9690	.9655	.9618	.9581	.9543
5.10	.9862	.9837	.9811	.9784	.9755	.9725	.9694	.9661	.9628	.9593
5.15	.9878	.9856	.9833	.9809	.9783	.9757	.9729	.9700	.9670	.9639
5.20	.9893	.9874	.9853	.9832	.9809	.9785	.9760	.9735	.9708	.9681
5.25	0.9906	0.9889	0.9871	0.9852	0.9832	0.9811	0.9789	0.9766	0.9742	0.9718
5.30	.9917	.9903	.9887	.9870	.9852	.9833	.9814	.9794	.9773	.9751
5.35	.9928	.9915	.9901	.9886	.9870	.9854	.9836	.9819	.9800	.9781
5.40	.9937	.9925	.9913	.9900	.9886	.9872	.9856	.9841	.9824	.9807
5.45	.9945	.9935	.9924	.9913	.9900	.9888	.9874	.9860	.9846	.9831
5.50	0.9952	0.9943	0.9934	0.9924	0.9913	0.9902	0.9890	0.9878	0.9865	0.9852
5.55	.9958	.9951	.9942	.9933	.9924	.9914	.9904	.9893	.9882	.9870
5.60	.9964	.9957	.9950	.9942	.9934	.9925	.9916	.9907	.9897	.9887
5.65	.9969	.9963	.9956	.9950	.9943	.9935	.9927	.9919	.9910	.9901
5.70	.9973	.9968	.9962	.9956	.9950	.9944	.9937	.9930	.9922	.9914
5.75	0.9976	0.9972	0.9967	0.9962	0.9957	0.9951	0.9945	0.9939	0.9932	0.9925
5.80	.9980	.9976	.9972	.9967	.9963	.9958	.9952	.9947	.9941	.9935
5.85	.9982	.9979	.9976	.9972	.9968	.9963	.9959	.9954	.9949	.9944
5.90	.9985	.9982	.9979	.9976	.9972	.9968	.9964	.9960	.9956	.9952
5.95	.9987	.9985	.9982	.9979	.9976	.9973	.9969	.9966	.9962	.9958
6.00	0.9989	0.9987	0.9984	0.9982	0.9979	0.9977	0.9974	0.9971	0.9967	0.9964

PROBABILITY INTEGRAL OF THE RANGE

W \ n	2	3	4	5	6	7	8	9	10
6.00		0.9999	0.9999	0.9998	0.9997	0.9996	0.9994	0.9993	0.9991
6.05		0.9999	.9999	.9998	.9997	.9996	.9995	.9994	.9992
6.10		1.0000	.9999	.9998	.9998	.9997	.9996	.9995	.9993
6.15			.9999	.9999	.9998	.9997	.9996	.9995	.9994
6.20			.9999	.9999	.9998	.9998	.9997	.9996	.9995
6.25			0.9999	0.9999	0.9999	0.9998	0.9997	0.9997	0.9996
6.30			1.0000	.9999	.9999	.9998	.9998	.9997	.9996
6.35				.9999	.9999	.9999	.9998	.9998	.9997
6.40				0.9999	.9999	.9999	.9998	.9998	.9997
6.45				0.9999	.9999	.9999	.9999	.9998	.9998
6.50				1.0000	0.9999	0.9999	0.9999	0.9999	0.9998
6.55					0.9999	.9999	.9999	.9999	.9998
6.60					1.0000	.9999	.9999	.9999	.9999
6.65						0.9999	.9999	.9999	.9999
6.70						1.0000	0.9999	.9999	.9999
6.75							1.0000	0.9999	0.9999
6.80								0.9999	.9999
6.85								1.0000	0.9999
6.90									1.0000
6.95									
7.00									
7.05									
7.10									
7.15									
7.20									
7.25									

PROBABILITY INTEGRAL OF THE RANGE

W \ n	11	12	13	14	15	16	17	18	19	20
6.00	0.9989	0.9987	0.9984	0.9982	0.9979	0.9977	0.9974	0.9971	0.9967	0.9964
6.05	.9990	.9989	.9987	.9985	.9982	.9980	.9977	.9975	.9972	.9969
6.10	.9992	.9990	.9989	.9987	.9985	.9983	.9981	.9978	.9976	9973
6.15	.9993	.9992	.9990	.9989	.9987	.9985	.9983	.9981	.9979	9977
6.20	.9994	.9993	.9992	.9990	.9989	.9987	.9986	.9984	.9982	.9980
6.25	0.9995	0.9994	0.9993	0.9992	0.9990	0.9989	0.9988	0.9986	0.9985	0.9983
6.30	.9996	.9995	.9994	.9993	.9992	.9991	.9990	.9988	.9987	.9986
6.35	.9996	.9996	.9995	.9994	.9993	.9992	.9991	.9990	.9989	.9988
6.40	.9997	.9996	.9996	.9995	.9994	.9993	.9992	.9992	.9991	.9990
6.45	.9997	.9997	.9996	.9996	.9995	.9994	.9994	.9993	.9992	.9991
6.50	0.9998	0.9997	0.9997	0.9996	0.9996	0.9995	0.9995	0.9994	0.9993	0.9993
6.55	.9998	.9998	.9997	.9997	.9996	.9996	.9995	.9995	.9994	.9994
6.60	.9998	.9998	.9998	.9997	.9997	.9997	.9996	.9996	.9995	.9995
6.65	.9999	.9998	.9998	.9998	.9997	.9997	.9997	.9996	.9996	.9995
6.70	.9999	.9999	.9998	.9998	.9998	.9998	.9997	.9997	.9997	.9996
6.75	0.9999	0.9999	0.9999	0.9998	0.9998	0.9998	0.9998	0.9997	0.9997	0.9997
6.80	.9999	.9999	.9999	.9999	.9998	.9998	.9998	.9998	.9998	.9997
6.85	.9999	.9999	.9999	.9999	.9999	.9999	.9998	.9998	.9998	.9998
6.90	0.9999	.9999	.9999	.9999	.9999	.9999	.9999	.9998	.9998	.9998
6.95	1.0000	0.9999	.9999	.9999	.9999	.9999	.9999	.9999	.9999	.9998
7.00		1.0000	0.9999	0.9999	0.9999	0.9999	0.9999	0.9999	0.9999	0.9999
7.05			1.0000	0.9999	.9999	.9999	.9999	.9999	.9999	.9999
7.10				1.0000	0.9999	0.9999	.9999	.9999	.9999	.9999
7.15					1.0000	1.0000	0.9999	0.9999	.9999	.9999
7.20							0.9999	0.9999	0.9999	0.9999
7.25							1.0000	1.0000	1.0000	0.9999
7.26										1.0000

VIII.2 PERCENTAGE POINTS, DISTRIBUTION OF THE RANGE

Percentage points of the range are found by the use of inverse interpolation in the table for the probability integral of the range.

Size of sample n	Factor $1/d_n$	Lower percentage points						Upper percentage points					
		0.1	**0.5**	**1.0**	**2.5**	**5.0**	**10.0**	**10.0**	**5.0**	**2.5**	**1.0**	**0.5**	**0.1**
2	0.8862	0.00	0.01	0.02	0.04	0.09	0.18	2.33	2.77	3.17	3.64	3.97	4.65
3	.5908	0.06	0.13	0.19	0.30	0.43	0.62	2.90	3.31	3.68	4.12	4.42	5.06
4	.4857	0.20	0.34	0.43	0.59	0.76	0.98	3.24	3.63	3.98	4.40	4.69	5.31
5	.4299	0.37	0.55	0.67	0.85	1.03	1.26	3.48	3.86	4.20	4.60	4.89	5.48
6	0.3946	0.53	0.75	0.87	1.07	1.25	1.49	3.66	4.03	4.36	4.76	5.03	5.62
7	.3698	0.69	0.92	1.05	1.25	1.44	1.68	3.81	4.17	4.49	4.88	5.15	5.73
8	.3512	0.83	1.08	1.20	1.41	1.60	1.84	3.93	4.29	4.60	4.99	5.25	5.82
9	.3367	0.97	1.21	1.34	1.55	1.74	1.97	4.04	4.39	4.70	5.08	5.34	5.90
10	0.3249	1.08	1.33	1.47	1.67	1.86	2.09	4.13	4.47	4.78	5.16	5.42	5.97
11	.3152	1.19	1.45	1.58	1.78	1.97	2.20	4.21	4.55	4.86	5.23	5.49	6.04
12	.3069	1.29	1.55	1.68	1.88	2.07	2.30	4.28	4.62	4.92	5.29	5.55	6.09
13	.2998	1.39	1.64	1.77	1.98	2.16	2.39	4.35	4.68	4.99	5.35	5.60	6.14
14	.2935	1.47	1.72	1.86	2.06	2.24	2.47	4.41	4.74	5.04	5.40	5.65	6.19
15	0.2880	1.55	1.80	1.93	2.14	2.32	2.54	4.47	4.80	5.09	5.45	5.70	6.23
16	.2831	1.63	1.88	2.01	2.21	2.39	2.61	4.52	4.85	5.14	5.49	5.74	6.27
17	.2787	1.69	1.94	2.07	2.27	2.45	2.67	4.57	4.89	5.18	5.54	5.78	6.31
18	.2747	1.76	2.01	2.14	2.34	2.52	2.73	4.61	4.93	5.22	5.57	5.82	6.35
19	.2711	1.82	2.07	2.20	2.39	2.57	2.79	4.65	4.97	5.26	5.61	5.86	6.38
20	0.2677	1.88	2.12	2.25	2.45	2.63	2.84	4.69	5.01	5.30	5.65	5.89	6.41

The unit is the population standard deviation.
Estimate of σ = range (or mean range) in a sample of n observations $\times 1/d_n$.

VIII.3 PERCENTAGE POINTS, STUDENTIZED RANGE

If in the standardized range $W = \frac{w}{\sigma}$, the unknown population standard deviation σ is replaced by s, the sample standard deviation computed from another sample from the same population, then the studentized range q is given by

$$q = \frac{w}{s},$$

where w is the range from a sample of size n and s is independent of w and is based on ν degrees of freedom. The probability integral of the studentized range is given by

$$\Pr\left\{\frac{w}{s} \le q\right\} = \int_0^\infty \left[\Gamma\left(\frac{\nu}{2}\right)\right]^{-1} 2^{-\frac{1}{2}\nu+1}\nu^{\nu/2}s^{\nu-1}e^{-\frac{1}{2}\nu s^2}f(qs)\,ds$$

where $f(qs)$ is the probability integral of the range for samples of size n.

UPPER 1 PER CENT POINTS OF THE STUDENTIZED RANGE

The entries are $q_{.01}$, where $P(q < q_{.01}) = .99$

ν \ n	2	3	4	5	6	7	8	9	10
1	90.03	135.0	164.3	185.6	202.2	215.8	227.2	237.0	245.6
2	14.04	19.02	22.29	24.72	26.63	28.20	29.53	30.68	31.69
3	8.26	10.62	12.17	13.33	14.24	15.00	15.64	16.20	16.69
4	6.51	8.12	9.17	9.96	10.58	11.10	11.55	11.93	12.27
5	5.70	6.98	7.80	8.42	8.91	9.32	9.67	9.97	10.24
6	5.24	6.33	7.03	7.56	7.97	8.32	8.61	8.87	9.10
7	4.95	5.92	6.54	7.01	7.37	7.68	7.94	8.17	8.37
8	4.75	5.64	6.20	6.62	6.96	7.24	7.47	7.68	7.86
9	4.60	5.43	5.96	6.35	6.66	6.91	7.13	7.33	7.49
10	4.48	5.27	5.77	6.14	6.43	6.67	6.87	7.05	7.21
11	4.39	5.15	5.62	5.97	6.25	6.48	6.67	6.84	6.99
12	4.32	5.05	5.50	5.84	6.10	6.32	6.51	6.67	6.81
13	4.26	4.96	5.40	5.73	5.98	6.19	6.37	6.53	6.67
14	4.21	4.89	5.32	5.63	5.88	6.08	6.26	6.41	6.54
15	4.17	4.84	5.25	5.56	5.80	5.99	6.16	6.31	6.44
16	4.13	4.79	5.19	5.49	5.72	5.92	6.08	6.22	6.35
17	4.10	4.74	5.14	5.43	5.66	5.85	6.01	6.15	6.27
18	4.07	4.70	5.09	5.38	5.60	5.79	5.94	6.08	6.20
19	4.05	4.67	5.05	5.33	5.55	5.73	5.89	6.02	6.14
20	4.02	4.64	5.02	5.29	5.51	5.69	5.84	5.97	6.09
24	3.96	4.55	4.91	5.17	5.37	5.54	5.69	5.81	5.92
30	3.89	4.45	4.80	5.05	5.24	5.40	5.54	5.65	5.76
40	3.82	4.37	4.70	4.93	5.11	5.26	5.39	5.50	5.60
60	3.76	4.28	4.59	4.82	4.99	5.13	5.25	5.36	5.45
120	3.70	4.20	4.50	4.71	4.87	5.01	5.12	5.21	5.30
∞	3.64	4.12	4.40	4.60	4.76	4.88	4.99	5.08	5.16

UPPER 1 PER CENT POINTS OF THE STUDENTIZED RANGE

ν \ n	11	12	13	14	15	16	17	18	19	20
1	253.2	260.0	266.2	271.8	277.0	281.8	286.3	290.4	294.3	298.0
2	32.59	33.40	34.13	34.81	35.43	36.00	36.53	37.03	37.50	37.95
3	17.13	17.53	17.89	18.22	18.52	18.81	19.07	19.32	19.55	19.77
4	12.57	12.84	13.09	13.32	13.53	13.73	13.91	14.08	14.24	14.40
5	10.48	10.70	10.89	11.08	11.24	11.40	11.55	11.68	11.81	11.93
6	9.30	9.48	9.65	9.81	9.95	10.08	10.21	10.32	10.43	10.54
7	8.55	8.71	8.86	9.00	9.12	9.24	9.35	9.46	9.55	9.65
8	8.03	8.18	8.31	8.44	8.55	8.66	8.76	8.85	8.94	9.03
9	7.65	7.78	7.91	8.03	8.13	8.23	8.33	8.41	8.49	8.57
10	7.36	7.49	7.60	7.71	7.81	7.91	7.99	8.08	8.15	8.23
11	7.13	7.25	7.36	7.46	7.56	7.65	7.73	7.81	7.88	7.95
12	6.94	7.06	7.17	7.26	7.36	7.44	7.52	7.59	7.66	7.73
13	6.79	6.90	7.01	7.10	7.19	7.27	7.35	7.42	7.48	7.55
14	6.66	6.77	6.87	6.96	7.05	7.13	7.20	7.27	7.33	7.39
15	6.55	6.66	6.76	6.84	6.93	7.00	7.07	7.14	7.20	7.26
16	6.46	6.56	6.66	6.74	6.82	6.90	6.97	7.03	7.09	7.15
17	6.38	6.48	6.57	6.66	6.73	6.81	6.87	6.94	7.00	7.05
18	6.31	6.41	6.50	6.58	6.65	6.73	6.79	6.85	6.91	6.97
19	6.25	6.34	6.43	6.51	6.58	6.65	6.72	6.78	6.84	6.89
20	6.19	6.28	6.37	6.45	6.52	6.59	6.65	6.71	6.77	6.82
24	6.02	6.11	6.19	6.26	6.33	6.39	6.45	6.51	6.56	6.61
30	5.85	5.93	6.01	6.08	6.14	6.20	6.26	6.31	6.36	6.41
40	5.69	5.76	5.83	5.90	5.96	6.02	6.07	6.12	6.16	6.21
60	5.53	5.60	5.67	5.73	5.78	5.84	5.89	5.93	5.97	6.01
120	5.37	5.44	5.50	5.56	5.61	5.66	5.71	5.75	5.79	5.83
∞	5.23	5.29	5.35	5.40	5.45	5.49	5.54	5.57	5.61	5.65

UPPER 5 PER CENT POINTS OF THE STUDENTIZED RANGE

The entries are $q_{.05}$, where $P(q < q_{.05}) = .95$

ν \ n	2	3	4	5	6	7	8	9	10
1	17.97	26.98	32.82	37.08	40.41	43.12	45.40	47.36	49.07
2	6.08	8.33	9.80	10.88	11.74	12.44	13.03	13.54	13.99
3	4.50	5.91	6.82	7.50	8.04	8.48	8.85	9.18	9.46
4	3.93	5.04	5.76	6.29	6.71	7.05	7.35	7.60	7.83
5	3.64	4.60	5.22	5.67	6.03	6.33	6.58	6.80	6.99
6	3.46	4.34	4.90	5.30	5.63	5.90	6.12	6.32	6.49
7	3.34	4.16	4.68	5.06	5.36	5.61	5.82	6.00	6.16
8	3.26	4.04	4.53	4.89	5.17	5.40	5.60	5.77	5.92
9	3.20	3.95	4.41	4.76	5.02	5.24	5.43	5.59	5.74
10	3.15	3.88	4.33	4.65	4.91	5.12	5.30	5.46	5.60
11	3.11	3.82	4.26	4.57	4.82	5.03	5.20	5.35	5.49
12	3.08	3.77	4.20	4.51	4.75	4.95	5.12	5.27	5.39
13	3.06	3.73	4.15	4.45	4.69	4.88	5.05	5.19	5.32
14	3.03	3.70	4.11	4.41	4.64	4.83	4.99	5.13	5.25
15	3.01	3.67	4.08	4.37	4.59	4.78	4.94	5.08	5.20
16	3.00	3.65	4.05	4.33	4.56	4.74	4.90	5.03	5.15
17	2.98	3.63	4.02	4.30	4.52	4.70	4.86	4.99	5.11
18	2.97	3.61	4.00	4.28	4.49	4.67	4.82	4.96	5.07
19	2.96	3.59	3.98	4.25	4.47	4.65	4.79	4.92	5.04
20	2.95	3.58	3.96	4.23	4.45	4.62	4.77	4.90	5.01
24	2.92	3.53	3.90	4.17	4.37	4.54	4.68	4.81	4.92
30	2.89	3.49	3.85	4.10	4.30	4.46	4.60	4.72	4.82
40	2.86	3.44	3.79	4.04	4.23	4.39	4.52	4.63	4.73
60	2.83	3.40	3.74	3.98	4.16	4.31	4.44	4.55	4.65
120	2.80	3.36	3.68	3.92	4.10	4.24	4.36	4.47	4.56
∞	2.77	3.31	3.63	3.86	4.03	4.17	4.29	4.39	4.47

UPPER 5 PER CENT POINTS OF THE STUDENTIZED RANGE

ν \ n	11	12	13	14	15	16	17	18	19	20
1	50.59	51.96	53.20	54.33	55.36	56.32	57.22	58.04	58.83	59.56
2	14.39	14.75	15.08	15.38	15.65	15.91	16.14	16.37	16.57	16.77
3	9.72	9.95	10.15	10.35	10.53	10.69	10.84	10.98	11.11	11.24
4	8.03	8.21	8.37	8.52	8.66	8.79	8.91	9.03	9.13	9.23
5	7.17	7.32	7.47	7.60	7.72	7.83	7.93	8.03	8.12	8.21
6	6.65	6.79	6.92	7.03	7.14	7.24	7.34	7.43	7.51	7.59
7	6.30	6.43	6.55	6.66	6.76	6.85	6.94	7.02	7.10	7.17
8	6.05	6.18	6.29	6.39	6.48	6.57	6.65	6.73	6.80	6.87
9	5.87	5.98	6.09	6.19	6.28	6.36	6.44	6.51	6.58	6.64
10	5.72	5.83	5.93	6.03	6.11	6.19	6.27	6.34	6.40	6.47
11	5.61	5.71	5.81	5.90	5.98	6.06	6.13	6.20	6.27	6.33
12	5.51	5.61	5.71	5.80	5.88	5.95	6.02	6.09	6.15	6.21
13	5.43	5.53	5.63	5.71	5.79	5.86	5.93	5.99	6.05	6.11
14	5.36	5.46	5.55	5.64	5.71	5.79	5.85	5.91	5.97	6.03
15	5.31	5.40	5.49	5.57	5.65	5.72	5.78	5.85	5.90	5.96
16	5.26	5.35	5.44	5.52	5.59	5.66	5.73	5.79	5.84	5.90
17	5.21	5.31	5.39	5.47	5.54	5.61	5.67	5.73	5.79	5.84
18	5.17	5.27	5.35	5.43	5.50	5.57	5.63	5.69	5.74	5.79
19	5.14	5.23	5.31	5.39	5.46	5.53	5.59	5.65	5.70	5.75
20	5.11	5.20	5.28	5.36	5.43	5.49	5.55	5.61	5.66	5.71
24	5.01	5.10	5.18	5.25	5.32	5.38	5.44	5.49	5.55	5.59
30	4.92	5.00	5.08	5.15	5.21	5.27	5.33	5.38	5.43	5.47
40	4.82	4.90	4.98	5.04	5.11	5.16	5.22	5.27	5.31	5.36
60	4.73	4.81	4.88	4.94	5.00	5.06	5.11	5.15	5.20	5.24
120	4.64	4.71	4.78	4.84	4.90	4.95	5.00	5.04	5.09	5.13
∞	4.55	4.62	4.68	4.74	4.80	4.85	4.89	4.93	4.97	5.01

UPPER 10 PER CENT POINTS OF THE STUDENTIZED RANGE

The entries are $q_{.10}$, where $P(q < q_{.10}) = .90$

ν \ n	2	3	4	5	6	7	8	9	10
1	8.93	13.44	16.36	18.49	20.15	21.51	22.64	23.62	24.48
2	4.13	5.73	6.77	7.54	8.14	8.63	9.05	9.41	9.72
3	3.33	4.47	5.20	5.74	6.16	6.51	6.81	7.06	7.29
4	3.01	3.98	4.59	5.03	5.39	5.68	5.93	6.14	6.33
5	2.85	3.72	4.26	4.66	4.98	5.24	5.46	5.65	5.82
6	2.75	3.56	4.07	4.44	4.73	4.97	5.17	5.34	5.50
7	2.68	3.45	3.93	4.28	4.55	4.78	4.97	5.14	5.28
8	2.63	3.37	3.83	4.17	4.43	4.65	4.83	4.99	5.13
9	2.59	3.32	3.76	4.08	4.34	4.54	4.72	4.87	5.01
10	2.56	3.27	3.70	4.02	4.26	4.47	4.64	4.78	4.91
11	2.54	3.23	3.66	3.96	4.20	4.40	4.57	4.71	4.84
12	2.52	3.20	3.62	3.92	4.16	4.35	4.51	4.65	4.78
13	2.50	3.18	3.59	3.88	4.12	4.30	4.46	4.60	4.72
14	2.49	3.16	3.56	3.85	4.08	4.27	4.42	4.56	4.68
15	2.48	3.14	3.54	3.83	4.05	4.23	4.39	4.52	4.64
16	2.47	3.12	3.52	3.80	4.03	4.21	4.36	4.49	4.61
17	2.46	3.11	3.50	3.78	4.00	4.18	4.33	4.46	4.58
18	2.45	3.10	3.49	3.77	3.98	4.16	4.31	4.44	4.55
19	2.45	3.09	3.47	3.75	3.97	4.14	4.29	4.42	4.53
20	2.44	3.08	3.46	3.74	3.95	4.12	4.27	4.40	4.51
24	2.42	3.05	3.42	3.69	3.90	4.07	4.21	4.34	4.44
30	2.40	3.02	3.39	3.65	3.85	4.02	4.16	4.28	4.38
40	2.38	2.99	3.35	3.60	3.80	3.96	4.10	4.21	4.32
60	2.36	2.96	3.31	3.56	3.75	3.91	4.04	4.16	4.25
120	2.34	2.93	3.28	3.52	3.71	3.86	3.99	4.10	4.19
∞	2.33	2.90	3.24	3.48	3.66	3.81	3.93	4.04	4.13

UPPER 10 PER CENT POINTS OF THE STUDENTIZED RANGE

ν \ n	11	12	13	14	15	16	17	18	19	20
1	25.24	25.92	26.54	27.10	27.62	28.10	28.54	28.96	29.35	29.71
2	10.01	10.26	10.49	10.70	10.89	11.07	11.24	11.39	11.54	11.68
3	7.49	7.67	7.83	7.98	8.12	8.25	8.37	8.48	8.58	8.68
4	6.49	6.65	6.78	6.91	7.02	7.13	7.23	7.33	7.41	7.50
5	5.97	6.10	6.22	6.34	6.44	6.54	6.63	6.71	6.79	6.86
6	5.64	5.76	5.87	5.98	6.07	6.16	6.25	6.32	6.40	6.47
7	5.41	5.53	5.64	5.74	5.83	5.91	5.99	6.06	6.13	6.19
8	5.25	5.36	5.46	5.56	5.64	5.72	5.80	5.87	5.93	6.00
9	5.13	5.23	5.33	5.42	5.51	5.58	5.66	5.72	5.79	5.85
10	5.03	5.13	5.23	5.32	5.40	5.47	5.54	5.61	5.67	5.73
11	4.95	5.05	5.15	5.23	5.31	5.38	5.45	5.51	5.57	5.63
12	4.89	4.99	5.08	5.16	5.24	5.31	5.37	5.44	5.49	5.55
13	4.83	4.93	5.02	5.10	5.18	5.25	5.31	5.37	5.43	5.48
14	4.79	4.88	4.97	5.05	5.12	5.19	5.26	5.32	5.37	5.43
15	4.75	4.84	4.93	5.01	5.08	5.15	5.21	5.27	5.32	5.38
16	4.71	4.81	4.89	4.97	5.04	5.11	5.17	5.23	5.28	5.33
17	4.68	4.77	4.86	4.93	5.01	5.07	5.13	5.19	5.24	5.30
18	4.65	4.75	4.83	4.90	4.98	5.04	5.10	5.16	5.21	5.26
19	4.63	4.72	4.80	4.88	4.95	5.01	5.07	5.13	5.18	5.23
20	4.61	4.70	4.78	4.85	4.92	4.99	5.05	5.10	5.16	5.20
24	4.54	4.63	4.71	4.78	4.85	4.91	4.97	5.02	5.07	5.12
30	4.47	4.56	4.64	4.71	4.77	4.83	4.89	4.94	4.99	5.03
40	4.41	4.49	4.56	4.63	4.69	4.75	4.81	4.86	4.90	4.95
60	4.34	4.42	4.49	4.56	4.62	4.67	4.73	4.78	4.82	4.86
120	4.28	4.35	4.42	4.48	4.54	4.60	4.65	4.69	4.74	4.78
∞	4.21	4.28	4.35	4.41	4.47	4.52	4.57	4.61	4.65	4.69

VIII.4 CRITICAL VALUES FOR DUNCAN'S NEW MULTIPLE RANGE TEST

Let $q = \frac{w}{s}$, where w is the range of n independent normal variables having the same mean and unit standard deviation, and νs^2 is distributed as chi-square with ν degrees of freedom. This table lists the critical values for Duncan's New Multiple Range Test corresponding to protection level $P = \gamma_{p,\alpha} = (1 - \alpha)^{p-1}$ (Significance level α) for testing p successive values out of an ordered arrangement of m means of samples from a normal population, with ν degrees of freedom for the independent estimate s^2 of the population variance. The critical values for Duncan's test are percentage points of the studentized range of $n = p$ observations corresponding to cumulative probability $P = (1 - \alpha)^{p-1}$.

CRITICAL VALUES FOR DUNCAN'S NEW MULTIPLE RANGE TEST

PROTECTION LEVEL $P = (.90)^{p-1}$ SIGNIFICANCE LEVEL $\alpha = .10$

ν \ p	2	3	4	5	6	7	8	9	10
1	8.929	8.929	8.929	8.929	8.929	8.929	8.929	8.929	8.929
2	4.130	4.130	4.130	4.130	4.130	4.130	4.130	4.130	4.130
3	3.328	3.330	3.330	3.330	3.330	3.330	3.330	3.330	3.330
4	3.015	3.074	3.081	3.081	3.081	3.081	3.081	3.081	3.081
5	2.850	2.934	2.964	2.970	2.970	2.970	2.970	2.970	2.970
6	2.748	2.846	2.890	2.908	2.911	2.911	2.911	2.911	2.911
7	2.680	2.785	2.838	2.864	2.876	2.878	2.878	2.878	2.878
8	2.630	2.742	2.800	2.832	2.849	2.857	2.858	2.858	2.858
9	2.592	2.708	2.771	2.808	2.829	2.840	2.845	2.847	2.847
10	2.563	2.682	2.748	2.788	2.813	2.827	2.835	2.839	2.839
11	2.540	2.660	2.730	2.772	2.799	2.817	2.827	2.833	2.835
12	2.521	2.643	2.714	2.759	2.789	2.808	2.821	2.828	2.832
13	2.505	2.628	2.701	2.748	2.779	2.800	2.815	2.824	2.829
14	2.491	2.616	2.690	2.739	2.771	2.794	2.810	2.820	2.827
15	2.479	2.605	2.681	2.731	2.765	2.789	2.805	2.817	2.825
16	2.469	2.596	2.673	2.723	2.759	2.784	2.802	2.815	2.824
17	2.460	2.588	2.665	2.717	2.753	2.780	2.798	2.812	2.822
18	2.452	2.580	2.659	2.712	2.749	2.776	2.796	2.810	2.821
19	2.445	2.574	2.653	2.707	2.745	2.773	2.793	2.808	2.820
20	2.439	2.568	2.648	2.702	2.741	2.770	2.791	2.807	2.819
24	2.420	2.550	2.632	2.688	2.729	2.760	2.783	2.801	2.816
30	2.400	2.532	2.615	2.674	2.717	2.750	2.776	2.796	2.813
40	2.381	2.514	2.600	2.660	2.705	2.741	2.769	2.791	2.810
60	2.363	2.497	2.584	2.646	2.694	2.731	2.761	2.786	2.807
120	2.344	2.479	2.568	2.632	2.682	2.722	2.754	2.781	2.804
∞	2.326	2.462	2.552	2.619	2.670	2.712	2.746	2.776	2.801

ν \ p	11	12	13	14	15	16	17	18	19
1	8.929	8.929	8.929	8.929	8.929	8.929	8.929	8.929	8.929
2	4.130	4.130	4.130	4.130	4.130	4.130	4.130	4.130	4.130
3	3.330	3.330	3.330	3.330	3.330	3.330	3.330	3.330	3.330
4	3.081	3.081	3.081	3.081	3.081	3.081	3.081	3.081	3.081
5	2.970	2.970	2.970	2.970	2.970	2.970	2.970	2.970	2.970
6	2.911	2.911	2.911	2.911	2.911	2.911	2.911	2.911	2.911
7	2.878	2.878	2.878	2.878	2.878	2.878	2.878	2.878	2.878
8	2.858	2.858	2.858	2.858	2.858	2.858	2.858	2.858	2.858
9	2.847	2.847	2.847	2.847	2.847	2.847	2.847	2.847	2.847
10	2.839	2.839	2.839	2.839	2.839	2.839	2.839	2.839	2.839
11	2.835	2.835	2.835	2.835	2.835	2.835	2.835	2.835	2.835
12	2.833	2.833	2.833	2.833	2.833	2.833	2.833	2.833	2.833
13	2.832	2.832	2.832	2.832	2.832	2.832	2.832	2.832	2.832
14	2.831	2.832	2.833	2.833	2.833	2.833	2.833	2.833	2.833
15	2.830	2.833	2.834	2.834	2.834	2.834	2.834	2.834	2.834
16	2.829	2.833	2.835	2.836	2.836	2.836	2.836	2.836	2.836
17	2.829	2.834	2.836	2.838	2.838	2.838	2.838	2.838	2.838
18	2.828	2.834	2.838	2.840	2.840	2.840	2.840	2.840	2.840
19	2.828	2.834	2.839	2.841	2.842	2.843	2.843	2.843	2.843
20	2.828	2.834	2.839	2.843	2.845	2.845	2.845	2.845	2.845
24	2.827	2.835	2.842	2.848	2.851	2.854	2.856	2.857	2.857
30	2.826	2.837	2.846	2.853	2.859	2.863	2.867	2.869	2.871
40	2.825	2.838	2.849	2.858	2.866	2.873	2.878	2.883	2.887
60	2.825	2.839	2.853	2.864	2.874	2.883	2.890	2.897	2.903
120	2.824	2.842	2.857	2.871	2.883	2.893	2.903	2.912	2.920
∞	2.824	2.844	2.861	2.877	2.892	2.905	2.918	2.929	2.939

CRITICAL VALUES FOR DUNCAN'S NEW MULTIPLE RANGE TEST

PROTECTION LEVEL $P = (.90)^{p-1}$ SIGNIFICANCE LEVEL $\alpha = .10$

ν \ p	20	22	24	26	28	30	32	34	36
1	8.929	8.929	8.929	8.929	8.929	8.929	8.929	8.929	8.929
2	4.130	4.130	4.130	4.130	4.130	4.130	4.130	4.130	4.130
3	3.330	3.330	3.330	3.330	3.330	3.330	3.330	3.330	3.330
4	3.081	3.081	3.081	3.081	3.081	3.081	3.081	3.081	3.081
5	2.970	2.970	2.970	2.970	2.970	2.970	2.970	2.970	2.970
6	2.911	2.911	2.911	2.911	2.911	2.911	2.911	2.911	2.911
7	2.878	2.878	2.878	2.878	2.878	2.878	2.878	2.878	2.878
8	2.858	2.858	2.858	2.858	2.858	2.858	2.858	2.858	2.858
9	2.847	2.847	2.847	2.847	2.847	2.847	2.847	2.847	2.847
10	2.839	2.839	2.839	2.839	2.839	2.839	2.839	2.839	2.839
11	2.835	2.835	2.835	2.835	2.835	2.835	2.835	2.835	2.835
12	2.833	2.833	2.833	2.833	2.833	2.833	2.833	2.833	2.833
13	2.832	2.832	2.832	2.832	2.832	2.832	2.832	2.832	2.832
14	2.833	2.833	2.833	2.833	2.833	2.833	2.833	2.833	2.833
15	2.834	2.834	2.834	2.834	2.834	2.834	2.834	2.834	2.834
16	2.836	2.836	2.836	2.836	2.836	2.836	2.836	2.836	2.836
17	2.838	2.838	2.838	2.838	2.838	2.838	2.838	2.838	2.838
18	2.840	2.840	2.840	2.840	2.840	2.840	2.840	2.840	2.840
19	2.843	2.843	2.843	2.843	2.843	2.843	2.843	2.843	2.843
20	2.845	2.845	2.845	2.845	2.845	2.845	2.845	2.845	2.845
24	2.857	2.857	2.857	2.857	2.857	2.857	2.857	2.857	2.857
30	2.873	2.873	2.873	2.873	2.873	2.873	2.873	2.873	2.873
40	2.890	2.894	2.897	2.898	2.898	2.898	2.898	2.898	2.898
60	2.908	2.916	2.923	2.927	2.931	2.933	3.935	2.935	2.936
120	2.928	2.940	2.951	2.960	2.967	2.974	2.979	2.984	2.988
∞	2.949	2.966	2.982	2.995	3.008	3.019	3.029	3.038	3.047

ν \ p	38	40	50	60	70	80	90	100	
1	8.929	8.929	8.929	8.929	8.929	8.929	8.929	8.929	
2	4.130	4.130	4.130	4.130	4.130	4.130	4.130	4.130	
3	3.330	3.330	3.330	3.330	3.330	3.330	3.330	3.330	
4	3.081	3.081	3.081	3.081	3.081	3.081	3.081	3.081	
5	2.970	2.970	2.970	2.970	2.970	2.970	2.970	2.970	
6	2.911	2.911	2.911	2.911	2.911	2.911	2.911	2.911	
7	2.878	2.878	2.878	2.878	2.878	2.878	2.878	2.878	
7	2.858	2.858	2.858	2.858	2.858	2.858	2.858	2.858	
9	2.847	2.847	2.847	2.847	2.847	2.847	2.847	2.847	
10	2.839	2.839	2.839	2.839	2.839	2.839	2.839	2.839	
11	2.835	2.835	2.835	2.835	2.835	2.835	2.835	2.835	
12	2.833	2.833	2.833	2.833	2.833	2.833	2.833	2.833	
13	2.832	2.832	2.832	2.832	2.832	2.832	2.832	2.832	
14	2.833	2.833	2.833	2.833	2.833	2.833	2.833	2.833	
15	2.834	2.834	2.834	2.834	2.834	2.834	2.834	2.834	
16	2.836	2.836	2.836	2.836	2.836	2.836	2.836	2.836	
17	2.838	2.838	2.838	2.838	2.838	2.838	2.838	2.838	
18	2.840	2.840	2.840	2.840	2.840	2.840	2.840	2.840	
19	2.843	2.843	2.843	2.843	2.843	2.843	2.843	2.843	
20	2.845	2.845	2.845	2.845	2.845	2.845	2.845	2.845	
24	2.857	2.857	2.857	2.857	2.857	2.857	2.857	2.857	
30	2.873	2.873	2.873	2.873	2.873	2.873	2.873	2.873	
40	2.898	2.898	2.898	2.898	2.898	2.898	2.898	2.898	
60	2.936	2.936	2.936	2.936	2.936	2.936	2.936	2.936	
120	2.991	2.994	3.001	3.001	3.001	3.001	3.001	3.001	
∞	3.054	3.062	3.091	3.113	3.129	3.143	3.154	3.163	

CRITICAL VALUES FOR DUNCAN'S NEW MULTIPLE RANGE TEST

PROTECTION LEVEL $P = (.95)^{p-1}$ SIGNIFICANCE LEVEL $\alpha = .05$

ν \ p	2	3	4	5	6	7	8	9	10
1	17.97	17.97	17.97	17.97	17.97	17.97	17.97	17.97	17.97
2	6.085	6.085	6.085	6.085	6.085	6.085	6.085	6.085	6.085
3	4.501	4.516	4.516	4.516	4.516	4.516	4.516	4.516	4.516
4	3.927	4.013	4.033	4.033	4.033	4.033	4.033	4.033	4.033
5	3.635	3.749	3.797	3.814	3.814	3.814	3.814	3.814	3.814
6	3.461	3.587	3.649	3.680	3.694	3.697	3.697	3.697	3.697
7	3.344	3.477	3.548	3.588	3.611	3.622	3.626	3.626	3.626
8	3.261	3.399	3.475	3.521	3.549	3.566	3.575	3.579	3.579
9	3.199	3.339	3.420	3.470	3.502	3.523	3.536	3.544	3.547
10	3.151	3.293	3.376	3.430	3.465	3.489	3.505	3.516	3.522
11	3.113	3.256	3.342	3.397	3.435	3.462	3.480	3.493	3.501
12	3.082	3.225	3.313	3.370	3.410	3.439	3.459	3.474	3.484
13	3.055	3.200	3.289	3.348	3.389	3.419	3.442	3.458	3.470
14	3.033	3.178	3.268	3.329	3.372	3.403	3.426	3.444	3.457
15	3.014	3.160	3.250	3.312	3.356	3.389	3.413	3.432	3.446
16	2.998	3.144	3.235	3.298	3.343	3.376	3.402	3.422	3.437
17	2.984	3.130	3.222	3.285	3.331	3.366	3.392	3.412	3.429
18	2.971	3.118	3.210	3.274	3.321	3.356	3.383	3.405	3.421
19	2.960	3.107	3.199	3.264	3.311	3.347	3.375	3.397	3.415
20	2.950	3.097	3.190	3.255	3.303	3.339	3.368	3.391	3.409
24	2.919	3.066	3.160	3.226	3.276	3.315	3.345	3.370	3.390
30	2.888	3.035	3.131	3.199	3.250	3.290	3.322	3.349	3.371
40	2.858	3.006	3.102	3.171	3.224	3.266	3.300	3.328	3.352
60	2.829	2.976	3.073	3.143	3.198	3.241	3.277	3.307	3.333
120	2.800	2.947	3.045	3.116	3.172	3.217	3.254	3.287	3.314
∞	2.772	2.918	3.017	3.089	3.146	3.193	3.232	3.265	3.294

ν \ p	11	12	13	14	15	16	17	18	19
1	17.97	17.97	17.97	17.97	17.97	17.97	17.97	17.97	17.97
2	6.085	6.085	6.085	6.085	6.085	6.085	6.085	6.085	6.085
3	4.516	4.516	4.516	4.516	4.516	4.516	4.516	4.516	4.516
4	4.033	4.033	4.033	4.033	4.033	4.033	4.033	4.033	4.033
5	3.814	3.814	3.814	3.814	3.814	3.814	3.814	3.814	3.814
6	3.697	3.697	3.697	3.697	3.697	3.697	3.697	3.697	3.697
7	3.626	3.626	3.626	3.626	3.626	3.626	3.626	3.626	3.626
8	3.579	3.579	3.579	3.579	3.579	3.579	3.579	3.579	3.579
9	3.547	3.547	3.547	3.547	3.547	3.547	3.547	3.547	3.547
10	3.525	3.526	3.526	3.526	3.526	3.526	3.526	3.526	3.526
11	3.506	3.509	3.510	3.510	3.510	3.510	3.510	3.510	3.510
12	3.491	3.496	3.498	3.499	3.499	3.499	3.499	3.499	3.499
13	3.478	3.484	3.488	3.490	3.490	3.490	3.490	3.490	3.490
14	3.467	3.474	3.479	3.482	3.484	3.484	3.485	3.485	3.485
15	3.457	3.465	3.471	3.476	3.478	3.480	3.481	3.481	3.481
16	3.449	3.458	3.465	3.470	3.473	3.477	3.478	3.478	3.478
17	3.441	3.451	3.459	3.465	3.469	3.473	3.475	3.476	3.476
18	3.435	3.445	3.454	3.460	3.465	3.470	3.472	3.474	3.474
19	3.429	3.440	3.449	3.456	3.462	3.467	3.470	3.472	3.473
20	3.424	3.436	3.445	3.453	3.459	3.464	3.467	3.470	3.472
24	3.406	3.420	3.432	3.441	3.449	3.456	3.461	3.465	3.469
30	3.389	3.405	3.418	3.430	3.439	3.447	3.454	3.460	3.466
40	3.373	3.390	3.405	3.418	3.429	3.439	3.448	3.456	3.463
60	3.355	3.374	3.391	3.406	3.419	3.431	3.442	3.451	3.460
120	3.337	3.359	3.377	3.394	3.409	3.423	3.435	3.446	3.457
∞	3.320	3.343	3.363	3.382	3.399	3.414	3.428	3.442	3.454

CRITICAL VALUES FOR DUNCAN'S NEW MULTIPLE RANGE TEST

PROTECTION LEVEL $P = (.95)^{p-1}$ SIGNIFICANCE LEVEL $\alpha = .05$

ν \ p	20	22	24	26	28	30	32	34	36
1	17.97	17.97	17.97	17.97	17.97	17.97	17.97	17.97	17.97
2	6.085	6.085	6.085	6.085	6.085	6.085	6.085	6.085	6.085
3	4.516	4.516	4.516	4.516	4.516	4.516	4.516	4.516	4.516
4	4.033	4.033	4.033	4.033	4.033	4.033	3.033	4.033	4.033
5	3.814	3.814	3.814	3.814	3.814	3.814	3.814	3.814	3.814
6	3.697	3.697	3.697	3.697	3.697	3.697	3.697	3.697	3.697
7	3.626	3.626	3.626	3.626	3.626	3.626	3.626	3.626	3.626
8	3.579	3.579	3.579	3.579	3.579	3.579	3.579	3.579	3.579
9	3.547	3.547	3.547	3.547	3.547	3.547	3.547	3.547	3.547
10	3.526	3.526	3.526	3.526	3.526	3.526	3.526	3.526	3.526
11	3.510	3.510	3.510	3.510	3.510	3.510	3.510	3.510	3.510
12	3.499	3.499	3.499	3.499	3.499	3.499	3.499	3.499	3.499
13	3.490	3.490	3.490	3.490	3.490	3.490	3.490	3.490	3.490
14	3.485	3.485	3.485	3.485	3.485	3.485	3.485	3.485	3.485
15	3.481	3.481	3.481	3.481	3.481	3.481	3.481	3.481	3.481
16	3.478	3.478	3.478	3.478	3.478	3.478	3.478	3.478	3.478
17	3.476	3.476	3.476	3.476	3.476	3.476	3.476	3.476	3.476
18	3.474	3.474	3.474	3.474	3.474	3.474	3.474	3.474	3.474
19	3.474	3.474	3.474	3.474	3.474	3.474	3.474	3.474	3.474
20	3.473	3.474	3.474	3.474	3.474	3.474	3.474	3.474	3.474
24	3.471	3.475	3.477	3.477	3.477	3.477	3.477	3.477	3.477
30	3.470	3.477	3.481	3.484	3.486	3.486	3.486	3.486	3.486
40	3.469	3.479	3.486	3.492	3.497	3.500	3.503	3.504	3.504
60	3.467	3.481	3.492	3.501	3.509	3.515	3.521	3.525	3.529
120	3.466	3.483	3.498	3.511	3.522	3.532	3.541	3.548	3.555
∞	3.466	3.486	3.505	3.522	3.536	3.550	3.562	3.574	3.584

ν \ p	38	40	50	60	70	80	90	100	
1	17.97	17.97	17.97	17.97	17.97	17.97	17.97	17.97	
2	6.085	6.085	6.085	6.085	6.085	6.085	6.085	6.085	
3	4.516	4.516	4.516	4.516	4.516	4.516	4.516	4.516	
4	4.033	4.033	4.033	4.033	4.033	4.033	4.033	4.033	
5	3.814	3.814	3.814	3.814	3.814	3.814	3.814	3.814	
6	3.697	3.697	3.697	3.697	3.697	3.697	3.697	3.697	
7	3.626	3.626	3.626	3.626	3.626	3.626	3.626	3.626	
8	3.579	3.579	3.579	3.579	3.579	3.579	3.579	3.579	
9	3.547	3.547	3.547	3.547	3.547	3.547	3.547	3.547	
10	3.526	3.526	3.526	3.526	3.526	3.526	3.526	3.526	
11	3.510	3.510	3.510	3.510	3.510	3.510	3.510	3.510	
12	3.499	3.499	3.499	3.499	3.499	3.499	3.499	3.499	
13	3.490	3.490	3.490	3.490	3.490	3.490	3.490	3.490	
14	3.485	3.485	3.485	3.485	3.485	3.485	3.485	3.485	
15	3.481	3.481	3.481	3.481	3.481	3.481	3.481	3.481	
16	3.478	3.478	3.478	3.478	3.478	3.478	3.478	3.478	
17	3.476	3.476	3.476	3.476	3.476	3.476	3.476	3.476	
18	3.474	3.474	3.474	3.474	3.474	3.474	3.474	3.474	
19	3.474	3.474	3.474	3.474	3.474	3.474	3.474	3.474	
20	3.474	3.474	3.474	3.474	3.474	3.474	3.474	3.474	
24	3.477	3.477	3.477	3.477	3.477	3.477	3.477	3.477	
30	3.486	3.486	3.486	3.486	3.486	3.486	3.486	3.486	
40	3.504	3.504	3.504	3.504	3.504	3.504	3.504	3.504	
60	3.531	3.534	3.537	3.537	3.537	3.537	3.537	3.537	
120	3.561	3.566	3.585	3.596	3.600	3.601	3.601	3.601	
∞	3.594	3.603	3.640	3.668	3.690	3.708	3.722	3.735	

CRITICAL VALUES FOR DUNCAN'S NEW MULTIPLE RANGE TEST

PROTECTION LEVEL $P = (.99)^{p-1}$ SIGNIFICANCE LEVEL $\alpha = .01$

ν \ p	2	3	4	5	6	7	8	9	10
1	90.03	90.03	90.03	90.03	90.03	90.03	90.03	90.03	90.03
2	14.04	14.04	14.04	14.04	14.04	14.04	14.04	14.04	14.04
3	8.261	8.321	8.321	8.321	8.321	8.321	8.321	8.321	8.321
4	6.512	6.677	6.740	6.756	6.756	6.756	6.756	6.756	6.756
5	5.702	5.893	5.989	6.040	6.065	6.074	6.074	6.074	6.074
6	5.243	5.439	5.549	5.614	5.655	5.680	5.694	5.701	5.703
7	4.949	5.145	5.260	5.334	5.383	5.416	5.439	5.454	5.464
8	4.746	4.939	5.057	5.135	5.189	5.227	5.256	5.276	5.291
9	4.596	4.787	4.906	4.986	5.043	5.086	5.118	5.142	5.160
10	4.482	4.671	4.790	4.871	4.931	4.975	5.010	5.037	5.058
11	4.392	4.579	4.697	4.780	4.841	4.887	4.924	4.952	4.975
12	4.320	4.504	4.622	4.706	4.767	4.815	4.852	4.883	4.907
13	4.260	4.442	4.560	4.644	4.706	4.755	4.793	4.824	4.850
14	4.210	4.391	4.508	4.591	4.654	4.704	4.743	4.775	4.802
15	4.168	4.347	4.463	4.547	4.610	4.660	4.700	4.733	4.760
16	4.131	4.309	4.425	4.509	4.572	4.622	4.663	4.696	4.724
17	4.099	4.275	4.391	4.475	4.539	4.589	4.630	4.664	4.693
18	4.071	4.246	4.362	4.445	4.509	4.560	4.601	4.635	4.664
19	4.046	4.220	4.335	4.419	4.483	4.534	4.575	4.610	4.639
20	4.024	4.197	4.312	4.395	4.459	4.510	4.552	4.587	4.617
24	3.956	4.126	4.239	4.322	4.386	4.437	4.480	4.516	4.546
30	3.889	4.056	4.168	4.250	4.314	4.366	4.409	4.445	4.477
40	3.825	3.988	4.098	4.180	4.244	4.296	4.339	4.376	4.408
60	3.762	3.922	4.031	4.111	4.174	4.226	4.270	4.307	4.340
120	3.702	3.858	3.965	4.044	4.107	4.158	4.202	4.239	4.272
∞	3.643	3.796	3.900	3.978	4.040	4.091	4.135	4.172	4.205

ν \ p	11	12	13	14	15	16	17	18	19
1	90.03	90.03	90.03	90.03	90.03	90.03	90.03	90.03	90.03
2	14.04	14.04	14.04	14.04	14.04	14.04	14.04	14.04	14.04
3	8.321	8.321	8.321	8.321	8.321	8.321	8.321	8.321	8.321
4	6.756	6.756	6.756	6.756	6.756	6.756	6.756	6.756	6.756
5	6.074	6.074	6.074	6.074	6.074	6.074	6.074	6.074	6.074
6	5.703	5.703	5.703	5.703	5.703	5.703	5.703	5.703	5.703
7	5.470	5.472	5.472	5.472	5.472	5.472	5.472	5.742	5.472
8	5.302	5.309	5.314	5.316	5.317	5.317	5.317	5.317	5.317
9	5.174	5.185	5.193	5.199	5.203	5.205	5.206	5.206	5.206
10	5.074	5.088	5.098	5.106	5.112	5.117	5.120	5.122	5.124
11	4.994	5.009	5.021	5.031	5.039	5.045	5.050	5.054	5.057
12	4.927	4.944	4.958	4.969	4.978	4.986	4.993	4.998	5.002
13	4.872	4.889	4.904	4.917	4.928	4.937	4.944	4.950	4.956
14	4.824	4.843	4.859	4.872	4.884	4.894	4.902	4.910	4.916
15	4.783	4.803	4.820	4.834	4.846	4.857	4.866	4.874	4.881
16	4.748	4.768	4.786	4.800	4.813	4.825	4.835	4.844	4.851
17	4.717	4.738	4.756	4.771	4.785	4.797	4.807	4.816	4.824
18	4.689	4.711	4.729	4.745	4.759	4.772	4.783	4.792	4.801
19	4.665	4.686	4.705	4.722	4.736	4.749	4.761	4.771	4.780
20	4.642	4.664	4.684	4.701	4.716	4.729	4.741	4.751	4.761
24	4.573	4.596	4.616	4.634	4.651	4.665	4.678	4.690	4.700
30	4.504	4.528	4.550	4.569	4.586	4.601	4.615	4.628	4.640
40	4.436	4.461	4.483	4.503	4.521	4.537	4.553	4.566	4.579
60	4.368	4.394	4.417	4.438	4.456	4.474	4.490	4.504	4.518
120	4.301	4.327	4.351	4.372	4.392	4.410	4.426	4.442	4.456
∞	4.235	4.261	4.285	4.307	4.327	4.345	4.363	4.379	4.394

CRITICAL VALUES FOR DUNCAN'S NEW MULTIPLE RANGE TEST

PROTECTION LEVEL $P = (.99)^{p-1}$ SIGNIFICANCE LEVEL $\alpha = .01$

ν \ p	20	22	24	26	28	30	32	34	36
1	90.03	90.03	90.03	90.03	90.03	90.03	90.03	90.03	90.03
2	14.04	14.04	14.04	14.04	14.04	14.04	14.04	14.04	14.04
3	8.321	8.321	8.321	8.321	8.321	8.321	8.321	8.321	8.321
4	6.756	6.756	6.756	6.756	6.756	6.756	6.756	6.756	6.756
5	6.074	6.074	6.074	6.074	6.074	6.074	6.074	6.074	6.074
6	5.703	5.703	5.703	5.703	5.703	5.703	5.703	5.703	5.703
7	5.472	5.472	5.472	5.472	5.472	5.472	5.472	5.472	5.472
8	5.317	5.317	5.317	5.317	5.317	5.317	5.317	5.317	5.317
9	5.206	5.206	5.206	5.206	5.206	5.206	5.206	5.206	5.206
10	5.124	5.124	5.124	5.124	5.124	5.124	5.124	5.124	5.124
11	5.059	5.061	5.061	5.061	5.061	5.061	5.061	5.061	5.061
12	5.006	5.010	5.011	5.011	5.011	5.011	5.011	5.011	5.011
13	4.960	4.966	4.970	4.972	4.972	4.972	4.972	4.972	4.972
14	4.921	4.929	4.935	4.938	4.940	4.940	4.940	4.940	4.940
15	4.887	4.897	4.904	4.909	4.912	4.914	4.914	4.914	4.914
16	4.858	4.869	4.877	4.883	4.887	4.890	4.892	4.892	4.892
17	4.832	4.844	4.853	4.860	4.865	4.869	4.872	4.873	4.874
18	4.808	4.821	4.832	4.839	4.846	4.850	4.854	4.856	4.857
19	4.788	4.802	4.812	4.821	4.828	4.833	4.838	4.841	4.843
20	4.769	4.784	4.795	4.805	4.813	4.818	4.823	4.827	4.830
24	4.710	4.727	4.741	4.752	4.762	4.770	4.777	4.783	4.788
30	4.650	4.669	4.685	4.699	4.711	4.721	4.730	4.738	4.744
40	4.591	4.611	4.630	4.645	4.659	4.671	4.682	4.692	4.700
60	4.530	4.553	4.573	4.591	4.607	4.620	4.633	4.645	4.655
120	4.469	4.494	4.516	4.535	4.552	4.568	4.583	4.596	4.609
∞	4.408	4.434	4.457	4.478	4.497	4.514	4.530	4.545	4.559

ν \ p	38	40	50	60	70	80	90	100
1	90.03	90.03	90.03	90.03	90.03	90.03	90.03	90.03
2	14.04	14.04	14.04	14.04	14.04	14.04	14.04	14.04
3	8.321	8.321	8.321	8.321	8.321	8.321	8.321	8.321
4	6.756	6.756	6.756	6.756	6.756	6.756	6.756	6.756
5	6.074	6.074	6.074	6.074	6.074	6.074	6.074	6.074
6	5.703	5.703	5.703	5.703	5.703	5.703	5.703	5.703
7	5.472	5.472	5.472	5.472	5.472	5.472	5.472	5.472
8	5.317	5.317	5.317	5.317	5.317	5.317	5.317	5.317
9	5.206	5.206	5.206	5.206	5.206	5.206	5.206	5.206
10	5.124	5.124	5.124	5.124	5.124	5.124	5.124	5.124
11	5.061	5.061	5.061	5.061	5.061	5.061	5.061	5.061
12	5.011	5.011	5.011	5.011	5.011	5.011	5.011	5.011
13	4.972	4.972	4.972	4.972	4.972	4.972	4.972	4.972
14	4.940	4.940	4.940	4.940	4.940	4.940	4.940	4.940
15	4.914	4.914	4.914	4.914	4.914	4.914	4.914	4.914
16	4.892	4.892	4.892	4.892	4.892	4.892	4.892	4.892
17	4.874	4.874	4.874	4.874	4.874	4.874	4.874	4.874
18	4.858	4.858	4.858	4.858	4.858	4.858	4.858	4.858
19	4.844	4.845	4.845	4.845	4.845	4.845	4.845	4.845
20	4.832	4.833	4.833	4.833	4.833	4.833	4.833	4.833
24	4.791	4.794	4.802	4.802	4.802	4.802	4.802	4.802
30	4.750	4.755	4.772	4.777	4.777	4.777	4.777	4.777
40	4.708	4.715	4.740	4.754	4.761	4.764	4.764	4.764
60	4.665	4.673	4.707	4.730	4.745	4.755	4.761	4.765
120	4.619	4.630	4.673	4.703	4.727	4.745	4.759	4.770
∞	4.572	4.584	4.635	4.675	4.707	4.734	4.756	4.776

CRITICAL VALUES FOR DUNCAN'S NEW MULTIPLE RANGE TEST

PROTECTION LEVEL $P = (.995)^{p-1}$ SIGNIFICANCE LEVEL $\alpha = .005$

ν \ p	2	3	4	5	6	7	8	9	10
1	180.1	180.1	180.1	180.1	180.1	180.1	180.1	180.1	180.1
2	19.93	19.93	19.93	19.93	19.93	19.93	19.93	19.93	19.93
3	10.55	10.63	10.63	10.63	10.63	10.63	10.63	10.63	10.63
4	7.916	8.126	8.210	8.238	8.238	8.238	8.238	8.238	8.238
5	6.751	6.980	7.100	7.167	7.204	7.222	7.228	7.228	7.228
6	6.105	6.334	6.466	6.547	6.600	6.635	6.658	6.672	6.679
7	5.699	5.922	6.057	6.145	6.207	6.250	6.281	6.304	6.320
8	5.420	5.638	5.773	5.864	5.930	5.978	6.014	6.042	6.064
9	5.218	5.430	5.565	5.657	5.725	5.776	5.815	5.846	5.871
10	5.065	5.273	5.405	5.498	5.567	5.620	5.662	5.695	5.722
11	4.945	5.149	5.280	5.372	5.442	5.496	5.539	5.574	5.603
12	4.849	5.048	5.178	5.270	5.341	5.396	5.439	5.475	5.505
13	4.770	4.966	5.094	5.186	5.256	5.312	5.356	5.393	5.424
14	4.704	4.897	5.023	5.116	5.185	5.241	5.286	5.324	5.355
15	4.647	4.838	4.964	5.055	5.125	5.181	5.226	5.264	5.297
16	4.599	4.787	4.912	5.003	5.073	5.129	5.175	5.213	5.245
17	4.557	4.744	4.867	4.958	5.027	5.084	5.130	5.168	5.201
18	4.521	4.705	4.828	4.918	4.987	5.043	5.090	5.129	5.162
19	4.488	4.671	4.793	4.883	4.952	5.008	5.054	5.093	5.127
20	4.460	4.641	4.762	4.851	4.920	4.976	5.022	5.061	5.095
24	4.371	4.547	4.666	4.753	4.822	4.877	4.924	4.963	4.997
30	4.285	4.456	4.572	4.658	4.726	4.781	4.827	4.867	4.901
40	4.202	4.369	4.482	4.566	4.632	4.687	4.733	4.772	4.806
60	4.122	4.284	4.394	4.476	4.541	4.595	4.640	4.679	4.713
120	4.045	4.201	4.308	4.388	4.452	4.505	4.550	4.588	4.622
∞	3.970	4.121	4.225	4.303	4.365	4.417	4.461	4.499	4.532

ν \ p	11	12	13	14	15	16	17	18	19
1	180.1	180.1	180.1	180.1	180.1	180.1	180.1	180.1	180.1
2	19.93	19.93	19.93	19.93	19.93	19.93	19.93	19.93	19.93
3	10.63	10.63	10.63	10.63	10.63	10.63	10.63	10.63	10.63
4	8.238	8.238	8.238	8.238	8.238	8.238	8.238	8.238	8.238
5	7.228	7.228	7.228	7.228	7.228	7.228	7.228	7.228	7.228
6	6.682	6.682	6.682	6.682	6.682	6.682	6.682	6.682	6.682
7	6.331	6.339	6.343	6.345	6.345	6.345	6.345	6.345	6.345
8	6.080	6.092	6.101	6.108	6.113	6.116	6.118	6.119	6.119
9	5.891	5.907	5.920	5.930	5.938	5.944	5.949	5.952	5.955
10	5.744	5.762	5.777	5.790	5.800	5.809	5.816	5.821	5.826
11	5.626	5.646	5.663	5.678	5.690	5.700	5.709	5.716	5.722
12	5.531	5.552	5.570	5.585	5.599	5.610	5.620	5.629	5.636
13	5.450	5.472	5.492	5.508	5.523	5.535	5.546	5.556	5.564
14	5.382	5.405	5.425	5.442	5.458	5.471	5.483	5.494	5.503
15	5.324	5.348	5.368	5.386	5.402	5.416	5.429	5.440	5.450
16	5.273	5.298	5.319	5.338	5.354	5.368	5.381	5.393	5.404
17	5.229	5.254	5.275	5.295	5.311	5.327	5.340	5.352	5.363
18	5.190	5.215	5.237	5.256	5.274	5.289	5.303	5.316	5.327
19	5.156	5.181	5.203	5.222	5.240	5.256	5.270	5.283	5.295
20	5.124	5.150	5.172	5.193	5.210	5.226	5.241	5.254	5.266
24	5.027	5.053	5.076	5.097	5.116	5.133	5.148	5.162	5.175
30	4.931	4.958	4.981	5.003	5.022	5.040	5.056	5.071	5.085
40	4.837	4.864	4.888	4.910	4.930	4.948	4.965	4.980	4.995
60	4.744	4.771	4.796	4.818	4.838	4.857	4.874	4.890	4.905
120	4.652	4.679	4.704	4.726	4.747	4.766	4.784	4.800	4.815
∞	4.562	4.589	4.614	4.636	4.657	4.676	4.694	4.710	4.726

CRITICAL VALUES FOR DUNCAN'S NEW MULTIPLE RANGE TEST

PROTECTION LEVEL $P = (.995)^{p-1}$ **SIGNIFICANCE LEVEL** $\alpha = .005$

ν \ p	20	22	24	26	28	30	32	34	36
1	180.1	180.1	180.1	180.1	180.1	180.1	180.1	180.1	180.1
2	19.93	19.93	19.93	19.93	19.93	19.93	19.93	19.93	19.93
3	10.63	10.63	10.63	10.63	10.63	10.63	10.63	10.63	10.63
4	8.238	8.238	8.238	8.238	8.238	8.238	8.238	8.238	8.238
5	7.228	7.228	7.228	7.228	7.228	7.228	7.228	7.228	7.228
6	6.682	6.682	6.682	6.682	6.682	6.682	6.682	6.682	6.682
7	6.345	6.345	6.345	6.345	6.345	6.345	6.345	6.345	6.345
8	6.119	6.119	6.119	6.119	6.119	6.119	6.119	6.119	6.119
9	5.956	5.957	5.957	5.957	5.957	5.957	5.957	5.957	5.957
10	5.829	5.834	5.836	5.836	5.836	5.836	5.836	5.836	5.836
11	5.727	5.735	5.740	5.743	5.744	5.744	5.744	5.744	5.744
12	5.642	5.653	5.660	5.665	5.668	5.670	5.670	5.670	5.670
13	5.571	5.583	5.593	5.600	5.605	5.608	5.610	5.611	5.611
14	5.511	5.525	5.535	5.544	5.550	5.555	5.559	5.561	5.563
15	5.459	5.474	5.486	5.495	5.503	5.509	5.514	5.518	5.520
16	5.413	5.429	5.442	5.453	5.462	5.469	5.475	5.479	5.483
17	5.373	5.390	5.404	5.416	5.425	5.433	5.440	5.445	5.450
18	5.338	5.355	5.370	5.383	5.393	5.402	5.409	5.415	5.420
19	5.306	5.325	5.340	5.353	5.364	5.374	5.382	5.388	5.395
20	5.277	5.296	5.313	5.326	5.338	5.348	5.357	5.364	5.370
24	5.187	5.209	5.226	5.242	5.255	5.267	5.278	5.287	5.295
30	5.098	5.120	5.140	5.157	5.172	5.186	5.198	5.209	5.218
40	5.008	5.032	5.054	5.072	5.089	5.104	5.118	5.130	5.141
60	4.919	4.944	4.967	4.987	5.005	5.021	5.036	5.050	5.062
120	4.830	4.856	4.880	4.901	4.920	4.937	4.953	4.968	4.982
∞	4.740	4.767	4.792	4.813	4.833	4.852	4.869	4.885	4.899

ν \ p	38	40	50	60	70	80	90	100
1	180.1	180.1	180.1	180.1	180.1	180.1	180.0	180.1
2	19.93	19.93	19.93	19.93	19.93	19.93	19.93	19.93
3	10.63	10.63	10.63	10.63	10.63	10.63	10.63	10.63
4	8.238	8.238	8.238	8.238	8.238	8.238	8.238	8.238
5	7.228	7.228	7.228	7.228	7.228	7.228	7.228	7.228
6	6.682	6.682	6.682	6.682	6.682	6.682	6.682	6.682
7	6.345	6.345	6.345	6.345	6.345	6.345	6.345	6.345
8	6.119	6.119	6.119	6.119	6.119	6.119	6.119	6.119
9	5.957	5.957	5.957	5.957	5.957	5.957	5.957	5.957
10	5.836	5.836	5.836	5.836	5.836	5.836	5.836	5.836
11	5.744	5.744	5.744	5.744	5.744	5.744	5.744	5.744
12	5.670	5.670	5.670	5.670	5.670	5.670	5.670	5.670
13	5.611	5.611	5.611	5.611	5.611	5.611	5.611	5.611
14	5.563	5.563	5.563	5.563	5.563	5.563	5.563	5.563
15	5.522	5.523	5.523	5.523	5.523	5.523	5.523	5.523
16	5.485	5.488	5.489	5.489	5.489	5.489	5.489	5.489
17	5.453	5.456	5.461	5.461	5.461	5.461	5.461	5.461
18	5.425	5.428	5.436	5.436	5.436	5.436	5.436	5.436
19	5.399	5.403	5.414	5.415	5.415	5.415	5.415	5.415
20	5.376	5.380	5.394	5.397	5.397	5.397	5.397	5.397
24	5.302	5.308	5.329	5.340	5.343	5.343	5.343	5.343
30	5.227	5.235	5.264	5.281	5.292	5.297	5.298	5.298
40	5.151	5.160	5.197	5.221	5.238	5.249	5.257	5.261
60	5.074	5.084	5.128	5.159	5.182	5.199	5.213	5.223
120	4.995	5.007	5.056	5.094	5.123	5.146	5.166	5.182
∞	4.913	4.926	4.981	5.024	5.059	5.088	5.114	5.136

CRITICAL VALUES FOR DUNCAN'S NEW MULTIPLE RANGE TEST

PROTECTION LEVEL $P = (.999)^{p-1}$ SIGNIFICANCE LEVEL $\alpha = .001$

ν \ p	2	3	4	5	6	7	8	9	10
1	900.3	900.3	900.3	900.3	900.3	900.3	900.3	900.3	900.3
2	44.69	44.69	44.69	44.69	44.69	44.69	44.69	44.69	44.69
3	18.28	18.45	18.45	18.45	18.45	18.45	18.45	18.45	18.45
4	12.18	12.52	12.67	12.73	12.75	12.75	12.75	12.75	12.75
5	9.714	10.05	10.24	10.35	10.42	10.46	10.48	10.49	10.49
6	8.427	8.743	8.932	9.055	9.139	9.198	9.241	9.272	9.294
7	7.648	7.943	8.127	8.252	8.342	8.409	8.460	8.500	8.530
8	7.130	7.407	7.584	7.708	7.799	7.869	7.924	7.968	8.004
9	6.762	7.024	7.195	7.316	7.407	7.478	7.535	7.582	7.619
10	6.487	6.738	6.902	7.021	7.111	7.182	7.240	7.287	7.327
11	6.275	6.516	6.676	6.791	6.880	6.950	7.008	7.056	7.097
12	6.106	6.340	6.494	6.607	6.695	6.765	6.822	6.870	6.911
13	5.970	6.195	6.346	6.457	6.543	6.612	6.670	6.718	6.759
14	5.856	6.075	6.223	6.332	6.416	6.485	6.542	6.590	6.631
15	5.760	5.974	6.119	6.225	6.309	6.377	6.433	6.481	6.522
16	5.678	5.888	6.030	6.135	6.217	6.284	6.340	6.388	6.429
17	5.608	5.813	5.953	6.056	6.138	6.204	6.260	6.307	6.348
18	5.546	5.748	5.886	5.988	6.068	6.134	6.189	6.236	6.277
19	5.492	5.691	5.826	5.927	6.007	6.072	6.127	6.174	6.214
20	5.444	5.640	5.774	5.873	5.952	6.017	6.071	6.117	6.158
24	5.297	5.484	5.612	5.708	5.784	5.846	5.899	5.945	5.984
30	5.156	5.335	5.457	5.549	5.622	5.682	5.734	5.778	5.817
40	5.022	5.191	5.308	5.396	5.466	5.524	5.574	5.617	5.654
60	4.894	5.055	5.166	5.249	5.317	5.372	5.420	5.461	5.498
120	4.771	4.924	5.029	5.109	5.173	5.226	5.271	5.311	5.346
∞	4.654	4.798	4.898	4.974	5.034	5.085	5.128	5.166	5.199

ν \ p	11	12	13	14	15	16	17	18	19
1	900.3	900.3	900.3	900.3	900.3	900.3	900.3	900.3	900.3
2	44.69	44.69	44.69	44.69	44.69	44.69	44.69	44.69	44.69
3	18.45	18.45	18.45	18.45	18.45	18.45	18.45	18.45	18.45
4	12.75	12.75	12.75	12.75	12.75	12.75	12.75	12.75	12.75
5	10.49	10.49	10.49	10.49	10.49	10.49	10.49	10.49	10.49
6	9.309	9.319	9.325	9.328	9.329	9.329	9.329	9.329	9.329
7	8.555	8.574	8.589	8.600	8.609	8.616	8.621	8.624	8.626
8	8.033	8.057	8.078	8.094	8.108	8.119	8.129	8.137	8.143
9	7.652	7.679	7.702	7.722	7.739	7.753	7.766	7.777	7.786
10	7.361	7.390	7.415	7.437	7.456	7.472	7.487	7.500	7.511
11	7.132	7.162	7.188	7.211	7.231	7.250	7.266	7.280	7.293
12	6.947	6.978	7.005	7.029	7.050	7.069	7.086	7.102	7.116
13	6.795	6.826	6.854	6.878	6.900	6.920	6.937	6.954	6.968
14	6.667	6.699	6.727	6.752	6.774	6.794	6.812	6.829	6.844
15	6.558	6.590	6.619	6.644	6.666	6.687	6.706	6.723	6.739
16	6.465	6.497	6.525	6.551	6.574	6.595	6.614	6.631	6.647
17	6.384	6.416	6.444	6.470	6.493	6.514	6.533	6.551	6.567
18	6.313	6.345	6.373	6.399	6.422	6.443	6.462	6.480	6.497
19	6.250	6.281	6.310	6.336	6.359	6.380	6.400	6.418	6.434
20	6.193	6.225	6.254	6.279	6.303	6.324	6.344	6.362	6.379
24	6.020	6.051	6.079	6.105	6.129	6.150	6.170	6.188	6.205
30	5.851	5.882	5.910	5.935	5.958	5.980	6.000	6.018	6.036
40	5.688	5.718	5.745	5.770	5.793	5.814	5.834	5.852	5.869
60	5.530	5.559	5.586	5.610	5.632	5.653	5.672	5.690	5.707
120	5.377	5.405	5.341	5.454	5.476	5.496	5.515	5.532	5.549
∞	5.229	5.256	5.280	5.303	5.324	5.343	5.361	5.378	5.394

CRITICAL VALUES FOR DUNCAN'S NEW MULTIPLE RANGE TEST

PROTECTION LEVEL $P = (.999)^{p-1}$ SIGNIFICANCE LEVEL $\alpha = .001$

ν \ p	20	22	24	26	28	30	32	34	36
1	900.3	900.3	900.3	900.3	900.3	900.3	900.3	900.3	900.3
2	44.69	44.69	44.69	44.69	44.69	44.69	44.69	44.69	44.69
3	18.45	18.45	18.45	18.45	18.45	18.45	18.45	18.45	18.45
4	12.75	12.75	12.75	12.75	12.75	12.75	12.75	12.75	12.75
5	10.49	10.49	10.49	10.49	10.49	10.49	10.49	10.49	10.49
6	9.329	9.329	9.329	9.329	9.329	9.329	9.329	9.329	9.329
7	8.627	8.627	8.627	8.627	8.627	8.627	8.627	8.627	8.627
8	8.149	8.156	8.160	8.161	8.161	8.161	8.161	8.161	8.161
9	7.794	7.808	7.817	7.824	7.828	7.831	7.832	7.832	7.832
10	7.522	7.538	7.552	7.562	7.570	7.577	7.582	7.585	7.587
11	7.304	7.324	7.340	7.354	7.364	7.373	7.380	7.386	7.391
12	7.128	7.150	7.168	7.184	7.196	7.207	7.216	7.223	7.230
13	6.982	7.005	7.025	7.042	7.056	7.068	7.079	7.088	7.096
14	6.858	6.883	6.904	6.922	6.937	6.951	6.962	6.973	6.982
15	6.753	6.778	6.800	6.819	6.836	6.850	6.863	6.874	6.883
16	6.661	6.688	6.711	6.730	6.748	6.763	6.776	6.788	6.799
17	6.582	6.609	6.632	6.653	6.670	6.686	6.701	6.713	6.724
18	6.512	6.539	6.563	6.584	6.602	6.619	6.633	6.647	6.658
19	6.450	6.477	6.501	6.523	6.542	6.559	6.574	6.587	6.600
20	6.394	6.422	6.447	6.468	6.487	6.505	6.520	6.534	6.547
24	6.221	6.250	6.275	6.298	6.318	6.336	6.353	6.368	6.381
30	6.051	6.081	6.106	6.130	6.151	6.169	6.187	6.203	6.217
40	5.885	5.915	5.941	5.964	5.986	6.005	6.023	6.040	6.055
60	5.723	5.752	5.778	5.802	5.823	5.843	5.862	5.878	5.894
120	5.565	5.593	5.619	5.642	5.664	5.683	5.702	5.718	5.734
∞	5.409	5.437	5.462	5.485	5.506	5.525	5.543	5.560	5.576

ν \ p	38	40	50	60	70	80	90	100
1	900.3	900.3	900.3	900.3	900.3	900.3	900.3	900.3
2	44.69	44.69	44.69	44.69	44.69	44.69	44.69	44.69
3	18.45	18.45	18.45	18.45	18.45	18.45	18.45	18.45
4	12.75	12.75	12.75	12.75	12.75	12.75	12.75	12.75
5	10.49	10.49	10.49	10.49	10.49	10.49	10.49	10.49
6	9.329	9.329	9.329	9.329	9.329	9.329	9.329	9.329
7	8.627	8.627	8.627	8.627	8.627	8.627	8.627	8.627
8	8.161	8.161	8.161	8.161	8.161	8.161	8.161	8.161
9	7.832	7.832	7.832	7.832	7.832	7.832	7.832	7.832
10	7.588	7.588	7.588	7.588	7.588	7.588	7.588	7.588
11	7.394	7.397	7.400	7.400	7.400	7.400	7.400	7.400
12	7.235	7.239	7.251	7.251	7.251	7.251	7.251	7.251
13	7.102	7.108	7.126	7.132	7.132	7.132	7.132	7.132
14	6.989	6.996	7.019	7.030	7.034	7.034	7.034	7.034
15	6.892	6.900	6.927	6.942	6.949	6.951	6.951	6.951
16	6.808	6.816	6.848	6.865	6.875	6.880	6.881	6.881
17	6.734	6.743	6.777	6.798	6.811	6.818	6.821	6.821
18	6.669	6.679	6.715	6.738	6.753	6.762	6.767	6.770
19	6.611	6.621	6.660	6.685	6.702	6.713	6.719	6.723
20	6.558	6.569	6.610	6.637	6.655	6.668	6.676	6.681
24	6.394	6.405	6.451	6.484	6.507	6.525	6.538	6.547
30	6.231	6.243	6.294	6.331	6.360	6.381	6.399	6.412
40	6.069	6.082	6.137	6.178	6.210	6.236	6.257	6.274
60	5.909	5.922	5.980	6.024	6.059	6.088	6.113	6.134
120	5.749	5.763	5.822	5.868	5.906	5.938	5.965	5.988
∞	5.590	5.604	5.663	5.711	5.750	5.783	5.811	5.837

VIII.5 SUBSTITUTE *t*-RATIOS

A. The statistic $\tau_1 = \frac{\bar{x} - \mu}{w}$, where w is the range of the observations can be used to test hypotheses about μ. This table gives percentage points of the distribution of τ_1 for sample sizes up to 20. The percentage points at the top of the table are upper percentage points. Lower percentage points are obtained by entering the bottom of the table and prefixing the tabulated value with a minus sign.

B. The statistic $\tau_d = \frac{\bar{x}_1 - \bar{x}_2}{\frac{1}{2}(w_1 + w_2)}$ may be used to test hypotheses about the differences between means. Percentage points of the distribution of τ_d are given for samples of equal size up to 20.

C. The statistic $\tau_2 = \frac{\frac{1}{2}[x_{(1)} + x_{(n)}] - \mu}{w}$ can be used to test hypotheses about μ. This table gives percentage points of the distribution of τ_2 for samples of size 10 or less.

SUBSTITUTE *t*-RATIOS

A. Percentiles* for $\tau_1 = \dfrac{\bar{x} - \mu}{w}$

Sample size	P_{95}	$P_{97.5}$	P_{99}	$P_{99.5}$	$P_{99.9}$	$P_{99.95}$
2	3.175	6.353	15.910	31.828	159.16	318.31
3	.885	1.304	2.111	3.008	6.77	9.58
4	.529	.717	1.023	1.316	2.29	2.85
5	.388	.507	.685	.843	1.32	1.58
6	.312	.399	.523	.628	.92	1.07
7	.263	.333	.429	.507	.71	.82
8	.230	.288	.366	.429	.59	.67
9	.205	.255	.322	.374	.50	.57
10	.186	.230	.288	.333	.44	.50
11	.170	.210	.262	.302	.40	.44
12	.158	.194	.241	.277	.36	.40
13	.147	.181	.224	.256	.33	.37
14	.138	.170	.209	.239	.31	.34
15	.131	.160	.197	.224	.29	.32
16	.124	.151	.186	.212	.27	.30
17	.118	.144	.177	.201	.26	.28
18	.113	.137	.168	.191	.24	.26
19	.108	.131	.161	.182	.23	.25
20	.104	.126	.154	.175	.22	.24
	$-P_{05}$	$-P_{02.5}$	$-P_{01}$	$-P_{0.5}$	$-P_{0.1}$	$-P_{0.05}$

* When the table is read from the foot, the tabled values are to be prefixed with a negative sign.

SUBSTITUTE *t*-RATIOS

B. Percentiles* for $\tau_d = \dfrac{\bar{x}_1 - \bar{x}_2}{\frac{1}{2}(w_1 + w_2)}$

Sample sizes $N_1 = N_2$	P_{95}	$P_{97.5}$	P_{99}	$P_{99.5}$	$P_{99.9}$	$P_{99.95}$
2	2.322	3.427	5.553	7.916	17.81	25.23
3	.974	1.272	1.715	2.093	3.27	4.18
4	.644	.813	1.047	1.237	1.74	1.99
5	.493	.613	.772	.896	1.21	1.35
6	.405	.499	.621	.714	.94	1.03
7	.347	.426	.525	.600	.77	.85
8	.306	.373	.459	.521	.67	.73
9	.275	.334	.409	.464	.59	.64
10	.250	.304	.371	.419	.53	.58
11	.233	.280	.340	.384	.48	.52
12	.214	.260	.315	.355	.44	.48
13	.201	.243	.294	.331	.41	.45
14	.189	.228	.276	.311	.39	.42
15	.179	.216	.261	.293	.36	.39
16	.170	.205	.247	.278	.34	.37
17	.162	.195	.236	.264	.33	.35
18	.155	.187	.225	.252	.31	.34
19	.149	.179	.216	.242	.30	.32
20	.143	.172	.207	.232	.29	.31
	$-P_{05}$	$-P_{02.5}$	$-P_{01}$	$-P_{0.5}$	$-P_{0.1}$	$-P_{0.05}$

* When the table is read from the foot, the tabled values are to be prefixed with a negative sign.

C. Percentiles for $\tau_2 = \dfrac{\frac{1}{2}[x_{(1)} + x_{(n)}] - \mu}{w}$

Sample size	P_{95}	$P_{97.5}$	P_{99}	$P_{99.5}$
2	3.16	6.35	15.91	31.83
3	.90	1.30	2.11	3.02
4	.55	.74	1.04	1.37
5	.42	.52	.71	.85
6	.35	.43	.56	.66
7	.30	.37	.47	.55
8	.26	.33	.42	.47
9	.24	.30	.38	.42
10	.22	.27	.35	.39
	$-P_{05}$	$-P_{02.5}$	$-P_{01}$	$-P_{0.5}$

VIII.6 SUBSTITUTE F-RATIO

The ratio $F' = w_1/w_2$ of two ranges can be used as a substitute for the ratio of two variances. This table gives percentage points of the ratio of two ranges for respective sample sizes n_1 and n_2 less than or equal to 10. The hypothesis $\sigma_1 = \sigma_2$ is rejected if F' is significantly large or small. To test the hypothesis $\sigma_1 = \sigma_2$ at the α-level of significance, use the critical region $F' < F'_{\frac{1}{2}\alpha}$ and $F' > F'_{1-\frac{1}{2}\alpha}$. For a one-sided test $\sigma_1 \leq \sigma_2$ the α-critical region is $F' > F'_{1-\alpha}$.

SUBSTITUTE *F*-RATIO

Sample size for denominator	Cum. prop.	Sample size for numerator								
		2	3	4	5	6	7	8	9	10
2	.005	.0078	.096	.21	.30	.38	.44	.49	.54	.57
	.01	.0157	.136	.26	.38	.46	.53	.59	.64	.68
	.025	.039	.217	.37	.50	.60	.68	.74	.79	.83
	.05	.079	.31	.50	.62	.74	.80	.86	.91	.95
	.95	12.7	19.1	23	26	29	30	32	34	35
	.975	25.5	38.2	52	57	60	62	64	67	68
	.99	63.7	95	116	132	142	153	160	168	174
	.995	127	191	230	250	260	270	280	290	290
3	.005	.0052	.071	.16	.24	.32	.38	.43	.47	.50
	.01	.0105	.100	.20	.30	.37	.43	.49	.53	.57
	.025	.026	.160	.28	.39	.47	.54	.59	.64	.68
	.05	.052	.23	.37	.49	.57	.64	.70	.75	.80
	.95	3.19	4.4	5.0	5.7	6.2	6.6	6.9	7.2	7.4
	.975	4.61	6.3	7.3	8.0	8.7	9.3	9.8	10.2	10.5
	.99	7.37	10	12	13	14	15	15	16	17
	.995	10.4	14	17	18	20	21	22	23	25
4	.005	.0043	.059	.14	.22	.28	.34	.39	.43	.46
	.01	.0086	.084	.18	.26	.33	.39	.44	.48	.52
	.025	.019	.137	.25	.34	.42	.48	.53	.57	.61
	.05	.043	.20	.32	.42	.50	.57	.62	.67	.70
	.95	2.02	2.7	3.1	3.4	3.6	3.8	4.0	4.2	4.4
	.975	2.72	3.5	4.0	4.4	4.7	5.0	5.2	5.4	5.6
	.99	3.83	5.0	5.5	6.0	6.4	6.7	7.0	7.2	7.5
	.995	4.85	6.1	7.0	7.6	8.1	8.5	8.8	9.3	9.6
5	.005	.0039	.054	.13	.20	.26	.32	.36	.40	.44
	.01	.0076	.079	.17	.24	.31	.36	.41	.45	.49
	.025	.018	.124	.23	.32	.38	.44	.49	.53	.57
	.05	.038	.18	.29	.40	.46	.52	.57	.61	.65
	.95	1.61	2.1	2.4	2.6	2.8	2.9	3.0	3.1	3.2
	.975	2.01	2.6	2.9	3.2	3.4	3.6	3.7	3.8	3.9
	.99	2.64	3.4	3.8	4.1	4.3	4.6	4.7	4.9	5.0
	.995	3.36	4.1	4.6	4.9	5.2	5.5	5.7	5.9	6.1
6	.005	.0038	.051	.12	.19	.25	.30	.35	.38	.42
	.01	.0070	.073	.16	.23	.29	.34	.39	.43	.46
	.025	.017	.115	.21	.30	.36	.42	.46	.50	.54
	.05	.035	.16	.27	.36	.43	.49	.54	.58	.61
	.95	1.36	1.8	2.0	2.2	2.3	2.4	2.5	2.6	2.7
	.975	1.67	2.1	2.4	2.6	2.8	2.9	3.0	3.1	3.2
	.99	2.16	2.7	3.0	3.2	3.4	3.6	3.7	3.8	3.9
	.995	2.67	3.1	3.5	3.8	4.0	4.1	4.3	4.5	4.6

SUBSTITUTE *F*-RATIO

Sample size for denominator	Cum. prop.	Sample size for numerator								
		2	3	4	5	6	7	8	9	10
7	.005	.0037	.048	.12	.18	.24	.29	.33	.37	.40
	.01	.0066	.069	.15	.22	.28	.33	.37	.41	.45
	.025	.016	.107	.20	.28	.34	.40	.44	.48	.52
	.05	.032	.15	.26	.35	.41	.47	.51	.55	.59
	.95	1.26	1.6	1.8	1.9	2.0	2.1	2.2	2.3	2.4
	.975	1.48	1.9	2.1	2.3	2.4	2.5	2.6	2.7	2.8
	.99	1.87	2.3	2.6	2.8	2.9	3.0	3.1	3.2	3.3
	.995	2.28	2.7	2.9	2.9	3.3	3.5	3.6	3.7	3.8
8	.005	.0036	.045	.11	.18	.23	.28	.32	.36	.39
	.01	.0063	.065	.14	.21	.27	.32	.36	.40	.43
	.025	.016	.102	.19	.27	.33	.38	.43	.47	.50
	.05	.031	.14	.25	.33	.40	.45	.50	.53	.57
	.95	1.17	1.4	1.6	1.8	1.9	1.9	2.0	2.1	2.1
	.975	1.36	1.7	1.9	2.0	2.2	2.3	2.3	2.4	2.5
	.99	1.69	2.1	2.3	2.4	2.6	2.7	2.8	2.8	2.9
	.995	2.03	2.3	2.6	2.7	2.9	3.0	3.1	3.2	3.3
9	.005	.0035	.042	.11	.17	.22	.27	.31	.35	.38
	.01	.0060	.062	.14	.21	.26	.31	.35	.39	.42
	.025	.015	.098	.18	.26	.32	.37	.42	.46	.49
	.05	.030	.14	.24	.32	.38	.44	.48	.52	.55
	.95	1.10	1.3	1.5	1.6	1.7	1.8	1.9	1.9	2.0
	.975	1.27	1.6	1.8	1.9	2.0	2.1	2.1	2.2	2.3
	.99	1.56	1.9	2.1	2.2	2.3	2.4	2.5	2.6	2.6
	.995	1.87	2.1	2.3	2.5	2.6	2.7	2.8	2.9	3.0
10	.005	.0034	.041	.10	.16	.22	.26	.30	.34	.37
	.01	.0058	.060	.13	.20	.26	.30	.34	.38	.41
	.025	.015	.095	.18	.25	.31	.36	.41	.44	.48
	.05	.029	.13	.23	.31	.37	.43	.47	.51	.54
	.95	1.05	1.3	1.4	1.5	1.6	1.7	1.8	1.8	1.9
	.975	1.21	1.5	1.6	1.8	1.9	1.9	2.0	2.0	2.1
	.99	1.47	1.8	1.9	2.1	2.2	2.2	2.3	2.4	2.4
	.995	1.75	2.0	2.2	2.3	2.4	2.5	2.6	2.6	2.7

VIII.7 ANALYSIS OF VARIANCE BASED ON RANGE

Standard tests of significance in the analysis of variance are often F-tests based on the ratio of a "treatment" mean square to an error mean square s^2. If the treatment means $\bar{x}_t$, $(t = 1, 2, \ldots, k)$, are all calculated from the same number of observations n, a possible alternative criterion is

$$\sqrt{n} \text{ range } \bar{x}_t / s \ . \tag{1}$$

The independence of numerator and denominator may be proved, so that (1) is a studentized range q. In an overall analysis of variance its use would save very little work; however in procedures for ranking treatment means it plays a fundamental role.

For the case of a one-way classification a computationally simple criterion is obtained if s in (1) is replaced by $\frac{\bar{w}}{c}$. The ratio

$$c\sqrt{n} \text{ range } \bar{x}_t / \bar{w} \tag{2}$$

is then distributed approximately as q with degrees of freedom and scale factor c obtained from table (ii). Simpler still, an immediate test can be made with the help of table (i) which gives upper 5% and 1% points of

$$Q = \text{range } X_t / W,$$

where

$$X_t = \sum_{i=1}^{n} x_{ti} \quad \text{and} \quad W = \sum_{t=1}^{k} w_t \ .$$

ANALYSIS OF VARIANCE BASED ON RANGE

(i) UPPER PERCENTAGE POINTS OF Q = RANGE OF GROUP TOTALS/SUM OF GROUP RANGES IN A ONE-WAY CLASSIFICATION INTO k GROUPS OF n OBSERVATIONS

k \ n	2		3		4		5		6		7		8		9		10	
	5%	1%	5%	1%	5%	1%	5%	1%	5%	1%	5%	1%	5%	1%	5%	1%	5%	1%
2	3.5	8.3	1.91	3.2	1.63	2.5	1.54	2.3	1.50	2.2	1.49	2.1	1.49	2.1	1.51	2.1	1.52	2.1
3	2.4	4.4	1.44	2.1	1.26	1.74	1.19	1.61	1.17	1.55	1.17	1.53	1.17	1.53	1.19	1.54	1.20	1.55
4	1.75	2.9	1.14	1.57	1.01	1.33	0.97	1.24	0.95	1.21	0.95	1.20	0.96	1.20	0.97	1.21	0.98	1.22
5	1.40	2.1	0.94	1.25	0.84	1.07	.81	1.01	.80	1.00	.80	0.99	.81	0.99	.82	1.00	.83	1.01
6	1.16	1.68	.80	1.04	.72	0.90	.70	0.86	.69	0.84	.69	.84	.70	.84	.71	0.85	.72	0.86
7	1.00	1.39	.70	0.89	.64	.78	.61	.75	.61	.74	.61	.74	.62	.74	.62	.74	.63	.75
8	0.87	1.18	.62	.78	.57	.69	.55	.66	.55	.65	.55	.66	.56	.66	.56	.67	.57	.67
9	.78	1.03	.56	.69	.51	.62	.50	.59	.50	.59	.50	.59	.50	.59	.51	.60	.52	.61
10	.70	0.91	.51	.62	.47	.56	.46	.54	.45	.53	.45	.53	.46	.54	.47	.55	.47	.55

(ii) SCALE FACTOR, c, AND EQUIVALENT DEGREES OF FREEDOM, ν, APPROPRIATE TO A ONE-WAY CLASSIFICATION INTO k GROUPS OF n OBSERVATIONS

k \ n	2		3		4		5		6		7		8		9		10	
	ν	c	ν	c	ν	c	ν	c	ν	c	ν	c	ν	c	ν	c	ν	c
1	1.00	1.41	1.98	1.91	2.93	2.24	3.83	2.48	4.68	2.67	5.48	2.83	6.25	2.96	6.98	3.08	7.68	3.18
2	1.92	1.28	3.83	1.81	5.69	2.15	7.47	2.40	9.16	2.60	10.8	2.77	12.3	2.91	13.8	3.02	15.1	3.13
3	2.82	1.23	5.66	1.77	8.44	2.12	11.1	2.38	13.6	2.58	16.0	2.75	18.3	2.89	20.5	3.01	22.6	3.11
4	3.71	1.21	7.49	1.75	11.2	2.11	14.7	2.37	18.1	2.57	21.3	2.74	24.4	2.88	27.3	3.00	30.1	3.10
5	4.59	1.19	9.30	1.74	13.9	2.10	18.4	2.36	22.6	2.56	26.6	2.73	30.4	2.87	34.0	2.99	37.5	3.10
6	5.47	1.18	11.1	1.73	16.7	2.09	22.0	2.35	27.0	2.56	31.8	2.73	36.4	2.87	40.8	2.99	45.0	3.09
7	6.35	1.17	12.9	1.73	19.4	2.09	25.6	2.35	31.5	2.55	37.1	2.72	42.5	2.86	47.6	2.99	52.4	3.09
8	7.23	1.17	14.8	1.72	22.1	2.08	29.2	2.35	36.0	2.55	42.4	2.72	48.5	2.86	54.3	2.98	59.9	3.09
9	8.11	1.16	16.6	1.72	24.9	2.08	32.9	2.34	40.4	2.55	47.6	2.72	54.5	2.86	61.1	2.98	67.3	3.09
10	8.99	1.16	18.4	1.72	27.6	2.08	36.5	2.34	44.9	2.55	52.9	2.72	60.6	2.86	67.8	2.98	74.8	3.09
d_n		1.13		1.69		2.06		2.33		2.53		2.70		2.85		2.97		3.08
C.D.	0.88		1.82		2.74		3.62		4.47		5.27		6.03		6.76		7.45	

N.B.: C.D. = constant difference

IX. CORRELATION COEFFICIENT

IX.1 PERCENTAGE POINTS, DISTRIBUTION OF THE CORRELATION COEFFICIENT, WHEN $\rho = 0$

The bivariate normal probability function is given by

$$f(x,y) = \frac{1}{2\pi\sigma_x\sigma_y\sqrt{1-\rho^2}} \exp\left\{-\frac{1}{2(1-\rho^2)}\left[\left(\frac{x-\mu_x}{\sigma_x}\right)^2 - 2\rho\left(\frac{x-\mu_x}{\sigma_x}\right)\left(\frac{y-\mu_y}{\sigma_y}\right) + \left(\frac{y-\mu_y}{\sigma_y}\right)^2\right]\right\},$$

where μ_x = mean of x
μ_y = mean of y
σ_x = standard deviation of x
σ_y = standard deviation of y
ρ = correlation coefficient between x and y.

If (x_i,y_i) $(i = 1, 2, \ldots, n)$ denote a random sample of n ordered observations drawn from a bivariate normal distribution, then an estimate of ρ is given by the sample product-moment correlation coefficient r, given by

$$r = \frac{\sum_i (x_i - \bar{x})(y_i - \bar{y})}{\sqrt{\sum_i (x_i - \bar{x})^2 \cdot \sum_i (y_i - \bar{y})^2}}.$$

The frequency function of r is given by

$$f(r) = \frac{(1-\rho^2)^{\frac{n-1}{2}}}{\pi(n-3)!}(1-r^2)^{\frac{n-4}{2}} \frac{d^{n-2}}{d(r\rho)^{n-2}}\left[\frac{\operatorname{Arccos}(-r\rho)}{\sqrt{1-r^2\rho^2}}\right]$$

which can also be written as

$$f(r) = \frac{(1-\rho^2)^{\frac{n-1}{2}}(1-r^2)^{\frac{n-4}{2}}}{\sqrt{\pi}\,\Gamma\left(\frac{n-1}{2}\right)\Gamma\left(\frac{n-2}{2}\right)} \sum_{i=0}^{\infty} \frac{(2r\rho)^i}{i!}\Gamma^2\left(\frac{n-1+i}{2}\right).$$

In the special case where $\rho = 0$, the frequency function of r becomes

$$f(r) = \frac{\Gamma\left(\frac{n-1}{2}\right)}{\sqrt{\pi}\,\Gamma\left(\frac{n}{2}-1\right)}(1-r^2)^{\frac{n-4}{2}}.$$

Under the transformation

$$r^2 = \frac{t^2}{t^2+\nu},$$

$f(r)$ is transformed into the t-distribution with $\nu = n - 2$ degrees of freedom. This table gives percentage points of the distribution of the correlation coefficient when $\rho = 0$.

PERCENTAGE POINTS, DISTRIBUTION OF THE CORRELATION COEFFICIENT, WHEN $\rho = 0$

$\Pr\{r \le \text{tabular value} \mid \rho = 0\} = 1 - \alpha$

ν	$\alpha =$ 0.05	0.025	0.01	0.005	0.0025	0.0005	ν	$\alpha =$ 0.05	0.025	0.01	0.005	0.0025	0.0005
	$2\alpha =$ 0.1	0.05	0.02	0.01	0.005	0.001		$2\alpha =$ 0.1	0.05	0.02	0.01	0.005	0.001
1	0.9877	0.9^2692	0.9^3507	0.9^3877	0.9^4692	0.9^5877	16	0.400	0.468	0.543	0.590	0.631	0.708
2	.9000	.9500	.9800	$.9^2000$	$.9^2500$	$.9^3000$	17	.389	.456	.529	.575	.616	.693
3	.805	.878	.9343	.9587	.9740	$.9^2114$	18	.378	.444	.516	.561	.602	.679
4	.729	.811	.882	.9172	.9417	.9741	19	.369	.433	.503	.549	.589	.665
5	.669	.754	.833	.875	.9056	.9509	20	.360	.423	.492	.537	.576	.652
6	0.621	0.707	0.789	0.834	0.870	0.9249	25	0.323	0.381	0.445	0.487	0.524	0.597
7	.582	.666	.750	.798	.836	.898	30	.296	.349	.409	.449	.484	.554
8	.549	.632	.715	.765	.805	.872	35	.275	.325	.381	.418	.452	.519
9	.521	.602	.685	.735	.776	.847	40	.257	.304	.358	.393	.425	.490
10	.497	.576	.658	.708	.750	.823	45	.243	.288	.338	.372	.403	.465
11	0.476	0.553	0.634	0.684	0.726	0.801	50	0.231	0.273	0.322	0.354	0.384	0.443
12	.457	.532	.612	.661	.703	.780	60	.211	.250	.295	.325	.352	.408
13	.441	.514	.592	.641	.683	.760	70	.195	.232	.274	.302	.327	.380
14	.426	.497	.574	.623	.664	.742	80	.183	.217	.257	.283	.307	.357
15	.412	.482	.558	.606	.647	.725	90	.173	.205	.242	.267	.290	.338
							100	.164	.195	.230	.254	.276	.321

$\alpha = 1 - F(r \mid \nu, \rho = 0)$ is the upper-tail area of the distribution of r appropriate for use in a single-tail test. For a two-tail test, 2α must be used. If r is calculated from n paired observations, enter the table with $\nu = n - 2$. For partial correlations enter with $\nu = n - k - 2$, where k is the number of variables held constant.

IX.2 CONFIDENCE LIMITS FOR THE POPULATION CORRELATION COEFFICIENT

The cumulative distribution of the correlation coefficient is given by

$$F(r;n,\rho) = \int_{-1}^{r} \frac{(1-\rho^2)^{\frac{n-1}{2}}}{\pi(n-3)!} (1-u^2)^{\frac{n-4}{2}} \frac{d^{n-2}}{d(u\rho)^{n-2}} \left[\frac{\text{Arccos}\,(-u\rho)}{\sqrt{1-u^2\rho^2}}\right] du \ .$$

This table shows graphically the roots ρ_1 and $\rho_2 (\rho_2 > \rho_1)$ of

$$\alpha = F(r;n,\rho_2) \qquad \text{and} \qquad 1 - \alpha = F(r;n,\rho_1)$$

plotted against r for selected sample sizes n for the values $\alpha = 0.025$ and 0.005.

GRAPHS SHOWING CONFIDENCE LIMITS FOR THE POPULATION CORRELATION COEFFICIENT, ρ, GIVEN THE SAMPLE COEFFICIENT, *r*. CONFIDENCE COEFFICIENT, $1 - 2\alpha = 0.95$

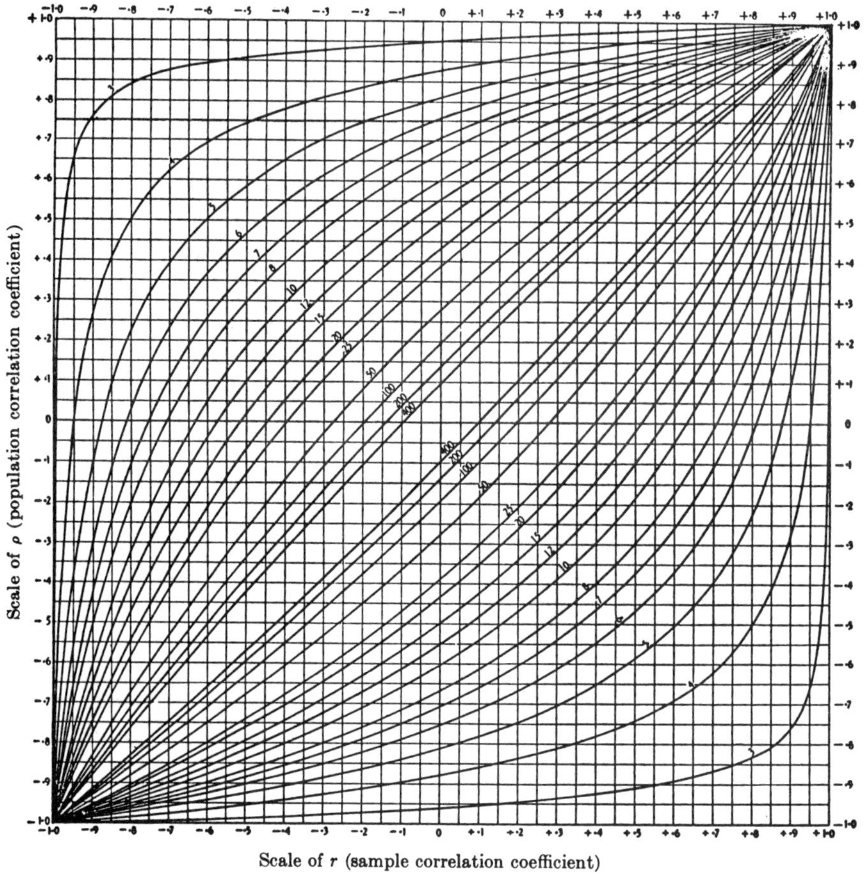

The numbers on the curves indicate sample size. The chart can also be used to determine upper and lower 2.5% significance points for *r*, given ρ.

GRAPHS SHOWING CONFIDENCE LIMITS FOR THE POPULATION CORRELATION COEFFICIENT, ρ, GIVEN THE SAMPLE COEFFICIENT, r. CONFIDENCE COEFFICIENT, $1 - 2\alpha = 0.99$

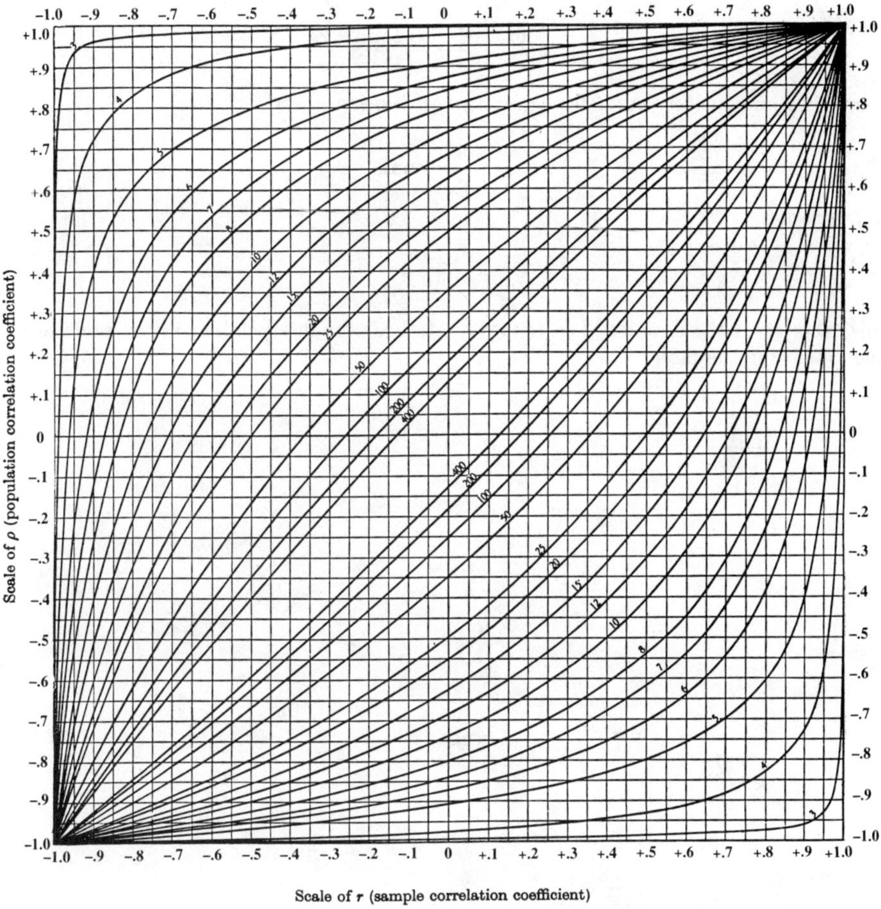

The numbers on the curves indicate sample size. The chart can also be used to determine upper and lower 0.5% significance points for r, given ρ.

IX.3 THE TRANSFORMATION $Z = \tanh^{-1} r$ FOR THE CORRELATION COEFFICIENT

If one introduces the transformation

$$Z = \frac{1}{2}\log_e \frac{1+r}{1-r} = \tanh^{-1} r,$$

then Z is approximately normally distributed with mean

$$\frac{1}{2}\log_e \frac{1+\rho}{1-\rho} = \tanh^{-1} \rho$$

and variance

$$\frac{1}{n-3}.$$

This table gives the function $Z = \tanh^{-1} r$. Methods for interpolation in the table are given following the table.

THE TRANSFORMATION $Z = \tanh^{-1} r$ FOR THE CORRELATION COEFFICIENT

	r (3rd decimal)					Proportional parts, for right side→										r (3rd decimal)					
r	.000	.002	.004	.006	.008	1	2	3	4	5	6	7	8	9	10	.000	.002	.004	.006	.008	r
.00	.0000	.0020	.0040	.0060	.0080	1	3	4	5	7	8	9	11	12	13	.5493	.5520	.5547	.5573	.5600	.50
1	.0100	.0120	.0140	.0160	.0180	1	3	4	5	7	8	10	11	12	14	.5627	.5654	.5682	.5709	.5736	1
2	.0200	.0220	.0240	.0260	.0280	1	3	4	6	7	8	10	11	13	14	.5763	.5791	.5818	.5846	.5874	2
3	.0300	.0320	.0340	.0360	.0380	1	3	4	6	7	8	10	11	13	14	.5901	.5929	.5957	.5985	.6013	3
4	.0400	.0420	.0440	.0460	.0480	1	3	4	6	7	9	10	11	13	14	.6042	.6070	.6098	.6127	.6155	4
.05	.0500	.0520	.0541	.0561	.0581	1	3	4	6	7	9	10	12	13	14	.6184	.6213	.6241	.6270	.6299	.55
6	.0601	.0621	.0641	.0661	.0681	1	3	4	6	7	9	10	12	13	15	.6328	.6358	.6387	.6416	.6446	6
7	.0701	.0721	.0741	.0761	.0782	1	3	4	6	7	9	10	12	14	15	.6475	.6505	.6535	.6565	.6595	7
8	.0802	.0822	.0842	.0862	.0882	2	3	5	6	8	9	11	12	14	15	.6625	.6655	.6685	.6716	.6746	8
9	.0902	.0923	.0943	.0963	.0983	2	3	5	6	8	9	11	12	14	15	.6777	.6807	.6838	.6869	.6900	9
.10	.1003	.1024	.1044	.1064	.1084	2	3	5	6	8	9	11	13	14	16	.6931	.6963	.6994	.7026	.7057	.60
1	.1104	.1125	.1145	.1165	.1186	2	3	5	6	8	10	11	13	14	16	.7089	.7121	.7153	.7185	.7218	1
2	.1206	.1226	.1246	.1267	.1287	2	3	5	7	8	10	11	13	15	16	.7250	.7283	.7315	.7348	.7381	2
3	.1307	.1328	.1348	.1368	.1389	2	3	5	7	8	10	12	13	15	17	.7414	.7447	.7481	.7514	.7548	3
4	.1409	.1430	.1450	.1471	.1491	2	3	5	7	9	10	12	14	15	17	.7582	.7616	.7650	.7684	.7718	4
.15	.1511	.1532	.1552	.1573	.1593	2	4	5	7	9	11	12	14	16	18	.7753	.7788	.7823	.7858	.7893	.65
6	.1614	.1634	.1655	.1676	.1696	2	4	5	7	9	11	13	14	16	18	.7928	.7964	.7999	.8035	.8071	6
7	.1717	.1737	.1758	.1779	.1799	2	4	6	7	9	11	13	15	17	18	.8107	.8144	.8180	.8217	.8254	7
8	.1820	.1841	.1861	.1882	.1903	2	4	6	8	9	11	13	15	17	19	.8291	.8328	.8366	.8404	.8441	8
9	.1923	.1944	.1965	.1986	.2007	2	4	6	8	10	12	14	15	17	19	.8480	.8518	.8556	.8595	.8634	9
.20	.2027	.2048	.2069	.2090	.2111	2	4	6	8	10	12	14	16	18	20	.8673	.8712	.8752	.8792	.8832	.70
1	.2132	.2153	.2174	.2195	.2216	2	4	6	8	10	12	15	16	18	20	.8872	.8912	.8953	.8994	.9035	1
2	.2237	.2258	.2279	.2300	.2321	2	4	6	8	11	13	15	17	19	21	.9076	.9118	.9160	.9202	.9245	2
3	.2342	.2363	.2384	.2405	.2427	2	4	7	9	11	13	15	17	20	22	.9287	.9330	.9373	.9417	.9461	3
4	.2448	.2469	.2490	.2512	.2533	2	4	7	9	11	13	16	18	20	22	.9505	.9549	.9594	.9639	.9684	4
r	.000	.002	.004	.006	.008	1	2	3	4	5	6	7	8	9	10	.000	.002	.004	.006	.008	r
	r (3rd decimal)					←Proportional parts, for left side										r (3rd decimal)					

Interpolation

(1) $0 \le r \le 0.25$: find argument r_0 nearest to r and form $z = z(r_0) + \Delta r$ (where $\Delta r = r - r_0$), e.g. for $r = 0.2042$, $z = 0.2069 + 0.0002 = 0.2071$.

(2) $0.25 \le r \le 0.75$: find argument r_0 nearest to r and form $z = z(r_0) \pm P$, where P is the proportional part for $\Delta r = r - r_0$, e.g. for $r = 0.5146$, $z = 0.5682 + 0.0008 = 0.5690$; for $r = 0.5372$, $z = 0.6013 - 0.0011 = 0.6002$.

(3) $0.75 \le r \le 0.98$: use linear interpolation to get 3-decimal place accuracy.

(4) $0.98 \le r < 1$: form $z = -\frac{1}{2}\log_e (1 - r) + 0.097 + \frac{1}{4}r$, with the help of table of natural logarithms.

THE TRANSFORMATION $Z = \text{TANH}^{-1}\ r$ FOR THE CORRELATION COEFFICIENT

	r (3rd decimal)					Proportional parts, for right side→										*r* (3rd decimal)					
r	.000	.002	.004	.006	.008	1	2	3	4	5	6	7	8	9	10	.000	.002	.004	.006	.008	*r*
.25	.2554	.2575	.2597	.2618	.2640	1	2	3	4	5	6	7	9	10	11	0.973	0.978	0.982	0.987	0.991	.75
6	.2661	.2683	.2704	.2726	.2747	1	2	3	4	5	6	8	9	10	11	0.996	1.001	1.006	1.011	1.015	6
7	.2769	.2790	.2812	.2833	.2855	1	2	3	4	5	6	8	9	10	11	1.020	1.025	1.030	1.035	1.040	7
8	.2877	.2899	.2920	.2942	.2964	1	2	3	4	5	7	8	9	10	11	1.045	1.050	1.056	1.061	1.066	8
9	.2986	.3008	.3029	.3051	.3073	1	2	3	4	5	7	8	9	10	11	1.071	1.077	1.082	1.088	1.093	9
.30	.3095	.3117	.3139	.3161	.3183	1	2	3	4	6	7	8	9	10	11	1.099	1.104	1.110	1.116	1.121	.80
1	.3205	.3228	.3250	.3272	.3294	1	2	3	4	6	7	8	9	10	11	1.127	1.133	1.139	1.145	1.151	1
2	.3316	.3339	.3361	.3383	.3406	1	2	3	4	6	7	8	9	10	11	1.157	1.163	1.169	1.175	1.182	2
3	.3428	.3451	.3473	.3496	.3518	1	2	3	5	6	7	8	9	10	11	1.188	1.195	1.201	1.208	1.214	3
4	.3541	.3564	.3586	.3609	.3632	1	2	3	5	6	7	8	9	10	11	1.221	1.228	1.235	1.242	1.249	4
.35	.3654	.3677	.3700	.3723	.3746	1	2	3	5	6	7	8	9	10	11	1.256	1.263	1.271	1.278	1.286	.85
6	.3769	.3792	.3815	.3838	.3861	1	2	3	5	6	7	8	9	10	12	1.293	1.301	1.309	1.317	1.325	6
7	.3884	.3907	.3931	.3954	.3977	1	2	3	5	6	7	8	9	10	12	1.333	1.341	1.350	1.358	1.367	7
8	.4001	.4024	.4047	.4071	.4094	1	2	4	5	6	7	8	9	11	12	1.376	1.385	1.394	1.403	1.412	8
9	.4118	.4142	.4165	.4189	.4213	1	2	4	5	6	7	8	9	11	12	1.422	1.432	1.442	1.452	1.462	9
.40	.4236	.4260	.4284	.4308	.4332	1	2	4	5	6	7	8	10	11	12	1.472	1.483	1.494	1.505	1.516	.90
1	.4356	.4380	.4404	.4428	.4453	1	2	4	5	6	7	8	10	11	12	1.528	1.539	1.551	1.564	1.576	1
2	.4477	.4501	.4526	.4550	.4574	1	2	4	5	6	7	9	10	11	12	1.589	1.602	1.616	1.630	1.644	2
3	.4599	.4624	.4648	.4673	.4698	1	2	4	5	6	7	9	10	11	12	1.658	1.673	1.689	1.705	1.721	3
4	.4722	.4747	.4772	.4797	.4822	1	2	4	5	6	7	9	10	11	12	1.738	1.756	1.774	1.792	1.812	4
.45	.4847	.4872	.4897	.4922	.4948	1	3	4	5	6	8	9	10	11	13	1.832	1.853	1.874	1.897	1.921	.95
6	.4973	.4999	.5024	.5049	.5075	1	3	4	5	6	8	9	10	11	13	1.946	1.972	2.000	2.029	2.060	6
7	.5101	.5126	.5152	.5178	.5204	1	3	4	5	6	8	9	10	12	13	2.092	2.127	2.165	2.205	2.249	7
8	.5230	.5256	.5282	.5308	.5334	1	3	4	5	7	8	9	10	12	13	2.298	2.351	2.410	2.477	2.555	8
9	.5361	.5387	.5413	.5440	.5466	1	3	4	5	7	8	9	11	12	13	2.647	2.759	2.903	3.106	3.453	9
r	.000	.002	.004	.006	.008	1	2	3	4	5	6	7	8	9	10	.000	.002	.004	.006	.008	*r*
	r (3rd decimal)					←Proportional parts, for left side										*r* (3rd decimal)					

Interpolation

(1) $0 \le r \le 0.25$: find argument r_0 nearest to r and form $z = z(r_0) + \Delta r$ (where $\Delta r = r - r_0$), e.g. for $r = 0.2042$, $z = 0.2069 + 0.0002 = 0.2071$.

(2) $0.25 \le r \le 0.75$: find argument r_0 nearest to r and form $z = z(r_0) \pm P$, where P is the proportional part for $\Delta r = r - r_0$, e.g. for $r = 0.5146$, $z = 0.5682 + 0.0008 = 0.5690$; for $r = 0.5372$, $z = 0.6013 - 0.0011 = 0.6002$.

(3) $0.75 \le r \le 0.98$: use linear interpolation to get 3-decimal place accuracy.

(4) $0.98 \le r < 1$: form $z = -\frac{1}{2}\log_e(1 - r) + 0.097 + \frac{1}{4}r$, with the help of table of natural logarithms.

X. NON-PARAMETRIC STATISTICS

X.1 CRITICAL VALUES FOR THE SIGN TEST

The observations in a random sample of size n from X and those of the same size from Y are paired according to the order of observation: (X_i, Y_i), $i = 1, 2, \ldots, n$. The differences $d_i = X_i - Y_i$ are calculated for each of the n pairs. The null hypothesis is that the difference d_i has a distribution with median zero, i.e., the true proportion of positive (negative) signs is equal to $p = \frac{1}{2}$. Thus the test is whether X and Y have the same median. The probability of x positive (negative) signs is given by the binomial probability function

$$f(x) = f(x; n, p = \tfrac{1}{2}) = \binom{n}{x}\left(\frac{1}{2}\right)^n .$$

This table gives the critical value k such that

$$P(x \leq k) = \sum_{x=0}^{k} \binom{n}{x}\left(\frac{1}{2}\right)^n < \frac{\alpha}{2} .$$

For a one-tailed test with significance level α enter the table in the column headed by 2α.

CRITICAL VALUES FOR THE SIGN TEST

(Two-tail percentage points for the binomial for $p = .5$)

n	1%	5%	10%	25%	n	1%	5%	10%	25%
1					46	13	15	16	18
2					47	14	16	17	19
3				0	48	14	16	17	19
4				0	49	15	17	18	19
5			0	0	50	15	17	18	20
6		0	0	1	51	15	18	19	20
7		0	0	1	52	16	18	19	21
8	0	0	1	1	53	16	18	20	21
9	0	1	1	2	54	17	19	20	22
10	0	1	1	2	55	17	19	20	22
11	0	1	2	3	56	17	20	21	23
12	1	2	2	3	57	18	20	21	23
13	1	2	3	3	58	18	21	22	24
14	1	2	3	4	59	19	21	22	24
15	2	3	3	4	60	19	21	23	25
16	2	3	4	5	61	20	22	23	25
17	2	4	4	5	62	20	22	24	25
18	3	4	5	6	63	20	23	24	26
19	3	4	5	6	64	21	23	24	26
20	3	5	5	6	65	21	24	25	27
21	4	5	6	7	66	22	24	25	27
22	4	5	6	7	67	22	25	26	28
23	4	6	7	8	68	22	25	26	28
24	5	6	7	8	69	23	25	27	29
25	5	7	7	9	70	23	26	27	29
26	6	7	8	9	71	24	26	28	30
27	6	7	8	10	72	24	27	28	30
28	6	8	9	10	73	25	27	28	31
29	7	8	9	10	74	25	28	29	31
30	7	9	10	11	75	25	28	29	32
31	7	9	10	11	76	26	28	30	32
32	8	9	10	12	77	26	29	30	32
33	8	10	11	12	78	27	29	31	33
34	9	10	11	13	79	27	30	31	33
35	9	11	12	13	80	28	30	32	34
36	9	11	12	14	81	28	31	32	34
37	10	12	13	14	82	28	31	33	35
38	10	12	13	14	83	29	32	33	35
39	11	12	13	15	84	29	32	33	36
40	11	13	14	15	85	30	32	34	36
41	11	13	14	16	86	30	33	34	37
42	12	14	15	16	87	31	33	35	37
43	12	14	15	17	88	31	34	35	38
44	13	15	16	17	89	31	34	36	38
45	13	15	16	18	90	32	35	36	39

For values of n larger than 90, approximate values of r may be found by taking the nearest integer less than $(n - 1)/2 - k\sqrt{n+1}$, where k is 1.2879, 0.9800, 0.8224, 0.5752 for the 1, 5, 10, 25% values, respectively.

X.2 CRITICAL VALUES OF T IN THE WILCOXON MATCHED-PAIRS SIGNED-RANKS TEST

Let d_i denote the difference score for any matched pair of a set of n pairs of observations: $d_i = x_i - y_i$. Rank all the d_i's without regard to sign: give the rank of 1 to the smallest d_i, the rank of 2 to the next smallest, etc. After the ranking is completed, affix the sign of the difference to each rank. Let T equal the smaller sum of the like-signed ranks. This table gives approximate 1%, 2%, and 5% points of T for various values of n. The hypothesis tested is that there is no difference between the distributions of x and y. The table is adapted for use with both one-tailed and two-tailed tests.

CRITICAL VALUES OF *T* IN THE WILCOXON MATCHED-PAIRS SIGNED-RANKS TEST

$n = 5(1)50$

One-sided	Two-sided	$n = 5$	$n = 6$	$n = 7$	$n = 8$	$n = 9$	$n = 10$
$P = .05$	$P = .10$	1	2	4	6	8	11
$P = .025$	$P = .05$		1	2	4	6	8
$P = .01$	$P = .02$			0	2	3	5
$P = .005$	$P = .01$				0	2	3
One-sided	**Two-sided**	$n = 11$	$n = 12$	$n = 13$	$n = 14$	$n = 15$	$n = 16$
$P = .05$	$P = .10$	14	17	21	26	30	36
$P = .025$	$P = .05$	11	14	17	21	25	30
$P = .01$	$P = .02$	7	10	13	16	20	24
$P = .005$	$P = .01$	5	7	10	13	16	19
One-sided	**Two-sided**	$n = 17$	$n = 18$	$n = 19$	$n = 20$	$n = 21$	$n = 22$
$P = .05$	$P = .10$	41	47	54	60	68	75
$P = .025$	$P = .05$	35	40	46	52	59	66
$P = .01$	$P = .02$	28	33	38	43	49	56
$P = .005$	$P = .01$	23	28	32	37	43	49
One-sided	**Two-sided**	$n = 23$	$n = 24$	$n = 25$	$n = 26$	$n = 27$	$n = 28$
$P = .05$	$P = .10$	83	92	101	110	120	130
$P = .025$	$P = .05$	73	81	90	98	107	117
$P = .01$	$P = .02$	62	69	77	85	93	102
$P = .005$	$P = .01$	55	61	68	76	84	92
One-sided	**Two-sided**	$n = 29$	$n = 30$	$n = 31$	$n = 32$	$n = 33$	$n = 34$
$P = .05$	$P = .10$	141	152	163	175	188	201
$P = .025$	$P = .05$	127	137	148	159	171	183
$P = .01$	$P = .02$	111	120	130	141	151	162
$P = .005$	$P = .01$	100	109	118	128	138	149
One-sided	**Two-sided**	$n = 35$	$n = 36$	$n = 37$	$n = 38$	$n = 39$	
$P = .05$	$P = .10$	214	228	242	256	271	
$P = .025$	$P = .05$	195	208	222	235	250	
$P = .01$	$P = .02$	174	186	198	211	224	
$P = .005$	$P = .01$	160	171	183	195	208	
One-sided	**Two-sided**	$n = 40$	$n = 41$	$n = 42$	$n = 43$	$n = 44$	$n = 45$
$P = .05$	$P = .10$	287	303	319	336	353	371
$P = .025$	$P = .05$	264	279	295	311	327	344
$P = .01$	$P = .02$	238	252	267	281	297	313
$P = .005$	$P = .01$	221	234	248	262	277	292
One-sided	**Two-sided**	$n = 46$	$n = 47$	$n = 48$	$n = 49$	$n = 50$	
$P = .05$	$P = .10$	389	408	427	446	466	
$P = .025$	$P = .05$	361	379	397	415	434	
$P = .01$	$P = .02$	329	345	362	380	398	
$P = .005$	$P = .01$	307	323	339	356	373	

X.3 PROBABILITIES FOR THE WILCOXON (MANN-WHITNEY) TWO-SAMPLE STATISTIC

Given two samples of size m and n, $m \leq n$, the Mann-Whitney U-Statistic is used to test the hypothesis that the two samples are from populations with the same median. Rank all the observations in ascending order of magnitude. Let T be the sum of the ranks assigned to the sample of size m. Then U is defined as

$$U = mn + \frac{m(m+1)}{2} - T .$$

This table is used to determine the exact probability associated with the occurrence under the null hypothesis of any U as extreme as an observed value of U.

The probabilities given in this table are one-tailed. For a two-tailed test, the value of p given in the table should be doubled. The table is made up of six separate subtables, one for each value of n.

PROBABILITIES ASSOCIATED WITH VALUES AS SMALL AS OBSERVED VALUES OF U IN THE MANN-WHITNEY TEST

$n = 3$

U \ m	1	2	3
0	.250	.100	.050
1	.500	.200	.100
2	.750	.400	.200
3		.600	.350
4			.500
5			.650

$n = 4$

U \ m	1	2	3	4
0	.200	.067	.028	.014
1	.400	.133	.057	.029
2	.600	.267	.114	.057
3		.400	.200	.100
4		.600	.314	.171
5			.429	.243
6			.571	.343
7				.443
8				.557

$n = 5$

U \ m	1	2	3	4	5
0	.167	.047	.018	.008	.004
1	.333	.095	.036	.016	.008
2	.500	.190	.071	.032	.016
3	.667	.286	.125	.056	.028
4		.429	.196	.095	.048
5		.571	.286	.143	.075
6			.393	.206	.111
7			.500	.278	.155
8			.607	.365	.210
9				.452	.274
10				.548	.345
11					.421
12					.500
13					.579

$n = 6$

U \ m	1	2	3	4	5	6
0	.143	.036	.012	.005	.002	.001
1	.286	.071	.024	.010	.004	.002
2	.428	.143	.048	.019	.009	.004
3	.571	.214	.083	.033	.015	.008
4		.321	.131	.057	.026	.013
5		.429	.190	.086	.041	.021
6		.571	.274	.129	.063	.032
7			.357	.176	.089	.047
8			.452	.238	.123	.066
9			.548	.305	.165	.090
10				.381	.214	.120
11				.457	.268	.155
12				.545	.331	.197
13					.396	.242
14					.465	.294
15					.535	.350
16						.409
17						.469
18						.531

PROBABILITIES ASSOCIATED WITH VALUES AS SMALL AS OBSERVED VALUES OF *U* IN THE MANN-WHITNEY TEST

$n = 7$

U \ m	1	2	3	4	5	6	7
0	.125	.028	.008	.003	.001	.001	.000
1	.250	.056	.017	.006	.003	.001	.001
2	.375	.111	.033	.012	.005	.002	.001
3	.500	.167	.058	.021	.009	.004	.002
4	.625	.250	.092	.036	.015	.007	.003
5		.333	.133	.055	.024	.011	.006
6		.444	.192	.082	.037	.017	.009
7		.556	.258	.115	.053	.026	.013
8			.333	.158	.074	.037	.019
9			.417	.206	.101	.051	.027
10			.500	.264	.134	.069	.036
11			.583	.324	.172	.090	.049
12				.394	.216	.117	.064
13				.464	.265	.147	.082
14				.538	.319	.183	.104
15					.378	.223	.130
16					.438	.267	.159
17					.500	.314	.191
18					.562	.365	.228
19						.418	.267
20						.473	.310
21						.527	.355
22							.402
23							.451
24							.500
25							.549

PROBABILITIES ASSOCIATED WITH VALUES AS SMALL AS OBSERVED VALUES OF U IN THE MANN-WHITNEY TEST

$n = 8$

U \ m	1	2	3	4	5	6	7	8	t	Normal
0	.111	.022	.006	.002	.001	.000	.000	.000	3.308	.001
1	.222	.044	.012	.004	.002	.001	.000	.000	3.203	.001
2	.333	.089	.024	.008	.003	.001	.001	.000	3.098	.001
3	.444	.133	.042	.014	.005	.002	.001	.001	2.993	.001
4	.556	.200	.067	.024	.009	.004	.002	.001	2.888	.002
5		.267	.097	.036	.015	.006	.003	.001	2.783	.003
6		.356	.139	.055	.023	.010	.005	.002	2.678	.004
7		.444	.188	.077	.033	.015	.007	.003	2.573	.005
8		.556	.248	.107	.047	.021	.010	.005	2.468	.007
9			.315	.141	.064	.030	.014	.007	2.363	.009
10			.387	.184	.085	.041	.020	.010	2.258	.012
11			.461	.230	.111	.054	.027	.014	2.153	.016
12			.539	.285	.142	.071	.036	.019	2.048	.020
13				.341	.177	.091	.047	.025	1.943	.026
14				.404	.217	.114	.060	.032	1.838	.033
15				.467	.262	.141	.076	.041	1.733	.041
16				.533	.311	.172	.095	.052	1.628	.052
17					.362	.207	.116	.065	1.523	.064
18					.416	.245	.140	.080	1.418	.078
19					.472	.286	.168	.097	1.313	.094
20					.528	.331	.198	.117	1.208	.113
21						.377	.232	.139	1.102	.135
22						.426	.268	.164	.998	.159
23						.475	.306	.191	.893	.185
24						.525	.347	.221	.788	.215
25							.389	.253	.683	.247
26							.433	.287	.578	.282
27							.478	.323	.473	.318
28							.522	.360	.368	.356
29								.399	.263	.396
30								.439	.158	.437
31								.480	.052	.481
32								.520		

X.4 CRITICAL VALUES OF *U* IN THE WILCOXON (MANN-WHITNEY) TWO-SAMPLE STATISTIC

This table gives critical values of U for significance levels 0.001, 0.005, 0.01, 0.025, 0.05 and 0.10 for a one-tailed test. For a two-tailed test, the significance levels are 0.002, 0.01, 0.02, 0.05, 0.10 and 0.20. If an observed U is equal to or less than the tabular value, the null hypothesis may be rejected at the level of significance indicated at the head of that table.

CRITICAL VALUES OF U IN THE MANN-WHITNEY TEST

Critical Values of U for the .10 Level of Significance

m \ n	1	2	3	4	5	6	7	8	9	10	11	12	13	14	15	16	17	18	19	20
1									0	0	0	0	0	0	0	0	0	0	1	1
2			0	0	1	1	1	2	2	3	3	4	4	4	5	5	6	6	7	7
3		0	1	1	2	3	4	5	5	6	7	8	9	10	10	11	12	13	14	15
4		0	1	3	4	5	6	7	9	10	11	12	13	15	16	17	18	20	21	22
5		1	2	4	5	7	8	10	12	13	15	17	18	20	22	23	25	27	28	30
6		1	3	5	7	9	11	13	15	17	19	21	23	25	27	29	31	34	36	38
7		1	4	6	8	11	13	16	18	21	23	26	28	31	33	36	38	41	43	46
8		2	5	7	10	13	16	19	22	24	27	30	33	36	39	42	45	48	51	54
9	0	2	5	9	12	15	18	22	25	28	31	35	38	41	45	48	52	55	58	62
10	0	3	6	10	13	17	21	24	28	32	36	39	43	47	51	54	58	62	66	70
11	0	3	7	11	15	19	23	27	31	36	40	44	48	52	57	61	65	69	73	78
12	0	4	8	12	17	21	26	30	35	39	44	49	53	58	63	67	72	77	81	86
13	0	4	9	13	18	23	28	33	38	43	48	53	58	63	68	74	79	84	89	94
14	0	4	10	15	20	25	31	36	41	47	52	58	63	69	74	80	85	91	97	102
15	0	5	10	16	22	27	33	39	45	51	57	63	68	74	80	86	92	98	104	110
16	0	5	11	17	23	29	36	42	48	54	61	67	74	80	86	93	99	106	112	119
17	0	6	12	18	25	31	38	45	52	58	65	72	79	85	92	99	106	113	120	127
18	0	6	13	20	27	34	41	48	55	62	69	77	84	91	98	106	113	120	128	135
19	1	7	14	21	28	36	43	51	58	66	73	81	89	97	104	112	120	128	135	143
20	1	7	15	22	30	38	46	54	62	70	78	86	94	102	110	119	127	135	143	151

Critical Values of U for the .05 Level of Significance

m \ n	1	2	3	4	5	6	7	8	9	10	11	12	13	14	15	16	17	18	19	20
1																			0	0
2					0	0	0	1	1	1	1	2	2	2	3	3	3	4	4	4
3			0	0	1	2	2	3	3	4	5	5	6	7	7	8	9	9	10	11
4			0	1	2	3	4	5	6	7	8	9	10	11	12	14	15	16	17	18
5		0	1	2	4	5	6	8	9	11	12	13	15	16	18	19	20	22	23	25
6		0	2	3	5	7	8	10	12	14	16	17	19	21	23	25	26	28	30	32
7		0	2	4	6	8	11	13	15	17	19	21	24	26	28	30	33	35	37	39
8		1	3	5	8	10	13	15	18	20	23	26	28	31	33	36	39	41	44	47
9		1	3	6	9	12	15	18	21	24	27	30	33	36	39	42	45	48	51	54
10		1	4	7	11	14	17	20	24	27	31	34	37	41	44	48	51	55	58	62
11		1	5	8	12	16	19	23	27	31	34	38	42	46	50	54	57	61	65	69
12		2	5	9	13	17	21	26	30	34	38	42	47	51	55	60	64	68	72	77
13		2	6	10	15	19	24	28	33	37	42	47	51	56	61	65	70	75	80	84
14		2	7	11	16	21	26	31	36	41	46	51	56	61	66	71	77	82	87	92
15		3	7	12	18	23	28	33	39	44	50	55	61	66	72	77	83	88	94	100
16		3	8	14	19	25	30	36	42	48	54	60	65	71	77	83	89	95	101	107
17		3	9	15	20	26	33	39	45	51	57	64	70	77	83	89	96	102	109	115
18		4	9	16	22	28	35	41	48	55	61	68	75	82	88	95	102	109	116	123
19	0	4	10	17	23	30	37	44	51	58	65	72	80	87	94	101	109	116	123	130
20	0	4	11	18	25	32	39	47	54	62	69	77	84	92	100	107	115	123	130	138

CRITICAL VALUES OF U IN THE MANN-WHITNEY TEST

Critical Values of U for the .025 Level of Significance

m \ n	1	2	3	4	5	6	7	8	9	10	11	12	13	14	15	16	17	18	19	20
1																				
2								0	0	0	0	1	1	1	1	1	2	2	2	2
3					0	1	1	2	2	3	3	4	4	5	5	6	6	7	7	8
4				0	1	2	3	4	4	5	6	7	8	9	10	11	11	12	13	13
5			0	1	2	3	5	6	7	8	9	11	12	13	14	15	17	18	19	20
6			1	2	3	5	6	8	10	11	13	14	16	17	19	21	22	24	25	27
7			1	3	5	6	8	10	12	14	16	18	20	22	24	26	28	30	32	34
8		0	2	4	6	8	10	13	15	17	19	22	24	26	29	31	34	36	38	41
9		0	2	4	7	10	12	15	17	20	23	26	28	31	34	37	39	42	45	48
10		0	3	5	8	11	14	17	20	23	26	29	33	36	39	42	45	48	52	55
11		0	3	6	9	13	16	19	23	26	30	33	37	40	44	47	51	55	58	62
12		1	4	7	11	14	18	22	26	29	33	37	41	45	49	53	57	61	65	69
13		1	4	8	12	16	20	24	28	33	37	41	45	50	54	59	63	67	72	76
14		1	5	9	13	17	22	26	31	36	40	45	50	55	59	64	67	74	78	83
15		1	5	10	14	19	24	29	34	39	44	49	54	59	64	70	75	80	85	90
16		1	6	11	15	21	26	31	37	42	47	53	59	64	70	75	81	86	92	98
17		2	6	11	17	22	28	34	39	45	51	57	63	67	75	81	87	93	99	105
18		2	7	12	18	24	30	36	42	48	55	61	67	74	80	86	93	99	106	112
19		2	7	13	19	25	32	38	45	52	58	65	72	78	85	92	99	106	113	119
20		2	8	13	20	27	34	41	48	55	62	69	76	83	90	98	105	112	119	127

Critical Values of U for the .01 Level of Significance

m \ n	1	2	3	4	5	6	7	8	9	10	11	12	13	14	15	16	17	18	19	20
1																				
2													0	0	0	0	0	0	1	1
3							0	0	1	1	1	2	2	2	3	3	4	4	4	5
4					0	1	1	2	3	3	4	5	5	6	7	7	8	9	9	10
5				0	1	2	3	4	5	6	7	8	9	10	11	12	13	14	15	16
6				1	2	3	4	6	7	8	9	11	12	13	15	16	18	19	20	22
7			0	1	3	4	6	7	9	11	12	14	16	17	19	21	23	24	26	28
8			0	2	4	6	7	9	11	13	15	17	20	22	24	26	28	30	32	34
9			1	3	5	7	9	11	14	16	18	21	23	26	28	31	33	36	38	40
10			1	3	6	8	11	13	16	19	22	24	27	30	33	36	38	41	44	47
11			1	4	7	9	12	15	18	22	25	28	31	34	37	41	44	47	50	53
12			2	5	8	11	14	17	21	24	28	31	35	38	42	46	49	53	56	60
13		0	2	5	9	12	16	20	23	27	31	35	39	43	47	51	55	59	63	67
14		0	2	6	10	13	17	22	26	30	34	38	43	47	51	56	60	65	69	73
15		0	3	7	11	15	19	24	28	33	37	42	47	51	56	61	66	70	75	80
16		0	3	7	12	16	21	26	31	36	41	46	51	56	61	66	71	76	82	87
17		0	4	8	13	18	23	28	33	38	44	49	55	60	66	71	77	82	88	93
18		0	4	9	14	19	24	30	36	41	47	53	59	65	70	76	82	88	94	100
19		1	4	9	15	20	26	32	38	44	50	56	63	69	75	82	88	94	101	107
20		1	5	10	16	22	28	34	40	47	53	60	67	73	80	87	93	100	107	114

CRITICAL VALUES OF *U* IN THE MANN-WHITNEY TEST

Critical Values of *U* for the .005 Level of Significance

m \ n	1	2	3	4	5	6	7	8	9	10	11	12	13	14	15	16	17	18	19	20
1																				
2																			0	0
3									0	0	0	1	1	1	2	2	2	2	3	3
4						0	0	1	1	2	2	3	3	4	5	5	6	6	7	8
5					0	1	1	2	3	4	5	6	7	7	8	9	10	11	12	13
6				0	1	2	3	4	5	6	7	9	10	11	12	13	15	16	17	18
7				0	1	3	4	6	7	9	10	12	13	15	16	18	19	21	22	24
8				1	2	4	6	7	9	11	13	15	17	18	20	22	24	26	28	30
9			0	1	3	5	7	9	11	13	16	18	20	22	24	27	29	31	33	36
10			0	2	4	6	9	11	13	16	18	21	24	26	29	31	34	37	39	42
11			0	2	5	7	10	13	16	18	21	24	27	30	33	36	39	42	45	48
12			1	3	6	9	12	15	18	21	24	27	31	34	37	41	44	47	51	54
13			1	3	7	10	13	17	20	24	27	31	34	38	42	45	49	53	56	60
14			1	4	7	11	15	18	22	26	30	34	38	42	46	50	54	58	63	67
15			2	5	8	12	16	20	24	29	33	37	42	46	51	55	60	64	69	73
16			2	5	9	13	18	22	27	31	36	41	45	50	55	60	65	70	74	79
17			2	6	10	15	19	24	29	34	39	44	49	54	60	65	70	75	81	86
18			2	6	11	16	21	26	31	37	42	47	53	58	64	70	75	81	87	92
19		0	3	7	12	17	22	28	33	39	45	51	56	63	69	74	81	87	93	99
20		0	3	8	13	18	24	30	36	42	48	54	60	67	73	79	86	92	99	105

Critical Values of *U* for the .001 Level of Significance

m \ n	1	2	3	4	5	6	7	8	9	10	11	12	13	14	15	16	17	18	19	20
1																				
2																				
3																	0	0	0	0
4										0	0	0	1	1	1	2	2	3	3	3
5								0	1	1	2	2	3	3	4	5	5	6	7	7
6							0	1	2	3	4	4	5	6	7	8	9	10	11	12
7						0	1	2	3	5	6	7	8	9	10	11	13	14	15	16
8					0	1	2	4	5	6	8	9	11	12	14	15	17	18	20	21
9					1	2	3	5	7	8	10	12	14	15	17	19	21	23	25	26
10				0	1	3	5	6	8	10	12	14	17	19	21	23	25	27	29	32
11				0	2	4	6	8	10	12	15	17	20	22	24	27	29	32	34	37
12				0	2	4	7	9	12	14	17	20	23	25	28	31	34	37	40	42
13				1	3	5	8	11	14	17	20	23	26	29	32	35	38	42	45	48
14				1	3	6	9	12	15	19	22	25	29	32	36	39	43	46	50	54
15				1	4	7	10	14	17	21	24	28	32	36	40	43	47	51	55	59
16				2	5	8	11	15	19	23	27	31	35	39	43	48	52	56	60	65
17			0	2	5	9	13	17	21	25	29	34	38	43	47	52	57	61	66	70
18			0	3	6	10	14	18	23	27	32	37	42	46	51	56	61	66	71	76
19			0	3	7	11	15	20	25	29	34	40	45	50	55	60	66	71	77	82
20			0	3	7	12	16	21	26	32	37	42	48	54	59	65	70	76	82	88

X.5 CRITICAL VALUES FOR THE WILCOXON RANK SUM TEST

Given two samples of size m and n, $m \leq n$, the Wilcoxon rank sum test is used to test the hypothesis that the two samples are from populations with the same mean. Rank all the observations in ascending order of magnitude. Assigned tied values the average rank. Let T be the sum of the ranks assigned to the sample of size m. This table gives, for specified m and n, the critical upper and lower rank sums, T_u and T_l, respectively, associated with specific probabilities. If $T \geq T_u$, then the mean of the smaller sample is said to be significantly larger than the mean of the other sample at the specified probability level. If $T \leq T_l$, then the mean of the smaller sample is said to be significantly smaller than the mean of the other sample at the specified probability level. If $T_l \leq T \leq T_u$, then there is not sufficient evidence at the specified probability level to say that the means of the two samples differ.

The relationship between T and the Mann-Whitney U-Statistic is given by

$$U = mn + \frac{m(m+1)}{2} - T\,.$$

CRITICAL VALUES FOR THE WILCOXON RANK SUM TEST

$m = 3(1)25$ and $n = m(1)m + 25$
$P = .05$ one-sided; $P = .10$ two-sided

n	$m = 3$	$m = 4$	$m = 5$	$m = 6$	$m = 7$	$m = 8$	$m = 9$	$m = 10$	$m = 11$	$m = 12$	$m = 13$	$m = 14$
$n = m$	6,15	12,24	19,36	28,50	39,66	52,84	66,105	83,127	101,152	121,179	143,208	167,239
$n = m + 1$	7,17	13,27	20,40	30,54	41,71	54,90	69,111	86,134	105,159	125,187	148,216	172,248
$n = m + 2$	7,20	14,30	22,43	32,58	43,76	57,95	72,117	89,141	109,166	129,195	152,225	177,257
$n = m + 3$	8,22	15,33	24,46	33,63	46,80	60,100	75,123	93,147	112,174	134,202	157,233	182,266
$n = m + 4$	9,24	16,36	25,50	35,67	48,85	62,106	78,129	96,154	116,181	138,210	162,241	187,275
$n = m + 5$	9,27	17,39	26,54	37,71	50,90	65,111	81,135	100,160	120,188	142,218	166,250	192,284
$n = m + 6$	10,29	18,42	27,58	39,75	52,95	67,117	84,141	103,167	124,195	147,225	171,258	197,293
$n = m + 7$	11,31	19,45	29,61	41,79	54,100	70,122	87,147	107,173	128,202	151,233	176,266	203,301
$n = m + 8$	11,34	20,48	30,65	42,84	57,104	73,127	90,153	110,180	132,209	155,241	181,274	208,310
$n = m + 9$	12,36	21,51	32,68	44,88	59,109	75,133	93,159	114,186	136,216	159,249	185,283	213,319
$n = m + 10$	13,38	22,54	33,72	46,92	61,114	78,138	96,165	117,193	139,224	164,256	190,291	218,328
$n = m + 11$	13,41	23,57	34,76	48,96	63,119	80,144	100,170	120,200	143,231	168,264	195,299	223,337
$n = m + 12$	14,43	24,60	36,79	50,100	65,124	83,149	103,176	124,206	147,238	172,272	199,308	228,346
$n = m + 13$	15,45	25,63	37,83	52,104	68,128	86,154	106,182	127,213	151,245	177,279	204,316	234,354
$n = m + 14$	15,48	26,66	39,86	53,109	70,133	88,160	109,188	131,219	155,252	181,287	209,324	239,363
$n = m + 15$	16,50	27,69	40,90	55,113	72,138	91,165	112,194	134,226	159,259	185,295	214,332	244,372
$n = m + 16$	17,52	28,72	42,93	57,117	74,143	94,170	115,200	138,232	163,266	190,302	218,341	249,381
$n = m + 17$	17,55	29,75	43,97	59,121	77,147	96,176	118,206	141,239	167,273	194,310	223,349	254,390
$n = m + 18$	18,57	30,78	44,101	61,125	79,152	99,181	121,212	145,245	171,280	198,318	228,357	260,398
$n = m + 19$	19,59	31,81	46,104	62,130	81,157	102,186	124,218	148,252	175,287	203,325	233,365	265,407
$n = m + 20$	19,62	32,84	47,108	64,134	83,162	104,192	127,224	152,258	178,295	207,333	237,374	270,416
$n = m + 21$	20,64	33,87	49,111	66,138	86,166	107,197	130,230	155,265	182,302	211,341	242,382	275,425
$n = m + 22$	21,66	34,90	50,115	68,142	88,171	109,203	133,236	159,271	186,309	216,348	247,390	280,434
$n = m + 23$	21,69	35,93	52,118	70,146	90,176	112,208	136,242	162,278	190,316	220,356	252,398	285,443
$n = m + 24$	22,71	37,95	53,122	72,150	92,181	115,213	139,248	166,284	194,323	224,364	257,406	291,451
$n = m + 25$	23,73	38,98	54,126	73,155	94,186	117,219	142,254	169,291	198,330	229,371	261,415	296,460

$m = 3(1)25$ and $n = m(1)m + 25$
$P = .05$ one-sided; $P = .10$ two-sided

n	$m = 15$	$m = 16$	$m = 17$	$m = 18$	$m = 19$	$m = 20$	$m = 21$	$m = 22$	$m = 23$	$m = 24$	$m = 25$
$n = m$	192,273	220,308	249,346	280,386	314,427	349,471	386,517	424,566	465,616	508,668	552,723
$n = m + 1$	198,282	226,318	256,356	287,397	321,439	356,484	394,530	433,579	474,630	517,683	562,738
$n = m + 2$	203,292	232,328	262,367	294,408	328,451	364,496	402,543	442,592	483,644	527,697	572.753
$n = m + 3$	209,301	238,338	268,378	301,419	336,462	372,508	410,556	450,606	492,658	536,712	582,768
$n = m + 4$	215,310	244,348	275,388	308,430	343,474	380,520	418,569	459,619	501,672	546,726	592,783
$n = m + 5$	220,320	250,358	281,399	315,441	350,486	387,533	427,581	468,632	511,685	555,741	602,798
$n = m + 6$	226,329	256,368	288,409	322,452	358,497	395,545	435,594	476,646	520,699	565,755	612,813
$n = m + 7$	231,339	262,378	294,420	329,463	365,509	403,557	443,607	485,659	529,713	574,770	622,828
$n = m + 8$	237,348	268,388	301,430	336,474	372,521	411,569	451,620	494,672	538,727	584,784	632,843
$n = m + 9$	242,358	274,398	307,441	342,486	380,532	419,581	459,633	502,686	547,741	594,798	642,858
$n = m + 10$	248,367	280,408	314,451	349,497	387,544	426,594	468,645	511,699	556,755	603,813	652,873
$n = m + 11$	254,376	286,418	320,462	356,508	394,556	434,606	476,658	520,712	565,769	613,827	662,888
$n = m + 12$	259,386	292,428	327,472	363,519	402,567	442,618	484,671	528,726	574,783	622,842	672,903
$n = m + 13$	265,395	298,438	333,483	370,530	409,579	450,630	492,684	537,739	584,796	632,856	682,918
$n = m + 14$	270,405	304,448	340,493	377,541	416,591	458,642	501,696	546,752	593,810	642,870	692,933
$n = m + 15$	276,414	310,458	346,504	384,552	424,602	465,655	509,709	554,766	602,824	651,885	702,948
$n = m + 16$	282,423	316,468	353,514	391,563	431,614	473,667	517,722	563,779	611,838	661,899	712,963
$n = m + 17$	287,433	322,478	359,525	398,574	438,626	481,679	526,734	572,792	620,852	670,914	723,977
$n = m + 18$	293,442	328,488	366,535	405,585	446,637	489,691	534,747	581,805	629,866	680,928	733,992
$n = m + 19$	299,451	334,498	372,546	412,596	453,649	497,703	542,760	589,819	639,879	690,942	743,1007
$n = m + 20$	304,461	340,508	379,556	419,607	461,660	505,715	550,773	598,832	648,893	699,957	753,1022
$n = m + 21$	310,470	347,517	385,568	426,618	468,672	512,728	559,785	607,845	657,907	709,971	763,1037
$n = m + 22$	315,480	353,527	392,577	433,629	475,684	520,740	567,798	615,859	666,921	718,986	773,1052
$n = m + 23$	321,489	359,537	398,588	439,641	483,695	528,752	575,811	624,872	675,935	728,1000	783,1067
$n = m + 24$	327,498	365,547	405,598	446,652	490,707	536,764	583,824	633,885	684,949	738,1014	793,1082
$n = m + 25$	332,508	371,557	411,609	453,663	498,718	544,776	592,836	642,898	694,962	747,1029	803,1097

CRITICAL VALUES FOR THE WILCOXON RANK SUM TEST

$m = 3(1)25$ and $n = m(1)m + 25$
$P = .025$ one-sided; $P = .05$ two-sided

n	$m = 3$	$m = 4$	$m = 5$	$m = 6$	$m = 7$	$m = 8$	$m = 9$	$m = 10$	$m = 11$	$m = 12$	$m = 13$	$m = 14$
$n = m$	5,16	11,25	18,37	26,52	37,68	49,87	63,108	79,131	96,157	116,184	137,214	160,246
$n = m + 1$	6,18	12,28	19,41	28,56	39,73	51,93	66,114	82,138	100,164	120,192	141,223	165,255
$n = m + 2$	6,21	12,32	20,45	29,61	41,78	54,98	68,121	85,145	103,172	124,200	146,231	170,264
$n = m + 3$	7,23	13,35	21,49	31,65	43,83	56,104	71,127	88,152	107,179	128,208	150,240	174,274
$n = m + 4$	7,26	14,38	22,53	32,70	45,88	58,110	74,133	91,159	110,187	131,217	154,249	179,283
$n = m + 5$	8,28	15,41	24,56	34,74	46,94	61,115	77,139	94,166	114,194	135,225	159,257	184,292
$n = m + 6$	8,31	16,44	25,60	36,78	48,99	63,121	79,146	97,173	118,201	139,233	163,266	189,301
$n = m + 7$	9,33	17,47	26,64	37,83	50,104	65,127	82,152	101,179	121,209	143,241	168,274	194,310
$n = m + 8$	10,35	17,51	27,68	39,87	52,109	68,132	85,158	104,186	125,216	147,249	172,283	198,320
$n = m + 9$	10,38	18,54	29,71	41,91	54,114	70,138	88,164	107,193	128,224	151,257	176,292	203,329
$n = m + 10$	11,40	19,57	30,75	42,96	56,119	72,144	90,171	110,200	132,231	155,265	181,300	208,338
$n = m + 11$	11,43	20,60	31,79	44,100	58,124	75,149	93,177	113,207	135,239	159,273	185,309	213,347
$n = m + 12$	12,45	21,63	32,83	45,105	60,129	77,155	96,183	117,213	139,246	163,281	190,317	218,356
$n = m + 13$	12,48	22,66	33,87	47,109	62,134	80,160	99,189	120,220	143,253	167,289	194,326	222,366
$n = m + 14$	13,50	23,69	35,90	49,113	64,139	82,166	101,196	123,227	146,261	171,297	198,335	227,375
$n = m + 15$	13,53	24,72	36,94	50,118	66,144	84,172	104,202	126,234	150,268	175,305	203,343	232,384
$n = m + 16$	14,55	24,76	37,98	52,122	68,149	87,177	107,208	129,241	153,276	179,313	207,352	237,393
$n = m + 17$	14,58	25,79	38,102	53,127	70,154	89,183	110,214	132,248	157,283	183,321	212,360	242,402
$n = m + 18$	15,60	26,82	40,105	55,131	72,159	92,188	113,220	136,254	161,290	187,329	216,369	247,411
$n = m + 19$	15,63	27,85	41,109	57,135	74,164	94,194	115,227	139,261	164,298	191,337	221,377	252,420
$n = m + 20$	16,65	28,88	42,113	58,140	76,169	96,200	118,233	142,268	168,305	195,345	225,386	256,430
$n = m + 21$	16,68	29,91	43,117	60,144	78,174	99,205	121,239	145,275	171,313	199,353	229,395	261,439
$n = m + 22$	17,70	30,94	45,120	61,149	80,179	101,211	124,245	148,282	175,320	203,361	234,403	266,448
$n = m + 23$	17,73	31,97	46,124	63,153	82,184	103,217	127,251	152,288	179,327	207,369	238,412	271,457
$n = m + 24$	18,75	31,101	47,128	65,157	84,189	106,222	129,258	155,295	182,335	211,377	243,420	276,466
$n = m + 25$	18,78	32,104	48,132	66,162	86,194	108,228	132,264	158,302	186,342	216,384	247,429	281,475

$m = 3(1)25$ and $n = m(1)m + 25$
$P = .025$ one-sided; $P = .05$ two-sided

n	$m = 15$	$m = 16$	$m = 17$	$m = 18$	$m = 19$	$m = 20$	$m = 21$	$m = 22$	$m = 23$	$m = 24$	$m = 25$
$n = m$	185,280	212,316	240,355	271,395	303,438	337,483	373,530	411,579	451,630	493,683	536,739
$n = m + 1$	190,290	217,327	246,366	277,407	310,450	345,495	381,543	419,593	460,644	502,698	546,754
$n = m + 2$	195,300	223,337	252,377	284,418	317,462	352,508	389,556	428,606	468,659	511,713	555,770
$n = m + 3$	201,309	229,347	258,388	290,430	324,474	359,521	397,569	436,620	477,673	520,728	565,785
$n = m + 4$	206,319	234,358	264,399	297,441	331,486	367,533	404,583	444,634	486,687	529,743	574,801
$n = m + 5$	211,329	240,368	271,409	303,453	338,498	374,546	412,596	452,648	494,702	538,758	584,816
$n = m + 6$	216,339	245,379	277,420	310,464	345,510	381,559	420,609	460,662	503,716	547,773	593,832
$n = m + 7$	221,349	251,389	283,431	316,476	351,523	389,571	428,622	469,675	512,730	556,788	603,847
$n = m + 8$	227,358	257,399	289,442	323,487	358,535	396,584	436,635	477,689	520,745	565,803	612,863
$n = m + 9$	232,368	262,410	295,453	329,499	365,547	403,597	443,649	485,703	529,759	575,817	622,878
$n = m + 10$	237,378	268,420	301,464	336,510	372,559	411,609	451,662	493,717	538,773	584,832	632,893
$n = m + 11$	242,388	274,430	307,475	342,522	379,571	418,622	459,675	502,730	546,788	593,847	641,909
$n = m + 12$	248,397	279,441	313,486	349,533	386,583	426,634	467,688	510,744	555,802	602,862	651,924
$n = m + 13$	253,407	285,451	319,497	355,545	393,595	433,647	475,701	518,758	564,816	611,877	660,940
$n = m + 14$	258,417	291,461	325,508	362,556	400,607	440,660	482,715	526,772	572,831	620,892	670,955
$n = m + 15$	263,427	296,472	331,519	368,568	407,619	448,672	490,728	535,785	581,845	629,907	679,971
$n = m + 16$	269,436	302,482	338,529	375,579	414,631	455,685	498,741	543,799	590,859	638,922	689,986
$n = m + 17$	274,446	308,492	344,540	381,591	421,643	463,697	506,754	551,813	599,873	648,936	699,1001
$n = m + 18$	279,456	314,502	350,551	388,602	428,655	470,710	514,767	560,826	607,888	657,951	708,1017
$n = m + 19$	284,466	319,513	356,562	395,613	435,667	477,723	522,780	568,840	616,902	666,966	718,1032
$n = m + 20$	290,475	325,523	362,573	401,625	442,679	485,735	530,793	576,854	625,916	675,981	727,1048
$n = m + 21$	295,485	331,533	368,584	408,636	449,691	492,748	537,807	584,868	633,931	684,996	737,1063
$n = m + 22$	300,495	336,544	374,595	414,648	456,703	500,760	545,820	593,881	642,945	693,1011	747,1078
$n = m + 23$	306,504	342,554	380,606	421,659	463,715	507,773	553,833	601,895	651,959	703,1025	756,1094
$n = m + 24$	311,514	348,564	387,616	427,671	470,727	515,785	561,846	609,909	660,973	712,1040	766,1109
$n = m + 25$	316,524	353,575	393,627	434,682	477,739	522,798	569,859	618,922	668,988	721,1055	775,1125

CRITICAL VALUES FOR THE WILCOXON RANK SUM TEST

$m = 3(1)25$ and $n = m(1)m + 25$
$P = .01$ one-sided; $P = .02$ two-sided

n	$m = 3$	$m = 4$	$m = 5$	$m = 6$	$m = 7$	$m = 8$	$m = 9$	$m = 10$	$m = 11$	$m = 12$	$m = 13$	$m = 14$
$n = m$	5,16	10,26	16,39	24,54	34,71	46,90	59,112	74,136	91,162	110,190	130,221	153,253
$n = m + 1$	5,19	10,30	17,43	26,58	36,76	48,96	62,118	77,143	94,170	113,199	134,230	157,263
$n = m + 2$	6,21	11,33	18,47	27,63	38,81	50,102	64,125	80,150	97,178	117,207	138,239	161,273
$n = m + 3$	6,24	12,36	19,51	28,68	39,87	52,108	66,132	83,157	101,185	120,216	142,248	166,282
$n = m + 4$	6,27	12,40	20,55	30,72	41,92	54,114	69,138	85,165	104,193	124,224	146,257	170,292
$n = m + 5$	7,29	13,43	21,59	31,77	43,97	56,120	71,145	88,172	107,201	128,232	150,266	174,302
$n = m + 6$	7,32	14,46	22,63	32,82	44,103	58,126	74,151	91,179	110,209	131,241	154;275	179,311
$n = m + 7$	7,35	14,50	23,67	34,86	46,108	60,132	76,158	94,186	113,217	135,249	158,284	183,321
$n = m + 8$	8,37	15,53	24,71	35,91	48,113	62,138	79,164	97,193	117,224	138,258	162,293	188,330
$n = m + 9$	8,40	16,56	25,75	36,96	49,119	64,144	81,171	100,200	120,232	142,266	166,302	192,340
$n = m + 10$	9,42	16,60	26,79	38,100	51,124	66,150	83,178	102,208	123,240	146,274	170,311	196,350
$n = m + 11$	9,45	17,63	27,83	39,105	53,129	68,156	86,184	105,215	126,248	149,283	174,320	201,359
$n = m + 12$	9,48	18,66	28,87	40,110	55,134	71,161	88,191	108,222	130,255	153,291	178,329	205,369
$n = m + 13$	10,50	18,70	29,91	42,114	56,140	73,167	91,197	111,229	133,263	157,299	182,338	210,378
$n = m + 14$	10,53	19,73	30,95	43,119	58,145	75,173	93,204	114,236	136,271	160,308	186,347	214,388
$n = m + 15$	10,56	20,76	31,99	45,123	60,150	77,179	96,210	117,243	139,279	164,316	190,356	219,397
$n = m + 16$	11,58	20,80	32,103	46,128	61,156	79,185	98,217	120,250	143,286	168,324	194,365	223,407
$n = m + 17$	11,61	21,83	33,107	47,133	63,161	81,191	101,223	122,258	146,294	171,333	198,374	228,416
$n = m + 18$	12,63	22,86	34,111	49,137	65,166	83,197	103,230	125,265	149,302	175,341	203,382	232,426
$n = m + 19$	12,66	23,89	35,115	50,142	67,171	85,203	106,236	128,272	152,310	179,349	207,391	236,436
$n = m + 20$	12,69	23,93	36,119	51,147	68,177	87,209	108,243	131,279	156,317	182,358	211,400	241,445
$n = m + 21$	13,71	24,96	37,123	53,151	70,182	90,214	111,249	134,286	159,325	186,366	215,409	245,455
$n = m + 22$	13,74	25,99	38,127	54,156	72;187	92,220	113,256	137,293	162,333	190,374	219,418	250,464
$n = m + 23$	14,76	25,103	39,131	56,160	74,192	94,226	116,262	140,300	165,341	193,383	223,427	254,474
$n = m + 24$	14,79	26,106	40,135	57,165	75,198	96,232	118,269	143,307	169,348	197,391	227,436	259,483
$n = m + 25$	14,82	27,109	41,139	58,170	77,203	98,238	121,275	145,315	172,356	201,399	231,445	263,493

$m = 3(1)25$ and $n = m(1)m + 25$
$P = .01$ one-sided; $P = .02$ two-sided

n	$m = 15$	$m = 16$	$m = 17$	$m = 18$	$m = 19$	$m = 20$	$m = 21$	$m = 22$	$m = 23$	$m = 24$	$m = 25$
$n = m$	177,288	202,326	230,365	260,406	291,450	324,496	359,544	396,594	435,646	476,700	518,757
$n = m + 1$	181,299	208,336	236,376	266,418	297,463	331,509	367,557	404,608	443,661	484,716	527,773
$n = m + 2$	186,309	213,347	241,388	272,430	304,475	338,522	374,571	412,622	451,676	493,731	536,789
$n = m + 3$	191,319	218,358	247,399	278,442	310,488	345,535	381,585	419,637	459,691	501,747	545,805
$n = m + 4$	196,329	223,369	253,410	284,454	317,500	352,548	388,599	427,651	467,706	510,762	554,821
$n = m + 5$	200,340	228,380	258,422	290,466	323,513	359,561	396,612	435,665	476,720	518,778	563,837
$n = m + 6$	205,350	234,390	264,433	296,478	330,525	365,575	403,626	442,680	484,735	527,793	572,853
$n = m + 7$	210,360	239,401	269,445	302,490	336,538	372,588	410,640	450,694	492,750	535,809	581,869
$n = m + 8$	215,370	244,412	275,456	308,502	343,550	379,601	418,653	458,708	500,765	544,824	590,885
$n = m + 9$	220,380	249,423	281,467	314,514	349,563	386,614	425,667	466,722	508,780	553,839	599,901
$n = m + 10$	225,390	255,433	286,479	320,526	356,575	393,627	432,681	473,737	516,795	561,855	608,917
$n = m + 11$	229,401	260,444	292,490	326,538	362,588	400,640	440,694	481,751	524,810	570,870	617,933
$n = m + 12$	234,411	265,455	298,501	332,550	369,600	407,653	447,708	489,765	533,824	578,886	626,949
$n = m + 13$	239,421	270,466	303,513	338,562	375,613	414,666	454,722	497,779	541,839	587,901	635,965
$n = m + 14$	244,431	276,476	309,524	344,574	382,625	421,679	462,735	504,794	549,854	596,916	644,981
$n = m + 15$	249,441	281,487	315,535	350,586	388,638	428,692	469,749	512,808	557,869	604,932	653,997
$n = m + 16$	254,451	286,498	320,547	357,597	395,650	434,706	476,763	520,822	565,884	613,947	662,1013
$n = m + 17$	259,461	291,509	326,558	363,609	401,663	441,719	484,776	528,836	574,898	621,963	671,1029
$n = m + 18$	263,472	297,519	332,569	369,621	408,675	448,732	491,790	535,851	582,913	630,978	680,1045
$n = m + 19$	268,482	302,530	337,581	375,633	414,688	455,745	498,804	543,865	590,928	639,993	689,1061
$n = m + 20$	273,492	307,541	343,592	381,645	421,700	462,758	506,817	551,879	598,943	647,1009	698,1077
$n = m + 21$	278,502	312,552	349,603	387,657	427,713	469,771	513,831	559,893	606,958	656,1024	707,1093
$n = m + 22$	283,512	318,562	355,614	393,669	434,725	476,784	520,845	567,907	615,972	665,1039	716,1109
$n = m + 23$	288,522	323,573	360,626	399,681	440,738	483,797	528,858	574,922	623,987	673,1055	726,1124
$n = m + 24$	293,532	328,584	366,637	405,693	447,750	490,810	535,872	582,936	631,1002	682,1070	735,1140
$n = m + 25$	298,542	334,594	372,648	412,704	453,763	497,823	543,885	590,950	639,1017	691,1085	744,1156

CRITICAL VALUES FOR THE WILCOXON RANK SUM TEST

$m = 3(1)25$ and $n = m(1)m + 25$
$P = .005$ one-sided; $P = .01$ two-sided

n	$m = 3$	$m = 4$	$m = 5$	$m = 6$	$m = 7$	$m = 8$	$m = 9$	$m = 10$	$m = 11$	$m = 12$	$m = 13$	$m = 14$
$n = m$	5,16	9,27	15,40	23,55	33,72	44,92	57,114	71,139	88,165	106,194	126,225	148,258
$n = m + 1$	5,19	10,30	16,44	24,60	34,78	46,98	59,121	74,146	91,173	109,203	130,234	152,268
$n = m + 2$	5,22	10,34	17,48	25,65	36,83	47,105	61,128	76,154	94,181	113,211	133,244	156,278
$n = m + 3$	5,25	11,37	18,52	27,69	37,89	49,111	63,135	79,161	97,189	116,220	137,253	160,288
$n = m + 4$	6,27	11,41	19,56	28,74	39,94	51,117	65,142	82,168	100,197	119,229	141,262	164,298
$n = m + 5$	6,30	12,44	19,61	29,79	40,100	53,123	68,148	84,176	102,206	123,237	144,272	168,308
$n = m + 6$	6,33	12,48	20,65	30,84	42,105	55,129	70,155	87,183	105,214	126,246	148,281	172,318
$n = m + 7$	6,36	13,51	21,69	31,89	43,111	57,135	72,162	89,191	108,222	129,255	152,290	176,328
$n = m + 8$	7,38	13,55	22,73	32,94	45,116	59,141	74,169	92,198	111,230	133,263	156,299	180,338
$n = m + 9$	7,41	14,58	23,77	34,98	46,122	61,147	77,175	95,205	114,238	136,272	159,309	185,347
$n = m + 10$	7,44	15,61	24,81	35,103	48,127	62,154	79,182	97,213	117,246	139,281	163,318	189,357
$n = m + 11$	8,46	15,65	25,85	36,108	49,133	64,160	81,189	100,220	120,254	143,289	167,327	193,367
$n = m + 12$	8,49	16,68	26,89	37,113	51,138	66,166	83,196	103,227	123,262	146,298	171,336	197,377
$n = m + 13$	8,52	16,72	26,94	38,118	52,144	68,172	86,202	105,235	126,270	150,306	175,345	201,387
$n = m + 14$	9,54	17,75	27,98	40,122	54,149	70,178	88,209	108,242	129,278	153,315	178,355	205,397
$n = m + 15$	9,57	17,79	28,102	41,127	55,155	72,184	90,216	110,250	132,286	156,324	182,364	210,406
$n = m + 16$	9,60	18,82	29,106	42,132	57,160	74,190	93,222	113,257	136,293	160,332	186,373	214,416
$n = m + 17$	9,63	19,85	30,110	43,137	59,165	76,196	95,229	116,264	139,301	163,341	190,382	218,426
$n = m + 18$	10,65	19,89	31,114	45,141	60,171	78,202	97,236	118,272	142,309	167,349	194,391	222,436
$n = m + 19$	10,68	20,92	32,118	46,146	62,176	80,208	99,243	121,279	145,317	170,358	197,401	226,446
$n = m + 20$	10,71	20,96	33,122	47,151	63,182	82,214	102,249	124,286	148,325	173,367	201,410	231,455
$n = m + 21$	11,73	21,99	33,127	48,156	65,187	83,221	104,256	126,294	151,333	177,375	205,419	235,465
$n = m + 22$	11,76	21,103	34,131	49,161	66,193	85,227	106,263	129,301	154,341	180,384	209,428	239,475
$n = m + 23$	11,79	22,106	35,135	51,165	68,198	87,233	109,269	132,308	157,349	184,392	213,437	243,485
$n = m + 24$	12,81	23,109	36,139	52,170	70,203	89,239	111,276	134,316	160,357	187,401	216,447	247,495
$n = m + 25$	12,84	23,113	37,143	53,175	71,209	91,245	113,283	137,323	163,365	191,409	220,456	252,504

$m = 3(1)25$ and $n = m(1)m + 25$
$P = .005$ one-sided; $P = .01$ two-sided

n	$m = 15$	$m = 16$	$m = 17$	$m = 18$	$m = 19$	$m = 20$	$m = 21$	$m = 22$	$m = 23$	$m = 24$	$m = 25$
$n = m$	171,294	196,332	223,372	252,414	283,458	316,504	350,553	386,604	424,657	464,712	506,769
$n = m + 1$	176,304	201,343	229,383	258,426	289,471	322,518	357,567	393,619	432,672	472,728	514,786
$n = m + 2$	180,315	206,354	234,395	264,438	295,484	329,531	364,581	401,633	440,687	480,744	523,802
$n = m + 3$	184,326	211,365	239,407	269,451	301,497	335,545	371,595	408,648	447,703	489,759	531,819
$n = m + 4$	189,336	216,376	245,418	275,463	307,510	342,558	378,609	415,663	455,718	497,775	540,835
$n = m + 5$	194,346	221,387	250,430	281,475	314,522	348,572	385,623	423,677	463,733	505,791	549,851
$n = m + 6$	198,357	226,398	255,442	287,487	320,535	355,585	392,637	430,692	471,748	513,807	557,868
$n = m + 7$	203,367	231,409	261,453	292,500	326,548	361,599	399,651	438,706	479,763	521,823	566,884
$n = m + 8$	207,378	236,420	266,465	298,512	332,561	368,612	405,666	445,721	486,779	530,838	575,900
$n = m + 9$	212,388	241,431	271,477	304,524	338,574	374,626	412,680	452,736	494,794	538,854	583,917
$n = m + 10$	216,399	245,443	277,488	310,536	344,587	381,639	419,694	460,750	502,809	546,870	592,933
$n = m + 11$	221,409	250,454	282,500	315,549	351,599	388,652	426,708	467,765	510,824	554,886	601,949
$n = m + 12$	225,420	255,465	287,512	321,561	357,612	394,666	433,722	475,779	518,839	563,901	609,966
$n = m + 13$	230,430	260,476	293,523	327,573	363,625	401,679	440,736	482,794	526,854	571,917	618,982
$n = m + 14$	235,440	265,487	298,535	333,585	369,638	407,693	447,750	490,808	533,870	579,933	627,998
$n = m + 15$	239,451	270,498	303,547	338,598	375,651	414,706	454,764	497,823	541,885	587,949	635,1015
$n = m + 16$	244,461	275,509	309,558	344,610	381,664	421,719	462,777	504,838	549,900	596,964	644,1031
$n = m + 17$	248,472	280,520	314,570	350,622	388,676	427,733	469,791	512,852	557,915	604,980	653,1047
$n = m + 18$	253,482	285,531	320,581	356,634	394,689	434,746	476,805	519,867	565,930	612,996	661,1064
$n = m + 19$	257,493	290,542	325,593	362,646	400,702	440,760	483,819	527,881	573,945	620,1012	670,1080
$n = m + 20$	262,503	295,553	330,605	367,659	406,715	447,773	490,833	534,896	580,961	629,1027	679,1096
$n = m + 21$	267,513	300,564	336,616	373,671	413,727	454,786	497,847	542,910	588,976	637,1043	687,1113
$n = m + 22$	271,524	305,575	341,628	379,683	419,740	460,800	504,861	549,925	596,991	645,1059	696,1129
$n = m + 23$	276,534	310,586	347,639	385,695	425,753	467,813	511,875	556,940	604,1006	654,1074	705,1145
$n = m + 24$	280,545	315,597	352,651	391,707	431,766	474,826	518,889	564,954	612,1021	662,1090	714,1161
$n = m + 25$	285,555	320,608	357,663	397,719	438,778	480,840	525,903	571,969	620,1036	670,1106	722,1178

X.6 DISTRIBUTION OF THE TOTAL NUMBER OF RUNS FOR UNEQUAL-SIZE SAMPLES

The theory of runs can be used to test data for randomness or to test the hypothesis that two samples come from the same population. A run is defined as a succession of identical elements which are followed and preceded by different elements or by no elements at all. Let N_1 be the number of elements of one kind and N_2 be the number of elements of the other kind. Let u equal the total number of runs among the $N_1 + N_2$ elements. Table (a) gives the sampling distribution for u for values of N_1 and N_2 less than or equal to 20 and Table (b) gives a number of percentage points of the distribution for larger sample sizes. The values listed in Table (a) give the probability that u or fewer runs will occur. In Table (b), the columns headed 0.5, 1, 2.5, 5 gives values of u such that u or fewer runs occur with probability less than that indicated; the columns headed 95, 97.5, 99, 99.5 gives values of u for which the probability of u or more runs is less than 0.05, 0.025, 0.01, 0.005. For large values of N_1 and N_2, particularly for $N_1 = N_2$ greater than 10, a normal approximation may be used, with

$$\text{mean} = \frac{2N_1N_2}{N_1 + N_2} + 1$$

and

$$\text{variance} = \frac{2N_1N_2(2N_1N_2 - N_1 - N_2)}{(N_1 + N_2)^2(N_1 + N_2 - 1)}$$

a) DISTRIBUTION OF THE TOTAL NUMBER OF RUNS u IN SAMPLES OF SIZE (N_1,N_2)

N_1,N_2 \ u	2	3	4	5	6	7	8	9	10
2,2	0.3333	0.6667	1.0000						
2,3	.2000	.5000	0.9000	1.0000					
2,4	.1333	.4000	.8000	1.0000					
2,5	.0952	.3333	.7143	1.0000					
2,6	.0714	.2857	.6429	1.0000					
2,7	.0556	.2500	.5833	1.0000					
2,8	.0444	.2222	.5333	1.0000					
2,9	.0364	.2000	.4909	1.0000					
2,10	.0303	.1818	.4545	1.0000					
2,11	.0256	.1667	.4231	1.0000					
2,12	.0220	.1538	.3956	1.0000					
2,13	.0190	.1429	.3714	1.0000					
2,14	.0167	.1333	.3500	1.0000					
2,15	.0147	.1250	.3309	1.0000					
2,16	.0131	.1176	.3137	1.0000					
2,17	.0117	.1111	.2982	1.0000					
2,18	.0105	.1053	.2842	1.0000					
2,19	.0095	.1000	.2714	1.0000					
2,20	.0087	.0952	.2597	1.0000					
3,3	0.1000	0.3000	0.7000	0.9000	1.0000				
3,4	.0571	.2000	.5429	.8000	0.9714	1.0000			
3,5	.0357	.1429	.4286	.7143	.9286	1.0000			
3,6	.0238	.1071	.3452	.6429	.8810	1.0000			
3,7	.0167	.0833	.2833	.5833	.8333	1.0000			
3,8	.0121	.0667	.2364	.5333	.7879	1.0000			
3,9	.0091	.0545	.2000	.4909	.7454	1.0000			
3,10	.0070	.0454	.1713	.4545	.7063	1.0000			
3,11	.0055	.0385	.1484	.4231	.6703	1.0000			
3,12	.0044	.0330	.1297	.3956	.6374	1.0000			
3,13	.0036	.0286	.1143	.3714	.6071	1.0000			
3,14	.0029	.0250	.1015	.3500	.5794	1.0000			
3,15	.0024	.0221	.0907	.3309	.5539	1.0000			
3,16	.0021	.0196	.0815	.3137	.5304	1.0000			
3,17	.0018	.0175	.0737	.2982	.5088	1.0000			
3,18	.0015	.0158	.0669	.2842	.4887	1.0000			
3,19	.0013	.0143	.0610	.2714	.4701	1.0000			
3,20	.0011	.0130	.0559	.2597	.4528	1.0000			

a) DISTRIBUTION OF THE TOTAL NUMBER OF RUNS u IN SAMPLES OF SIZE (N_1,N_2)

N_1,N_2 \ u	2	3	4	5	6	7	8	9	10
4,4	0.0286	0.1143	0.3714	0.6286	0.8857	0.9714	1.0000		
4,5	.0159	.0714	.2619	.5000	.7857	.9286	0.9921	1.0000	
4,6	.0095	.0476	.1905	.4048	.6905	.8810	.9762	1.0000	
4,7	.0061	.0333	.1424	.3333	.6061	.8333	.9545	1.0000	
4,8	.0040	.0242	.1091	.2788	.5333	.7879	.9293	1.0000	
4,9	.0028	.0182	.0853	.2364	.4713	.7454	.9021	1.0000	
4,10	.0020	.0140	.0679	.2028	.4186	.7063	.8741	1.0000	
4,11	.0015	.0110	.0549	.1758	.3736	.6703	.8462	1.0000	
4,12	.0011	.0088	.0451	.1538	.3352	.6374	.8187	1.0000	
4,13	$.0^{3}840$	.0071	.0374	.1357	.3021	.6071	.7920	1.0000	
4,14	$.0^{3}654$	.0059	.0314	.1206	.2735	.5794	.7663	1.0000	
4,15	$.0^{3}516$	.0049	.0266	.1078	.2487	.5539	.7417	1.0000	
4,16	$.0^{3}413$	.0041	.0227	.0970	.2270	.5304	.7183	1.0000	
4,17	$.0^{3}334$	.0035	.0195	.0877	.2080	.5088	.6959	1.0000	
4,18	$.0^{3}273$	.0030	.0170	.0797	.1912	.4887	.6746	1.0000	
4,19	$.0^{3}226$	.0026	.0148	.0727	.1764	.4701	.6544	1.0000	
4,20	$.0^{3}188$	.0023	.0130	.0666	.1632	.4528	.6352	1.0000	
5,5	$0.0^{2}794$	0.0397	0.1667	0.3571	0.6429	0.8333	0.9603	0.9921	1.0000
5,6	$.0^{2}433$	.0238	.1104	.2619	.5216	.7381	.9112	.9762	0.9978
5,7	$.0^{2}252$	.0152	.0758	.1970	.4242	.6515	.8535	.9545	.9924
5,8	$.0^{2}155$	.0101	.0536	.1515	.3473	.5758	.7933	.9293	.9837
5,9	$.0^{3}999$	$.0^{2}699$	.0390	.1189	.2867	.5105	.7343	.9021	.9720
5,10	$.0^{3}666$	$.0^{2}500$	.0290	.0949	.2388	.4545	.6783	.8741	.9580
5,11	$.0^{3}458$	$.0^{2}366$	.0220	.0769	.2005	.4066	.6264	.8462	.9423
5,12	$.0^{3}323$	$.0^{2}275$	.0170	.0632	.1698	.3654	.5787	.8187	.9253
5,13	$.0^{3}233$	$.0^{2}210$	.0133	.0525	.1450	.3298	.5352	.7920	.9076
5,14	$.0^{3}172$	$.0^{2}163$	.0106	.0441	.1246	.2990	.4958	.7663	.8893
5,15	$.0^{3}129$	$.0^{2}129$	$.0^{2}851$	.0374	.1078	.2722	.4600	.7417	.8709
5,16	$.0^{4}983$	$.0^{2}103$	$.0^{2}693$	.0320	.0939	.2487	.4276	.7183	.8524
5,17	$.0^{4}759$	$.0^{3}835$	$.0^{2}570$	.0276	.0822	.2281	.3982	.6959	.8341
5,18	$.0^{4}594$	$.0^{3}684$	$.0^{2}472$	.0239	.0724	.2098	.3715	.6746	.8161
5,19	$.0^{4}471$	$.0^{3}565$	$.0^{2}395$	.0209	.0641	.1937	.3473	.6544	.7984
5,20	$.0^{4}376$	$.0^{3}470$	$.0^{2}333$	.0184	.0570	.1793	.3252	.6352	.7811
6,6	$0.0^{2}216$	0.0130	0.0671	0.1753	0.3918	0.6082	0.8247	0.9329	0.9870
6,7	$.0^{2}117$	$.0^{2}758$	.0425	.1212	.2960	.5000	.7331	.8788	.9662
6,8	$.0^{3}666$	$.0^{2}466$	.0280	.0862	.2261	.4126	.6457	.8205	.9371
6,9	$.0^{3}400$	$.0^{2}300$	.0190	.0629	.1748	.3427	.5664	.7622	.9021
6,10	$.0^{3}250$	$.0^{2}200$	.0132	.0470	.1369	.2867	.4965	.7063	.8636
6,11	$.0^{3}162$	$.0^{2}137$	$.0^{2}945$	.0357	.1084	.2418	.4357	.6538	.8235
6,12	$.0^{3}108$	$.0^{3}970$	$.0^{2}690$	.0276	.0869	.2054	.3832	.6054	.7831
6,13	$.0^{4}737$	$.0^{3}700$	$.0^{2}512$	.0217	.0704	.1758	.3379	.5609	.7434
6,14	$.0^{4}516$	$.0^{3}516$	$.0^{2}387$	.0173	.0575	.1514	.2990	.5204	.7048
6,15	$.0^{4}369$	$.0^{3}387$	$.0^{2}297$	.0139	.0475	.1313	.2655	.4835	.6680
6,16	$.0^{4}268$	$.0^{3}295$	$.0^{2}230$	.0114	.0395	.1146	.2365	.4500	.6329
6,17	$.0^{4}198$	$.0^{3}228$	$.0^{2}181$	$.0^{2}934$	.0331	.1005	.2114	.4195	.5998
6,18	$.0^{4}149$	$.0^{3}178$	$.0^{2}144$	$.0^{2}776$	.0280	.0886	.1896	.3917	.5685
6,19	$.0^{4}113$	$.0^{3}141$	$.0^{2}116$	$.0^{2}649$	.0238	.0785	.1706	.3665	.5392
6,20	$.0^{5}087$	$.0^{3}113$	$.0^{3}938$	$.0^{2}548$	.0203	.0698	.1540	.3434	.5118

a) **DISTRIBUTION OF THE TOTAL NUMBER OF RUNS** u **IN SAMPLES OF SIZE** (N_1, N_2)

11	12	13	14	15	16	17	18	19	20	21
1.0000										
1.0000										
1.0000										
1.0000										
1.0000										
1.0000										
1.0000										
1.0000										
1.0000										
1.0000										
1.0000										
1.0000										
1.0000										
1.0000										
1.0000										
0.9978	1.0000									
.9924	0.9994	1.0000								
.9837	.9977	1.0000								
.9720	.9944	1.0000								
.9580	.9895	1.0000								
.9423	.9830	1.0000								
.9253	.9751	1.0000								
.9076	.9659	1.0000								
.8893	.9557	1.0000								
.8709	.9447	1.0000								
.8524	.9329	1.0000								
.8341	.9207	1.0000								
.8161	.9080	1.0000								
.7984	.8952	1.0000								
.7811	.8822	1.0000								

a) **DISTRIBUTION OF THE TOTAL NUMBER OF RUNS** u **IN SAMPLES OF SIZE** (N_1, N_2)

N_1, N_2 \ u	2	3	4	5	6	7	8	9	10
7,7	$0.0^{3}583$	$0.0^{2}408$	0.0251	0.0775	0.2086	0.3834	0.6166	0.7914	0.9225
7,8	$.0^{3}311$	$.0^{2}233$	.0154	.0513	.1492	.2960	.5136	.7040	.8671
7,9	$.0^{3}175$	$.0^{2}140$	$.0^{2}979$	.0350	.1084	.2308	.4266	.6224	.8059
7,10	$.0^{3}103$	$.0^{3}874$	$.0^{2}643$	.0245	.0800	.1818	.3546	.5490	.7433
7,11	$.0^{4}628$	$.0^{3}566$	$.0^{2}434$	.0175	.0600	.1448	.2956	.4842	.6821
7,12	$.0^{4}397$	$.0^{3}377$	$.0^{2}300$	.0128	.0456	.1165	.2475	.4276	.6241
7,13	$.0^{4}258$	$.0^{3}258$	$.0^{2}212$	$.0^{2}955$	.0351	.0947	.2082	.3785	.5700
7,14	$.0^{4}172$	$.0^{3}181$	$.0^{2}152$	$.0^{2}722$	.0273	.0777	.1760	.3359	.5204
7,15	$.0^{4}117$	$.0^{3}129$	$.0^{2}111$	$.0^{2}555$	.0216	.0642	.1496	.2990	.4751
7,16	$.0^{4}082$	$.0^{4}938$	$.0^{3}828$	$.0^{2}432$	.0172	.0536	.1278	.2670	.4340
7,17	$.0^{4}058$	$.0^{4}693$	$.0^{3}624$	$.0^{2}340$	.0138	.0450	.1097	.2392	.3969
7,18	$.0^{4}042$	$.0^{4}520$	$.0^{3}476$	$.0^{2}270$	.0112	.0381	.0946	.2149	.3634
7,19	$.0^{4}030$	$.0^{4}395$	$.0^{3}368$	$.0^{2}217$	$.0^{2}915$	.0324	.0820	.1937	.3332
7,20	$.0^{4}023$	$.0^{4}304$	$.0^{3}287$	$.0^{2}176$	$.0^{2}754$	.0278	.0714	.1751	.3060
8,8	$0.0^{3}155$	$0.0^{2}124$	$0.0^{2}886$	0.03170	0.1002	0.2144	0.4048	0.5952	0.7855
8,9	$.0^{4}823$	$.0^{3}6993$	$.0^{2}5306$	.02028	.06865	.1573	.3186	.5000	.7016
8,10	$.0^{4}457$	$.0^{3}4114$	$.0^{2}3291$	.01337	.04792	.1170	.2514	.4194	.6209
8,11	$.0^{4}265$	$.0^{3}2514$	$.0^{2}2104$	$.0^{2}9050$	.03406	.08824	.1994	.3522	.5467
8,12	$.0^{4}159$	$.0^{3}1588$	$.0^{2}1381$	$.0^{2}6271$	.02461	.06740	.1591	.2966	.4800
8,13	$.0^{4}098$	$.0^{3}1032$	$.0^{3}9288$	$.0^{2}4438$	.01806	.05212	.1278	.2508	.4210
8,14	$.0^{4}063$	$.0^{4}688$	$.0^{3}6380$	$.0^{2}3199$	.01344	.04076	.1034	.2129	.3694
8,15	$.0^{4}041$	$.0^{4}469$	$.0^{3}4467$	$.0^{2}2345$	.01014	.03223	.08419	.1816	.3245
8,16	$.0^{4}027$	$.0^{4}326$	$.0^{3}3182$	$.0^{2}1746$	$.0^{2}7742$	.02573	.06904	.1556	.2856
8,17	$.0^{4}018$	$.0^{4}231$	$.0^{3}2302$	$.0^{2}1318$	$.0^{2}5977$	.02073	.05698	.1340	.2518
8,18	$.0^{4}013$	$.0^{4}166$	$.0^{3}1690$	$.0^{2}1007$	$.0^{2}4663$	.01685	.04732	.1159	.2225
8,19	$.0^{4}009$	$.0^{4}122$	$.0^{3}1257$	$.0^{3}7784$	$.0^{2}3673$	.01380	.03953	.1006	.1971
8,20	$.0^{4}006$	$.0^{4}090$	$.0^{4}946$	$.0^{3}6081$	$.0^{2}2919$	.01139	.03322	.08777	.1751
9,9	$0.0^{4}411$	$0.0^{3}3702$	$0.0^{2}3003$	0.01222	0.04447	0.1090	0.2380	0.3992	0.6008
9,10	$.0^{4}217$	$.0^{3}2057$	$.0^{2}1764$	$.0^{2}7610$	.02943	.07672	.1786	.3186	.5095
9,11	$.0^{4}119$	$.0^{3}1191$	$.0^{2}1072$	$.0^{2}4882$	.01989	.05489	.1349	.2549	.4300
9,12	$.0^{4}068$	$.0^{4}714$	$.0^{3}6702$	$.0^{2}3215$	.01369	.03989	.1028	.2049	.3621
9,13	$.0^{4}040$	$.0^{4}442$	$.0^{3}4302$	$.0^{2}2167$	$.0^{2}9598$	.02941	.07895	.1656	.3050
9,14	$.0^{4}024$	$.0^{4}281$	$.0^{3}2827$	$.0^{2}1492$	$.0^{2}6837$	.02198	.06118	.1347	.2572
9,15	$.0^{4}015$	$.0^{4}184$	$.0^{3}1897$	$.0^{2}1046$	$.0^{2}4944$	.01664	.04782	.1102	.2174
9,16	$.0^{4}010$	$.0^{4}122$	$.0^{3}1297$	$.0^{3}7465$	$.0^{2}3625$	.01274	.03768	.09069	.1842
9,17	$.0^{4}006$	$.0^{4}083$	$.0^{4}903$	$.0^{3}5409$	$.0^{2}2692$	$.0^{2}9861$	.02993	.07510	.1566
9,18	$.0^{4}004$	$.0^{4}058$	$.0^{4}638$	$.0^{3}3975$	$.0^{2}2022$	$.0^{2}7710$	.02396	.06255	.1336
9,19	$.0^{4}003$	$.0^{4}041$	$.0^{4}458$	$.0^{3}2959$	$.0^{2}1536$	$.0^{2}6085$	.01932	.05240	.1144
9,20	$.0^{4}002$	$.0^{4}029$	$.0^{4}333$	$.0^{3}2230$	$.0^{2}1179$	$.0^{2}4844$	.01568	.04413	.09831
10,10	$0.0^{4}108$	$0.0^{3}1083$	$0.0^{3}9851$	$0.0^{2}4492$	0.01852	0.05126	0.1276	0.2422	0.4141
10,11	$.0^{4}057$	$.0^{4}595$	$.0^{3}5699$	$.0^{2}2739$	.01192	.03489	.09205	.1849	.3350
10,12	$.0^{4}031$	$.0^{4}340$	$.0^{3}3402$	$.0^{2}1718$	$.0^{2}7842$	.02417	.06704	.1421	.2707
10,13	$.0^{4}017$	$.0^{4}201$	$.0^{3}2089$	$.0^{2}1106$	$.0^{2}5259$	.01703	.04933	.1099	.2189
10,14	$.0^{4}010$	$.0^{4}122$	$.0^{3}1315$	$.0^{3}7281$	$.0^{2}3592$	.01218	.03668	.08568	.1775
10,15	$.0^{4}006$	$.0^{4}076$	$.0^{4}847$	$.0^{3}4895$	$.0^{2}2494$	$.0^{2}8841$	.02755	.06731	.1445
10,16	$.0^{4}004$	$.0^{4}049$	$.0^{4}557$	$.0^{3}3353$	$.0^{2}1759$	$.0^{2}6503$	.02089	.05327	.1180
10,17	$.0^{4}002$	$.0^{4}032$	$.0^{4}373$	$.0^{3}2336$	$.0^{2}1258$	$.0^{2}4842$	.01599	.04248	.09684
10,18	$.0^{4}002$	$.0^{4}021$	$.0^{4}255$	$.0^{3}1654$	$.0^{3}9115$	$.0^{2}3648$	.01235	.03412	.07982
10,19	$.0^{4}001$	$.0^{4}014$	$.0^{4}176$	$.0^{3}1187$	$.0^{3}6687$	$.0^{2}2777$	$.0^{2}9621$	.02759	.06608
10,20	$.0^{5}001$	$.0^{4}010$	$.0^{4}124$	$.0^{4}864$	$.0^{3}4962$	$.0^{2}2135$	$.0^{2}7554$	.02245	.05496

a) DISTRIBUTION OF THE TOTAL NUMBER OF RUNS u IN SAMPLES OF SIZE (N_1, N_2)

11	12	13	14	15	16	17	18	19	20	21
0.9749	0.9959	0.9994	1.0000							
.9487	.9879	.9977	0.9998	1.0000						
.9161	.9748	.9944	.9993	1.0000						
.8794	.9571	.9895	.9981	1.0000						
.8405	.9355	.9830	.9962	1.0000						
.8009	.9109	.9751	.9934	1.0000						
.7616	.8842	.9659	.9898	1.0000						
.7233	.8561	.9557	.9852	1.0000						
.6864	.8273	.9447	.9799	1.0000						
.6512	.7982	.9329	.9738	1.0000						
.6178	.7692	.9207	.9669	1.0000						
.5862	.7407	.9081	.9595	1.0000						
.5565	.7128	.8952	.9516	1.0000						
.5286	.6857	.8822	.9433	1.0000						
0.8998	0.9683	0.9911	0.9988	0.9998	1.0000					
.8427	.9394	.9797	.9958	.9993	0.99996	1.0000				
.7822	.9031	.9636	.9905	.9981	.99979	1.0000				
.7217	.8618	.9434	.9823	.9962	.99940	1.0000				
.6634	.8174	.9201	.9714	.9934	.99869	1.0000				
.6084	.7718	.8944	.9580	.9898	.99757	1.0000				
.5573	.7263	.8672	.9423	.9852	.99598	1.0000				
.5103	.6818	.8390	.9248	.9799	.99388	1.0000				
.4674	.6389	.8104	.9057	.9738	.99125	1.0000				
.4285	.5981	.7818	.8855	.9670	.9881	1.0000				
.3931	.5595	.7536	.8645	.9595	.9844	1.0000				
.3611	.5232	.7258	.8429	.9516	.9803	1.0000				
.3322	.4893	.6988	.8210	.9433	.9757	1.0000				
0.7620	0.8910	0.9555	0.9878	0.9970	0.9997	0.99996	1.0000			
.6814	.8342	.9233	.9742	.9924	.9986	.9998	0.99999	1.0000		
.6050	.7731	.8851	.9551	.9851	.9966	.9994	.99994	1.0000		
.5350	.7110	.8431	.9311	.9751	.9931	.9987	.99981	1.0000		
.4721	.6505	.7991	.9031	.9625	.9880	.9976	.99956	1.0000		
.4164	.5928	.7545	.8721	.9477	.9813	.9960	.99912	1.0000		
.3674	.5389	.7104	.8390	.9309	.9729	.9939	.99847	1.0000		
.3245	.4892	.6675	.8047	.9125	.9629	.9912	.99755	1.0000		
.2871	.4437	.6264	.7699	.8929	.9515	.9881	.99634	1.0000		
.2545	.4024	.5872	.7351	.8724	.9388	.9844	.99481	1.0000		
.2261	.3650	.5502	.7008	.8513	.9250	.9803	.99296	1.0000		
.2013	.3313	.5155	.6672	.8298	.9103	.9757	.99078	1.0000		
0.5859	0.7578	0.8724	0.9487	0.9815	0.9955	0.9990	0.9999	0.99999	1.0000	
.5000	.6800	.8151	.9151	.9651	.9896	.9973	.9996	.99994	0.999997	1.0000
.4250	.6050	.7551	.8751	.9437	.9804	.9942	.9988	.9998	.99998	1.0000
.3607	.5351	.6950	.8370	.9180	.9678	.9896	.9974	.9996	.99994	1.0000
.3062	.4715	.6369	.7839	.8889	.9519	.9834	.9952	.9991	.99985	1.0000
.2602	.4146	.5818	.7361	.8574	.9330	.9755	.9920	.9985	.99969	1.0000
.2216	.3641	.5303	.6886	.8243	.9115	.9660	.9879	.9976	.99943	1.0000
.1893	.3197	.4828	.6423	.7904	.8880	.9552	.9826	.9963	.99905	1.0000
.1621	.2809	.4393	.5978	.7562	.8629	.9429	.9763	.9948	.99852	1.0000
.1392	.2470	.3997	.5554	.7223	.8367	.9296	.9689	.9930	.99782	1.0000
.1200	.2175	.3638	.5155	.6889	.8096	.9153	.9606	.9908	.99692	1.0000

a) DISTRIBUTION OF THE TOTAL NUMBER OF RUNS u IN SAMPLES OF SIZE (N_1, N_2)

N_1,N_2 \ u	2	3	4	5	6	7	8	9	10
11,11	0.0^4028	0.0^4312	0.0^3147	0.0^21590	0.0^27332	0.02264	0.06347	0.1349	0.2599
11,12	$.0^4015$	$.0^4170$	$.0^31797$	$.0^39526$	$.0^24614$	.01499	.04427	.09919	.2017
11,13	$.0^4008$	$.0^4096$	$.0^31058$	$.0^35865$	$.0^22966$	.01010	.03126	.07356	.1568
11,14	$.0^4004$	$.0^4056$	$.0^4639$	$.0^33702$	$.0^21945$	$.0^26932$	.02233	.05505	.1224
11,15	$.0^4003$	$.0^4034$	$.0^4346$	$.0^32389$	$.0^21299$	$.0^24832$	.01614	.04158	.09600
11,16	$.0^4002$	$.0^4021$	$.0^4251$	$.0^31574$	$.0^38822$	$.0^23419$	.01180	.03169	.07566
11,17	$.0^4001$	$.0^4013$	$.0^4162$	$.0^31056$	$.0^36085$	$.0^22453$	$.0^28711$	.02436	.05995
11,18	$.0^4001$	$.0^4008$	$.0^4107$	$.0^4721$	$.0^34259$	$.0^21782$	$.0^26499$	.01888	.04777
11,19		$.0^4005$	$.0^4071$	$.0^4500$	$.0^33020$	$.0^21310$	$.0^24895$	.01475	.03828
11,20		$.0^4004$	$.0^4049$	$.0^4351$	$.0^32169$	$.0^39742$	$.0^23721$	.01162	.03084
12,12	0.0^4007	0.0^4089	0.0^4984	0.0^35458	0.0^22783	0.0^29495	0.02963	0.06990	0.1504
12,13	$.0^4004$	$.0^4048$	$.0^4556$	$.0^33221$	$.0^21718$	$.0^26139$	.02010	.04977	.1126
12,14	$.0^4002$	$.0^4027$	$.0^4323$	$.0^31952$	$.0^21084$	$.0^24045$	.01382	.03581	.08467
12,15	$.0^4001$	$.0^4016$	$.0^4193$	$.0^31211$	$.0^36970$	$.0^22712$	$.0^29622$	.02603	.06404
12,16	$.0^4001$	$.0^4009$	$.0^4118$	$.0^4769$	$.0^34565$	$.0^21849$	$.0^26784$	.01912	.04874
12,17		$.0^4006$	$.0^4073$	$.0^4497$	$.0^33041$	$.0^21279$	$.0^24840$	.01419	.03733
12,18		$.0^4003$	$.0^4047$	$.0^4328$	$.0^32057$	$.0^38976$	$.0^23492$	.01063	.02879
12,19		$.0^4002$	$.0^4030$	$.0^4220$	$.0^31412$	$.0^36381$	$.0^22546$	$.0^28032$	.02234
12,20		$.0^4001$	$.0^4020$	$.0^4150$	$.0^4983$	$.0^34593$	$.0^21876$	$.0^26124$	.01745
13,13	0.0^4002	0.0^4025	0.0^4302	0.0^31825	0.0^21020	0.0^23812	0.01312	0.03406	0.08118
13,14	$.0^4001$	$.0^4013$	$.0^4169$	$.0^31063$	$.0^36196$	$.0^22416$	$.0^28690$	.02359	.05888
13,15	$.0^4001$	$.0^4007$	$.0^4097$	$.0^4636$	$.0^33844$	$.0^21561$	$.0^25838$	.01653	.04300
13,16		$.0^4004$	$.0^4057$	$.0^4389$	$.0^32431$	$.0^21026$	$.0^23976$	.01172	.03168
13,17		$.0^4003$	$.0^4035$	$.0^4243$	$.0^31566$	$.0^36856$	$.0^22743$	$.0^28401$	.02345
13,18		$.0^4002$	$.0^4021$	$.0^4155$	$.0^31025$	$.0^34652$	$.0^21916$	$.0^26086$	.01751
13,19		$.0^4001$	$.0^4013$	$.0^4100$	$.0^4682$	$.0^33201$	$.0^21354$	$.0^24454$	.01318
13,20		$.0^4001$	$.0^4009$	$.0^4066$	$.0^4460$	$.0^32232$	$.0^39671$	$.0^23292$	$.0^29986$
14,14		0.0^4007	0.0^4095	0.0^4597	0.0^33630	0.0^21475	0.0^25553	0.01575	0.04123
14,15		$.0^4004$	$.0^4051$	$.0^4344$	$.0^32174$	$.0^39191$	$.0^23604$	.01065	.02911
14,16		$.0^4002$	$.0^4029$	$.0^4203$	$.0^31330$	$.0^35835$	$.0^22373$	$.0^27295$	.02072
14,17		$.0^4001$	$.0^4017$	$.0^4123$	$.0^4829$	$.0^33770$	$.0^21585$	$.0^25058$	.01487
14,18		$.0^4001$	$.0^4010$	$.0^4076$	$.0^4526$	$.0^32476$	$.0^21073$	$.0^23548$	.01077
14,19			$.0^4006$	$.0^4048$	$.0^4339$	$.0^31651$	$.0^37351$	$.0^22516$	$.0^27861$
14,20			$.0^4004$	$.0^4030$	$.0^4222$	$.0^31116$	$.0^35098$	$.0^21804$	$.0^25786$
15,15		0.0^4002	0.0^4027	0.0^4191	0.0^31259	0.0^35530	0.0^22261	0.0^26959	0.01988
15,16		$.0^4001$	$.0^4015$	$.0^4109$	$.0^4745$	$.0^33395$	$.0^21442$	$.0^24610$	.01370
15,17		$.0^4001$	$.0^4008$	$.0^4064$	$.0^4450$	$.0^32123$	$.0^39329$	$.0^23095$	$.0^29536$
15,18			$.0^4005$	$.0^4038$	$.0^4277$	$.0^31351$	$.0^36124$	$.0^22104$	$.0^26698$
15,19			$.0^4003$	$.0^4023$	$.0^4173$	$.0^4873$	$.0^34074$	$.0^21448$	$.0^24748$
15,20			$.0^4002$	$.0^4014$	$.0^4110$	$.0^4573$	$.0^32745$	$.0^21008$	$.0^23397$
16,16		0.0^4001	0.0^4008	0.0^4060	0.0^4427	0.0^32017	0.0^38905	0.0^22957	0.0^29157
16,17			$.0^4004$	$.0^4034$	$.0^4250$	$.0^31222$	$.0^35590$	0.0^21924	$.0^26182$
16,18			$.0^4002$	$.0^4020$	$.0^4149$	$.0^4754$	$.0^33562$	$.0^21269$	$.0^24217$
16,19			$.0^4001$	$.0^4012$	$.0^4091$	$.0^4473$	$.0^32302$	$.0^38475$	$.0^22905$
16,20			$.0^4001$	$.0^4007$	$.0^4056$	$.0^4302$	$.0^31509$	$.0^35732$	$.0^22021$
17,17			0.0^4002	0.0^4019	0.0^4142	0.0^4718	0.0^33406	0.0^21214	0.0^24053
17,18			$.0^4001$	$.0^4011$	$.0^4083$	$.0^4430$	$.0^32109$	$.0^37773$	$.0^22686$
17,19			$.0^4001$	$.0^4006$	$.0^4049$	$.0^4262$	$.0^31325$	$.0^35046$	$.0^21800$
17,20				$.0^4004$	$.0^4029$	$.0^4163$	$.0^4845$	$.0^33318$	$.0^21219$
18,18			0.0^4001	0.0^4006	0.0^4047	0.0^4250	0.0^31269	0.0^34836	0.0^21732
18,19				$.0^4003$	$.0^4027$	$.0^4148$	$.0^4776$	$.0^33053$	$.0^21130$
18,20				$.0^4002$	$.0^4016$	$.0^4090$	$.0^4482$	$.0^31954$	$.0^37448$
19,19				0.0^4002	0.0^4015	0.0^4086	0.0^4462	0.0^31875	0.0^37174
19,20				$.0^4001$	$.0^4009$	$.0^4050$	$.0^4280$	$.0^31169$	$.0^34611$
20,20				0.0^4001	0.0^4005	0.0^4029	0.0^4165	0.0^4710	0.0^32890

a) **DISTRIBUTION OF THE TOTAL NUMBER OF RUNS** u **IN SAMPLES OF SIZE** (N_1, N_2)

11	12	13	14	15	16	17	18	19	20	21
0.4100	0.5900	0.7401	0.8651	0.9365	0.9774	0.9927	0.9984	0.9997	0.99997	0.999997
.3350	.5072	.6650	.8086	.9008	.9594	.9850	.9960	.9990	.9999	.99998
.2735	.4335	.5933	.7488	.8598	.9360	.9740	.9919	.9978	.9996	.9999
.2235	.3690	.5266	.6883	.8154	.9078	.9598	.9857	.9958	.9990	.9998
.1831	.3137	.4660	.6293	.7692	.8758	.9424	.9774	.9930	.9981	.9997
.1504	.2665	.4116	.5728	.7225	.8410	.9224	.9669	.9891	.9967	.9994
.1240	.2265	.3632	.5199	.6765	.8043	.9002	.9542	.9841	.9948	.9990
.1027	.1928	.3205	.4708	.6317	.7666	.8763	.9395	.9781	.9922	.9985
.08533	.1644	.2830	.4257	.5888	.7286	.8510	.9230	.9711	.9890	.9978
.07122	.1404	.2500	.3846	.5480	.6908	.8247	.9051	.9631	.9849	.9969
0.2632	0.4211	0.5789	0.7368	0.8496	0.9301	0.9704	0.9905	0.9972	0.9994	0.9999
.2068	.3475	.5000	.6642	.7932	.8937	.9502	.9816	.9939	.9985	.9997
.1628	.2860	.4296	.5938	.7345	.8518	.9251	.9691	.9886	.9968	.9992
.1286	.2351	.3681	.5277	.6759	.8062	.8958	.9528	.9813	.9940	.9984
.1020	.1932	.3149	.4669	.6189	.7585	.8632	.9330	.9718	.9899	.9971
.08131	.1591	.2693	.4118	.5646	.7101	.8283	.9101	.9602	.9844	.9953
.06511	.1312	.2304	.3626	.5137	.6621	.7919	.8847	.9465	.9774	.9929
.05240	.1085	.1973	.3189	.4665	.6153	.7548	.8572	.9311	.9690	.9898
.04238	.08996	.1693	.2803	.4231	.5703	.7176	.8281	.9140	.9590	.9860
0.1566	0.2772	0.4179	0.5821	0.7228	0.8434	0.9188	0.9659	0.9869	0.9962	0.9990
.1189	.2205	.3475	.5056	.6524	.7880	.8811	.9446	.9764	.9921	.9976
.09064	.1753	.2883	.4365	.5847	.7299	.8388	.9182	.9623	.9858	.9952
.06947	.1396	.2389	.3751	.5212	.6714	.7934	.8873	.9446	.9771	.9917
.05354	.1113	.1980	.3215	.4628	.6141	.7465	.8529	.9238	.9658	.9868
.04150	.08902	.1643	.2752	.4098	.5592	.6692	.8159	.9001	.9520	.9805
.03236	.07143	.1366	.2353	.3623	.5074	.6525	.7772	.8742	.9358	.9728
.02538	.05752	.1138	.2012	.3200	.4592	.6072	.7377	.8465	.9174	.9635
0.08711	0.1697	0.2798	0.4266	0.5734	0.7202	0.8303	0.9129	0.9588	0.9842	0.9944
.06417	.1306	.2247	.3576	.5000	.6519	.7753	.8749	.9358	.9727	.9893
.04756	.1007	.1804	.2986	.4336	.5854	.7183	.8322	.9081	.9574	.9820
.03548	.07788	.1450	.2486	.3745	.5226	.6614	.7863	.8765	.9382	.9721
.02665	.06044	.1168	.2068	.3227	.4643	.6058	.7386	.8418	.9155	.9598
.02015	.04709	.09422	.1720	.2776	.4110	.5527	.6903	.8049	.8898	.9450
.01534	.03684	.07626	.1432	.2387	.3640	.5027	.6425	.7667	.8616	.9281
0.04572	0.09739	0.1749	0.2912	0.4241	0.5759	0.7088	0.8251	0.9026	0.9543	0.9801
.03280	.07281	.1362	.2362	.3576	.5046	.6424	.7710	.8638	.9305	.9672
.02370	.05462	.1062	.1912	.3005	.4393	.5781	.7147	.8210	.9020	.9505
.01726	.04115	.08296	.1546	.2519	.3806	.5174	.6581	.7754	.8693	.9303
.01267	.03115	.06504	.1251	.2109	.3286	.4610	.6026	.7285	.8334	.9068
$.0^{2}9370$	.02370	.05118	.1014	.1766	.2831	.4095	.5493	.6813	.7952	.8806
0.02280	0.05280	0.1028	0.1862	0.2933	0.4311	0.5689	0.7067	0.8138	0.8972	0.9472
.01598	.03846	.07781	.1465	.2397	.3659	.5000	.6420	.7603	.8584	.9222
.01129	.02816	.05907	.1153	.1956	.3091	.4369	.5789	.7050	.8155	.8928
$.0^{2}8049$	.02072	.04502	.09079	.1594	.2603	.3801	.5188	.6498	.7697	.8596
$.0^{2}5786$	.01534	.03446	.07162	.1300	.2188	.3297	.4628	.5959	.7224	.8237
0.01087	0.02722	0.05720	0.1122	0.1907	0.3028	0.4290	0.5710	0.6972	0.8093	0.8878
$.0^{2}7460$	.01937	.04221	.08589	.1514	.2495	.3659	.5038	.6341	.7566	.8486
$.0^{2}5168$	.01388	.03129	.06587	.1202	.2049	.3108	.4418	.5728	.7022	.8057
$.0^{2}3614$	.01000	.02331	.05063	.09551	.1680	.2631	.3854	.5146	.6474	.7604
$0.0^{2}4978$	0.01342	0.03029	0.06405	0.1171	0.2004	0.3046	0.4349	0.5651	0.6954	0.7996
$.0^{2}3355$	$.0^{2}9355$	.02186	.04786	.09057	.1606	.2525	.3729	.5000	.6338	.7475
$.0^{2}2283$	$.0^{2}6569$	.01586	.03586	.07014	.1285	.2088	.3182	.4398	.5736	.6940
$0.0^{2}2201$	$0.0^{2}6355$	0.01536	0.03486	0.06828	0.1256	0.2044	0.3127	0.4331	0.5669	0.6873
$.0^{2}1459$	$.0^{2}4350$	.01086	.02547	.05157	.09810	.1650	.2610	.3729	.5033	.6271
$0.0^{3}9429$	$0.0^{2}2905$	$0.0^{2}7482$	0.01816	0.03800	0.07484	0.1301	0.2130	0.3143	0.4381	0.5619

a) DISTRIBUTION OF THE TOTAL NUMBER OF RUNS u IN SAMPLES OF SIZE (N_1, N_2)

N_1, N_2 \ u	22	23	24	25	26	27	28	29
11,11	1.0000							
11,12	0.999999	1.0000						
11,13	.99999	1.0000						
11,14	.99998	1.0000						
11,15	.99995	1.0000						
11,16	.99989	1.0000						
11,17	.9998	1.0000						
11,18	.9996	1.0000						
11,19	.9994	1.0000						
11,20	.9991	1.0000						
12,12	0.99999	0.999999	1.0000					
12,13	.99996	.99999	0.999999	1.0000				
12,14	.99986	.99998	.999999	1.0000				
12,15	.99966	.99995	.999995	1.0000				
12,16	.99930	.9999	.999985	1.0000				
12,17	.99872	.9998	.99996	1.0000				
12,18	.9978	.9996	.99993	1.0000				
12,19	.9966	.9994	.99987	1.0000				
12,20	.9950	.9991	.99978	1.0000				
13,13	0.9998	0.99997	0.999998	0.9999998	1.0000			
13,14	.9995	.9999	.99999	.999999	0.9999999	1.0000		
13,15	.9988	.9997	.99996	.999995	.9999996	1.0000		
13,16	.9975	.9994	.99988	.99999	.999998	1.0000		
13,17	.9957	.9989	.99975	.99996	.999995	1.0000		
13,18	.9930	.9981	.99951	.99993	.99999	1.0000		
13,19	.9894	.9969	.99914	.99987	.99998	1.0000		
13,20	.9848	.9954	.9986	.99978	.99995	1.0000		
14,14	0.9985	0.9996	0.9999	0.99999	0.999999	0.9999999	1.0000	
14,15	.9967	.9991	.9998	.99997	.999996	.9999996	0.99999999	1.0000
14,16	.9938	.9981	.9995	.99990	.999986	.9999985	.9999999	1.0000
14,17	.9894	.9965	.9990	.99978	.999961	.9999953	.9999995	1.0000
14,18	.9834	.9941	.9982	.99957	.999910	.9999885	.9999986	1.0000
14,19	.9756	.9909	.9970	.99923	.999817	.9999753	.9999963	1.0000
14,20	.9660	.9867	.9952	.99872	.999663	.9999527	.9999916	1.0000
15,15	0.9930	0.9977	0.9994	0.9999	0.99998	0.999997	0.9999998	0.9999999
15,16	.9872	.9954	.9987	.9997	.99994	.999989	.9999988	.9999999
15,17	.9789	.9918	.9974	.9992	.99983	.999968	.9999956	.9999995
15,18	.9678	.9866	.9953	.9985	.99963	.999923	.9999871	.9999986
15,19	.9540	.9798	.9923	.9975	.99928	.999839	.9999686	.9999963
15,20	.9375	.9712	.9881	.9959	.99872	.999699	.9999332	.9999916
16,16	0.9772	0.9908	0.9970	0.9991	0.9998	0.99996	0.99999	0.999999
16,17	.9634	.9840	.9942	.9981	.9995	.99988	.99998	.999997
16,18	.9457	.9747	.9900	.9964	.9989	.99971	.99994	.999989
16,19	.9244	.9626	.9840	.9938	.9980	.99942	.99986	.999973
16,20	.8996	.9479	.9761	.9902	.9965	.99894	.99972	.999942
17,17	0.9428	0.9728	0.9891	0.9959	0.9988	0.9997	0.9999	0.99999
17,18	.9172	.9578	.9816	.9925	.9975	.9992	.9998	.99996
17,19	.8872	.9391	.9714	.9876	.9954	.9985	.9996	.99989
17,20	.8534	.9168	.9584	.9808	.9924	.9972	.9992	.99977
18,18	0.8829	0.9360	0.9697	0.9866	0.9950	0.9983	0.9995	0.9999
18,19	.8438	.9094	.9540	.9782	.9911	.9966	.9990	.9997
18,20	.8010	.8788	.9345	.9670	.9856	.9941	.9980	.9994
19,19	0.7956	0.8744	0.9317	0.9651	0.9846	0.9936	0.9978	0.9993
19,20	.7444	.8350	.9048	.9484	.9756	.9891	.9959	.9985
20,20	0.6857	0.7870	0.8699	0.9252	0.9620	0.9818	0.9925	0.9971

a) **DISTRIBUTION OF THE TOTAL NUMBER OF RUNS** u **IN SAMPLES OF SIZE** (N_1, N_2)

30	31	32	33	34	35	36	37
1.0000							
1.0000							
1.0000							
0.9999999	1.0000						
.9999996	1.0000						
.9999988	1.0000						
0.9999999	1.0000						
.9999997	1.0000						
.9999986	0.9999999	1.0000					
.9999958	.9999996	1.0000					
.9999893	.9999988	0.9999999	1.0000				
0.9999981	0.9999998	1.0000					
.9999929	.9999989	0.9999999	1.0000				
.9999795	.9999965	.9999996	1.0000				
.9999499	.9999909	.9999986	0.9999999	1.0000			
0.99998	0.999995	0.999999	0.9999999	1.0000			
.99993	.999985	.999998	.9999997	1.0000			
.99984	.999962	.999993	.9999989	0.9999999	0.9999999	1.0000	
0.9998	0.99995	0.99999	0.999999	.9999998	0.9999999	1.0000	
.9996	.99988	.99997	.999995	.9999993	.9999999	1.0000	
0.9990	0.9997	0.99993	0.99998	0.999997	0.9999995	0.9999999	1.0000

b) DISTRIBUTION OF THE TOTAL NUMBER OF RUNS u IN SAMPLES OF SIZE (N_1, N_2)

The values listed on the previous pages give the chance that u or fewer runs will occur. For example, for two samples of size 4, the chance of three or fewer runs is .114. For sample sizes $N_1 = N_2$ larger than 10 the following table can be used. The columns headed 0.5, 1, 2.5, 5 give values of u such that u or fewer-runs occur with chance less than the indicated percentage. For example, for $N_1 = N_2 = 12$ the chance of 8 or fewer runs is about .05. The columns headed 95, 97.5, 99, 99.5 give values of u for which the chance of u or more runs is less than 5, 2.5, 1, 0.5 per cent.

$N_1 = N_2$	0.5	1	2.5	5	95	97.5	99	99.5	Mean	Var.	s.d.
11	5	6	7	7	16	16	17	18	12	5.24	2.29
12	6	7	7	8	17	18	18	19	13	5.74	2.40
13	7	7	8	9	18	19	20	20	14	6.24	2.50
14	7	8	9	10	19	20	21	22	15	6.74	2.60
15	8	9	10	11	20	21	22	23	16	7.24	2.69
16	9	10	11	11	22	22	23	24	17	7.74	2.78
17	10	10	11	12	23	24	25	25	18	8.24	2.87
18	10	11	12	13	24	25	26	27	19	8.74	2.96
19	11	12	13	14	25	26	27	28	20	9.24	3.04
20	12	13	14	15	26	27	28	29	21	9.74	3.12
25	16	17	18	19	32	33	34	35	26	12.24	3.50
30	20	21	22	24	37	39	40	41	31	14.75	3.84
35	24	25	27	28	43	44	46	47	36	17.25	4.15
40	29	30	31	33	48	50	51	52	41	19.75	4.44
45	33	34	36	37	54	55	57	58	46	22.25	4.72
50	37	38	40	42	59	61	63	64	51	24.75	4.97
55	42	43	45	46	65	66	68	69	56	27.25	5.22
60	46	47	49	51	70	72	74	75	61	29.75	5.45
65	50	52	54	56	75	77	79	81	66	32.25	5.68
70	55	56	58	60	81	83	85	86	71	34.75	5.89
75	59	61	63	65	86	88	90	92	76	37.25	6.10
80	64	65	68	70	91	93	96	97	81	39.75	6.30
85	68	70	72	74	97	99	101	103	86	42.25	6.50
90	73	74	77	79	102	104	107	108	91	44.75	6.69
95	77	79	82	84	107	109	112	114	96	47.25	6.87
100	82	84	86	88	113	115	117	119	101	49.75	7.05

X.7 CRITICAL VALUES FOR THE KOLMOGOROV-SMIRNOV ONE-SAMPLE STATISTIC

A sample of size n is drawn from a population with cumulative distribution function $F(x)$. Define the empirical distribution function $F_n(x)$ to be the step function

$$F_n(x) = \frac{k}{n} \qquad \text{for} \qquad x_{(i)} \leq x \leq x_{(i+1)} \ ,$$

where k is the number of observations not greater than x. $x_{(1)}\ .\ .\ .\ , x_{(n)}$ denote the sample values arranged in ascending order. Under the null hypothesis that the sample has been drawn from the specified distribution, $F_n(x)$ should be fairly close to $F(x)$. Define

$$D = \max |F_n(x) - F(x)| \ .$$

For a two-tailed test this table gives critical values of the sampling distribution of D under the null hypothesis. Reject the hypothetical distribution if D exceeds the tabulated value. If n is over 35, determine the critical values of D by the divisions indicated in the table.

A one-tailed test is provided by the statistic

$$D^+ = \max\,[F_n(x) - F(x)] \ .$$

CRITICAL VALUES FOR THE KOLMOGOROV-SMIRNOV TEST OF GOODNESS OF FIT

One-sided test Two-sided test	p = 0.90 p = 0.80	0.95 0.90	0.975 0.95	0.99 0.98	0.995 0.99
n = 1	0.900	0.950	0.975	0.990	0.995
2	0.684	0.776	0.842	0.900	0.929
3	0.565	0.636	0.708	0.785	0.829
4	0.493	0.565	0.624	0.689	0.734
5	0.447	0.509	0.563	0.627	0.669
6	0.410	0.468	0.519	0.577	0.617
7	0.381	0.436	0.483	0.538	0.576
8	0.358	0.410	0.454	0.507	0.542
9	0.339	0.387	0.430	0.480	0.513
10	0.323	0.369	0.409	0.457	0.489
11	0.308	0.352	0.391	0.437	0.468
12	0.296	0.338	0.375	0.419	0.449
13	0.285	0.325	0.361	0.404	0.432
14	0.275	0.314	0.349	0.390	0.418
15	0.266	0.304	0.338	0.377	0.404
16	0.258	0.295	0.327	0.366	0.392
17	0.250	0.286	0.318	0.355	0.381
18	0.244	0.279	0.309	0.346	0.371
19	0.237	0.271	0.301	0.337	0.361
20	0.232	0.265	0.294	0.329	0.352
21	0.226	0.259	0.287	0.321	0.344
22	0.221	0.253	0.281	0.314	0.337
23	0.216	0.247	0.275	0.307	0.330
24	0.212	0.242	0.269	0.301	0.323
25	0.208	0.238	0.264	0.295	0.317
26	0.204	0.233	0.259	0.290	0.311
27	0.200	0.229	0.254	0.284	0.305
28	0.197	0.225	0.250	0.279	0.300
29	0.193	0.221	0.246	0.275	0.295
30	0.190	0.218	0.242	0.270	0.290
31	0.187	0.214	0.238	0.266	0.285
32	0.184	0.211	0.234	0.262	0.281
33	0.182	0.208	0.231	0.258	0.277
34	0.179	0.205	0.227	0.254	0.273
35	0.177	0.202	0.224	0.251	0.269
36	0.174	0.199	0.221	0.247	0.265
37	0.172	0.196	0.218	0.244	0.262
38	0.170	0.194	0.215	0.241	0.258
39	0.168	0.191	0.213	0.238	0.255
40	0.165	0.189	0.210	0.235	0.252
Approximation for $n > 40$:	$\frac{1.07}{\sqrt{n}}$	$\frac{1.22}{\sqrt{n}}$	$\frac{1.36}{\sqrt{n}}$	$\frac{1.52}{\sqrt{n}}$	$\frac{1.63}{\sqrt{n}}$

X.8 CRITICAL VALUES FOR THE KOLMOGOROV-SMIRNOV TWO-SAMPLE STATISTIC

A sample of size n_1 is drawn from a population with cumulative distribution function $F(x)$. Define the empirical distribution function $F_{n_1}(x)$ to be the step function

$$F_{n_1}(x) = \frac{k}{n_1} ,$$

where k is the number of observations not greater than x. A second sample of size n_2 is drawn with empirical distribution function $F_{n_2}(x)$. Define

$$D_{n_1,n_2} = \max |F_{n_1}(x) - F_{n_2}(x)|$$

for a two-tailed test. This table gives critical values of the sampling distribution of D under the null hypothesis that two independent samples have been drawn from the same population or from populations with the same distribution. Reject the null hypothesis if D exceeds the tabulated value.

A one-tailed test is provided by the statistic

$$D^+ = \max [F_{n_1}(x) - F_{n_2}(x)] .$$

For large values of n_1 and n_2, approximate formulas to be used are given at the bottom of the table.

CRITICAL VALUES FOR THE KOLMOGOROV-SMIRNOV TEST OF H_0: $F_1(x) = F_2(x)$

Sample size n_2	Sample size n_1: 1	2	3	4	5	6	7	8	9	10	12	15
1	* *	* *	* *	* *	* *	* *	* *	* *	* *	* *		
2		* *	* *	* *	* *	* *	* *	7/8 *	16/18 *	9/10 *		
3			* *	* *	12/15 *	5/6 *	18/21 *	18/24 *	7/9 8/9		9/12 11/12	
4				3/4 *	16/20 *	9/12 10/12	21/28 24/28	6/8 7/8	27/36 32/36	14/20 16/20	8/12 10/12	
5					4/5 4/5	20/30 25/30	25/35 30/35	27/40 32/40	31/45 36/45	7/10 8/10		10/15 11/15
6						4/6 5/6	29/42 35/42	16/24 18/24	12/18 14/18	19/30 22/30	7/12 9/12	
7							5/7 5/7	35/56 42/56	40/63 47/63	43/70 53/70		
8								5/8 6/8	45/72 54/72	23/40 28/40	14/24 16/24	
9									5/9 6/9	52/90 62/90	20/36 24/36	
10										6/10 7/10		15/30 19/30
12											6/12 7/12	30/60 35/60
15												7/15 8/15

Reject H_0 if

$$D = \max |F_{n_1}(x) - F_{n_2}(x)|$$

exceeds the tabulated value. The upper value gives a level at most .05 and the lower value gives a level at most .01.

Note 1: Where * appears, do not reject H_0 at the given level.
Note 2: For large values of n_1 and n_2, the following approximate formulas may be used:

$$\alpha = .05: \quad 1.36\sqrt{\frac{n_1 + n_2}{n_1 n_2}}$$

$$\alpha = .01: \quad 1.63\sqrt{\frac{n_1 + n_2}{n_1 n_2}}$$

CRITICAL VALUES OF D IN THE KOLMOGOROV-SMIRNOV TWO-SAMPLE TEST

(Large samples: two-tailed test)

Level of significance	Value of D so large as to call for rejection of H_0 at the indicated level of significance, where D = maximum $\lvert F_{n_1}(X) - F_{n_2}(X)\rvert$
.10	$1.22\sqrt{\frac{n_1+n_2}{n_1n_2}}$
.05	$1.36\sqrt{\frac{n_1+n_2}{n_1n_2}}$
.025	$1.48\sqrt{\frac{n_1+n_2}{n_1n_2}}$
.01	$1.63\sqrt{\frac{n_1+n_2}{n_1n_2}}$
.005	$1.73\sqrt{\frac{n_1+n_2}{n_1n_2}}$
.001	$1.95\sqrt{\frac{n_1+n_2}{n_1n_2}}$

X.9 KRUSKAL-WALLIS ONE-WAY ANALYSIS OF VARIANCE BY RANKS. PROBABILITIES ASSOCIATED WITH VALUES AS LARGE AS OBSERVED VALUES OF H

Three samples of sizes n_1, n_2, and n_3 are combined and ranked in ascending order of magnitude: numbers from 1 up to $N = n_1 + n_2 + n_3$ are attached to the ranks. To test whether the three samples come from the same population, the test statistic is

$$H = \frac{12}{N(N+1)} \sum_{j=1}^{3} \frac{R_j^2}{n_j} - 3(N+1),$$

where n_j = number of observations in j^{th} sample, $j = 1, 2, 3$,

$$N = \sum_{j=1}^{3} n_j = \text{number of observations in all samples combined} \ ,$$

R_j = sum of ranks in j^{th} sample.

Large values of H lead to rejection of the null hypothesis. If the three samples are from identical populations and the sample sizes are not too small, then H is approximately distributed as chi-square with two degrees of freedom. The first column in the table gives the sizes of the three samples. The second gives various values of H. The third gives the probability associated with the occurrence under the null hypothesis of values as large as an observed H.

PROBABILITIES ASSOCIATED WITH VALUES AS LARGE AS OBSERVED VALUES OF H IN THE KRUSKAL-WALLIS ONE-WAY ANALYSIS OF VARIANCE BY RANKS

Sample sizes			H	p
n_1	n_2	n_3		
2	1	1	2.7000	.500
2	2	1	3.6000	.200
2	2	2	4.5714	.067
			3.7143	.200
3	1	1	3.2000	.300
3	2	1	4.2857	.100
			3.8571	.133
3	2	2	5.3572	.029
			4.7143	.048
			4.5000	.067
			4.4643	.105
3	3	1	5.1429	.043
			4.5714	.100
			4.0000	.129
3	3	2	6.2500	.011
			5.3611	.032
			5.1389	.061
			4.5556	.100
			4.2500	.121
3	3	3	7.2000	.004
			6.4889	.011
			5.6889	.029
			5.6000	.050
			5.0667	.086
			4.6222	.100
4	1	1	3.5714	.200
4	2	1	4.8214	.057
			4.5000	.076
			4.0179	.114
4	2	2	6.0000	.014
			5.3333	.033
			5.1250	.052
			4.4583	.100
			4.1667	.105
4	3	1	5.8333	.021
			5.2083	.050
			5.0000	.057
			4.0556	.093
			3.8889	.129
4	3	2	6.4444	.008
			6.3000	.011
			5.4444	.046
			5.4000	.051
			4.5111	.098
			4.4444	.102
4	3	3	6.7455	.010
			6.7091	.013
			5.7909	.046
			5.7273	.050
			4.7091	.092
			4.7000	.101
4	4	1	6.6667	.010
			6.1667	.022
			4.9667	.048
			4.8667	.054
			4.1667	.082
			4.0667	.102
4	4	2	7.0364	.006
			6.8727	.011
			5.4545	.046
			5.2364	.052
			4.5545	.098
			4.4455	.103
4	4	3	7.1439	.010
			7.1364	.011
			5.5985	.049
			5.5758	.051
			4.5455	.099
			4.4773	.102
4	4	4	7.6538	.008
			7.5385	.011
			5.6923	.049
			5.6538	.054
			4.6539	.097
			4.5001	.104
5	1	1	3.8571	.143
5	2	1	5.2500	.036
			5.0000	.048
			4.4500	.071
			4.2000	.095
			4.0500	.119

PROBABILITIES ASSOCIATED WITH VALUES AS LARGE AS OBSERVED VALUES OF H IN THE KRUSKAL-WALLIS ONE-WAY ANALYSIS OF VARIANCE BY RANKS

Sample sizes			H	p
n_1	n_2	n_3		
5	2	2	6.5333	.008
			6.1333	.013
			5.1600	.034
			5.0400	.056
			4.3733	.090
			4.2933	.122
5	3	1	6.4000	.012
			4.9600	.048
			4.8711	.052
			4.0178	.095
			3.8400	.123
5	3	2	6.9091	.009
			6.8218	.010
			5.2509	.049
			5.1055	.052
			4.6509	.091
			4.4945	.101
5	3	3	7.0788	.009
			6.9818	.011
			5.6485	.049
			5.5152	.051
			4.5333	.097
			4.4121	.109
5	4	1	6.9545	.008
			6.8400	.011
			4.9855	.044
			4.8600	.056
			3.9873	.098
			3.9600	.102
5	4	2	7.2045	.009
			7.1182	.010
			5.2727	.049
			5.2682	.050
			4.5409	.098
			4.5182	.101
5	4	3	7.4449	.010
			7.3949	.011
			5.6564	.049
			5.6308	.050
			4.5487	.099
			4.5231	.103
5	4	4	7.7604	.009
			7.7440	.011
			5.6571	.049
			5.6176	.050
			4.6187	.100
			4.5527	.102
5	5	1	7.3091	.009
			6.8364	.011
			5.1273	.046
			4.9091	.053
			4.1091	.086
			4.0364	.105
5	5	2	7.3385	.010
			7.2692	.010
			5.3385	.047
			5.2462	.051
			4.6231	.097
			4.5077	.100
5	5	3	7.5780	.010
			7.5429	.010
			5.7055	.046
			5.6264	.051
			4.5451	.100
			4.5363	.102
5	5	4	7.8229	.010
			7.7914	.010
			5.6657	.049
			5.6429	.050
			4.5229	.099
			4.5200	.101
5	5	5	8.0000	.009
			7.9800	.010
			5.7800	.049
			5.6600	.051
			4.5600	.100
			4.5000	.102

X.10 CRITICAL VALUES OF SPEARMAN'S RANK CORRELATION COEFFICIENT

Spearman's coefficient of rank correlation, denoted by the letter ρ_s measures the correspondence between two rankings. If d_i is the difference between the ranks of the ith pair of a set of n pairs of elements, then Spearman's Rho is defined as

$$\rho_s = 1 - \frac{6 \sum_{i=1}^{n} d_i^2}{n^3 - n}$$

$$= 1 - \frac{6S_r}{n^3 - n}, \qquad \text{where } S_r = \sum_{i=1}^{n} d_i^2.$$

The exact distribution of S_r has been studied, and critical values when there is complete independence are given in Table X.12a).

Table X.12b) gives the distribution of Σd_i^2. These values are such that Σd_i^2 computed for a sample will equal or exceed the tabulated value with probability as given in the table.

n	*p* = 0.900	0.950	0.975	0.990	0.995	0.999
4	0.8000	0.8000				
5	0.7000	0.8000	0.9000	0.9000		
6	0.6000	0.7714	0.8286	0.8857	0.9429	
7	0.5357	0.6786	0.7450	0.8571	0.8929	0.9643
8	0.5000	0.6190	0.7143	0.8095	0.8571	0.9286
9	0.4667	0.5833	0.6833	0.7667	0.8167	0.9000
10	0.4424	0.5515	0.6364	0.7333	0.7818	0.8667
11	0.4182	0.5273	0.6091	0.7000	0.7545	0.8364
12	0.3986	0.4965	0.5804	0.6713	0.7273	0.8182
13	0.3791	0.4780	0.5549	0.6429	0.6978	0.7912
14	0.3626	0.4593	0.5341	0.6220	0.6747	0.7670
15	0.3500	0.4429	0.5179	0.6000	0.6536	0.7464
16	0.3382	0.4265	0.5000	0.5824	0.6324	0.7265
17	0.3260	0.4118	0.4853	0.5637	0.6152	0.7083
18	0.3148	0.3994	0.4716	0.5480	0.5975	0.6904
19	0.3070	0.3895	0.4579	0.5333	0.5825	0.6737
20	0.2977	0.3789	0.4451	0.5203	0.5684	0.6586
21	0.2909	0.3688	0.4351	0.5078	0.5545	0.6455
22	0.2829	0.3597	0.4241	0.4963	0.5426	0.6318
23	0.2767	0.3518	0.4150	0.4852	0.5306	0.6186
24	0.2704	0.3435	0.4061	0.4748	0.5200	0.6070
25	0.2646	0.3362	0.3977	0.4654	0.5100	0.5962
26	0.2588	0.3299	0.3894	0.4564	0.5002	0.5856
27	0.2540	0.3236	0.3822	0.4481	0.4915	0.5757
28	0.2490	0.3175	0.3749	0.4401	0.4828	0.5660
29	0.2443	0.3113	0.3685	0.4320	0.4744	0.5567
30	0.2400	0.3059	0.3620	0.4251	0.4665	0.5479

b) EXACT VALUES OF Σd_i^2 FOR SPEARMAN'S RANK CORRELATION

The probability that $\Sigma d^2 \geq S$ for $S \geq \Sigma m$, or that $\Sigma d^2 \leq S$ for $S \leq \Sigma m$
(where Σm represents mean value of sum of squares)

	n = 2	3	4	5	6	7	8	9	10
S \\ Σm	1	4	10	20	35	56	84	120	165
0	0.5000	0.1667	0.0417	0.0083	0.0014	0.0002	0.0003	0.0001	0.0000
2	.5000	.5000	.1667	.0417	.0083	.0014	.0006	.0002	.0001
4		.5000	.2083	.0667	.0167	.0034	.0011	.0003	.0001
6		.5000	.3750	.1167	.0292	.0062	.0018	.0005	.0001
8		.1667	.4583	.1750	.0514	.0119	.0028	.0007	.0002
10			0.5417	0.2250	0.0681	0.0171	0.0042	0.0010	0.0003
12			.4583	.2583	.0875	.0240	.0059	.0015	.0004
14			.3750	.3417	.1208	.0331	.0081	.0020	.0005
16			.2083	.3917	.1486	.0440	.0108	.0027	.0007
18			.1667	.4750	.1778	.0548	.0141	.0035	.0009
20			0.0417	0.5250	0.2097	0.0694	0.0179	0.0045	0.0011
22				.4750	.2486	.0833	.0224	.0057	.0014
24				.3917	.2819	.1000	.0275	.0071	.0018
26				.3417	.3292	.1179	.0331	.0087	.0022
28				.2583	.3569	.1333	.0396	.0106	.0027
30				0.2250	0.4014	0.1512	0.0469	0.0127	0.0032
32				.1750	.4597	.1768	.0550	.0152	.0039
34				.1167	.5000	.1978	.0639	.0179	.0046
36				.0667	.5000	.2222	.0736	.0210	.0054
38				.0417	.4597	.2488	.0841	.0244	.0064
40				0.0083	0.4014	0.2780	0.0956	0.0281	0.0075
42					.3569	.2974	.1078	.0323	.0086
44					.3292	.3308	.1207	.0368	.0100
46					.2819	.3565	.1345	.0417	.0114
48					.2486	.3913	.1491	.0470	.0130
50					0.2097	0.4198	0.1645	0.0528	0.0148
52					.1778	.4532	.1806	.0589	.0168
54					.1486	.4817	.1974	.0656	.0189
56					.1208	.5183	.2150	.0726	.0212
58					.0875	.4817	.2332	.0802	.0237
60					0.0681	0.4532	0.2520	0.0882	0.0264
62					.0514	.4198	.2715	.0966	.0293
64					.0292	.3913	.2915	.1056	.0324
66					.0167	.3565	.3120	.1149	.0358
68					.0083	.3308	.3330	.1248	.0394
70					0.0014	0.2974	0.3544	0.1351	0.0432
72						.2780	.3761	.1459	.0472
74						.2488	.3982	.1571	.0515
76						.2222	.4205	.1688	.0561
78						.1978	.4431	.1809	.0609

b) EXACT VALUES OF Σd_i^2 FOR SPEARMAN'S RANK CORRELATION

The probability that $\Sigma d^2 \geq S$ for $S \geq \Sigma m$, or that $\Sigma d^2 \leq S$ for $S \leq \Sigma m$
(where Σm represents mean value of sum of squares)

	n = 2	3	4	5	6	7	8	9	10
S \ Σm	1	4	10	20	35	56	84	120	165
80						0.1768	0.4657	0.1935	0.0659
82						.1512	.4885	.2065	.0713
84						.1333	.5113	.2198	.0769
86						.1179	.4885	.2336	.0828
88						.1000	. 4657	.2477	.0889
90						0.0833	0.4431	0.2622	0.0954
92						.0694	.4205	.2770	.1021
94						.0548	.3982	.2922	.1091
96						.0440	.3761	.3077	.1164
98						.0331	.3544	.3234	.1239
100						0.0240	0.3330	0.3394	0.1318
102						.0171	.3120	.3557	.1399
104						.0119	.2915	.3721	.1483
106						.0062	.2715	.3888	.1570
108						.0034	.2520	.4056	.1659
110						0.0014	0.2332	0.4226	0.1751
112						.0002	.2150	.4397	.1846
114							.1974	.4568	.1944
116							.1806	.4741	.2044
118							.1645	.4914	.2146
120							0.1491	0.5086	0.2251
122							.1345	.4914	.2358
124							.1207	.4741	.2468
126							.1078	.4568	.2580
128							.0956	.4397	.2694
130							0.0841	0.4226	0.2810
132							.0736	.4056	.2928
134							.0639	.3888	.3048
136							.0550	.3721	.3169
138							.0469	.3557	.3293
140							0.0396	0.3394	0.3418
142							.0331	.3234	.3545
144							.0275	.3077	.3673
146							.0224	.2922	.3802
148							.0179	.2770	.3932
150							0.0141	0.2622	0.4063
152							.0108	.2477	.4196
154							.0081	.2336	.4328
156							.0059	.2198	.4462
158							.0042	.2065	.4596
160							0.0028	0.1935	0.4731
162							.0018	.1809	.4865
164							.0011	.1688	.5000
166							.0006	.1571	.5000
168							.0003	.1459	.4865

(Tables for cases of $n = 9$ and $n = 10$ can be completed by symmetry)

X.11 DISTRIBUTION OF KENDALL'S RANK CORRELATION COEFFICIENT

Consider any one of the $\frac{n}{2}(n-1)$ possible pairs for two sets of ranked elements. Associate with this pair (*a*) a score of $+1$ if the ranking for both sets is the same order or (*b*) a score of -1 if the ranking is in different order. Kendall's score S_t is then defined as the total of these $\frac{n}{2}(n-1)$ individual pairs. S_t will have a maximum value of $\frac{n}{2}(n-1)$ if the two rankings are identical and a minimum value of $-\frac{n}{2}(n-1)$ if the sets are ranked in exactly opposite order. Kendall's Tau is defined as

$$\tau = \frac{S_t}{\frac{n}{2}(n-1)},$$

and has the range $-1 \leq \tau \leq 1$. This table may be used to determine the exact probability associated with the occurrence (one-tailed) under the null hypothesis that the observed value of Kendall's Tau indicates the existence of an association between the two sets of any value as extreme as an observed S_t. The tabled value is the probability that S_t is equalled or exceeded.

DISTRIBUTION OF KENDALL'S RANK CORRELATION COEFFICIENT, t_k, IN RANDOM RANKINGS

S_t	Values of n				S_t	Values of n		
	4	5	8	9		6	7	10
0	0.625	0.592	0.548	0.540	1	0.500	0.500	0.500
2	.375	.408	.452	.460	3	.360	.386	.431
4	.167	.242	.360	.381	5	.235	.281	.364
6	.042	.117	.274	.306	7	.136	.191	.300
8		.042	.199	.238	9	.068	.119	.242
10		0.0083	0.138	0.179	11	0.028	0.068	0.190
12			.089	.130	13	.0083	.035	.146
14			.054	.090	15	.0014	.015	.108
16			.031	.060	17		.0054	.078
18			.016	.038	19		.0014	.054
20			0.0071	0.022	21		0.0002	0.036
22			.0028	.012	23			.023
24			.0009	.0063	25			.014
26			.0002	.0029	27			.0083
28				.0012	29			.0046
30				0.0004	31			0.0023
					33			.0011
					35			.0005

The distribution of S_t is symmetrical so that values of the probability for negative S_t can be obtained by appropriate subtraction from unity; e.g. for $n = 9$,

$$\Pr\{S_t \geq -14\} = 1 - \Pr\{S_t \geq 16\} = 1 - 0.060 = 0.940 \ .$$

XI. QUALITY CONTROL

XI.1 FACTORS FOR COMPUTING CONTROL LIMITS

A. Control Charts for Measurement

If the process mean and standard deviation, μ and σ, are known, and it is assumed that the underlying distribution is normal, it is possible to assert with probability $1 - \alpha$ that the mean of a random sample of size n will fall between $\bar{x} - z_{\alpha/2}\frac{\sigma}{\sqrt{n}}$ and $\bar{x} + z_{\alpha/2}\frac{\sigma}{\sqrt{n}}$. These two limits on $\bar{x}$ provide upper and lower control limits. In actual practice, μ and σ are usually unknown and it is necessary to estimate their values from a large sample taken while the process is "in control". The central line of an $\bar{x}$-chart is given by μ and the lower and upper three-sigma control limits are given by $\mu - A\sigma$ and $\mu + A\sigma$, respectively, where $A = \frac{3}{\sqrt{n}}$ and n is the sample size. Where the population parameters are unknown, it is necessary to estimate these parameters on the basis of preliminary samples. If k samples are used, each of size n, denote the mean of the ith sample by $\bar{x}_i$ and the grand mean of the k sample means by $\bar{\bar{x}}$, i.e.

$$\bar{\bar{x}} = \frac{1}{k}\sum_{i=1}^{k} \bar{x}_i \ .$$

Denote the range of the ith sample by R_i and by $\bar{R}$ the mean of the k sample ranges, i.e.

$$\bar{R} = \frac{1}{k}\sum_{i=1}^{k} R_i \ .$$

Since $\bar{\bar{x}}$ is an unbiased estimate of the population mean μ, the central line for the $\bar{x}$-chart is given by $\bar{\bar{x}}$. The statistic R does not provide an unbiased estimate of σ, but $A_2\bar{R}$ is an unbiased estimate of $\frac{3\sigma}{\sqrt{n}}$. The constant multiplier A_2 depends on the assumption of normality. Thus, the central line and the lower and upper three sigma limits, LCL and UCL, for an $\bar{x}$-chart (with μ and σ estimated from past date) are given by

$$\begin{aligned} \text{central line} &= \bar{\bar{x}} \\ \text{LCL} &= \bar{\bar{x}} - A_2\bar{R} \\ \text{UCL} &= \bar{\bar{x}} + A_2\bar{R} \ . \end{aligned}$$

The central line and control limits of an R chart are based on the distribution of the range of samples of size n from a normal population. The mean and standard deviation of the sampling distribution of R are given by $d_2\sigma$ and $d_3\sigma$, respectively, when σ is known. Here d_2 and d_3 are constants which depend on the size of the sample. The set of control chart values for an R chart (with σ known) is given by

$$\begin{aligned} \text{central line} &= d_2\sigma \\ \text{LCL} &= D_1\sigma \\ \text{UCL} &= D_2\sigma, \end{aligned}$$

where $D_1 = d_2 - 3d_3$ and $D_2 = d_2 + 3d_3$.

If σ is unknown, the control chart values for an R chart are given by

$$\begin{aligned} \text{central line} &= \bar{R} \\ \text{LCL} &= D_3\bar{R} \\ \text{UCL} &= D_4\bar{R}, \end{aligned}$$

where $D_3 = \dfrac{D_1}{d_2}$ and $D_4 = \dfrac{D_2}{d_2}$.

The central line and control limits of an s-chart are based on estimates obtained from the samples. A pooled estimate of the population variance is obtained from the k samples, i.e.

$$s_p^2 = \frac{\sum_i (n_i - 1)s_i^2}{\sum_i (n_i - 1)}, \qquad i = 1, 2, \ldots, k .$$

If the sample sizes are all equal, the pooled estimate is

$$s_p^2 = \frac{1}{k}\sum_i s_i^2 .$$

The control chart values for an s-chart are given by

$$\begin{aligned} \text{central line} &= C_2' s_p \\ \text{LCL} &= B_2' s_p \\ \text{UCL} &= B_4' s_p . \end{aligned}$$

If one uses the biased estimator of the variance s_p', as is often done in quality control work, the control chart values are given by

$$\begin{aligned} \text{central line} &= c_2 s_p' \\ \text{LCL} &= B_2 s_p' \\ \text{UCL} &= B_4 s_p' . \end{aligned}$$

B. Control Charts for Attributes

Control limits for a fraction-defective chart are based on the sampling theory for proportions, using the normal curve approximation to the binomial. If k samples are taken, the estimator of p is given by

$$\bar{p} = \frac{\sum_i x_i}{\sum_i n_i}, \qquad i = 1, 2, \ldots, k$$

where x_i is the number of defectives in the ith sample of size n_i. The central line and control limits of a fraction defective chart based on analysis of past data are given by

$$\begin{aligned} \text{central line} &= \bar{p} \\ \text{LCL} &= \bar{p} - 3\sqrt{\frac{\bar{p}(1-\bar{p})}{n_i}} \\ \text{UCL} &= \bar{p} + 3\sqrt{\frac{\bar{p}(1-\bar{p})}{n_i}} . \end{aligned}$$

When the sample sizes are approximately equal, n_i is replaced by $\bar{n} = \frac{1}{k}\sum_i n_i$.

Equivalent to the p chart for the fraction defective is the control chart for the number of defective. Here, if p is estimated by $\bar{p}$, the control chart values for a number-of-defectives chart are given by

$$\begin{aligned} \text{central line} &= \bar{n}\bar{p} \\ \text{LCL} &= \bar{n}\bar{p} - 3\sqrt{\bar{n}\bar{p}(1-\bar{p})} \\ \text{UCL} &= \bar{n}\bar{p} + 3\sqrt{\bar{n}\bar{p}(1-\bar{p})}\ . \end{aligned}$$

In many cases it is necessary to control the number of defects per unit C, where C is taken to be a value of a random variable having a Poisson distribution. If k is the number of units available for estimating λ, the parameter of the Poisson distribution, and if C_i is the number of defects in the ith unit, then λ is estimated by

$$\bar{C} = \frac{1}{k}\sum_{i=1}^{k} C_i\ ,$$

and the control-chart values for the C-chart are

$$\begin{aligned} \text{central line} &= \bar{C} \\ \text{LCL} &= \bar{C} - 3\sqrt{\bar{C}} \\ \text{UCL} &= \bar{C} + 3\sqrt{\bar{C}} \end{aligned}$$

This table presents values of the factors for computing control limits for various sample sizes n.

FACTORS FOR COMPUTING CONTROL LIMITS

Number of observations in sample, n	$\bar{X}$ chart		R chart			s chart			$\hat{\sigma}$ chart (biased)		
	Factors for control limits		Factor for central line	Factors for control limits		Factor for central line	Factors for control limits		Factor for central line	Factors for control limits	
	A	A_2	d_2	D_3	D_4	c_2'	B_2'	B_4'	c_2	B_2	B_4
2	2.121	1.880	1.128	0	3.267	0.798	0	2.298	0.5642	0	3.267
3	1.732	1.023	1.693	0	2.575	0.886	0	2.111	0.7236	0	2.568
4	1.500	0.729	2.059	0	2.282	0.921	0	1.982	0.7979	0	2.266
5	1.342	0.577	2.326	0	2.115	0.940	0	1.889	0.8407	0	2.089
6	1.225	0.483	2.534	0	2.004	0.951	0.085	1.817	0.8686	0.030	1.970
7	1.134	0.419	2.704	0.076	1.924	0.960	0.158	1.762	0.8882	0.118	1.882
8	1.061	0.373	2.847	0.136	1.864	0.965	0.215	1.715	0.9027	0.185	1.815
9	1.000	0.337	2.970	0.184	1.816	0.969	0.262	1.676	0.9139	0.239	1.761
10	0.949	0.308	3.078	0.223	1.777	0.973	0.302	1.644	0.9227	0.284	1.716
11	0.905	0.285	3.173	0.256	1.744	0.976	0.336	1.616	0.9300	0.321	1.679
12	0.866	0.266	3.258	0.284	1.716	0.977	0.365	1.589	0.9359	0.354	1.646
13	0.832	0.249	3.336	0.308	1.692	0.980	0.392	1.568	0.9410	0.382	1.618
14	0.802	0.235	3.407	0.329	1.671	0.981	0.414	1.548	0.9453	0.406	1.594
15	0.775	0.223	3.472	0.348	1.652	0.982	0.434	1.530	0.9490	0.428	1.572
16	0.750	0.212	3.532	0.364	1.636	0.984	0.454	1.514	0.9523	0.448	1.552
17	0.728	0.203	3.588	0.379	1.621	0.984	0.469	1.499	0.9551	0.466	1.534
18	0.707	0.194	3.640	0.392	1.608	0.986	0.486	1.486	0.9576	0.482	1.518
19	0.688	0.187	3.689	0.404	1.596	0.986	0.500	1.472	0.9599	0.497	1.503
20	0.671	0.180	3.735	0.414	1.586	0.987	0.513	1.461	0.9619	0.510	1.490
21	0.655	0.173	3.778	0.425	1.575	0.988	0.525	1.451	0.9638	0.523	1.477
22	0.640	0.167	3.819	0.434	1.566	0.988	0.536	1.440	0.9655	0.534	1.466
23	0.626	0.162	3.858	0.443	1.557	0.989	0.546	1.432	0.9670	0.545	1.455
24	0.612	0.157	3.895	0.452	1.548	0.989	0.556	1.422	0.9684	0.555	1.445
25	0.600	0.153	3.931	0.459	1.541	0.990	0.566	1.414	0.9696	0.565	1.435

XI.2 PERCENTAGE POINTS OF THE DISTRIBUTION OF THE MEAN DEVIATION

If $x_1, x_2, \ldots, x_n$ is a random sample of n observations, the mean deviation is given by

$$\text{M.D.} = \frac{1}{n}\sum_{i=1}^{n} |x_i - \bar{x}|$$

where $\bar{x}$ is the sample mean. This table gives certain lower and upper percentage points of the standardized mean deviation $\frac{\text{M.D.}}{\sigma}$.

PERCENTAGE POINTS OF THE DISTRIBUTION OF THE MEAN DEVIATION

Lower percentage points						
Size of sample n	**0.1**	**0.5**	**1.0**	**2.5**	**5.0**	**10.0**
2	0.001	0.004	0.009	0.022	0.044	0.089
3	0.022	0.052	0.073	0.116	0.166	0.238
4	0.066	0.114	0.145	0.199	0.254	0.328
5	0.112	0.170	0.203	0.260	0.315	0.386
6	0.153	0.215	0.250	0.306	0.360	0.428
7	0.190	0.252	0.287	0.342	0.394	0.459
8	0.220	0.283	0.318	0.372	0.422	0.484
9	0.247	0.310	0.344	0.396	0.445	0.504
10	0.271	0.333	0.366	0.417	0.464	0.521
Normal approximation						
10	0.171	0.269	0.316	0.386	0.445	0.514

Upper percentage points						
Size of sample n	**10.0**	**5.0**	**2.5**	**1.0**	**0.5**	**0.1**
2	1.163	1.386	1.585	1.821	1.985	2.327
3	1.117	1.276	1.417	1.586	1.703	1.949
4	1.089	1.224	1.344	1.489	1.590	1.806
5	1.069	1.187	1.292	1.419	1.507	1.693
6	1.052	1.158	1.253	1.366	1.445	1.613
7	1.038	1.135	1.222	1.325	1.397	1.550
8	1.026	1.116	1.196	1.292	1.358	1.499
9	1.016	1.100	1.175	1.264	1.326	1.457
10	1.007	1.086	1.156	1.240	1.299	1.422
Normal approximation						
10	1.000	1.069	1.128	1.198	1.245	1.342

The unit is the population standard deviation.

XI.3 CUMULATIVE SUM CONTROL CHARTS (CSCC)

Another form of control chart which has gained wide applicability in the last few years is the cumulative sum control chart (CSCC). CSCC for means, ranges, variances, np, and c are presented here.

A. CSCC for the Mean

The mean of the ith sample of size n is denoted by $\bar{x}_i$. We plot on the control chart points with the coordinates (m, Y_m) where m is the sample number and

$$Y_m = \sigma_{\bar{x}}^{-1} \sum_i (\bar{x}_i - \mu_0)$$

with μ_0 equal to the proposed "target mean". The chart is interpreted by placing a mask, which is the shaded area of Figure a, over the chart with the point O over the last point

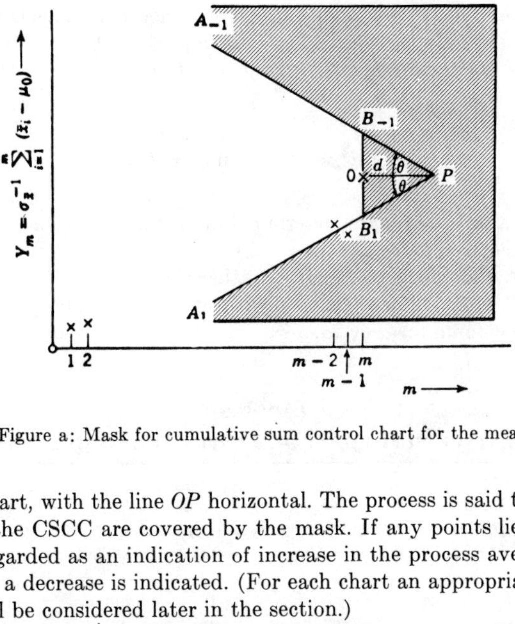

Figure a: Mask for cumulative sum control chart for the mean.

plotted on the chart, with the line OP horizontal. The process is said to be out of control if any points of the CSCC are covered by the mask. If any points lie below the straight line A_1B_1 it is regarded as an indication of increase in the process average; if any points lie above $A_{-1}B_{-1}$ a decrease is indicated. (For each chart an appropriate scaling factor is utilized. This will be considered later in the section.)

In order to determine the dimensions of the mask we must calculate the size 2θ of the angle $B_{-1}PB_1$, and the length, d, from O to the vertex, P, of this angle in Figure a. To do so we first decide on the size of errors of the first and second kind. (As long as β is very small, less than 0.01, say, this can be deleted from the exact formula.) The approximate formulas for θ and d are

$$(1) \qquad \begin{cases} \theta = \arctan(\delta/2) \\ d = -2\delta^{-2} \ln \alpha \end{cases}$$

where $\delta = D/\sigma_{\bar{x}}$ and "D" is the least size shift (in either direction) which it is desired to detect with fair certainty ($1 - \beta$, or power). The probability of error of the first kind for a *two-sided test* is taken here as 2α and for a *one-sided test* as α.

The procedure for a CSCC on means is as follows:

1. Decide on α (or 2α) and D.
2. Determine θ and d from equation (1).
3. Plot the sequential points Y_m moving the mask with each successive point.

4. At each step make a decision to
   a. continue the test
   b. accept a shift of $\mu_0 + D$, or
   c. accept a shift of $\mu_0 - D$.

If σ (and hence $\sigma_{\bar{x}}$) is not known or assumed before the test, this can be estimated by

$$s_p = \sqrt{\Sigma s_i^2/m}$$

where s_i^2 is the variance from sample i, and m is the number of samples. As long as the number of degrees of freedom $\nu = m(n - 1)$ is greater than 30 or 40, this estimate by s_p is quite reliable.

An alternative to calculating the values of θ and d is to make use of Table a. For selected values of δ and α, the values of θ and d can be taken directly from this table.

To attempt to calculate the dimensions of the mask is somewhat meaningless unless the appropriate *scaling factor* is brought into these dimensions. This is different from the Shewhart chart where only the vertical scale is important. Let k units for the ordinate be equal to one unit for the abscissa. Then the equations for θ^* and d^* become

$$\begin{cases} \theta^* = \arctan(D/2k) \\ d^* = -2\delta^{-2} \ln \alpha = d\,. \end{cases}$$

Note that if Table a be used for the determination of the dimensions of the mask for θ^* and d^*, it must be entered twice as follows:

1. To select θ^*, choose the row for D/k rather than δ.
2. To select d^* (for a designated α or 2α) choose the appropriate row for δ and appropriate column for α or 2α.

TABLE a

CUMULATIVE SUM CONTROL LIMITS FOR SAMPLE MEANS

		Values of d						
δ	θ	$2\alpha = 0.10$* $\alpha = 0.05$†	$2\alpha = 0.05$ $\alpha = 0.025$	$2\alpha = 0.02$ $\alpha = 0.01$	$2\alpha = 0.01$ $\alpha = 0.005$	$2\alpha = 0.0027$ $\alpha = 0.00135$‡	$2\alpha = 0.002$ $\alpha = 0.001$	$2\alpha = 0.001$ $\alpha = 0.0005$
0.2	5° 43′	149.8	184.4	230.6	264.9	330.4	345.4	380.0
0.4	11° 19′	37.4	46.1	57.6	66.2	82.6	86.3	95.0
0.6	16° 42′	16.6	20.5	25.6	29.4	36.7	38.4	42.2
0.8	21° 48′	9.36	11.5	14.4	16.6	20.6	21.6	23.8
1.0	26° 34′	5.99	7.38	9.21	10.6	13.2	13.8	15.2
1.2	30° 58′	4.16	5.12	6.40	7.36	9.18	9.59	10.6
1.4	35° 0′	3.06	3.76	4.70	5.41	6.74	7.05	7.76
1.6	38° 40′	2.34	2.88	3.60	4.14	5.16	5.40	5.94
1.8	41° 59′	1.85	2.28	2.84	3.27	4.08	4.26	4.69
2.0	45° 0′	1.50	1.84	2.30	2.65	3.30	3.45	3.80
2.2	47° 44′	1.24	1.52	1.90	2.19	2.73	2.85	3.14
2.4	50° 12′	1.04	1.28	1.60	1.84	2.29	2.40	2.64
2.6	52° 26′	0.89	1.09	1.36	1.57	1.95	2.04	2.25
2.8	54° 28′	0.76	0.94	1.17	1.35	1.69	1.76	1.94
3.0	56° 19′	0.67	0.82	1.02	1.18	1.47	1.54	1.69

* Two-sided test.
† One-sided test.
‡ These are comparable to the "3σ" limits used in the Shewhart chart, i.e. $2\alpha = 0.0027$ and $\alpha = 0.00135$.

B. CSCC for Sample Ranges

In constructing a CSCC on sample ranges, we utilize the distribution of the sample range, using two approximations for the distribution of the sample range from samples of size n from a normal population, with variance equal to 1. These are

(*a*) $c \times$ (χ with ν_1 degrees of freedom)
(*b*) $c' \times$ (χ^2 with ν_1' degrees of freedom)

The first of these is a better approximation if n is less than 10; otherwise (*b*) is better. Again we retain a constant sample size (n) with c, c', ν_1 and ν_1' dependent upon n.

For approximation (*a*) one plots the point

$$\left(m\nu_1, (\sigma c)^{-2} \sum_i R_i^2\right) .$$

The corresponding values of θ and d are

$$\begin{cases} \theta = \arctan\left[\dfrac{2 \ln \sigma_1/\sigma_0}{1 - (\sigma_0/\sigma_1)^2}\right] \\ d = -\ln \alpha / \ln (\sigma_1/\sigma_0) . \end{cases}$$

In approximation (*b*) the coordinates of the point and the values of d and θ as shown in Figure b.1, are

$$\begin{cases} \left(m\nu_1', (\sigma_0 c')^{-1} \sum_i R_i\right) \\ \theta = \arctan\left[\dfrac{\ln (\sigma_1/\sigma_0)}{1 - (\sigma_0/\sigma_1)}\right] \\ d = -2 \ln \alpha / \ln (\sigma_1/\sigma_0) . \end{cases}$$

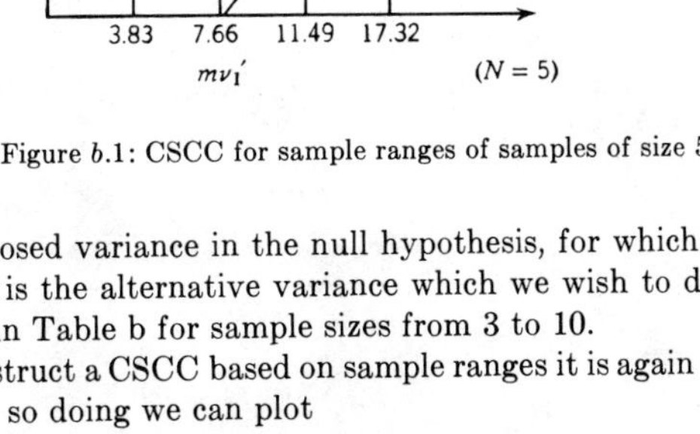

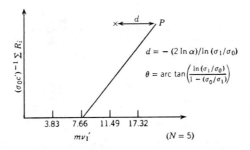

Figure *b*.1: CSCC for sample ranges of samples of size 5.

Here σ_0^2 is the proposed variance in the null hypothesis, for which the risk of rejection, if true, is α and σ_1^2 is the alternative variance which we wish to detect. Values of c, c', ν_1 and ν_1' are given in Table b for sample sizes from 3 to 10.

In order to construct a CSCC based on sample ranges it is again desirable to introduce a scaling factor. By so doing we can plot

$$m, \Sigma R_i$$

with a scale factor k (that is, k units on the ordinate is the same length as one unit on the abscissa). For approximation (*b*) the critical values for the mask as shown in Figure b.2 are

$$\begin{cases} \theta^* = \arctan\left[\dfrac{\sigma_0 c' \nu_1'}{k} \cdot \dfrac{\ln (\sigma_1/\sigma_0)}{1 - (\sigma_0/\sigma_1)}\right] \\ d^* = -2 \ln \alpha / [\nu_1' \ln (\sigma_1/\sigma_0)] = d/\nu_1' \end{cases}$$

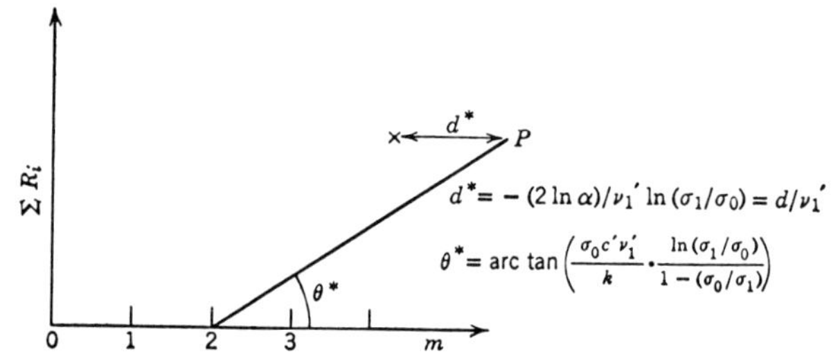

Figure b.2: Scaling in CSCC on sample ranges.

TABLE b

SCALE VALUES FOR CSCC ON SAMPLE RANGES*

Sample Size	Approximation (a)		Approximation (b)	
n	c	ν_1	c'	ν_1'
3	1.378	1.93	0.233	7.27
4	1.302	2.95	0.188	10.95
5	1.268	2.83	0.160	14.49
6	1.237	4.69	0.142	17.86
7	1.207	5.50	0.128	21.08
8	1.184	6.26	0.118	24.11
9	1.164	6.99	0.110	27.01
10	1.146	7.69	0.103	29.82

* c and ν are based on the work of P. B. Patnaik, "The Use of the Mean Range in Statistical Tests", *Biometrika*, **37** (1950). c' and ν' are based on the work of D. R. Cox, "The Use of Range in Sequential Analysis", *Journal of the Royal Statistical Society Series B*, **11** (1949).

C. CSCC for Sample Variances

Let us consider a two-sided control chart where H_0 is $\sigma^2 = \sigma_0^2$, H_1 is $\sigma^2 = \sigma_1^2$ $(> \sigma_0^2)$, and H_{-1} is $\sigma^2 = \sigma_1'^2$ $(< \sigma_0^2)$. Again let the probability of error of the first kind be α. If the scale of the control chart has length of k units on the ordinate equal to the length of 1 unit on the abscissa, then the values for θ^* and d^* are

$$\begin{cases} \theta^* = \arc\tan\left[\dfrac{2(\sigma_0^2/k)\ln(\sigma_1/\sigma_0)}{1-(\sigma_0/\sigma_1)^2}\right] \\ d^* = -\ln\alpha/\ln(\sigma_1/\sigma_0) \end{cases}$$

These values can be read directly from Table c for both a two-sided and one-sided test. In plotting the points on a CSCC chart for sample variances, the coordinates of each point are

$$\sum_{i=1}^{m} \nu_i, \sum_{i=1}^{m} \nu_i s_i^2$$

where ν_i and s_i^2 are the degrees of freedom and variance, respectively, of sample i. An illustration of a one-sided CSCC for variances is given in Figure c.1. A two-sided test is shown in Figure c.2, in which $d^{*\prime}$ and $\theta^{*\prime}$ are the critical values for acceptance of the hypothesis, H_{-1}. Note that if $\sigma_1/\sigma_0 < 1$, d is measured in the negative direction, that is, from right to left. Table d.2 can also be used to evaluate d, if

$$\frac{\sigma_1}{\sigma_0} = \frac{1-p_0}{1-p_1}.$$

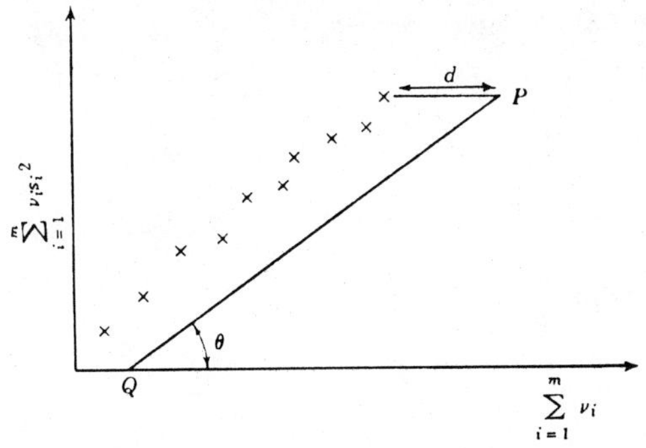

Figure c.1: CSCC for sample variances (one-sided limit to detect increase in variance).

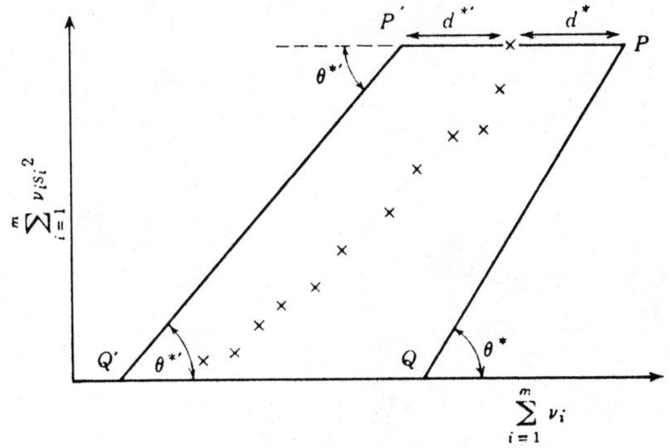

Figure c.2: CSCC for sample variances (two-sided limits).

TABLE c

CUMULATIVE SUM CONTROL LIMITS FOR SAMPLE VARIANCES

		Values of d						
σ_1/σ_0	θ	$2\alpha = 0.10$* $\alpha = 0.05$†	$2\alpha = 0.05$ $\alpha = 0.025$	$2\alpha = 0.02$ $\alpha = 0.01$	$2\alpha = 0.01$ $\alpha = 0.005$	$2\alpha = 0.0027$ $\alpha = 0.00135$‡	$2\alpha = 0.002$ $\alpha = 0.001$	$2\alpha = 0.001$ $\alpha = 0.0005$
0.25	10° 28′	2.16	2.66	3.32	3.82	4.77	4.98	5.48
0.5	24° 48′	4.32	5.32	6.64	7.64	9.53	9.93	11.0
0.75	36° 31′	10.4	12.8	16.0	18.4	23.0	24.0	26.4
1.2	50° 2′	16.4	20.2	25.3	29.1	36.2	37.9	41.7
1.4	52° 37′	8.90	11.0	13.7	15.7	19.6	20.5	22.6
1.6	57° 2′	6.37	7.85	9.80	11.3	14.1	14.7	16.2
1.8	59° 32′	5.10	6.28	7.83	9.01	11.2	11.8	12.9
2.0	61° 35′	4.32	5.32	6.64	7.64	9.53	9.97	11.0
2.5	65° 23′	3.27	4.03	5.03	5.78	7.21	7.54	8.30
3.0	67° 57′	2.73	3.36	4.19	4.82	6.01	6.29	6.92
3.5	69° 52′	2.39	2.94	3.68	4.23	5.27	5.51	6.07
4.0	71° 19′	2.16	2.66	3.32	3.82	4.77	4.98	5.48

Note that if $\sigma_1/\sigma_0 < 1$, d is measured in negative direction, that is, from right to left. Table d.2 can also be used to evaluate d, if $\frac{\sigma_1}{\sigma_0} = \frac{1 - p_0}{1 - p_1}$.

* Two-sided test.
† One-sided test.
‡ "3σ" limits.

D. CSCC for Number of Defectives, np, or Fraction Defective, p

The control limit diagram is similar in appearance to those for the range and variance. The line PQ in a figure similar to Figure d is inclined at an angle θ^* to the sample number axis, and P is at a distance d^* to the right of the last plotted point with

$$\begin{cases} \theta^* = \arc\tan\left[\dfrac{\ln[(1-p_0)/(1-p_1)]}{k\ln[p_1(1-p_0)/p_0(1-p_1)]}\right] \\ d^* = -\dfrac{\ln\alpha}{\ln[(1-p_0)/(1-p_1)]} \end{cases}$$

Again, k units on the ordinate are equal in length to one unit on the abscissa. The coordinates plotted on the CSCC chart are

$$\left(\sum_{i=1}^{m} n_i,\ X_m = \sum_{i=1}^{m} x_i\right)$$

where n_i and x_i are the sample size and number of defectives, respectively, of sample i. Figure d presents an illustration of a CSCC for fraction defective, p, where the coordinates of the point are

$$(m, \Sigma x_i)$$

and all of the sample sizes, n_i, are equal to n, say. Given this latter scale, the values of θ^{**} and d^{**} become

$$\begin{cases} \theta^{**} = \arc\tan(n\tan\theta^*) \\ d^{**} = d^*/n \end{cases}$$

In order to obtain 0^* and d^* we may make use of Tables d.1 (A and B) and d.2 and read off approximately the values of θ and d respectively. These are related to θ and d by the equations

$$\begin{cases} \theta^* = \arc\tan[(\tan\theta)/k] \\ d^* = d \end{cases}$$

or, in the case of θ^{**} and d^{**},

$$\begin{cases} \theta^{**} = \arc\tan[n(\tan\theta)/k] \\ d^{**} = d/n \end{cases}$$

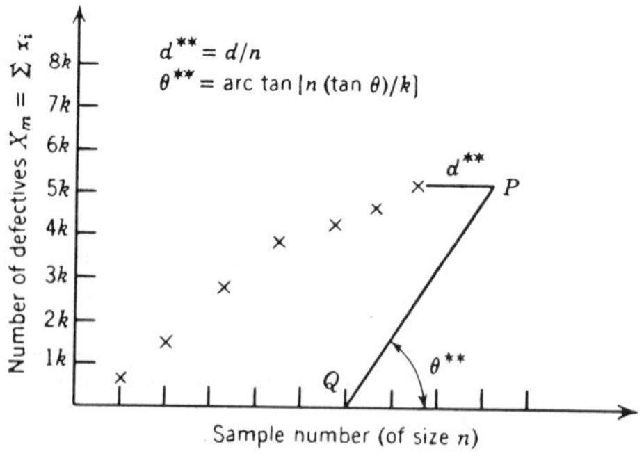

Figure d: CSCC for number of defectives.

TABLE *d*.1

CUMULATIVE SUM CONTROL LIMITS FOR BINOMIAL VARIABLES*

VALUES OF θ (FOR ANY α)

TABLE A

	p_1			
p_0	0.025	0.05	0.075	0.10
0.005	0° 43′	1° 8′	1° 30′	1° 51′
0.01	0° 56′	1° 26′	1° 52′	2° 17′
0.015	1° 7′	1° 40′	2° 9′	2° 36′
0.02	1° 17′	1° 53′	2° 24′	2° 53′
0.025	—	2° 4′	2° 37′	3° 8′
0.03	—	2° 15′	2° 49′	3° 21′
0.035	—	2° 25′	3° 1′	3° 34′
0.04	—	3° 34′	3° 12′	3° 46′
0.045	—	2° 43′	3° 22′	3° 58′
0.05	—	—	3° 32′	4° 8′
0.06	—	—	3° 51′	4° 29′
0.07	—	—	4° 9′	4° 49′
0.08	—	—	—	5° 8′
0.09	—	—	—	5° 25′

TABLE B

	p_1				
p_0	0.15	0.20	0.25	0.30	0.35
0.10	7° 3′	8° 16′	9° 25′	10° 33′	11° 39′
0.12	7° 40′	8° 56′	10° 8′	11° 18′	12° 26′
0.14	8° 15′	9° 34′	10° 49′	12° 0′	13° 10′
0.16	—	10° 10′	11° 27′	12° 40′	13° 52′
0.18	—	10° 45′	12° 3′	13° 18′	14° 31′
0.20	—	—	12° 39′	13° 55′	15° 9′
0.25	—	—	—	15° 21′	16° 38′

* p (or Np) charts.

TABLE d.2

CUMULATIVE SUM CONTROL LIMITS FOR BINOMIAL VARIABLES*

		Values of d						
		$2\alpha = 0.10$†	$2\alpha = 0.05$	$2\alpha = 0.02$	$2\alpha = 0.01$	$2\alpha = 0.0027$	$2\alpha = 0.002$	$2\alpha = 0.001$
p_0	p_1	$\alpha = 0.05$‡	$\alpha = 0.025$	$\alpha = 0.01$	$\alpha = 0.005$	$\alpha = 0.00135$§	$\alpha = 0.001$	$\alpha = 0.0005$
0.02	0.05	96.3	119	148	170	212	222	244
0.04	0.05	286	352	440	506	631	659	726
0.04	0.075	80.7	99.3	124	143	178	186	205
0.06	0.10	186	229	286	329	411	429	472
0.08	0.10	136	168	209	241	300	314	346
0.10	0.15	52.3	64.4	80.4	92.5	115	121	133
0.15	0.20	49.4	60.8	76.0	87.4	109	114	125
0.15	0.25	23.9	29.5	36.8	42.3	52.8	55.2	60.7
0.20	0.25	46.4	57.2	71.4	82.1	102	107	118
0.20	0.30	22.4	27.6	34.5	39.7	49.5	51.7	56.9
0.25	0.30	43.4	53.5	66.8	86.9	95.8	100	110
0.30	0.35	40.4	49.8	62.1	71.5	89.1	93.2	103

* Table c can also be used if $\frac{1 - p_0}{1 - p_1} = \frac{\sigma_1}{\sigma_0}$.

† Two sided test.
‡ One-sided test.
§ "3σ" limits.

E. CSCC for Number of Defects, c

The control limits for a CSCC for the number of defects are based on the constants

(1) $$\begin{cases} \theta = \arctan\left[(\mu_1 - \mu_0)/\ln(\mu_1/\mu_0)\right] \\ d = -\ln\alpha/(\mu_1 - \mu_0) \end{cases}$$

The coordinates of the points on the control chart are

$$\left(m, \sum_{i=1}^{m} x_i\right)$$

where x_i is the number of defects in sample i. Figure e presents an example of a CSCC for number of defects for a 2-sided test. In order to calculate θ' and d', we substitute μ_1' ($<\mu_0$) for μ_1 in equations (1) above. Tables e.1 and e.2 can be used to obtain the values of θ and d, respectively.

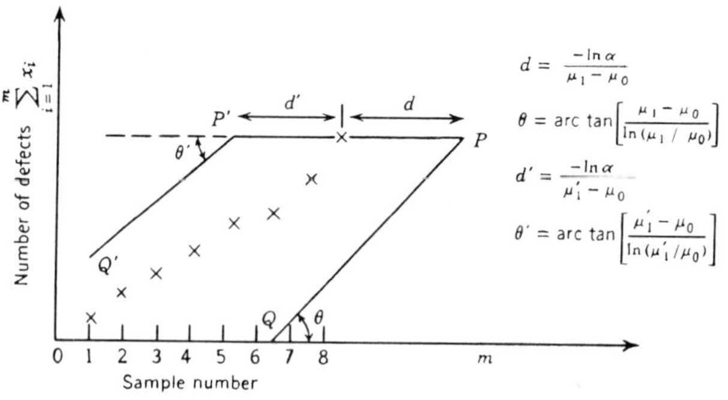

Figure e: CSCC for number of defects (c).

TABLE e.1

CUMULATIVE SUM CONTROL LIMITS FOR POISSON VARIABLE (c-CHARTS) VALUES OF θ (FOR ANY α)

μ_0	μ_1 1	2	3	4	5	6	8	10	12	15
0.5	35° 48′	47° 15′	54° 22′	59° 17′	62° 54′	65° 41′	69° 43′	72° 30′	74° 33′	76° 48′
1.0	—	55° 16′	61° 13′	65° 12′	68° 5′	70° 17′	73° 27′	75° 39′	77° 16′	79° 3′
1.5	—	60° 5′	65° 12′	68° 35′	71° 1′	72° 53′	75° 33′	77° 25′	78° 48′	80° 19′
2.0	—	—	67° 56′	70° 53′	73° 1′	74° 39′	76° 59′	78° 38′	79° 51′	81° 11′
2.5	—	—	69° 58′	72° 36′	74° 30′	75° 57′	78° 4′	79° 32′	80° 37′	81° 51′
3.0	—	—	—	73° 57′	75° 40′	76° 59′	78° 54′	80° 14′	81° 15′	82° 22′
3.5	—	—	—	75° 3′	76° 37′	77° 50′	79° 35′	80° 50′	81° 45′	82° 47′
4.0	—	—	—	—	77° 25′	78° 32′	80° 10′	81° 19′	82° 11′	83° 9′
4.5	—	—	—	—	78° 6′	79° 9′	80° 40′	81° 45′	82° 33′	83° 28′
5	—	—	—	—	—	79° 40′	81° 6′	82° 6′	82° 52′	83° 44′
6	—	—	—	—	—	—	81° 49′	82° 43′	83° 25′	84° 11′
7	—	—	—	—	—	—	82° 24′	83° 13′	83° 51′	84° 33′
8	—	—	—	—	—	—	—	83° 38′	84° 13′	84° 52′
9	—	—	—	—	—	—	—	83° 59′	84° 31′	85° 8′
10	—	—	—	—	—	—	—	—	84° 47′	85° 22′

TABLE e.2

CUMULATIVE SUM CONTROL LIMITS FOR POISSON VARIABLES (c-CHARTS) VALUES OF d

$\mu_1 - \mu_0$	$2\alpha_0 = 0.10$* $\alpha_0 = 0.05$†	$2\alpha = 0.05$ $\alpha_0 = 0.025$	$2\alpha_0 = 0.02$ $\alpha_0 = 0.01$	$2\alpha_0 = 0.01$ $\alpha_0 = 0.005$	$2\alpha_0 = 0.0027$ $\alpha_0 = 0.00135$‡	$2\alpha_0 = 0.002$ $\alpha_0 = 0.001$	$2\alpha_0 = 0.001$ $\alpha_0 = 0.0005$
0.5	6.00	7.38	9.21	10.6	13.2	13.8	15.2
1.0	3.00	3.69	4.61	5.30	6.61	6.91	7.60
1.5	2.00	2.46	3.07	3.53	4.40	4.61	5.07
2.0	1.50	1.84	2.30	2.65	3.30	3.45	3.80
2.5	1.20	1.48	1.84	2.12	2.64	2.76	3.04
3.0	1.00	1.23	1.54	1.77	2.20	2.30	2.53
3.5	0.86	1.05	1.32	1.51	1.89	1.97	2.03
4.0	0.75	0.92	1.15	1.32	1.65	1.73	1.90
4.5	0.68	0.82	1.02	1.18	1.47	1.53	1.69
5.0	0.60	0.74	0.92	1.06	1.32	1.38	1.52
6.0	0.50	0.61	0.77	0.88	1.10	1.15	1.27
7.0	0.43	0.53	0.66	0.76	0.94	0.99	1.09
8.0	0.37	0.46	0.58	0.66	0.83	0.86	0.95
9.0	0.33	0.41	0.51	0.59	0.73	0.77	0.84
10.0	0.30	0.37	0.46	0.53	0.66	0.69	0.76

* Two-sided test.
† One-sided test.
‡ These are comparable to the "3σ" limits used in the Shewhart chart.

F. Summary of CSCC Limits

The formulas for θ and α for the various CSCC are given in Table f for both the case of a scaling factor k and when no scaling factor is used.

TABLE f

FORMULAS FOR CSCC LIMITS (ONE-SIDED: α)

Sample Statistic	Coordinates (No Scaling Factor)	d (No Scaling Factor)	$\tan\theta$ (No Scaling Factor)	Coordinates (Including Scaling Factor, k)	d^* (Including Scaling Factor, k)	$\tan\theta^*$ (Including Scaling Factor, k)
Mean $\bar{x}$	$m,\ \sigma_{\bar{x}}^{-1}\Sigma(\bar{x}_i - \mu_0)$	$(-2\ln\alpha)/\delta^2$ $[\delta = (\mu_1 - \mu_0)/\sigma_{\bar{x}}]$	$\frac{1}{2}\delta$	$m,\ \Sigma(x_i - \mu_0)$	$(-2\ln\alpha)/\delta$	$D/2k$ $[D = \mu_1 - \mu_0]$
Variance s^2	$\Sigma\nu_i,\ \dfrac{\Sigma\nu_i s_i^2}{\sigma_0^2}$	$\dfrac{-\ln\alpha}{\ln(\sigma_1/\sigma_0)}$	$\dfrac{2\ln(\sigma_1/\sigma_0)}{1-(\sigma_0/\sigma_1)^2}$	$\Sigma\nu_i,\ \Sigma\nu_i s_i^2$	$\dfrac{-\ln\alpha}{\ln(\sigma_1/\sigma_0)}$	$\dfrac{2(\sigma_0^2/k)\ \ln(\sigma_1/\sigma_0)}{1-(\sigma_0/\sigma_1)^2}$
Range R*	$m\nu_1',\ (\sigma_0 c_1')^{-1}\Sigma R_i$	$\dfrac{-2\ln\alpha}{\ln(\sigma_1/\sigma_0)}$	$\dfrac{\ln(\sigma_1/\sigma_0)}{1-(\sigma_0/\sigma_1)}$	$m,\ \Sigma R_i$	$\dfrac{-2\ln\alpha}{\nu_1'\ln(\sigma_1/\sigma_0)}$	$\dfrac{\sigma_0 c'\nu_1'}{k}\cdot\dfrac{\ln(\sigma_1/\sigma_0)}{1-(\sigma_0/\sigma_1)}$
Number of Defects c	$m,\ \Sigma x_i$	$\dfrac{-\ln\alpha}{\mu_1-\mu_0}$	$\dfrac{(\mu_1-\mu_0)}{\ln(\mu_1/\mu_0)}$	$m,\ \Sigma x_i$ $(x_i = 0 \text{ or } 1)$	$\dfrac{-\ln\alpha}{\mu_1-\mu_0}$	$\dfrac{\mu_1-\mu_0}{k\ln(\mu_1/\mu_0)}$
Number of Defectives Np	$m,\ \Sigma x_i$ (sample of size 1)	$\dfrac{-\ln\alpha}{\ln\left(\dfrac{1-p_0}{1-p_1}\right)}$	$\dfrac{\ln\left(\dfrac{1-p_0}{1-p_1}\right)}{\ln\left(\dfrac{p_1(1-p_0)}{p_0(1-p_1)}\right)}$	$m,\ \Sigma x_i$ $(x_i = 0 \text{ or } 1)$ m = sample number n = fixed sample size	$\dfrac{-\ln\alpha}{n\ln\left(\dfrac{1-p_0}{1-p_1}\right)}$	$\dfrac{\ln\left(\dfrac{1-p_0}{1-p_1}\right)}{k\ln\left(\dfrac{p_1(1-p_0)}{p_0(1-p_1)}\right)}$
"Np" (unequal sample sizes)				$\Sigma n_i,\ \Sigma x_i$ $(x_i = 0 \text{ or } 1)$	$\dfrac{-\ln\alpha}{\ln\left(\dfrac{1-p_0}{1-p_1}\right)}$	$\dfrac{\ln\left(\dfrac{1-p_0}{1-p_1}\right)}{k\ln\left(\dfrac{p_1(1-p_0)}{p_0(1-p_1)}\right)}$

* Approximation b (see Section B).

XII. MISCELLANEOUS STATISTICAL TABLES

XII.1 NUMBER OF PERMUTATIONS $P(n,m)$

This table contains the number of permutations of n distinct things taken m at a time, given by

$$P(n,m) = \frac{n!}{(n-m)!} = n(n-1)\cdots(n-m+1)$$

n \ m	0	1	2	3	4	5	6	7	8	9	10
0	1										
1	1	1									
2	1	2	2								
3	1	3	6	6							
4	1	4	12	24	24						
5	1	5	20	60	120	120					
6	1	6	30	120	360	720	720				
7	1	7	42	210	840	2520	5040	5040			
8	1	8	56	336	1680	6720	20160	40320	40320		
9	1	9	72	504	3024	15120	60480	1 81440	3 62880	3 62880	
10	1	10	90	720	5040	30240	1 51200	6 04800	18 14400	36 28800	36 28800
11	1	11	110	990	7920	55440	3 32640	16 63200	66 52800	199 58400	399 16800
12	1	12	132	1320	11880	95040	6 65280	39 91680	199 58400	798 33600	2395 00800
13	1	13	156	1716	17160	1 54440	12 35520	86 48640	518 91840	2594 59200	10378 36800
14	1	14	182	2184	24024	2 40240	21 62160	172 97280	1210 80960	7264 85760	36324 28800
15	1	15	210	2730	32760	3 60360	36 03600	324 32400	2594 59200	18162 14400	1 08972 86400

n \ m	11	12	13	14	15
8					
9					
10					
11	399 16800				
12	4790 01600	4790 01600			
13	31135 10400	62270 20800	62270 20800		
14	1 45297 15200	4 35891 45600	8 71782 91200	8 71782 91200	
15	5 44864 32000	21 79457 28000	65 38371 84000	130 76743 68000	130 76743 68000

XII.2 NUMBER OF COMBINATIONS $c(n,m) = \binom{n}{m}$

This table contains the number of combinations of n distinct things taken m at a time, given by $\binom{n}{m} = C(n,m)$. For coefficients missing from the table, use the relation $\binom{n}{m} = \binom{n}{n-m}$.

n \ m	0	1	2	3	4	5	6	7	8
1	1	1							
2	1	2	1						
3	1	3	3	1					
4	1	4	6	4	1				
5	1	5	10	10	5	1			
6	1	6	15	20	15	6	1		
7	1	7	21	35	35	21	7	1	
8	1	8	28	56	70	56	28	8	1
9	1	9	36	84	126	126	84	36	9
10	1	10	45	120	210	252	210	120	45
11	1	11	55	165	330	462	462	330	165
12	1	12	66	220	495	792	924	792	495
13	1	13	78	286	715	1287	1716	1716	1287
14	1	14	91	364	1001	2002	3003	3432	3003
15	1	15	105	455	1365	3003	5005	6435	6435
16	1	16	120	560	1820	4368	8008	11440	12870
17	1	17	136	680	2380	6188	12376	19448	24310
18	1	18	153	816	3060	8568	18564	31824	43758
19	1	19	171	969	3876	11628	27132	50388	75582
20	1	20	190	1140	4845	15504	38760	77520	1 25970
21	1	21	210	1330	5985	20349	54264	1 16280	2 03490
22	1	22	231	1540	7315	26334	74613	1 70544	3 19770
23	1	23	253	1771	8855	33649	1 00947	2 45157	4 90314
24	1	24	276	2024	10626	42504	1 34596	3 46104	7 35471
25	1	25	300	2300	12650	53130	1 77100	4 80700	10 81575
26	1	26	325	2600	14950	65780	2 30230	6 57800	15 62275
27	1	27	351	2925	17550	80730	2 96010	8 88030	22 20075
28	1	28	378	3276	20475	98280	3 76740	11 84040	31 08105
29	1	29	406	3654	23751	1 18755	4 75020	15 60780	42 92145
30	1	30	435	4060	27405	1 42506	5 93775	20 35800	58 52925
31	1	31	465	4495	31465	1 69911	7 36281	26 29575	78 88725
32	1	32	496	4960	35960	2 01376	9 06192	33 65856	105 18300
33	1	33	528	5456	40920	2 37336	11 07568	42 72048	138 84156
34	1	34	561	5984	46376	2 78256	13 44904	53 79616	181 56204
35	1	35	595	6545	52360	3 24632	16 23160	67 24520	235 35820
36	1	36	630	7140	58905	3 76992	19 47792	83 47680	302 60340
37	1	37	666	7770	66045	4 35897	23 24784	102 95472	386 08020
38	1	38	703	8436	73815	5 01942	27 60681	126 20256	489 03492
39	1	39	741	9139	82251	5 75757	32 62623	153 80937	615 23748
40	1	40	780	9880	91390	6 58008	38 38380	186 43560	769 04685
41	1	41	820	10660	101270	7 49398	44 96388	224 81940	955 48245
42	1	42	861	11480	111930	8 50668	52 45786	269 78328	1180 30185
43	1	43	903	12341	123410	9 62598	60 96454	322 24114	1450 08513
44	1	44	946	13244	135751	10 86008	70 59052	383 20568	1772 32627
45	1	45	990	14190	148995	12 21759	81 45060	453 79620	2155 53195
46	1	46	1035	15180	163185	13 70754	93 66819	535 24680	2609 32815
47	1	47	1081	16215	178365	15 33939	107 37573	628 91499	3144 57495
48	1	48	1128	17296	194580	17 12304	122 71512	736 29072	3773 48994
49	1	49	1176	18424	211876	19 06884	139 83816	859 00584	4509 78066
50	1	50	1225	19600	230300	21 18760	158 90700	998 84400	5368 78650

NUMBER OF COMBINATIONS

$$\binom{n}{m} = C(n,m)$$

n \ m	9	10	11	12	13
9	1				
10	10	1			
11	55	11	1		
12	220	66	12	1	
13	715	286	78	13	1
14	2002	1001	364	91	14
15	5005	3003	1365	455	105
16	11440	8008	4368	1820	560
17	24310	19448	12376	6188	2380
18	48620	43758	31824	18564	8568
19	92378	92378	75582	50388	27132
20	1 67960	1 84756	1 67960	1 25970	77520
21	2 93930	3 52716	3 52716	2 93930	2 03490
22	4 97420	6 46646	7 05432	6 46646	4 97420
23	8 17190	11 44066	13 52078	13 52078	11 44066
24	13 07504	19 61256	24 96144	27 04156	24 96144
25	20 42975	32 68760	44 57400	52 00300	52 00300
26	31 24550	53 11735	77 26160	96 57700	104 00600
27	46 86825	84 36285	130 37895	173 83860	200 58300
28	69 06900	131 23110	214 74180	304 21755	374 42160
29	100 15005	200 30010	345 97290	518 95935	678 63915
30	143 07150	300 45015	546 27300	864 93225	1197 59850
31	201 60075	443 52165	846 72315	1411 20525	2062 53075
32	280 48800	645 12240	1290 24480	2257 92840	3473 73600
33	385 67100	925 61040	1935 36720	3548 17320	5731 66440
34	524 51256	1311 28140	2860 97760	5483 54040	9279 83760
35	706 07460	1835 79396	4172 25900	8344 51800	14763 37800
36	941 43280	2541 86856	6008 05296	12516 77700	23107 89600
37	1244 03620	3483 30136	8549 92152	18524 82996	35624 67300
38	1630 11640	4727 33756	12033 22288	27074 75148	54149 50296
39	2119 15132	6357 45396	16760 56044	39107 97436	81224 25444
40	2734 38880	8476 60528	23118 01440	55868 53480	1 20332 22880
41	3503 43565	11210 99408	31594 61968	78986 54920	1 76200 76360
42	4458 91810	14714 42973	42805 61376	1 10581 16888	2 55187 31280
43	5639 21995	19173 34783	57520 04349	1 53386 78264	3 65768 48168
44	7098 30508	24812 56778	76693 39132	2 10906 82613	5 19155 26432
45	8861 63135	31901 87286	1 01505 95910	2 87600 21745	7 30062 09045
46	11017 16330	40763 50421	1 33407 83196	3 89106 17655	10 17662 30790
47	13626 49145	51780 66751	1 74171 33617	5 22514 00851	14 06768 48445
48	16771 06640	65407 15896	2 25952 00368	6 96685 34468	19 29282 49296
49	20544 55634	82178 22536	2 91359 16264	9 22637 34836	26 25967 83764
50	25054 33700	1 02722 78170	3 73537 38800	12 13996 51100	35 48605 18600

NUMBER OF COMBINATIONS

$$\binom{n}{m} = C(n,m)$$

n \ m	14	15	16	17	18	19
14	1					
15	15	1				
16	120	16	1			
17	680	136	17	1		
18	3060	816	153	18	1	
19	11628	3876	969	171	19	1
20	38760	15504	4845	1140	190	20
21	1 16280	54264	20349	5985	1330	210
22	3 19770	1 70544	74613	26334	7315	1540
23	8 17190	4 90314	2 45157	1 00947	33649	8855
24	19 61256	13 07504	7 35471	3 46104	1 34596	42504
25	44 57400	32 68760	20 42975	10 81575	4 80700	1 77100
26	96 57700	77 26160	53 11735	31 24550	15 62275	6 57800
27	200 58300	173 83860	130 37895	84 36285	46 86825	22 20075
28	401 16600	374 42160	304 21755	214 74180	131 23110	69 06900
29	775 58760	775 58760	678 63915	518 95935	345 97290	200 30010
30	1454 22675	1551 17520	1454 22675	1197 59850	864 93225	546 27300
31	2651 82525	3005 40195	3005 40195	2651 82525	2062 53075	1411 20525
32	4714 35600	5657 22720	6010 80390	5657 22720	4714 35600	3473 73600
33	8188 09200	10371 58320	11668 03110	11668 03110	10371 58320	8188 09200
34	13919 75640	18559 67520	22039 61430	23336 06220	22039 61430	18559 67520
35	23199 59400	32479 43160	40599 28950	45375 67650	45375 67650	40599 28950
36	37962 97200	55679 02560	73078 72110	85974 96600	90751 35300	85974 96600
37	61070 86800	93641 99760	1 28757 74670	1 59053 68710	1 76726 31900	1 76726 31900
38	96695 54100	1 54712 86560	2 22399 74430	2 87811 43380	3 35780 00610	3 53452 63800
39	1 50845 04396	2 51408 40660	3 77112 60990	5 10211 17810	6 23591 43990	6 89232 64410
40	2 32069 29840	4 02253 45056	6 28521 01650	8 87323 78800	11 33802 61800	13 12824 08400
41	3 52401 52720	6 34322 74896	10 30774 46706	15 15844 80450	20 21126 40600	24 46626 70200
42	5 28602 29080	9 86724 27616	16 65097 21602	25 46619 27156	35 36971 21050	44 67753 10800
43	7 83789 60360	15 15326 56696	26 51821 49218	42 11716 48758	60 83590 48206	80 04724 31850
44	11 49558 08528	22 99116 17056	41 67148 05914	68 63537 97976	102 95306 96964	140 88314 80056
45	16 68713 34960	34 48674 25584	64 66264 22970	110 30686 03890	171 58844 94940	243 83621 77020
46	23 98775 44005	51 17387 60544	99 14938 48554	174 96950 26860	281 89530 98830	415 42466 71960
47	34 16437 74795	75 16163 04549	150 32326 09098	274 11888 75414	456 86481 25690	697 31997 70790
48	48 23206 23240	109 32600 79344	225 48489 13647	424 44214 84512	730 98370 01104	1154 18478 96480
49	67 52488 72536	157 55807 02584	334 81089 92991	649 92703 98159	1155 42584 85616	1885 16848 97584
50	93 78456 56300	225 08295 75120	492 36896 95575	984 73793 91150	1805 35288 83775	3040 59433 83200

NUMBER OF COMBINATIONS

$$\binom{n}{m} = C(n,m)$$

n \ m	20	21	22	23	24	25
20	1					
21	21	1				
22	231	22	1			
23	1771	253	23	1		
24	10626	2024	276	24	1	
25	53130	12650	2300	300	25	1
26	2 30230	65780	14950	2600	325	26
27	8 88030	2 96010	80730	17550	2925	351
28	31 08105	11 84040	3 76740	98280	20475	3276
29	100 15005	42 92145	15 60780	4 75020	1 18755	23751
30	300 45015	143 07150	58 52925	20 35800	5 93775	1 42506
31	846 72315	443 52165	201 60075	78 88725	26 29575	7 36281
32	2257 92840	1290 24480	645 12240	280 48800	105 18300	33 65856
33	5731 66440	3548 17320	1935 36720	925 61040	385 67100	138 84156
34	13919 75640	9279 83760	5483 54040	2860 97760	1311 28140	524 51256
35	32479 43160	23199 59400	14763 37800	8344 51800	4172 25900	1835 79396
36	73078 72110	55679 02560	37962 97200	23107 89600	12516 77700	6008 05296
37	1 59053 68710	1 28757 74670	93641 99760	61070 86800	35624 67300	18524 82996
38	3 35780 00610	2 87811 43380	2 22399 74430	1 54712 86560	96695 54100	54149 50296
39	6 89232 64410	6 23591 43990	5 10211 17810	3 77112 60990	2 51408 40660	1 50845 04396
40	13 78465 28820	13 12824 08400	11 33802 61800	8 87323 78800	6 28521 01650	4 02253 45056
41	26 91289 37220	26 91289 37220	24 46626 70200	20 21126 40600	15 15844 80450	10 30774 46706
42	51 37916 07420	53 82578 74440	51 37916 07420	44 67753 10800	35 36971 21050	25 46619 27156
43	96 05669 18220	105 20494 81860	105 20494 81860	96 05669 18220	80 04724 31850	60 83590 48206
44	176 10393 50070	201 26164 00080	210 40989 63720	201 26164 00080	176 10393 50070	140 88314 80056
45	316 98708 30126	377 36557 50150	411 67153 63800	411 67153 63800	377 36557 50150	316 98708 30126
46	560 82330 07146	694 35265 80276	789 03711 13950	823 34307 27600	789 03711 13950	694 35265 80276
47	976 24796 79106	1255 17595 87422	1483 38976 94226	1612 38018 41550	1612 38018 41550	1483 38976 94226
48	1673 56794 49896	2231 42392 66528	2738 56572 81648	3095 76995 35776	3224 76036 83100	3095 76995 35776
49	2827 75273 46376	3904 99187 16424	4969 98965 48176	5834 33568 17424	6320 53032 18876	6320 53032 18876
50	4712 92122 43960	6732 74460 62800	8874 98152 64600	10804 32533 65600	12154 86600 36300	12641 06064 37752

Properties of Binomial Coefficients

$$(1+x)^n = \binom{n}{0}x^0 + \binom{n}{1}x^n + \binom{n}{2}x^2 + \ldots + \binom{n}{n}x^n$$

$$\binom{n}{m} + \binom{n}{m+1} = \binom{n+1}{m+1}, \binom{n}{m} = \binom{n}{n-m}$$

This leads to Pascal's triangle

$$\binom{n}{0} + \binom{n}{1} + \binom{n}{2} + \ldots + \binom{n}{n} = 2^n$$

$$\binom{n}{0} - \binom{n}{1} + \binom{n}{2} - \ldots (-1)^n \binom{n}{n} = 0$$

$$\binom{n}{n} + \binom{n+1}{n} + \binom{n+2}{n} + \ldots + \binom{n+m}{n} = \binom{n+m+1}{n+1}$$

$$\binom{n}{0} + \binom{n}{2} + \binom{n}{4} + \ldots = 2^{n-1}$$

$$\binom{n}{1} + \binom{n}{3} + \binom{n}{5} + \ldots = 2^{n-1}$$

$$\binom{n}{0}^2 + \binom{n}{1}^2 + \binom{n}{2}^2 + \ldots + \binom{n}{n}^2 = \binom{2n}{n}$$

$$\binom{m}{0}\binom{n}{p} + \binom{m}{1}\binom{n}{p-1} + \ldots + \binom{m}{p}\binom{n}{0} = \binom{m+n}{p}$$

$$(1)\binom{n}{1} + (2)\binom{n}{2} + (3)\binom{n}{3} + \ldots + (n)\binom{n}{n} = n2^{n-1}$$

$$(1)\binom{n}{1} - (2)\binom{n}{2} + (3)\binom{n}{3} - \ldots (-1)^{n+1}(n)\binom{n}{n} = 0$$

XII.3 RANDOM UNITS

Use of Table. If one wishes to select a random sample of N items from a universe of M items, the following procedure may be applied. ($M > N$.)

1. Decide upon some arbitrary scheme of selecting entries from the table. For example, one may decide to use the entries in the first line, second column; second line, third column; third line, fourth column; etc.

2. Assign numbers to each of the items in the universe from 1 to M. Thus, if $M = 500$, the items would be numbered from 001 to 500, and therefore, each designated item is associated with a three digit number.

3. Decide upon some arbitrary scheme of selecting positional digits from each entry chosen according to Step 1. Thus, if $M = 500$, one may decide to use the first, third, and fourth digit of each entry selected, and as a consequence a three digit number is created for each entry choice.

4. If the number formed is $\leq M$, the correspondingly designated item in the universe is chosen for the random sample of N items. If a number formed is $> M$ or is a repeated number of one already chosen, it is passed over and the next desirable number is taken. This process is continued until the random sample of N items is selected.

Table of Random Units

A TABLE OF 14,000 RANDOM UNITS

Line/Col.	(1)	(2)	(3)	(4)	(5)	(6)	(7)	(8)	(9)	(10)	(11)	(12)	(13)	(14)
1	10480	15011	01536	02011	81647	91646	69179	14194	62590	36207	20969	99570	91291	90700
2	22368	46573	25595	85393	30995	89198	27982	53402	93965	34095	52666	19174	39615	99505
3	24130	48360	22527	97265	76393	64809	15179	24830	49340	32081	30680	19655	63348	58629
4	42167	93093	06243	61680	07856	16376	39440	53537	71341	57004	00849	74917	97758	16379
5	37570	39975	81837	16656	06121	91782	60468	81305	49684	60672	14110	06927	01263	54613
6	77921	06907	11008	42751	27756	53498	18602	70659	90655	15053	21916	81825	44394	42880
7	99562	72905	56420	69994	98872	31016	71194	18738	44013	48840	63213	21069	10634	12952
8	96301	91977	05463	07972	18876	20922	94595	56869	69014	60045	18425	84903	42508	32307
9	89579	14342	63661	10281	17453	18103	57740	84378	25331	12566	58678	44947	05585	56941
10	85475	36857	43342	53988	53060	59533	38867	62300	08158	17983	16439	11458	18593	64952
11	28918	69578	88231	33276	70997	79936	56865	05859	90106	31595	01547	85590	91610	78188
12	63553	40961	48235	03427	49626	69445	18663	72695	52180	20847	12234	90511	33703	90322
13	09429	93969	52636	92737	88974	33488	36320	17617	30015	08272	84115	27156	30613	74952
14	10365	61129	87529	85689	48237	52267	67689	93394	01511	26358	85104	20285	29975	89868
15	07119	97336	71048	08178	77233	13916	47564	81056	97735	85977	29372	74461	28551	90707
16	51085	12765	51821	51259	77452	16308	60756	92144	49442	53900	70960	63990	75601	40719
17	02368	21382	52404	60268	89368	19885	55322	44819	01188	65255	64835	44919	05944	55157
18	01011	54092	33362	94904	31273	04146	18594	29852	71585	85030	51132	01915	92747	64951
19	52162	53916	46369	58586	23216	14513	83149	98736	23495	64350	94738	17752	35156	35749
20	07056	97628	33787	09998	42698	06691	76988	13602	51851	46104	88916	19509	25625	58104
21	48663	91245	85828	14346	09172	30168	90229	04734	59193	22178	30421	61666	99904	32812
22	54164	58492	22421	74103	47070	25306	76468	26384	58151	06646	21524	15227	96909	44592
23	32639	32363	05597	24200	13363	38005	94342	28728	35806	06912	17012	64161	18296	22851
24	29334	27001	87637	87308	58731	00256	45834	15398	46557	41135	10367	07684	36188	18510
25	02488	33062	28834	07351	19731	92420	60952	61280	50001	67658	32586	86679	50720	94953
26	81525	72295	04839	96423	24878	82651	66566	14778	76797	14780	13300	87074	79666	95725
27	29676	20591	68086	26432	46901	20849	89768	81536	86645	12659	92259	57102	80428	25280
28	00742	57392	39064	66432	84673	40027	32832	61362	98947	96067	64760	64584	96096	98253
29	05366	04213	25669	26422	44407	44048	37937	63904	45766	66134	75470	66520	34693	90449
30	91921	26418	64117	94305	26766	25940	39972	22209	71500	64568	91402	42416	07844	69618
31	00582	04711	87917	77341	42206	35126	74087	99547	81817	42607	43808	76655	62028	76630
32	00725	69884	62797	56170	86324	88072	76222	36086	84637	93161	76038	65855	77919	88006
33	69011	65797	95876	55293	18988	27354	26575	08625	40801	59920	29841	80150	12777	48501
34	25976	57948	29888	88604	67917	48708	18912	82271	65424	69774	33611	54262	85963	03547
35	09763	83473	73577	12908	30883	18317	28290	35797	05998	41688	34952	37888	38917	88050
36	91567	42595	27958	30134	04024	86385	29880	99730	55536	84855	29080	09250	79656	73211
37	17955	56349	90999	49127	20044	59931	06115	20542	18059	02008	73708	83517	36103	42791
38	46503	18584	18845	49618	02304	51038	20655	58727	28168	15475	56942	53389	20562	87338
39	92157	89634	94824	78171	84610	82834	09922	25417	44137	48413	25555	21246	35509	20468
40	14577	62765	35605	81263	39667	47358	56873	56307	61607	49518	89656	20103	77490	18062
41	98427	07523	33362	64270	01638	92477	66969	98420	04880	45585	46565	04102	46880	45709
42	34914	63976	88720	82765	34476	17032	87589	40836	32427	70002	70663	88863	77775	69348
43	70060	28277	39475	46473	23219	53416	94970	25832	69975	94884	19661	72828	00102	66794
44	53976	54914	06990	67245	68350	82948	11398	42878	80287	88267	47363	46634	06541	97809
45	76072	29515	40980	07391	58745	25774	22987	80059	39911	96189	41151	14222	60697	59583
46	90725	52210	83974	29992	65831	38857	50490	83765	55657	14361	31720	57375	56228	41546
47	64364	67412	33339	31926	14883	24413	59744	92351	97473	89286	35931	04110	23726	51900
48	08962	00358	31662	25388	61642	34072	81249	35648	56891	69352	48373	45578	78547	81788
49	95012	68379	93526	70765	10593	04542	76463	54328	02349	17247	28865	14777	62730	92277
50	15664	10493	20492	38391	91132	21999	59516	81652	27195	48223	46751	22923	32261	85653

Table of Random Units

A TABLE OF 14,000 RANDOM UNITS (Continued)

Line/Col.	(1)	(2)	(3)	(4)	(5)	(6)	(7)	(8)	(9)	(10)	(11)	(12)	(13)	(14)
51	16408	81899	04153	53381	79401	21438	83035	92350	36693	31238	59649	91754	72772	02338
52	18629	81953	05520	91962	04739	13092	97662	24822	94730	06496	35090	04822	86772	98289
53	73115	35101	47498	87637	99016	71060	88824	71013	18735	20286	23153	72924	35165	43040
54	57491	16703	23167	49323	45021	33132	12544	41035	80780	45393	44812	12515	98931	91202
55	30405	83946	23792	14422	15059	45799	22716	19792	09983	74353	68668	30429	70735	25499
56	16631	35006	85900	98275	32388	52390	16815	69298	82732	38480	73817	32523	41961	44437
57	96773	20206	42559	78985	05300	22164	24369	54224	35083	19687	11052	91491	60383	19746
58	38935	64202	14349	82674	66523	44133	00697	35552	35970	19124	63318	29686	03387	59846
59	31624	76384	17403	53363	44167	64486	64758	75366	76554	31601	12614	33072	60332	92325
60	78919	19474	23632	27889	47914	02584	37680	20801	72152	39339	34806	08930	85001	87820
61	03931	33309	57047	74211	63445	17361	62825	39908	05607	91284	68833	25570	38818	46920
62	74426	33278	43972	10119	89917	15665	52872	73823	73144	88662	88970	74492	51805	99378
63	09066	00903	20795	95452	92648	45454	09552	88815	16553	51125	79375	97596	16296	66092
64	42238	12426	87025	14267	20979	04508	64535	31355	86064	29472	47689	05974	52468	16834
65	16153	08002	26504	41744	81959	65642	74240	56302	00033	67107	77510	70625	28725	34191
66	21457	40742	29820	96783	29400	21840	15035	34537	33310	06116	95240	15957	16572	06004
67	21581	57802	02050	89728	17937	37621	47075	42080	97403	48626	68995	43805	33386	21597
68	55612	78095	83197	33732	05810	24813	86902	60397	16489	03264	88525	42786	05269	92532
69	44657	66999	99324	51281	84463	60563	79312	93454	68876	25471	93911	25650	12682	73572
70	91340	84979	46949	81973	37949	61023	43997	15263	80644	43942	89203	71795	99533	50501
71	91227	21199	31935	27022	84067	05462	35216	14486	29891	68607	41867	14951	91696	85065
72	50001	38140	66321	19924	72163	09538	12151	06878	91903	18749	34405	56087	82790	70925
73	65390	05224	72958	28609	81406	39147	25549	48542	42627	45233	57202	94617	23772	07896
74	27504	96131	83944	41575	10573	08619	64482	73923	36152	05184	94142	25299	84387	34925
75	37169	94851	39117	89632	00959	16487	65536	49071	39782	17095	02330	74301	00275	48280
76	11508	70225	51111	38351	19444	66499	71945	05422	13442	78675	84081	66938	93654	59894
77	37449	30362	06694	54690	04052	53115	62757	95348	78662	11163	81651	50245	34971	52924
78	46515	70331	85922	38329	57015	15765	97161	17869	45349	61796	66345	81073	49106	79860
79	30986	81223	42416	58353	21532	30502	32305	86482	05174	07901	54339	58861	74818	46942
80	63798	64995	46583	09765	44160	78128	83991	42865	92520	83531	80377	35909	81250	54238
81	82486	84846	99254	67632	43218	50076	21361	64816	51202	88124	41870	52689	51275	83556
82	21885	32906	92431	09060	64297	51674	64126	62570	26123	05155	59194	52799	28225	85762
83	60336	98782	07408	53458	13564	59089	26445	29789	85205	41001	12535	12133	14645	23541
84	43937	46891	24010	25560	86355	33941	25786	54990	71899	15475	95434	98227	21824	19585
85	97656	63175	89303	16275	07100	92063	21942	18611	47348	20203	18534	03862	78095	50136
86	03299	01221	05418	38982	55758	92237	26759	86367	21216	98442	08303	56613	91511	75928
87	79626	06486	03574	17668	07785	76020	79924	25651	83325	88428	85076	72811	22717	50585
88	85636	68335	47539	03129	65651	11977	02510	26113	99447	68645	34327	15152	55230	93448
89	18039	14367	61337	06177	12143	46609	32989	74014	64708	00533	35398	58408	13261	47908
90	08362	15656	60627	36478	65648	16764	53412	09013	07832	41574	17639	82163	60859	75567
91	79556	29068	04142	16268	15387	12856	66227	38358	22478	73373	88732	09443	82558	05250
92	92608	82674	27072	32534	17075	27698	98204	63863	11951	34648	88022	56148	34925	57031
93	23982	25835	40055	67006	12293	02753	14827	22235	35071	99704	37543	11601	35503	85171
94	09915	96306	05908	97901	28395	14186	00821	80703	70426	75647	76310	88717	37890	40129
95	50937	33300	26695	62247	69927	76123	50842	43834	86654	70959	79725	93872	28117	19233
96	42488	78077	69882	61657	34136	79180	97526	43092	04098	73571	80799	76536	71255	64239
97	46764	86273	63003	93017	31204	36692	40202	35275	57306	55543	53203	18098	47625	88684
98	03237	45430	55417	63282	90816	17349	88298	90183	36600	78406	06216	95787	42579	90730
99	86591	81482	52667	61583	14972	90053	89534	76036	49199	43716	97548	04379	46370	28672
100	38534	01715	94964	87288	65680	43772	39560	12918	86537	62738	19636	51132	25739	56947

Table of Random Units

A TABLE OF 14,000 RANDOM UNITS (Continued)

Line/Col.	(1)	(2)	(3)	(4)	(5)	(6)	(7)	(8)	(9)	(10)	(11)	(12)	(13)	(14)
101	13284	16834	74151	92027	24670	36665	00770	22878	02179	51602	07270	76517	97275	45960
102	21224	00370	30420	03883	96648	89428	41583	17564	27395	63904	41548	49197	82277	24120
103	99052	47887	81085	64933	66279	80432	65793	83287	34142	13241	30590	97760	35848	91983
104	00199	50993	98603	38452	87890	94624	69721	57484	67501	77638	44331	11257	71131	11059
105	60578	06483	28733	37867	07936	98710	98539	27186	31237	80612	44488	97819	70401	95419
106	91240	18312	17441	01929	18163	69201	31211	54288	39296	37318	65724	90401	79017	62077
107	97458	14229	12063	59611	32249	90466	33216	19358	02591	54263	88449	01912	07436	50813
108	35249	38646	34475	72417	60514	69257	12489	51924	86871	92446	36607	11458	30440	52639
109	38980	46600	11759	11900	46743	27860	77940	39298	97838	95145	32378	68038	89351	37005
110	10750	52745	38749	87365	58959	53731	89295	59062	39404	13198	59960	70408	29812	83126
111	36247	27850	73958	20673	37800	63835	71051	84724	52492	22342	78071	17456	96104	18327
112	70994	66986	99744	72438	01174	42159	11392	20724	54322	36923	70009	23233	65438	59685
113	99638	94702	11463	18148	81386	80431	90628	52506	02016	85151	88598	47821	00265	82525
114	72055	15774	43857	99805	10419	76939	25993	03544	21560	83471	43989	90770	22965	44247
115	24038	65541	85788	55835	38835	59399	13790	35112	01324	39520	76210	22467	83275	32286
116	74976	14631	35908	28221	39470	91548	12854	30166	09073	75887	36782	00268	97121	57676
117	35553	71628	70189	26436	63407	91178	90348	55359	80392	41012	36270	77786	89578	21059
118	35676	12797	51434	82976	42010	26344	92920	92155	58807	54644	58581	95331	78629	73344
119	74815	67523	72985	23183	02446	63594	98924	20633	58842	85961	07648	70164	34994	67662
120	45246	88048	65173	50989	91060	89894	36063	32819	68559	99221	49475	50558	34698	71800
121	76509	47069	86378	41797	11910	49672	88575	97966	32466	10083	54728	81972	58975	30761
122	19689	90332	04315	21358	97248	11188	39062	63312	52496	07349	79178	33692	57352	72862
123	42751	35318	97513	61537	54955	08159	00337	80778	27507	95478	21252	12746	37554	97775
124	11946	22681	45045	13964	57517	59419	58045	44067	58716	58840	45557	96345	33271	53464
125	96518	48688	20996	11090	48396	57177	83867	86464	14342	21545	46717	72364	86954	55580
126	35726	58643	76869	84622	39098	36083	72505	92265	23107	60278	05822	46760	44294	07672
127	39737	42750	48968	70536	84864	64952	38404	94317	65402	13589	01055	79044	19308	83623
128	97025	66492	56177	04049	80312	48028	26408	43591	75528	65341	49044	95495	81256	53214
129	62814	08075	09788	56350	76787	51591	54509	49295	85830	59860	30883	89660	96142	18354
130	25578	22950	15227	83291	41737	79599	96191	71845	86899	70694	24290	01551	80092	82118
131	68763	69576	88991	49662	46704	63362	56625	00481	73323	91427	15264	06969	57048	54149
132	17900	00813	64361	60725	88974	61005	99709	30666	26451	11528	44323	34778	60342	60388
133	71944	60227	63551	71109	05624	43836	58254	26160	32116	63403	35404	57146	10909	07346
134	54684	93691	85132	64399	29182	44324	14491	55226	78793	34107	30374	48429	51376	09559
135	25946	27623	11258	65204	52832	50880	22273	05554	99521	73791	85744	29276	70326	60251
136	01353	39318	44961	44972	91766	90262	56073	06606	51826	18893	83448	31915	97764	75091
137	99083	88191	27662	99113	57174	35571	99884	13951	71057	53961	61448	74909	07322	80960
138	52021	45406	37945	75234	24327	86978	22644	87779	23753	99926	63898	54886	18051	96314
139	78755	47744	43776	83098	03225	14281	83637	55984	13300	52212	58781	14905	46502	04472
140	25282	69106	59180	16257	22810	43609	12224	25643	89884	31149	85423	32581	34374	70873
141	11959	94202	02743	86847	79725	51811	12998	76844	05320	54236	53891	70226	38632	84776
142	11644	13792	98190	01424	30078	28197	55583	05197	47714	68440	22016	79204	06862	94451
143	06307	97912	68110	59812	95448	43244	31262	88880	13040	16458	43813	89416	42482	33939
144	76285	75714	89585	99296	52640	46518	55486	90754	88932	19937	57119	23251	55619	23679
145	55322	07589	39600	60866	63007	20007	66819	84164	61131	81429	60676	42807	78286	29015
146	78017	90928	90220	92503	83375	26986	74399	30885	88567	29169	72816	53357	15428	86932
147	44768	43342	20696	26331	43140	69744	82928	24988	94237	46138	77426	39039	55596	12655
148	25100	19336	14605	86603	51680	97678	24261	02464	86563	74812	60069	71674	15478	47642
149	83612	46623	62876	85197	07824	91392	58317	37726	84628	42221	10268	20692	15699	29167
150	41347	81666	82961	60413	71020	83658	02415	33322	66036	98712	46795	16308	28413	05417

Table of Random Units

A TABLE OF 14,000 RANDOM UNITS (Continued)

Line/Col.	(1)	(2)	(3)	(4)	(5)	(6)	(7)	(8)	(9)	(10)	(11)	(12)	(13)	(14)
151	38128	51178	75096	13609	16110	73533	42564	59870	29399	67834	91055	89917	51096	89011
152	60950	00455	73254	96067	50717	13878	03216	78274	65863	37011	91283	33914	91303	49326
153	90524	17320	29832	96118	75792	25326	22940	24904	80523	38928	91374	55597	97567	38914
154	49897	18278	67160	39408	97056	43517	84426	59650	20247	19293	02019	14790	02852	05819
155	18494	99209	81060	19488	65596	59787	47939	91225	98768	43688	00438	05548	09443	82897
156	65373	72984	30171	37741	70203	94094	87261	30056	58124	70133	18936	02138	59372	09075
157	40653	12843	04213	70925	95360	55774	76439	61768	52817	81151	52188	31940	54273	49032
158	51638	22238	56344	44587	83231	50317	74541	07719	25472	41602	77318	15145	57515	07633
159	69742	99303	62578	83575	30337	07488	51941	84316	42067	49692	28616	29101	03013	73449
160	58012	74072	67488	74580	47992	69482	58624	17106	47538	13452	22620	24260	40155	74716
161	18348	19855	42887	08279	43206	47077	42637	45606	00011	20662	14642	49984	94509	56380
162	59614	09193	58064	29086	44385	45740	70752	05663	49081	26960	57454	99264	24142	74648
163	75688	28630	39210	52897	62748	72658	98059	67202	72789	01869	13496	14663	87645	89713
164	13941	77802	69101	70061	35460	34576	15412	81304	58757	35498	94830	75521	00603	97701
165	96656	86420	96475	86458	54463	96419	55417	41375	76886	19008	66877	35934	59801	00497
166	03363	82042	15942	14549	38324	87094	19069	67590	11087	68570	22591	65232	85915	91499
167	70366	08390	69155	25496	13240	57407	91407	49160	07379	34444	94567	66035	38918	65708
168	47870	36605	12927	16043	53257	93796	52721	73120	48025	76074	95605	67422	41646	14557
169	79504	77606	22761	30518	28373	73898	30550	76684	77366	32276	04690	61667	64798	66276
170	46967	74841	50923	15339	37755	98995	40162	89561	69199	42257	11647	47603	48779	97907
171	14558	50769	35444	59030	87516	48193	02945	00922	48189	04724	21263	20892	92955	90251
172	12440	25057	01132	38611	28135	68089	10954	10097	54243	06460	50856	65435	79377	53890
173	32293	29938	68653	10497	98919	46587	77701	99119	93165	67788	17638	23097	21468	36992
174	10640	21875	72462	77981	56550	55999	87310	69643	45124	00349	25748	00844	96831	30651
175	47615	23169	39571	56972	20628	21788	51736	33133	72696	32605	41569	76148	91544	21121
176	16948	11128	71624	72754	49084	96303	27830	45817	67867	18062	87453	17226	72904	71474
177	21258	61092	66634	70335	92448	17354	83432	49608	66520	06442	59664	20420	39201	69549
178	15072	48853	15178	30730	47481	48490	41436	25015	49932	20474	53821	51015	79841	32405
179	99154	57412	09858	65671	70655	71479	63520	31357	56968	06729	34465	70685	04184	25250
180	08759	61089	23706	32994	35426	36666	63988	98844	37533	08269	27021	45886	22835	78451
181	67323	57839	61114	62192	47547	58023	64630	34886	98777	75442	95592	06141	45096	73117
182	09255	13986	84834	20764	72206	89393	34548	93438	88730	61805	78955	18952	46436	58740
183	36304	74712	00374	10107	85061	69228	81969	92216	03568	39630	81869	52824	50937	27954
184	15884	67429	86612	47367	10242	44880	12060	44309	46629	55105	66793	93173	00480	13311
185	18745	32031	35303	08134	33925	03044	59929	95418	04917	57596	24878	61733	92834	64454
186	72934	40086	88292	65728	38300	42323	64068	98373	48971	09049	59943	36538	05976	82118
187	17626	02944	20910	57662	80181	38579	24580	90529	52303	50436	29401	57824	86039	81062
188	27117	61399	50967	41399	81636	16663	15634	79717	94696	59240	25543	97989	63306	90946
189	93995	18678	90012	63645	85701	85269	62263	68331	00389	72571	15210	20769	44686	96176
190	67392	89421	09623	80725	62620	84162	87368	29560	00519	84545	08004	24526	41252	14521
191	04910	12261	37566	80016	21245	69377	50420	85658	55263	68667	78770	04533	14513	18099
192	81453	20283	79929	59839	23875	13245	46808	74124	74703	35769	95588	21014	37078	39170
193	19480	75790	48539	23703	15537	48885	02861	86587	74539	65227	90799	58789	96257	02708
194	21456	13162	74608	81011	55512	07481	93551	72189	76261	91206	89941	15132	37738	59284
195	89406	20912	46189	76376	25538	87212	20748	12831	57166	35026	16817	79121	18929	40628
196	09866	07414	55977	16419	01101	69343	13305	94302	80703	57910	36933	57771	42546	03003
197	86541	24681	23421	13521	28000	94917	07423	57523	97234	63951	42876	46829	09781	58160
198	10414	96941	06205	72222	57167	83902	07460	69507	10600	08858	07685	44472	64220	27040
199	49942	06683	41479	58982	56288	42853	92196	20632	62045	78812	35895	51851	83534	10689
200	23995	68882	42291	23374	24299	27024	67460	94783	40937	16961	26053	78749	46704	21983

XII.4 RANDOM NORMAL NUMBERS, $\mu = 0$, $\sigma = 1$

01	02	03	04	05	06	07	08	09	10
0.464	0.137	2.455	−0.323	−0.068	0.296	−0.288	1.298	0.241	−0.957
0.060	−2.526	−0.531	−0.194	0.543	−1.558	0.187	−1.190	0.022	0.525
1.486	−0.354	−0.634	0.697	0.926	1.375	0.785	−0.963	−0.853	−1.865
1.022	−0.472	1.279	3.521	0.571	−1.851	0.194	1.192	−0.501	−0.273
1.394	−0.555	0.046	0.321	2.945	1.974	−0.258	0.412	0.439	−0.035
0.906	−0.513	−0.525	0.595	0.881	−0.934	1.579	0.161	−1.885	0.371
1.179	−1.055	0.007	0.769	0.971	0.712	1.090	−0.631	−0.255	−0.702
−1.501	−0.488	−0.162	−0.136	1.033	0.203	0.448	0.748	−0.423	−0.432
−0.690	0.756	−1.618	−0.345	−0.511	−2.051	−0.457	−0.218	0.857	−0.465
1.372	0.225	0.378	0.761	0.181	−0.736	0.960	−1.530	−0.260	0.120
−0.482	1.678	−0.057	−1.229	−0.486	0.856	−0.491	−1.983	−2.830	−0.238
−1.376	−0.150	1.356	−0.561	−0.256	−0.212	0.219	0.779	0.953	−0.869
−1.010	0.598	−0.918	1.598	0.065	0.415	−0.169	0.313	−0.973	−1.016
−0.005	−0.899	0.012	−0.725	1.147	−0.121	1.096	0.481	−1.691	0.417
1.393	−1.163	−0.911	1.231	−0.199	−0.246	1.239	−2.574	−0.558	0.056
−1.787	−0.261	1.237	1.046	−0.508	−1.630	−0.146	−0.392	−0.627	0.561
−0.105	−0.357	−1.384	0.360	−0.992	−0.116	−1.698	−2.832	−1.108	−2.357
−1.339	1.827	−0.959	0.424	0.969	−1.141	−1.041	0.362	−1.726	1.956
1.041	0.535	0.731	1.377	0.983	−1.330	1.620	−1.040	0.524	−0.281
0.279	−2.056	0.717	−0.873	−1.096	−1.396	1.047	0.089	−0.573	0.932
−1.805	−2.008	−1.633	0.542	0.250	−0.166	0.032	0.079	0.471	−1.029
−1.186	1.180	1.114	0.882	1.265	−0.202	0.151	−0.376	−0.310	0.479
0.658	−1.141	1.151	−1.210	−0.927	0.425	0.290	−0.902	0.610	2.709
−0.439	0.358	−1.939	0.891	−0.227	0.602	0.873	−0.437	−0.220	−0.057
−1.399	−0.230	0.385	−0.649	−0.577	0.237	−0.289	0.513	0.738	−0.300
0.199	0.208	−1.083	−0.219	−0.291	1.221	1.119	0.004	−2.015	−0.594
0.159	0.272	−0.313	0.084	−2.828	−0.439	−0.792	−1.275	−0.623	−1.047
2.273	0.606	0.606	−0.747	0.247	1.291	0.063	−1.793	−0.699	−1.347
0.041	−0.307	0.121	0.790	−0.584	0.541	0.484	−0.986	0.481	0.996
−1.132	−2.098	0.921	0.145	0.446	−1.661	1.045	−1.363	−0.586	−1.023
0.768	0.079	−1.473	0.034	−2.127	0.665	0.084	−0.880	−0.579	0.551
0.375	−1.658	−0.851	0.234	−0.656	0.340	−0.086	−0.158	−0.120	0.418
−0.513	−0.344	0.210	−0.735	1.041	0.008	0.427	−0.831	0.191	0.074
0.292	−0.521	1.266	−1.206	−0.899	0.110	−0.528	−0.813	0.071	0.524
1.026	2.990	−0.574	−0.491	−1.114	1.297	−1.433	−1.345	−3.001	0.479
−1.334	1.278	−0.568	−0.109	−0.515	−0.566	2.923	0.500	0.359	0.326
−0.287	−0.144	−0.254	0.574	−0.451	−1.181	−1.190	−0.318	−0.094	1.114
0.161	−0.886	−0.921	−0.509	1.410	−0.518	0.192	−0.432	1.501	1.068
−1.346	0.193	−1.202	0.394	−1.045	0.843	0.942	1.045	0.031	0.772
1.250	−0.199	−0.288	1.810	1.378	0.584	1.216	0.733	0.402	0.226
0.630	−0.537	0.782	0.060	0.499	−0.431	1.705	1.164	0.884	−0.298
0.375	−1.941	0.247	−0.491	−0.665	−0.135	−0.145	−0.498	0.457	1.064
−1.420	0.489	−1.711	−1.186	0.754	−0.732	−0.066	1.006	−0.798	0.162
−0.151	−0.243	−0.430	−0.762	0.298	1.049	1.810	2.885	−0.768	−0.129
−0.309	0.531	0.416	−1.541	1.456	2.040	−0.124	0.196	0.023	−1.204
0.424	−0.444	0.593	0.993	−0.106	0.116	0.484	−1.272	1.066	1.097
0.593	0.658	−1.127	−1.407	−1.579	−1.616	1.458	1.262	0.736	−0.916
0.862	−0.885	−0.142	−0.504	0.532	1.381	0.022	−0.281	−0.342	1.222
0.235	−0.628	−0.023	−0.463	−0.899	−0.394	−0.538	1.707	−0.188	−1.153
−0.853	0.402	0.777	0.833	0.410	−0.349	−1.094	0.580	1.395	1.298

RANDOM NORMAL NUMBERS, $\mu = 0$, $\sigma = 1$

11	12	13	14	15	16	17	18	19	20
−1.329	−0.238	−0.838	−0.988	−0.445	0.964	−0.266	−0.322	−1.726	2.252
1.284	−0.229	1.058	0.090	0.050	0.523	0.016	0.277	1.639	0.554
0.619	0.628	0.005	0.973	−0.058	0.150	−0.635	−0.917	0.313	−1.203
0.699	−0.269	0.722	−0.994	−0.807	−1.203	1.163	1.244	1.306	−1.210
0.101	0.202	−0.150	0.731	0.420	0.116	−0.496	−0.037	−2.466	0.794
−1.381	0.301	0.522	0.233	0.791	−1.017	−0.182	0.926	−1.096	1.001
−0.574	1.366	−1.843	0.746	0.890	0.824	−1.249	−0.806	−0.240	0.217
0.096	0.210	1.091	0.990	0.900	−0.837	−1.097	−1.238	0.030	−0.311
1.389	−0.236	0.094	3.282	0.295	−0.416	0.313	0.720	0.007	0.354
1.249	0.706	1.453	0.366	−2.654	−1.400	0.212	0.307	−1.145	0.639
0.756	−0.397	−1.772	−0.257	1.120	1.188	−0.527	0.709	0.479	0.317
−0.860	0.412	−0.327	0.178	0.524	−0.672	−0.831	0.758	0.131	0.771
−0.778	−0.979	0.236	−1.033	1.497	−0.661	0.906	1.169	−1.582	1.303
0.037	0.062	0.426	1.220	0.471	0.784	−0.719	0.465	1.559	−1.326
2.619	−0.440	0.477	1.063	0.320	1.406	−0.701	−0.128	0.518	−0.676
−0.420	−0.287	−0.050	−0.481	1.521	−1.367	0.609	0.292	0.048	0.592
1.048	0.220	1.121	−1.789	−1.211	−0.871	−0.740	0.513	−0.558	−0.395
1.000	−0.638	1.261	0.510	−0.150	0.034	0.054	−0.055	0.639	−0.825
0.170	−1.131	−0.985	0.102	−0.939	−1.457	1.766	1.087	−1.275	2.362
0.389	−0.435	0.171	0.891	1.158	1.041	1.048	−0.324	−0.404	1.060
−0.305	0.838	−2.019	−0.540	0.905	1.195	−1.190	0.106	0.571	0.298
−0.321	−0.039	1.799	−1.032	−2.225	−0.148	0.758	−0.862	0.158	−0.726
1.900	1.572	−0.244	−1.721	1.130	0.495	−0.484	0.014	−0.778	−1.483
−0.778	−0.288	−0.224	−1.324	−0.072	0.890	−0.410	0.752	0.376	−0.224
0.617	−1.718	−0.183	−0.100	1.719	0.696	−1.339	−0.614	1.071	−0.386
−1.430	−0.953	0.770	−0.007	−1.872	1.075	−0.913	−1.168	1.775	0.238
0.267	−0.048	0.972	0.734	−1.408	−1.955	−0.848	2.002	0.232	−1.273
0.978	−0.520	−0.368	1.690	−1.479	0.985	1.475	−0.098	−1.633	2.399
−1.235	−1.168	0.325	1.421	2.652	−0.486	−1.253	0.270	−1.103	0.118
−0.258	0.638	2.309	0.741	−0.161	−0.679	0.336	1.973	0.370	−2.277
0.243	0.629	−1.516	−0.157	0.693	1.710	0.800	−0.265	1.218	0.655
−0.292	−1.455	−1.451	1.492	−0.713	0.821	−0.031	−0.780	1.330	0.977
−0.505	0.389	0.544	−0.042	1.615	−1.440	−0.989	−0.580	0.156	0.052
0.397	−0.287	1.712	0.289	−0.904	0.259	−0.600	−1.635	−0.009	−0.799
−0.605	−0.470	0.007	0.721	−1.117	0.635	0.592	−1.362	−1.441	0.672
1.360	0.182	−1.476	−0.599	−0.875	0.292	−0.700	0.058	−0.340	−0.639
0.480	−0.699	1.615	−0.225	1.014	−1.370	−1.097	0.294	0.309	−1.389
−0.027	−0.487	−1.000	−0.015	0.119	−1.990	−0.687	−1.964	−0.366	1.759
−1.482	−0.815	−0.121	1.884	−0.185	0.601	0.793	0.430	−1.181	0.426
−1.256	−0.567	−0.994	1.011	−1.071	−0.623	−0.420	−0.309	1.362	0.863
−1.132	2.039	1.934	−0.222	0.386	1.100	0.284	1.597	−1.718	−0.560
−0.780	−0.239	−0.497	−0.434	−0.284	−0.241	−0.333	1.348	−0.478	−0.169
−0.859	−0.215	0.241	1.471	0.389	−0.952	0.245	0.781	1.093	−0.240
0.447	1.479	0.067	0.426	−0.370	−0.675	−0.972	0.225	0.815	0.389
0.269	0.735	−0.066	−0.271	−1.439	1.036	−0.306	−1.439	−0.122	−0.336
0.097	−1.883	−0.218	0.202	−0.357	0.019	1.631	1.400	0.223	−0.793
−0.686	1.596	−0.286	0.722	0.655	−0.275	1.245	−1.504	0.066	−1.280
0.957	0.057	−1.153	0.701	−0.280	1.747	−0.745	1.338	−1.421	0.386
−0.976	−1.789	−0.696	−1.799	−0.354	0.071	2.355	0.135	−0.598	1.883
0.274	0.226	−0.909	−0.572	0.181	1.115	0.406	0.453	−1.218	−0.115

RANDOM NORMAL NUMBERS, $\mu = 0$, $\sigma = 1$

21	22	23	24	25	26	27	28	29	30
−1.752	−0.329	−1.256	0.318	1.531	0.349	−0.958	−0.059	0.415	−1.084
−0.291	0.085	1.701	−1.087	−0.443	−0.292	0.248	−0.539	−1.382	0.318
−0.933	0.130	0.634	0.899	1.409	−0.883	−0.095	0.229	0.129	0.367
−0.450	−0.244	0.072	1.028	1.730	−0.056	−1.488	−0.078	−2.361	−0.992
0.512	−0.882	0.490	−1.304	−0.266	0.757	−0.361	0.194	−1.078	0.529
−0.702	0.472	0.429	−0.664	−0.592	1.443	−1.515	−1.209	−1.043	0.278
0.284	0.039	−0.518	1.351	1.473	0.889	0.300	0.339	−0.206	1.392
−0.509	1.420	−0.782	−0.429	−1.266	0.627	−1.165	0.819	−0.261	0.409
−1.776	−1.033	1.977	0.014	0.702	−0.435	−0.816	1.131	0.656	0.061
−0.044	1.807	0.342	−2.510	1.071	−1.220	−0.060	−0.764	0.079	−0.964
0.263	−0.578	1.612	−0.148	−0.383	−1.007	−0.414	0.638	−0.186	0.507
0.986	0.439	−0.192	−0.132	0.167	0.883	−0.400	−1.440	−0.385	−1.414
−0.441	−0.852	−1.446	−0.605	−0.348	1.018	0.963	−0.004	2.504	−0.847
−0.866	0.489	0.097	0.379	0.192	−0.842	0.065	1.420	0.426	−1.191
−1.215	0.675	1.621	0.394	−1.447	2.199	−0.321	−0.540	−0.037	0.185
−0.475	−1.210	0.183	0.526	0.495	1.297	−1.613	1.241	−1.016	−0.090
1.200	0.131	2.502	0.344	−1.060	−0.909	−1.695	−0.666	−0.838	−0.866
−0.498	−1.202	−0.057	−1.354	−1.441	−1.590	0.987	0.441	0.637	−1.116
−0.743	0.894	−0.028	1.119	−0.598	0.279	2.241	0.830	0.267	−0.156
0.779	−0.780	−0.954	0.705	−0.361	−0.734	1.365	1.297	−0.142	−1.387
−0.206	−0.195	1.017	−1.167	−0.079	−0.452	0.058	−1.068	−0.394	−0.406
−0.092	−0.927	−0.439	0.256	0.503	0.338	1.511	−0.465	−0.118	−0.454
−1.222	−1.582	1.786	−0.517	−1.080	−0.409	−0.474	−1.890	0.247	0.575
0.068	0.075	−1.383	−0.084	0.159	1.276	1.141	0.186	−0.973	−0.266
0.183	1.600	−0.335	1.553	0.889	0.896	−0.035	0.461	0.486	1.246
−0.811	−2.904	0.618	0.588	0.533	0.803	−0.696	0.690	0.820	0.557
−1.010	1.149	1.033	0.336	1.306	0.835	1.523	0.296	−0.426	0.004
1.453	1.210	−0.043	0.220	−0.256	−1.161	−2.030	−0.046	0.243	1.082
0.759	−0.838	−0.877	−0.177	1.183	−0.218	−3.154	−0.963	−0.822	−1.114
0.287	0.278	−0.454	0.897	−0.122	0.013	0.346	0.921	0.238	−0.586
−0.669	0.035	−2.077	1.077	0.525	−0.154	−1.036	0.015	−0.220	0.882
0.392	0.106	−1.430	−0.204	−0.326	0.825	−0.432	−0.094	−1.566	0.679
−0.337	0.199	−0.160	0.625	−0.891	−1.464	−0.318	1.297	0.932	−0.032
0.369	−1.990	−1.190	0.666	−1.614	0.082	0.922	−0.139	−0.833	0.091
−1.694	0.710	−0.655	−0.546	1.654	0.134	0.466	0.033	−0.039	0.838
0.985	0.340	0.276	0.911	−0.170	−0.551	1.000	−0.838	0.275	−0.304
−1.063	−0.594	−1.526	−0.787	0.873	−0.405	−1.324	0.162	−0.163	−2.716
0.033	−1.527	1.422	0.308	0.845	−0.151	0.741	0.064	1.212	0.823
0.597	0.362	−3.760	1.159	0.874	−0.794	−0.915	1.215	1.627	−1.248
−1.601	−0.570	0.133	−0.660	1.485	0.682	−0.898	0.686	0.658	0.346
−0.266	−1.309	0.597	0.989	0.934	1.079	−0.656	−0.999	−0.036	−0.537
0.901	1.531	−0.889	−1.019	0.084	1.531	−0.144	−1.920	0.678	−0.402
−1.433	−1.008	−0.990	0.090	0.940	0.207	−0.745	0.638	1.469	1.214
1.327	0.763	−1.724	−0.709	−1.100	−1.346	−0.946	−0.157	0.522	−1.264
−0.248	0.788	−0.577	0.122	−0.536	0.293	1.207	−2.243	1.642	1.353
−0.401	−0.679	0.921	0.476	1.121	−0.864	0.128	−0.551	−0.872	1.511
0.344	−0.324	0.686	−1.487	−0.126	0.803	−0.961	0.183	−0.358	−0.184
0.441	−0.372	−1.336	0.062	1.506	−0.315	−0.112	−0.452	1.594	−0.264
0.824	0.040	−1.734	0.251	0.054	−0.379	1.298	−0.126	0.104	−0.529
1.385	1.320	−0.509	−0.381	−1.671	−0.524	−0.805	1.348	0.676	0.799

RANDOM NORMAL NUMBERS, $\mu = 0$, $\sigma = 1$

31	32	33	34	35	36	37	38	39	40
1.556	0.119	−0.078	0.164	−0.455	0.077	−0.043	−0.299	0.249	−0.182
0.647	1.029	1.186	0.887	1.204	−0.657	0.644	−0.410	−0.652	−0.165
0.329	0.407	1.169	−2.072	1.661	0.891	0.233	−1.628	−0.762	−0.717
−1.188	1.171	−1.170	−0.291	0.863	−0.045	−0.205	0.574	−0.926	1.407
−0.917	−0.616	−1.589	1.184	0.266	0.559	−1.833	−0.572	−0.648	−1.090
0.414	0.469	−0.182	0.397	1.649	1.198	0.067	−1.526	−0.081	−0.192
0.107	−0.187	1.343	0.472	−0.112	1.182	0.548	2.748	0.249	0.154
−0.497	1.907	0.191	0.136	−0.475	0.458	0.183	−1.640	−0.058	1.278
0.501	0.083	−0.321	1.133	1.126	−0.299	1.299	1.617	1.581	2.455
−1.382	−0.738	1.225	1.564	−0.363	−0.548	1.070	0.390	−1.398	0.524
−0.590	0.699	−0.162	−0.011	1.049	−0.689	1.225	0.339	−0.539	−0.445
−1.125	1.111	−1.065	0.534	0.102	0.425	−1.026	0.695	−0.057	0.795
0.849	0.169	−0.351	0.584	2.177	0.009	−0.696	−0.426	−0.692	−1.638
−1.233	−0.585	0.306	0.773	1.304	−1.304	0.282	−1.705	0.187	−0.880
0.104	−0.468	0.185	0.498	−0.624	−0.322	−0.875	1.478	−0.691	−0.281
0.261	−1.883	−0.181	1.675	−0.324	−1.029	−0.185	0.004	−0.101	−1.187
−0.007	1.280	0.568	−1.270	1.405	1.731	2.072	1.686	0.728	−0.417
0.794	−0.111	0.040	−0.536	−0.976	2.192	1.609	−0.190	−0.279	−1.611
0.431	−2.300	−1.081	−1.370	2.943	0.653	−2.523	0.756	0.886	−0.983
−0.149	1.294	−0.580	0.482	−1.449	−1.067	1.996	−0.274	0.721	0.490
−0.216	−1.647	1.043	0.481	−0.011	−0.587	−0.916	−1.016	−1.040	−1.117
1.604	−0.851	−0.317	−0.686	−0.008	1.939	0.078	−0.465	0.533	0.652
−0.212	0.005	0.535	0.837	0.362	1.103	0.219	0.488	1.332	−0.200
0.007	−0.076	1.484	0.455	−0.207	−0.554	1.120	0.913	−0.681	1.751
−0.217	0.937	0.860	0.323	1.321	−0.492	−1.386	−0.003	−0.230	0.539
−0.649	0.300	−0.698	0.900	0.569	0.842	0.804	1.025	0.603	−1.546
−1.541	0.193	2.047	−0.552	1.190	−0.087	2.062	−2.173	−0.791	−0.520
0.274	−0.530	0.112	0.385	0.656	0.436	0.882	0.312	−2.265	−0.218
0.876	−1.498	−0.128	−0.387	−1.259	−0.856	−0.353	0.714	0.863	1.169
−0.859	−1.083	1.288	−0.078	−0.081	0.210	0.572	1.194	−1.118	−1.543
−0.015	−0.567	0.113	2.127	−0.719	3.256	−0.721	−0.663	−0.779	−0.930
−1.529	−0.231	1.223	0.300	−0.995	−0.651	0.505	0.138	−0.064	1.341
0.278	−0.058	−2.740	−0.296	−1.180	0.574	1.452	0.846	−0.243	−1.208
1.428	0.322	2.302	−0.852	0.782	−1.322	−0.092	−0.546	0.560	−1.430
0.770	−1.874	0.347	0.994	−0.485	−1.179	0.048	−1.324	1.061	0.449
−0.303	−0.629	0.764	0.013	−1.192	−0.475	−1.085	−0.880	1.738	−1.225
−0.263	−2.105	0.509	−0.645	1.362	0.504	−0.755	1.274	1.448	0.604
0.997	−1.187	−0.242	0.121	2.510	−1.935	0.350	0.073	0.458	−0.446
−0.063	−0.475	−1.802	−0.476	0.193	−1.199	0.339	0.364	−0.684	1.353
−0.168	1.904	−0.485	−0.032	−0.554	0.056	−0.710	−0.778	0.722	−0.024
0.366	−0.491	0.301	−0.008	−0.894	−0.945	0.384	−1.748	−1.118	0.394
0.436	−0.464	0.539	0.942	−0.458	0.445	−1.883	1.228	1.113	−0.218
0.597	−1.471	−0.434	0.705	−0.788	0.575	0.086	0.504	1.445	−0.513
−0.805	−0.624	1.344	0.649	−1.124	0.680	−0.986	1.845	−1.152	−0.393
1.681	−1.910	0.440	0.067	−1.502	−0.755	−0.989	−0.054	−2.320	0.474
−0.007	−0.459	1.940	0.220	−1.259	−1.729	0.137	−0.520	−0.412	2.847
0.209	−0.633	0.299	0.174	1.975	−0.271	0.119	−0.199	0.007	2.315
1.254	1.672	−1.186	−1.310	0.474	0.878	−0.725	−0.191	0.642	−1.212
−1.016	−0.697	0.017	−0.263	−0.047	−1.294	−0.339	2.257	−0.078	−0.049
−1.169	−0.355	1.086	−0.199	0.031	0.396	−0.143	1.572	0.276	0.027

RANDOM NORMAL NUMBERS, $\mu = 0$, $\sigma = 1$

41	42	43	44	45	46	47	48	49	50
−0.856	−0.063	0.787	−2.052	−1.192	−0.831	1.623	1.135	0.759	−0.189
−0.276	−1.110	0.752	−1.378	−0.583	0.360	0.365	1.587	0.621	1.344
0.379	−0.440	0.858	1.453	−1.356	0.503	−1.134	1.950	−1.816	−0.283
1.468	0.131	0.047	0.355	0.162	−1.491	−0.739	−1.182	−0.533	−0.497
−1.805	−0.772	1.286	−0.636	−1.312	−1.045	1.559	−0.871	−0.102	−0.123
2.285	0.554	0.418	−0.577	−1.489	−1.255	0.092	−0.597	−1.051	−0.980
−0.602	0.399	1.121	−1.026	0.087	1.018	−1.437	0.661	0.091	−0.637
0.229	−0.584	0.705	0.124	0.341	1.320	−0.824	−1.541	−0.163	2.329
1.382	−1.454	1.537	−1.299	0.363	−0.356	−0.025	0.294	2.194	−0.395
0.978	0.109	1.434	−1.094	−0.265	−0.857	−1.421	−1.773	0.570	−0.053
−0.678	−2.335	1.202	−1.697	0.547	−0.201	−0.373	−1.363	−0.081	0.958
−0.366	−1.084	−0.626	0.798	1.706	−1.160	−0.838	1.462	0.636	0.570
−1.074	−1.379	0.086	−0.331	−0.288	−0.309	−1.527	−0.408	0.183	0.856
−0.600	−0.096	0.696	0.446	1.417	−2.140	0.599	−0.157	1.485	1.387
0.918	1.163	−1.445	0.759	0.878	−1.781	−0.056	−2.141	−0.234	0.975
−0.791	−0.528	0.946	1.673	−0.680	−0.784	1.494	−0.086	−1.071	−1.196
0.598	−0.352	0.719	−0.341	0.056	−1.041	1.429	0.235	0.314	−1.693
0.567	−1.156	−0.125	−0.534	0.711	−0.511	0.187	−0.644	−1.090	−1.281
0.963	0.052	0.037	0.637	−1.335	0.055	0.010	−0.860	−0.621	0.713
0.489	−0.209	1.659	0.054	1.635	0.169	0.794	−1.550	1.845	−0.388
−1.627	−0.017	0.699	0.661	−0.073	0.188	1.183	−1.054	−1.615	−0.765
−1.096	1.215	0.320	0.738	1.865	−1.169	−0.667	−0.674	−0.062	1.378
−2.532	1.031	−0.799	1.665	−2.756	−0.151	−0.704	0.602	−0.672	1.264
0.024	−1.183	−0.927	−0.629	0.204	−0.825	0.496	2.543	0.262	−0.785
0.192	0.125	0.373	−0.931	−0.079	0.186	−0.306	0.621	−0.292	1.131
−1.324	−1.229	−0.648	−0.430	0.811	0.868	0.787	1.845	−0.374	−0.651
−0.726	−0.746	1.572	−1.420	1.509	−0.361	−0.310	−3.117	1.637	0.642
−1.618	1.082	−0.319	0.300	1.524	−0.418	−1.712	0.358	−1.032	0.537
1.695	0.843	2.049	0.388	−0.297	1.077	−0.462	0.655	0.940	−0.354
0.790	0.605	−3.077	1.009	−0.906	−1.004	0.693	−1.098	1.300	0.549
1.792	−0.895	−0.136	−1.765	1.077	0.418	−0.150	0.808	0.697	0.435
0.771	−0.741	−0.492	−0.770	−0.458	−0.021	1.385	−1.225	−0.066	−1.471
−1.438	0.423	−1.211	0.723	−0.731	0.883	−2.109	−2.455	−0.210	1.644
−0.294	1.266	−1.994	−0.730	0.545	0.397	1.069	−0.383	−0.097	−0.985
−1.966	0.909	0.400	0.685	−0.800	1.759	0.268	1.387	−0.414	1.615
0.999	1.587	1.423	0.937	−0.943	0.090	1.185	−1.204	0.300	−1.354
0.581	0.481	−2.400	0.000	0.231	0.079	−2.842	−0.846	−0.508	−0.516
0.370	−1.452	−0.580	−1.462	−0.972	1.116	−0.994	0.374	−3.336	−0.058
0.834	−1.227	−0.709	−1.039	−0.014	−0.383	−0.512	−0.347	0.881	−0.638
−0.376	−0.813	0.660	−1.029	−0.137	0.371	0.376	0.968	1.338	−0.786
−1.621	0.815	−0.544	−0.376	−0.852	0.436	1.562	0.815	−1.048	0.188
0.163	−0.161	2.501	−0.265	−0.285	1.934	1.070	0.215	−0.876	0.073
1.786	−0.538	−0.437	0.324	0.105	−0.421	−0.410	−0.947	0.700	−1.006
2.140	1.218	−0.351	−0.068	0.254	0.448	−1.461	0.784	0.317	1.013
0.064	0.410	0.368	0.419	−0.982	1.371	0.100	−0.505	0.856	0.890
0.789	−0.131	1.330	0.506	−0.645	−1.414	2.426	1.389	−0.169	−0.194
−0.011	−0.372	−0.699	2.382	−1.395	−0.467	1.256	−0.585	−1.359	−1.804
−0.463	0.003	−1.470	1.493	0.960	0.364	−1.267	−0.007	0.616	0.624
−1.210	−0.669	0.009	1.284	−0.617	0.355	−0.589	−0.243	−0.015	−0.712
−1.157	0.481	0.560	1.287	1.129	−0.126	0.006	1.532	1.328	0.980

RANDOM NORMAL NUMBERS, $\mu = 0$, $\sigma = 1$

51	52	53	54	55	56	57	58	59	60
0.240	1.774	0.210	−1.471	1.167	−1.114	0.182	−0.485	−0.318	1.156
0.627	−0.758	−0.930	1.641	0.162	−0.874	−0.235	0.203	−0.724	−0.155
−0.594	0.098	0.158	−0.722	1.385	−0.985	−1.707	0.175	0.449	0.654
1.082	−0.753	−1.944	−1.964	−2.131	−2.796	−1.286	0.807	−0.122	0.527
0.060	−0.014	1.577	−0.814	−0.633	0.275	−0.087	0.517	0.474	−1.432
−0.013	0.402	−0.086	−0.394	0.292	−2.862	−1.660	−1.658	1.610	−2.205
1.586	−0.833	1.444	−0.615	−1.157	−0.220	−0.517	−1.668	−2.036	−0.850
−0.405	−1.315	−1.355	−1.331	1.394	−0.381	−0.729	−0.447	−0.906	0.622
−0.329	1.701	0.427	0.627	−0.271	−0.971	−1.010	1.182	−0.143	0.844
0.992	0.708	−0.115	−1.630	0.596	0.499	−0.862	0.508	0.474	−0.974
0.296	−0.390	2.047	−0.363	0.724	0.788	−0.089	0.930	−0.497	0.058
−2.069	−1.422	−0.948	−1.742	−1.173	0.215	0.661	0.842	−0.984	−0.577
−0.211	−1.727	−0.277	1.592	−0.707	0.327	−0.527	0.912	0.571	−0.525
−0.467	1.848	−0.263	−0.862	0.706	−0.533	0.626	−0.200	−2.221	0.368
1.284	0.412	1.512	0.328	0.203	−1.231	−1.480	−0.400	−0.491	0.913
0.821	−1.503	−1.066	1.624	1.345	0.440	−1.416	0.301	−0.355	0.106
1.056	1.224	0.281	−0.098	1.868	−0.395	0.610	−1.173	−1.449	1.171
1.090	−0.790	0.882	1.687	−0.009	−2.053	−0.030	−0.421	1.253	−0.081
0.574	0.129	1.203	0.280	1.438	−2.052	−0.443	0.522	0.468	−1.211
−0.531	2.155	0.334	0.898	−1.114	0.243	1.026	0.391	−0.011	−0.024
0.896	0.181	−0.941	−0.511	0.648	−0.710	−0.181	−1.417	−0.585	0.087
0.042	0.579	−0.316	0.394	1.133	−0.305	−0.683	−1.318	−0.050	0.993
2.328	−0.243	0.534	0.241	0.275	0.060	0.727	−1.459	0.174	−1.072
0.486	−0.558	0.426	0.728	−0.360	−0.068	0.058	1.471	−0.051	0.337
−0.304	−0.309	0.646	0.309	−1.320	0.311	−1.407	−0.011	0.387	0.128
−2.319	−0.129	0.866	−0.424	0.236	0.419	−1.359	−1.088	−0.045	1.096
1.098	−0.875	0.659	−1.086	−0.424	−1.462	0.743	−0.787	1.472	1.677
−0.038	−0.118	−1.285	−0.545	−0.140	1.244	−1.104	0.146	0.058	1.245
−0.207	−0.746	1.681	0.137	0.104	−0.491	−0.935	0.671	−0.448	−0.129
0.333	−1.386	1.840	1.089	0.837	−1.642	−0.273	−0.798	0.067	0.334
1.190	−0.547	−1.016	0.540	−0.993	0.443	−0.190	1.019	−1.021	−1.276
−1.416	−0.749	0.325	0.846	2.417	−0.479	−0.655	−1.326	−1.952	1.234
0.622	0.661	0.028	1.302	−0.032	−0.157	1.470	−0.766	0.697	−0.303
−1.134	0.499	0.538	0.564	−2.392	−1.398	0.010	1.874	1.386	0.000
0.725	−0.242	0.281	1.355	−0.036	0.204	−0.345	0.395	−0.753	1.645
−0.210	0.611	−0.219	0.450	0.308	0.993	−0.146	0.225	−1.496	0.246
0.219	0.302	0.000	−0.437	−2.127	0.883	−0.599	−1.516	0.826	1.242
−1.098	−0.252	−2.480	−0.973	0.712	−1.430	−0.167	−1.237	0.750	−0.763
0.144	0.489	−0.637	1.990	0.411	−0.563	0.027	1.278	2.105	−1.130
−1.738	−1.295	0.431	−0.503	2.327	−0.007	−1.293	−1.206	−0.066	1.370
−0.487	−0.097	−1.361	−0.340	0.204	0.938	−0.148	−1.099	−0.252	−0.384
−0.636	−0.626	1.967	1.677	−0.331	−0.440	−1.440	1.281	1.070	−1.167
−1.464	−1.493	0.945	0.180	−0.672	−0.035	−0.293	−0.905	0.196	−1.122
0.561	−0.375	−0.657	1.304	0.833	−1.159	1.501	1.265	0.438	−0.437
−0.525	−0.017	1.815	0.789	−1.908	−0.353	1.383	−1.208	−1.135	1.082
0.980	−0.111	−0.804	−1.078	−1.930	0.171	−1.318	2.377	−0.303	1.062
0.501	0.835	−0.518	−1.034	−1.493	0.712	0.421	−1.165	0.782	−1.484
1.081	−1.176	−0.542	0.321	0.688	0.670	−0.771	−0.090	−0.611	−0.813
−0.148	−1.203	−1.553	1.244	0.826	0.077	0.128	−0.772	1.683	0.318
0.096	−0.286	0.362	0.888	0.551	1.782	0.335	2.083	0.350	0.260

RANDOM NORMAL NUMBERS, $\mu = 0$, $\sigma = 1$

61	62	63	64	65	66	67	68	69	70
0.052	1.504	−1.350	−1.124	−0.521	0.515	0.839	0.778	0.438	−0.550
−0.315	−0.865	0.851	0.127	−0.379	1.640	−0.441	0.717	0.670	−0.301
0.938	−0.055	0.947	1.275	1.557	−1.484	−1.137	0.398	1.333	1.988
0.497	0.502	0.385	−0.467	2.468	−1.810	−1.438	0.283	1.740	0.420
2.308	−0.399	−1.798	0.018	0.780	1.030	0.806	−0.408	−0.547	−0.280
1.815	0.101	−0.561	0.236	0.166	0.227	−0.309	0.056	0.610	0.732
−0.421	0.432	0.586	1.059	0.278	−1.672	1.859	1.433	−0.919	−1.770
0.008	0.555	−1.310	−1.440	−0.142	−0.295	−0.630	−0.911	0.133	−0.308
1.191	−0.114	1.039	1.083	0.185	−0.492	0.419	−0.433	−1.019	−2.260
1.299	1.918	0.318	1.348	0.935	1.250	−0.175	−0.828	−0.336	0.726
0.012	−0.739	−1.181	−0.645	−0.736	1.801	−0.209	−0.389	0.867	−0.555
−0.586	−0.044	−0.983	0.332	0.371	−0.072	−1.212	1.047	−1.930	0.812
−0.122	1.515	0.338	−1.040	−0.008	0.467	−0.600	0.923	1.126	−0.752
0.879	0.516	−0.920	2.121	0.674	1.481	0.660	−0.986	1.644	−2.159
0.435	1.149	−0.065	1.391	0.707	0.548	−0.490	−1.139	0.249	−0.933
0.645	0.878	−0.904	0.896	−1.284	0.237	−0.378	−0.510	−1.123	−0.129
−0.514	−1.017	0.529	0.973	−1.202	0.005	−0.644	−0.167	−0.664	0.167
0.242	−0.427	−0.727	−1.150	−1.092	−0.736	0.925	−0.050	−0.200	−0.770
0.443	0.445	−1.287	−1.463	−0.650	0.412	−2.714	−0.903	−0.341	0.957
0.273	0.203	0.423	1.423	0.508	1.058	−0.828	0.143	−1.059	0.345
0.255	1.036	1.471	0.476	0.592	−0.658	0.677	0.155	1.068	−0.759
0.858	−0.370	0.522	−1.890	−0.389	0.609	1.210	0.489	−0.006	0.834
0.097	−1.709	1.790	−0.929	0.405	0.024	−0.036	0.580	−0.642	−1.121
0.520	0.889	−0.540	0.266	−0.354	0.524	−0.788	−0.497	−0.973	1.481
−0.311	−1.772	−0.496	1.275	−0.904	0.147	1.497	0.657	−0.469	−0.783
−0.604	0.857	−0.695	0.397	0.296	−0.285	0.191	0.158	1.672	1.190
−0.001	0.287	−0.868	−0.013	−1.576	−0.168	0.047	−0.159	0.086	−1.077
1.160	0.989	0.205	0.937	−0.099	−1.281	−0.276	0.845	0.752	0.663
1.579	−0.303	−1.174	−0.960	−0.470	−0.556	−0.689	1.535	−0.711	−0.743
−0.615	−0.154	0.008	1.353	−0.381	1.137	0.022	0.175	0.586	2.941
1.578	1.529	−0.294	−1.301	0.614	0.099	−0.700	−0.003	1.052	1.643
0.626	−0.447	−1.261	−2.029	0.182	−1.176	0.083	1.868	0.872	0.965
−0.493	−0.020	0.920	1.473	1.873	−0.289	0.410	0.394	0.881	0.054
−0.217	0.342	1.423	0.364	−0.119	0.509	−2.266	0.189	0.149	1.041
−0.792	0.347	−1.367	−0.632	−1.238	−0.136	−0.352	−0.157	−1.163	1.305
0.568	−0.226	0.391	−0.074	−0.312	0.400	1.583	0.481	−1.048	0.759
0.051	0.549	−2.192	1.257	−1.460	0.363	0.127	−1.020	−1.192	0.449
−0.891	0.490	0.279	0.372	−0.578	−0.836	2.285	−0.448	0.720	0.510
0.622	−0.126	−0.637	1.255	−0.354	0.032	−1.076	0.352	0.103	−0.496
0.623	0.819	−0.489	0.354	−0.943	−0.694	0.248	0.092	−0.673	−1.428
−1.208	−1.038	0.140	−0.762	−0.854	−0.249	2.431	0.067	−0.317	−0.874
−0.487	−2.117	0.195	2.154	1.041	−1.314	−0.785	−0.414	−0.695	2.310
0.522	0.314	−1.003	0.134	−1.748	−0.107	0.459	1.550	1.118	−1.004
0.838	0.613	0.227	0.308	−0.757	0.912	2.272	0.556	−0.041	0.008
−1.534	−0.407	1.202	1.251	−0.891	−1.588	−2.380	0.059	0.682	−0.878
−0.099	2.391	1.067	−2.060	−0.464	−0.103	3.486	1.121	0.632	−1.626
0.070	1.465	−0.080	−0.526	−1.090	−1.002	0.132	1.504	0.050	−0.393
0.115	−0.601	1.751	1.956	−0.196	0.400	−0.522	0.571	−0.101	−2.160
0.252	−0.329	−0.586	−0.118	−0.242	−0.521	0.818	−0.167	−0.469	0.430
0.017	0.185	0.377	1.883	−0.443	−0.039	−1.244	−0.820	−1.171	0.104

RANDOM NORMAL NUMBERS, $\mu = 0$, $\sigma = 1$

71	72	73	74	75	76	77	78	79	80
2.988	0.423	−1.261	−1.893	0.187	−0.412	−0.228	0.002	−0.384	−1.032
0.760	0.995	−0.256	−0.505	0.750	−0.654	0.647	0.613	0.086	−0.118
−0.650	−0.927	−1.071	−0.796	1.130	−1.042	−0.181	−1.020	1.648	−1.327
−0.394	−0.452	0.893	1.410	1.133	0.319	0.537	−0.789	0.078	−0.062
−1.168	1.902	0.206	0.303	1.413	2.012	0.278	−0.566	−0.900	0.200
1.343	−0.377	−0.131	−0.585	0.053	0.137	−1.371	−0.175	−0.878	0.118
−0.733	−1.921	0.471	−1.394	−0.885	−0.523	0.553	0.344	−0.775	1.545
−0.172	−0.575	0.066	−0.310	1.795	−1.148	0.772	−1.063	0.818	0.302
1.457	0.862	1.677	−0.507	−1.691	−0.034	0.270	0.075	−0.554	1.420
−0.087	0.744	1.829	1.203	−0.436	−0.618	−0.200	−1.134	−1.352	−0.098
−0.092	1.043	−0.255	0.189	0.270	−1.034	−0.571	−0.336	−0.742	2.141
0.441	−0.379	−1.757	0.608	0.527	−0.338	−1.995	0.573	−0.034	−0.056
0.073	−0.250	0.531	−0.695	1.402	−0.462	−0.938	1.130	1.453	−0.106
0.637	0.276	−0.013	1.968	−0.205	0.486	0.727	1.416	0.963	1.349
−0.792	−1.778	1.284	−0.452	0.602	0.668	0.516	−0.210	0.040	−0.103
−1.223	1.561	−2.099	1.419	0.223	−0.482	1.098	0.513	0.418	−1.686
−0.407	1.587	0.335	−2.475	−0.284	1.567	−0.248	−0.759	1.792	−2.319
−0.462	−0.193	−0.012	−1.208	2.151	1.336	−1.968	−1.767	−0.374	0.783
1.457	0.883	1.001	−0.169	0.836	−1.236	1.632	−0.142	−0.222	0.340
−1.918	−1.246	−0.209	0.780	−0.330	−2.953	−0.447	−0.094	1.344	−0.196
−0.126	1.094	−1.206	−1.426	1.474	−1.080	0.000	0.764	1.476	−0.016
−0.306	−0.847	0.639	−0.262	−0.427	0.391	−1.298	−1.013	2.024	−0.539
0.477	1.595	−0.762	0.424	0.799	0.312	1.151	−1.095	1.199	−0.765
0.369	−0.709	1.283	−0.007	−1.440	−0.782	0.061	1.427	1.656	0.974
−0.579	0.606	−0.866	−0.715	−0.301	−0.180	0.188	0.668	−1.091	1.476
−0.418	−0.588	0.919	−0.083	1.084	0.944	0.253	−1.833	1.305	0.171
0.128	−0.834	0.009	0.742	0.539	−0.948	−1.055	−0.689	−0.338	1.091
−0.291	0.235	−0.971	−1.696	1.119	0.272	0.635	−0.792	−1.355	1.291
−1.024	1.212	−1.100	−0.348	1.741	0.035	1.268	0.192	0.729	−0.467
−0.378	1.026	0.093	0.468	−0.967	0.675	0.807	−2.109	−1.214	0.559
1.232	−0.815	0.608	1.429	−0.748	0.201	0.400	−1.230	−0.398	−0.674
1.793	−0.581	−1.076	0.512	−0.442	−1.488	−0.580	0.172	−0.891	0.311
0.766	0.310	−0.070	0.624	−0.389	1.035	−0.101	−0.926	0.816	−1.048
−0.606	−1.224	1.465	0.012	1.061	0.491	−1.023	1.948	0.866	−0.737
0.106	−2.715	0.363	0.343	−0.159	2.672	1.119	0.731	−1.012	−0.889
−0.060	0.444	1.596	−0.630	0.362	−0.306	1.163	−0.974	0.486	−0.373
2.081	1.161	−1.167	0.021	0.053	−0.094	0.381	−0.628	−2.581	−1.243
−1.727	−1.266	0.088	0.936	0.368	0.648	−0.799	1.115	−0.968	−2.588
0.001	1.364	1.677	0.644	1.505	0.440	−0.329	0.498	0.869	−0.965
−1.114	−0.239	−0.409	−0.334	−0.605	0.501	−1.921	−0.470	2.354	−0.660
0.189	−0.547	−1.758	−0.295	−0.279	−0.515	−1.053	0.553	−0.297	0.496
−0.065	−0.023	−0.267	−0.247	1.318	0.904	−0.712	−1.152	−0.543	0.176
−1.742	−0.599	0.430	−0.615	1.165	0.084	2.017	−1.207	2.614	1.490
0.732	0.188	2.343	0.526	−0.812	0.389	1.036	−0.023	0.229	−2.262
−1.490	0.014	0.167	1.422	0.015	0.069	0.133	0.897	−1.678	0.323
1.507	−0.571	−0.724	1.741	−0.152	−0.147	−0.158	−0.076	0.652	0.447
0.513	0.168	−0.076	−0.171	0.428	0.205	−0.865	0.107	1.023	0.077
−0.834	−1.121	1.441	0.492	0.559	1.724	−1.659	0.245	1.354	−0.041
0.258	1.880	−0.536	1.246	−0.188	0.746	1.097	0.258	1.547	1.238
−0.818	0.273	0.159	−0.765	0.526	1.281	1.154	−0.687	−0.793	0.795

RANDOM NORMAL NUMBERS, μ = 0, σ = 1

81	82	83	84	85	86	87	88	89	90
−0.713	−0.541	−0.571	−0.807	−1.560	1.000	0.140	−0.549	0.887	2.237
−0.117	0.530	−1.599	−1.602	0.412	−1.450	−1.217	1.074	−1.021	−0.424
1.187	−1.523	1.437	0.051	1.237	−0.798	1.616	−0.823	−1.207	1.258
−0.182	−0.186	0.517	1.438	0.831	−1.319	−0.539	−0.192	0.150	2.127
1.964	−0.629	−0.944	−0.028	0.948	1.005	0.242	−0.432	−0.329	0.113
0.230	1.523	1.658	0.753	0.724	0.183	−0.147	0.505	0.448	−0.053
0.839	−0.849	−0.145	−1.843	−1.276	0.481	−0.142	−0.534	0.403	0.370
−0.801	0.343	−1.822	0.447	−0.931	−0.824	−0.484	0.864	−1.069	0.860
−0.124	0.727	1.654	−0.182	−1.381	−1.146	−0.572	0.159	0.186	1.221
−0.088	0.032	−0.564	0.654	1.141	−0.056	−0.343	0.067	−0.267	−0.219
0.912	−1.114	−1.035	−1.070	−0.297	1.195	0.030	0.022	0.406	−0.414
1.397	−0.473	0.433	0.023	−1.204	1.254	0.551	−1.012	−0.789	0.906
−0.652	−0.029	0.064	0.511	1.117	−0.465	0.523	−0.083	0.386	0.259
1.236	−0.457	−1.354	−0.898	−0.270	−1.837	1.641	−0.657	−0.753	−1.686
−0.498	1.302	0.816	−0.936	1.404	0.555	2.450	−0.789	−0.120	0.505
−0.005	2.174	1.893	−1.361	−0.991	0.508	−0.823	0.918	0.524	0.488
0.115	−1.373	−0.900	−1.010	0.624	0.946	0.312	−1.384	0.224	2.343
0.167	0.254	1.219	1.153	−0.510	−0.007	−0.285	−0.631	−0.356	0.254
0.976	1.158	−0.469	1.099	0.509	−1.324	−0.102	−0.296	−0.907	0.449
0.653	−0.366	0.450	−2.653	−0.592	−0.510	0.983	0.023	−0.881	0.876
−0.150	−0.088	0.457	−0.448	0.605	0.668	−0.613	0.261	0.023	−0.050
0.060	0.276	0.229	−1.527	−0.316	−0.834	−1.652	−0.387	0.632	0.895
−0.678	0.547	0.243	−2.183	−0.368	1.158	−0.996	−0.705	−0.314	1.464
2.139	0.395	−0.376	−0.175	0.406	0.309	−1.021	−0.460	−0.217	0.307
0.091	1.793	0.822	0.054	0.573	−0.729	−0.517	0.589	1.927	0.940
−0.003	0.344	1.242	−1.105	0.234	−1.222	−0.474	1.831	0.124	−0.840
−0.965	0.268	−1.543	0.690	0.917	2.017	−0.297	1.087	0.371	1.495
−0.076	−0.495	−0.103	0.646	2.427	−2.172	0.660	−1.541	−0.852	0.583
−0.365	−3.305	0.805	−0.418	−1.201	0.623	−0.223	0.109	0.205	−0.663
0.578	0.145	−1.438	1.122	−1.406	1.172	0.272	−2.245	1.207	1.227
−0.398	−0.304	0.529	−0.514	−0.681	−0.366	0.338	0.801	−0.301	−0.790
−0.951	−1.483	−0.613	−0.171	−0.459	1.231	−1.232	−0.497	−0.779	0.247
1.025	−0.039	−0.721	0.813	1.203	0.245	0.402	1.541	0.691	−1.420
−0.958	0.791	0.948	0.222	−0.704	−0.375	−0.246	−0.682	−0.871	0.056
1.097	−1.428	1.402	−1.425	−0.877	0.536	0.988	2.529	0.768	−1.321
0.377	2.240	0.854	−1.158	0.066	−1.222	0.821	−1.602	−0.760	−0.871
1.729	0.073	1.022	0.891	0.659	−1.040	0.251	−0.710	−1.734	−0.038
−1.329	−0.381	−0.515	1.484	−0.430	−0.466	−0.167	−0.788	−0.660	0.003
−0.132	0.391	2.205	−1.165	0.200	0.415	−0.765	0.239	−1.182	1.135
0.336	0.657	−0.805	0.150	−0.938	1.057	−1.090	1.604	−0.598	−0.760
0.124	−1.812	1.750	0.270	−0.114	0.517	−0.226	0.127	0.129	−0.751
−0.036	0.365	0.766	0.877	−0.804	−0.140	0.182	−0.483	−0.376	−0.564
−0.609	−0.019	−0.992	−1.193	−0.516	0.517	1.677	0.839	−1.134	0.675
−0.894	0.318	0.607	−0.865	0.526	−0.971	1.365	0.319	1.804	1.740
−0.357	−0.802	0.635	−0.491	−1.110	0.785	−0.042	−1.042	−0.572	0.243
−0.258	−0.383	−1.013	0.001	−1.673	0.561	−1.054	−0.106	−0.760	−1.009
2.245	−0.431	−0.496	0.796	0.193	1.202	−0.429	−0.217	0.333	−0.643
1.956	0.477	0.812	−0.117	0.606	−0.330	0.425	−0.232	0.802	0.656
1.358	0.139	0.199	−0.475	−0.120	0.184	−0.020	−1.326	0.517	−1.708
0.656	1.081	0.180	0.145	0.376	−1.363	−0.491	0.352	−1.477	1.280

RANDOM NORMAL NUMBERS, $\mu = 0$, $\sigma = 1$

91	92	93	94	95	96	97	98	99	100
−0.181	0.583	−1.478	−0.181	0.281	−0.559	1.985	−1.122	−1.106	1.441
1.549	−1.183	−2.089	−1.997	−0.343	1.275	0.676	−0.212	1.252	0.163
0.978	−1.067	−2.640	0.134	0.328	−0.052	−0.030	−0.273	−0.570	1.026
−0.596	−0.420	−0.318	−0.057	−0.695	−1.148	0.333	−0.531	−2.037	−1.587
−0.440	0.032	0.163	1.029	0.079	1.148	0.762	−1.961	−0.674	−0.486
0.443	−1.100	0.728	−2.397	−0.543	0.872	−0.568	0.980	−0.174	0.728
−2.401	−1.375	−1.332	−2.177	−2.064	−0.245	−0.039	0.585	1.344	1.386
0.311	0.322	−0.158	0.359	0.103	0.371	0.735	0.011	2.091	0.490
−1.209	0.241	−1.488	−0.667	−1.772	−0.197	0.741	−1.303	−1.149	2.251
0.575	−1.227	−1.674	1.400	0.289	0.005	0.185	−1.072	0.431	−1.096
−0.190	0.272	1.216	0.227	1.358	0.215	−2.306	−1.301	−0.597	−1.401
−0.817	−0.769	−0.470	−0.633	0.187	−0.517	−0.888	−1.712	1.774	−0.162
0.265	−0.676	0.244	1.897	−0.629	−0.206	−1.419	1.049	0.266	−0.438
−0.221	0.678	2.149	1.486	−1.361	1.402	−0.028	0.493	0.744	0.195
−0.436	0.358	−0.602	0.107	0.085	0.573	0.529	1.577	0.239	1.898
−0.010	0.475	0.655	0.659	−0.029	−0.029	0.126	−1.335	−1.261	2.036
−0.244	1.654	1.335	−0.610	0.617	0.642	0.371	0.241	0.001	−1.799
−0.932	−1.275	−1.134	−1.246	−1.508	0.949	1.743	−0.271	−1.333	−1.875
−0.199	−1.285	−0.387	0.191	0.726	−0.151	0.064	−0.803	−0.062	0.780
−0.251	−0.431	−0.831	0.036	−0.464	−1.089	0.284	−0.451	1.693	1.004
1.074	−1.323	−1.659	−0.186	−0.612	1.612	−2.159	−1.210	0.596	−1.421
1.518	2.101	0.397	0.516	−1.169	−1.821	1.346	2.435	1.165	−0.428
0.935	−0.206	1.117	−0.241	−0.963	−0.099	0.412	−1.344	0.411	0.583
1.360	−0.380	0.031	1.066	0.893	0.431	−0.081	0.099	0.500	−2.441
0.115	−0.211	1.471	0.332	0.750	0.652	−0.812	1.383	−0.355	−0.638
0.082	−0.309	−0.355	−0.402	0.774	0.150	0.015	2.539	−0.756	−1.049
−1.492	0.259	0.323	0.697	−0.509	0.968	−0.053	1.033	−0.220	−2.322
−0.203	0.548	1.494	1.185	0.083	−1.196	−0.749	−1.105	1.324	0.689
1.857	−0.167	−1.531	1.551	0.848	0.120	0.415	−0.317	1.446	1.002
0.669	−1.017	−2.437	−0.558	−0.657	0.940	0.985	0.483	−0.361	0.095
0.128	1.463	−0.436	−0.239	−1.443	0.732	0.168	−0.144	−0.392	0.989
1.879	−2.456	0.029	0.429	0.618	−1.683	−2.262	0.034	−0.002	1.914
0.680	0.252	0.130	1.658	−1.023	0.407	−0.235	−0.224	−0.434	0.253
−0.631	0.225	−0.951	1.072	−0.285	−1.731	−0.427	−1.446	−0.873	0.619
−1.273	0.723	0.201	0.505	−0.370	−0.421	−0.015	−0.463	0.288	1.734
−0.643	−1.485	0.403	0.003	−0.243	0.000	0.964	−0.703	0.844	−0.686
−0.435	−2.162	−0.169	−1.311	−1.639	0.193	2.692	−1.994	0.326	0.562
−1.706	0.119	−1.566	0.637	−1.948	−1.068	0.935	0.738	0.650	0.491
−0.498	1.640	0.384	−0.945	−1.272	0.945	−1.013	−0.913	−0.469	2.250
−0.065	−0.005	0.618	−0.523	−0.055	1.071	0.758	−0.736	−0.959	0.598
0.190	−1.020	−1.104	0.936	−0.029	−1.004	−0.657	1.270	−0.060	−0.809
0.879	−0.642	1.155	−0.523	−0.757	−1.027	0.985	−1.222	1.078	0.163
0.559	1.094	1.587	−0.384	−1.701	0.418	0.327	0.669	0.019	0.782
−0.261	1.234	−0.505	−0.664	−0.446	−0.747	0.427	−0.369	0.089	−1.302
3.136	1.120	−0.591	2.515	−2.853	1.375	2.421	0.672	1.817	−0.067
−1.307	−0.586	−0.311	−0.026	1.633	−1.340	−1.209	0.110	−0.126	−0.288
1.455	1.099	−1.225	−0.817	0.667	−0.212	0.684	0.349	−1.161	−2.432
−0.443	−0.415	−0.660	0.098	0.435	−0.846	−0.375	−0.410	−1.747	−0.790
−0.326	0.798	0.349	0.524	0.690	−0.520	−0.522	0.602	−0.193	−0.535
−1.027	−1.459	−0.840	−1.637	−0.462	0.607	−0.760	1.342	−1.916	0.424

XII.5 RANDOM NORMAL NUMBERS, $\mu = 2$, $\sigma = 1$

01	02	03	04	05	06	07	08	09	10
2.422	0.130	2.232	1.700	1.903	0.725	2.031	0.515	−0.684	2.788
0.694	2.556	1.868	1.263	2.115	1.516	1.972	3.627	1.482	3.263
1.875	2.273	0.655	2.299	0.055	1.955	−0.147	2.168	2.193	1.879
1.017	0.757	1.288	1.322	2.080	2.170	1.502	2.953	0.171	1.951
2.453	4.199	1.403	2.017	3.496	0.165	2.556	1.003	1.973	2.159
2.274	1.767	1.564	2.412	2.207	0.475	2.656	1.579	0.394	1.225
3.000	1.618	1.530	2.224	2.881	2.715	3.103	1.941	2.179	3.748
2.510	2.256	1.146	5.177	1.931	1.693	1.021	3.337	2.137	1.839
1.233	2.085	2.251	1.578	3.796	3.017	2.863	2.514	1.615	1.548
3.075	1.730	2.427	2.990	1.680	3.250	3.050	3.243	1.846	1.798
1.344	−0.095	2.166	4.116	2.500	1.939	1.567	3.047	1.385	−0.831
1.246	3.860	1.253	1.876	4.373	1.993	1.262	2.319	2.488	2.406
0.889	2.299	2.458	1.790	1.048	2.302	0.138	2.383	1.170	2.204
1.154	1.401	1.935	3.106	1.548	−0.096	2.153	2.333	1.761	3.728
3.031	1.048	0.719	1.474	2.779	0.292	2.341	2.707	1.741	2.353
0.534	1.155	1.705	1.662	0.457	0.602	1.365	2.663	3.755	1.900
2.230	3.096	0.045	3.639	0.680	0.970	1.593	2.117	2.395	1.935
2.355	1.761	1.816	1.822	1.434	2.259	3.788	3.280	1.317	2.940
1.461	0.947	0.717	2.923	2.133	2.526	2.687	2.144	1.692	1.469
3.034	1.778	2.122	2.025	3.008	1.447	−0.305	2.452	1.726	0.870
2.761	0.473	3.726	1.893	2.455	1.633	1.654	3.006	3.523	2.317
1.961	0.965	1.481	1.402	2.106	2.214	1.727	3.670	3.795	2.258
2.639	4.010	1.915	1.713	1.484	1.443	1.444	2.394	1.688	0.793
1.349	2.225	0.644	1.404	2.583	2.149	2.359	2.274	1.432	1.610
2.959	2.797	4.635	3.268	2.889	2.349	0.933	3.403	2.206	−0.214
2.440	2.919	1.455	0.695	1.466	1.124	1.257	1.265	0.096	3.412
3.078	3.279	0.352	2.583	1.690	0.729	2.072	1.332	1.158	1.827
1.736	1.968	0.011	2.418	1.026	1.342	2.103	1.792	2.175	1.646
3.275	3.147	2.800	2.172	0.004	1.763	3.801	2.510	2.517	−0.117
2.579	2.297	2.030	2.725	3.721	2.545	1.631	−0.346	−0.011	1.961
2.549	3.546	2.805	1.250	0.769	2.238	2.284	3.722	2.085	2.653
2.954	1.990	1.249	1.028	3.241	1.926	3.056	1.732	2.116	1.825
1.442	2.542	2.557	1.741	0.630	2.117	1.662	2.237	−0.046	3.132
4.039	2.030	2.859	3.538	2.424	2.169	3.643	3.290	2.742	1.336
2.127	0.288	2.921	0.175	1.670	3.151	1.443	0.935	1.125	2.872
1.102	2.536	1.476	2.980	0.416	1.784	2.521	1.867	1.709	1.558
2.938	2.112	1.350	2.115	1.164	1.761	1.350	1.798	3.160	2.593
2.975	2.681	0.721	1.291	2.276	2.131	2.187	2.752	1.380	0.676
1.386	1.712	1.692	2.844	1.559	0.418	3.020	0.785	1.962	3.184
2.834	1.485	0.632	0.872	0.735	1.934	1.221	2.544	1.797	1.410
3.346	1.147	1.766	1.862	2.595	1.524	3.499	2.652	2.139	2.533
2.243	3.881	2.846	2.670	3.377	1.380	4.183	0.883	1.373	1.992
2.705	2.661	1.521	1.290	2.280	1.638	0.884	2.636	2.077	1.012
2.760	1.182	1.152	3.074	1.073	2.917	2.150	2.866	1.688	1.684
2.086	1.250	1.577	2.871	2.985	2.585	2.897	2.398	0.999	1.764
0.802	1.421	4.793	0.268	2.838	2.227	3.331	2.395	2.064	2.916
4.165	2.014	0.616	1.929	0.641	2.304	1.263	2.125	0.908	1.768
2.291	2.549	0.851	1.856	2.452	3.282	0.978	2.255	1.683	1.926
1.428	4.194	2.262	2.957	1.991	2.759	1.553	3.538	1.272	3.417
2.051	2.455	2.759	2.267	2.794	4.106	2.373	1.401	2.562	2.502

RANDOM NORMAL NUMBERS, μ = 2, σ = 1

11	12	13	14	15	16	17	18	19	20
1.911	0.626	2.289	1.628	1.638	2.676	0.900	1.685	1.605	1.366
3.196	2.979	2.447	2.099	1.273	2.733	2.653	2.219	1.318	3.129
0.398	2.304	1.019	0.363	1.286	2.428	0.677	1.684	1.267	0.651
1.228	2.134	0.300	1.785	2.547	1.566	2.545	2.428	1.702	2.276
1.190	3.020	0.954	2.907	2.916	1.279	3.403	2.698	1.629	1.448
0.953	2.127	1.723	2.302	1.474	0.826	1.644	2.035	2.359	2.930
1.479	1.956	1.280	1.722	0.938	0.922	2.734	3.484	1.659	2.789
1.509	0.952	1.258	−0.864	1.620	1.789	2.931	2.616	1.622	1.566
0.627	2.404	0.571	2.940	2.705	1.709	2.404	1.456	2.486	2.869
1.923	2.765	2.422	1.725	1.009	2.372	1.925	1.083	3.314	1.961
2.760	2.633	3.011	2.277	1.539	0.873	2.379	2.610	1.635	−0.625
2.009	3.204	1.114	2.269	0.912	0.831	2.485	2.076	1.230	3.607
0.876	1.124	2.137	1.448	1.236	1.699	1.408	1.454	2.018	1.514
1.430	1.920	2.969	1.518	1.543	1.509	4.071	3.444	0.907	2.478
3.422	2.307	2.919	1.833	1.792	3.090	2.212	0.814	1.661	0.865
3.304	1.292	1.863	2.785	1.666	0.323	2.384	3.133	3.393	2.814
2.329	2.671	3.353	1.166	1.016	3.036	2.024	1.439	2.203	1.128
1.402	1.964	1.505	1.746	1.912	1.202	0.595	0.527	1.881	3.456
2.274	1.209	1.450	2.241	1.678	1.565	2.746	2.149	1.829	1.520
1.205	0.531	2.975	3.024	3.357	2.558	1.450	2.192	1.665	3.373
2.462	1.328	1.301	3.312	1.959	2.010	2.482	1.530	1.909	3.171
0.227	3.166	1.989	2.976	2.188	1.399	1.407	2.610	1.903	0.624
2.142	2.926	1.634	1.940	0.785	2.331	1.663	0.847	2.533	1.166
2.558	0.903	0.082	1.299	2.366	2.554	1.948	1.055	1.559	1.787
0.818	3.174	0.123	−1.149	1.606	2.118	−0.044	0.022	0.866	2.336
3.083	2.287	2.379	2.909	2.520	0.708	1.600	0.790	1.751	2.480
2.517	1.470	2.621	0.880	1.931	1.495	1.943	1.868	2.048	3.879
2.594	1.571	1.218	2.346	2.267	0.946	2.840	1.753	2.237	0.687
0.411	0.760	1.114	1.842	1.756	3.951	2.110	2.251	2.116	1.042
2.853	3.054	2.421	2.418	1.542	2.070	0.641	0.753	1.040	0.702
1.262	−0.591	1.320	2.049	2.705	3.826	3.272	1.054	2.494	2.050
0.540	1.678	2.534	1.944	1.939	2.544	1.582	1.333	1.895	1.746
2.381	2.968	1.656	3.152	1.730	3.927	3.183	3.211	3.765	2.035
2.225	1.420	1.334	1.923	1.664	1.939	0.680	2.785	1.569	1.701
1.953	2.779	2.584	2.228	0.221	1.378	1.381	2.209	2.979	2.906
3.413	2.229	2.976	2.535	3.589	0.615	3.425	1.187	2.748	0.906
1.610	2.376	2.086	0.610	2.532	3.083	1.332	1.776	0.407	0.721
0.984	2.243	2.939	1.704	2.277	1.026	1.879	0.405	1.003	0.755
1.808	2.362	1.717	0.831	2.160	0.546	2.686	1.924	1.756	1.829
−0.766	3.529	2.361	0.955	2.148	1.104	0.541	1.460	1.840	1.579
2.643	2.051	1.384	2.229	2.952	2.203	0.765	4.381	1.611	1.936
1.952	2.752	3.588	2.481	1.911	3.753	1.428	3.223	1.873	2.034
2.590	2.306	3.280	1.664	2.281	1.443	2.024	2.126	3.250	1.384
0.622	2.617	1.969	2.231	−0.079	0.768	2.547	1.365	1.163	1.280
0.433	−0.560	3.292	1.987	1.065	2.766	1.425	0.846	2.520	0.981
3.146	3.323	1.713	1.887	2.010	1.277	0.491	2.489	1.503	1.974
4.021	1.744	0.598	2.954	2.633	1.960	1.539	2.393	4.012	3.356
1.188	0.450	2.958	1.177	1.482	1.090	1.671	3.021	0.386	3.560
1.211	2.575	0.158	3.124	3.632	2.647	3.029	3.526	2.237	0.671
3.750	2.362	1.407	0.642	1.274	1.632	2.378	2.601	0.003	1.261

RANDOM NORMAL NUMBERS, $\mu = 2$, $\sigma = 1$

21	22	23	24	25	26	27	28	29	30
1.707	2.089	1.315	0.278	3.045	2.968	1.396	1.534	2.365	2.746
1.113	1.779	1.935	0.971	4.024	0.847	1.382	2.342	2.110	0.316
1.847	0.547	3.697	1.250	1.586	2.036	2.924	0.585	0.456	2.859
2.713	2.761	1.664	2.461	2.158	3.453	2.078	1.113	1.769	1.263
0.676	0.432	2.667	2.515	1.369	3.196	2.979	2.447	2.099	1.273
2.167	1.828	2.867	1.178	2.078	1.500	2.622	2.341	1.504	2.468
3.445	3.323	2.558	1.789	1.595	1.191	1.175	2.872	1.257	1.062
1.284	3.180	3.315	1.210	1.842	3.384	2.942	2.550	0.727	1.736
2.135	2.590	2.533	1.635	1.983	0.614	0.377	−0.663	0.427	2.445
2.944	2.043	2.220	1.987	2.859	3.029	2.091	1.052	1.532	1.956
3.654	2.333	1.468	3.126	1.241	2.936	1.557	2.020	1.423	2.701
0.821	1.542	2.365	2.199	3.479	3.111	−0.107	1.644	1.337	1.442
2.483	2.583	2.075	1.026	0.668	2.281	1.566	1.255	2.020	1.135
0.715	1.384	2.080	2.542	2.368	0.019	2.906	2.325	2.175	5.197
4.638	2.662	1.012	2.941	1.336	0.574	3.034	2.937	2.553	0.174
2.327	2.152	3.057	2.077	2.321	0.861	2.892	1.394	−0.556	1.459
−0.082	0.676	3.038	2.470	1.394	2.131	1.262	3.207	1.810	0.322
2.051	1.576	2.087	3.030	2.030	2.827	2.183	1.182	1.507	−0.042
2.438	0.924	1.699	0.477	2.449	2.540	1.620	2.509	2.347	3.022
2.284	2.159	2.975	3.268	0.484	1.862	1.676	1.449	2.475	2.556
0.872	0.474	2.213	3.602	3 244	3.078	1.376	2.612	2.421	1.014
2.236	1.963	1.839	1.598	2.195	2.680	2.228	1.107	−0.661	1.041
2.425	2.412	1.500	2.278	2.328	2.102	2.087	3.098	2.697	0.765
1.511	2.431	1.434	1.558	1.020	2.864	0.871	2.523	1.878	1.370
1.600	2.040	2.993	0.873	0.568	2.703	2.578	1.515	3.627	2.097
3.076	1.939	0.682	3.085	2.877	2.696	−0.771	2.560	1.954	0.999
2.593	1.610	2.800	2.456	0.226	3.575	1.435	2.170	1.165	3.506
1.362	2.727	2.145	2.023	0.509	0.336	2.045	0.375	1.010	2.316
1.603	2.783	0.682	2.108	2.031	0.854	2.028	2.357	0.722	1.562
1.908	1.635	2.009	1.203	1.775	2.868	1.949	1.391	1.151	1.352
3.486	0.507	2.322	1.204	2.434	1.720	1.804	2.235	2.439	1.492
2.029	1.352	3.629	2.076	1.587	0.891	3.029	1.242	0.014	4.019
2.894	1.688	0.657	1.800	2.943	1.373	1.269	3.411	1.316	2.405
0.965	−0.028	1.904	2.241	2.563	1.149	2.375	1.386	1.562	2.882
2.191	2.133	2.676	0.229	2.319	1.114	3.197	2.588	3.163	2.423
2.115	2.418	2.741	1.839	2.416	1.452	0.319	0.853	2.774	0.929
1.120	2.126	0.773	0.798	3.436	2.374	2.173	−0.333	2.004	1.765
3.524	0.008	3.260	1.109	4.111	2.474	2.482	2.416	0.832	4.059
0.103	2.774	2.056	2.463	0.383	−0.962	2.458	2.388	1.556	1.088
1.573	2.519	2.153	3.188	1.618	2.477	2.185	1.851	0.498	2.066
1.138	3.032	2.390	2.436	2.655	1.484	2.378	3.166	2.531	2.082
2.665	2.960	2.518	1.940	0.026	2.570	2.703	2.592	3.094	1.862
1.397	1.859	2.208	2.559	1.749	0.624	0.074	1.398	0.996	2.910
1.875	2.250	0.183	2.214	1.356	4.282	2.370	3.006	1.413	2.412
3.195	2.671	1.918	3.305	3.722	1.372	2.564	2.106	1.871	1.792
1.464	2.055	3.045	2.367	1.992	0.919	3.006	2.713	4.049	4.618
3.328	1.781	2.565	1.304	2.041	1.597	0.225	2.309	−0.558	2.504
2.804	3.606	1.858	3.028	2.456	1.730	1.430	3.405	0.474	2.222
2.590	1.641	3.857	2.582	2.594	1.933	3.341	1.002	2.704	1.341
2.980	0.601	1.595	2.248	2.381	1.911	0.626	2.289	1.628	1.638

RANDOM NORMAL NUMBERS, $\mu = 2$, $\sigma = 1$

31	32	33	34	35	36	37	38	39	40
3.355	0.073	3.139	2.472	1.825	0.296	1.685	3.401	1.820	1.428
1.086	1.955	2.529	2.503	1.687	1.754	4.138	2.394	0.303	3.776
2.367	1.525	2.625	1.789	0.991	4.127	0.915	3.023	1.377	3.435
0.248	0.749	3.697	4.166	2.544	1.620	3.217	1.083	1.907	2.951
1.694	0.258	1.836	1.953	1.853	3.590	3.604	1.907	1.995	2.468
1.546	1.255	2.856	3.221	2.397	−0.010	2.169	2.781	3.001	2.536
1.266	2.089	2.974	1.305	2.376	−0.475	1.792	1.546	0.583	1.214
0.713	2.473	1.381	1.750	1.064	3.744	2.470	1.004	2.155	2.332
−0.001	1.600	2.166	0.561	0.898	2.587	0.580	−0.461	0.954	1.364
3.406	2.207	2.110	1.522	3.923	1.379	3.613	3.379	2.716	2.796
1.432	1.651	1.584	3.649	2.485	2.820	2.948	2.626	1.763	3.329
1.541	1.154	4.311	2.354	2.257	1.262	2.304	2.178	1.657	2.126
2.216	3.505	−0.056	1.332	0.980	1.675	1.850	2.487	2.051	1.433
1.602	2.225	2.949	3.945	3.753	3.855	2.769	0.760	2.095	1.419
2.211	1.804	2.642	0.975	1.646	2.552	2.291	1.277	2.341	−0.219
3.006	2.279	1.097	3.473	0.919	2.535	2.459	3.934	1.826	1.587
2.520	2.468	2.156	2.438	1.625	1.604	1.628	1.139	2.608	2.643
2.666	4.058	2.805	3.069	0.945	2.533	2.761	1.140	2.604	1.627
2.852	0.570	3.920	1.572	2.924	2.135	1.558	2.604	2.191	2.529
2.014	2.825	3.502	2.006	1.879	3.304	1.538	0.906	3.125	1.009
1.540	0.444	1.541	1.850	1.793	2.284	1.890	3.091	2.293	2.491
1.190	2.087	2.159	1.157	2.314	1.753	0.722	2.447	2.124	2.927
0.741	3.411	1.689	1.945	0.286	3.288	1.390	0.240	1.448	2.768
2.169	1.937	2.261	0.766	2.075	0.457	2.031	0.831	−0.009	4.316
0.979	1.935	2.232	1.812	3.290	2.031	3.222	2.520	4.105	0.705
1.405	0.166	0.137	3.246	4.142	2.808	2.526	2.687	−0.627	2.023
0.923	2.287	1.164	0.732	0.736	0.892	2.633	2.107	1.260	0.615
1.529	3.188	2.153	3.828	3.610	1.654	2.596	0.957	1.479	1.497
0.781	3.562	3.633	0.889	0.832	2.068	2.103	3.360	1.686	1.538
2.153	2.125	1.930	3.161	2.931	1.941	3.108	1.732	4.296	1.830
3.204	3.945	0.682	4.165	2.419	0.565	1.637	1.931	1.092	2.482
2.154	1.889	1.391	1.690	1.356	2.560	1.784	1.041	2.808	0.576
3.391	2.602	2.496	2.177	1.564	1.781	0.302	2.499	1.501	1.410
3.266	2.051	1.958	0.979	2.454	1.438	2.098	3.208	2.374	2.710
1.842	0.513	1.736	2.878	1.893	1.614	2.775	1.060	1.508	1.197
2.799	0.757	0.625	3.336	2.268	1.418	1.616	2.363	0.751	2.138
0.104	3.564	0.681	1.231	2.527	0.172	1.331	0.991	3.570	1.382
2.232	3.514	−0.433	2.932	3.245	2.778	2.196	−0.326	1.034	1.889
4.201	3.351	1.761	1.957	1.342	3.575	3.216	1.335	1.527	0.812
1.046	1.646	1.363	1.051	4.600	3.209	3.041	3.234	2.034	0.682
2.874	1.663	2.591	1.396	1.052	1.068	2.226	3.048	1.906	2.755
1.389	2.966	2.846	2.410	1.663	3.620	2.151	2.036	3.733	1.462
−0.144	1.641	1.693	1.599	2.704	3.083	1.387	0.593	1.191	2.707
2.177	0.829	2.094	1.737	1.625	1.766	1.415	2.238	0.549	1.887
2.595	2.094	2.851	1.175	0.425	2.242	1.477	3.237	2.614	1.226
1.655	3.804	0.607	1.958	4.251	1.457	3.369	2.077	1.511	1.458
2.601	2.255	1.787	1.136	2.912	3.060	2.562	3.137	3.248	1.382
2.308	2.422	3.081	2.185	1.963	3.855	2.389	4.057	2.428	3.054
1.196	4.160	2.841	1.550	0.919	1.884	1.911	1.386	2.607	1.625
0.843	1.330	1.678	2.198	1.398	0.709	1.810	2.269	4.242	0.777

RANDOM NORMAL NUMBERS, $\mu = 2$, $\sigma = 1$

41	42	43	44	45	46	47	48	49	50
1.017	2.773	3.278	2.557	1.003	4.181	0.946	3.464	1.945	2.929
0.723	0.781	1.546	1.649	2.723	4.542	1.819	0.511	2.580	3.707
1.681	1.200	0.335	3.391	2.382	3.080	0.685	1.924	1.085	1.459
0.622	0.742	2.495	1.860	1.145	2.040	2.103	−0.256	0.976	2.414
1.815	2.061	2.092	2.089	2.281	2.377	1.821	1.760	2.515	1.898
4.334	1.662	0.044	1.363	0.681	2.111	2.443	1.603	1.803	2.149
0.863	2.642	5.436	0.332	2.847	1.466	3.031	1.571	3.024	1.988
2.414	1.988	2.666	0.867	1.589	2.192	3.027	2.257	1.868	1.927
1.505	2.364	0.762	1.955	1.888	1.845	3.180	2.618	1.730	1.603
3.048	2.037	2.759	2.609	−0.042	1.215	1.292	1.582	1.522	2.097
2.347	4.816	1.535	1.367	0.385	2.013	2.557	2.041	3.070	1.934
2.637	2.563	1.892	2.131	0.191	2.484	1.788	2.762	2.166	1.211
4.176	2.393	1.075	3.911	0.959	2.438	3.201	1.810	2.049	3.476
0.814	1.055	0.395	2.185	1.741	2.742	2.228	2.151	1.997	3.302
2.972	3.710	4.682	4.813	0.468	2.311	2.382	0.810	0.155	1.685
3.210	2.294	1.751	2.719	3.103	2.459	3.656	4.862	3.724	3.457
4.647	2.777	2.450	4.247	3.151	0.197	3.602	1.754	1.739	2.646
2.398	2.318	1.071	4.416	1.063	1.568	3.057	0.985	3.425	1.924
2.846	1.300	1.631	2.344	1.073	1.049	2.743	0.365	1.949	0.378
2.654	1.044	4.907	3.688	2.752	2.365	2.083	1.669	2.538	2.617
2.522	2.231	1.380	1.734	2.419	1.313	2.226	2.524	2.073	3.032
0.711	1.460	1.175	2.244	0.929	−0.091	1.096	2.061	3.099	2.186
3.372	3.769	0.942	3.646	2.481	1.554	3.715	1.193	1.956	1.735
2.854	1.464	3.607	2.428	1.384	1.977	1.504	0.492	2.102	2.624
1.851	0.855	2.913	2.684	3.043	2.595	1.803	1.303	0.233	−0.429
0.851	0.943	2.635	1.671	0.778	2.899	2.145	2.747	1.342	2.313
2.348	2.970	1.982	3.217	1.025	2.626	2.164	2.568	1.080	2.814
2.284	2.458	3.307	0.374	1.370	2.631	−0.649	1.111	1.296	2.403
0.983	2.360	1.880	4.331	3.672	−0.018	3.053	2.068	2.051	2.506
3.603	1.047	1.433	3.600	2.465	2.472	1.190	3.504	2.205	0.793
1.809	3.479	1.013	3.249	3.934	1.432	2.893	1.707	3.498	1.429
1.277	2.925	2.783	1.597	2.619	2.000	1.513	2.888	1.421	0.639
0.303	3.879	2.063	2.132	2.682	2.316	1.718	2.201	4.431	3.085
2.498	3.072	3.567	2.302	3.157	1.860	2.802	2.098	0.902	1.945
−0.542	0.666	3.987	2.668	2.360	2.762	1.351	2.835	2.972	1.796
1.640	2.193	0.976	1.777	1.383	3.100	1.663	1.609	2.503	1.596
2.248	1.911	0.620	2.295	1.884	3.421	1.086	2.085	1.861	−0.191
1.900	0.623	3.047	1.127	−0.199	3.653	0.976	−0.088	−0.966	2.626
1.536	0.718	−0.513	2.675	3.145	1.838	1.609	0.857	1.854	3.839
2.503	3.434	2.290	2.397	1.162	1.932	2.626	0.816	1.229	1.753
1.142	1.628	1.783	2.148	−0.105	3.072	2.312	3.666	2.784	2.102
1.877	3.107	0.960	1.363	1.139	1.135	2.370	4.245	3.284	0.188
3.632	2.586	1.531	1.613	1.645	0.963	4.596	1.979	2.649	1.435
4.072	0.554	1.319	2.224	1.879	1.806	1.606	3.049	0.099	2.996
1.564	1.624	1.014	1.414	1.796	1.244	1.712	2.319	2.166	2.727
2.876	0.772	−0.646	1.254	3.797	1.827	2.039	4.280	2.208	1.842
2.833	3.289	1.977	1.568	2.582	0.198	1.190	2.708	3.264	2.876
1.108	2.332	1.546	0.872	4.085	2.583	3.384	3.934	3.073	1.029
2.644	1.766	1.846	3.098	2.757	3.840	2.353	3.384	2.716	2.435
2.105	1.828	1.899	0.854	2.878	1.569	4.151	0.821	2.818	2.038

XII.6 RANDOM NORMAL NUMBERS, $\mu = 0, \sigma = 2$

01	02	03	04	05	06	07	08	09	10
−0.221	−0.540	−0.701	5.511	−2.404	−0.987	−0.158	−0.578	−1.893	0.854
−2.454	−2.816	0.580	−1.068	1.010	1.209	2.234	3.224	3.750	1.285
0.089	0.418	−0.421	2.448	−0.279	1.916	−3.166	−0.773	−0.818	−1.411
0.931	1.345	3.164	0.019	0.767	0.439	−3.412	−0.982	0.520	−0.473
0.361	0.794	0.120	−0.347	2.785	0.980	1.003	−1.796	−1.778	−0.783
−0.559	−2.111	−3.396	4.236	2.764	−1.990	−0.060	−2.488	−0.503	−4.406
−4.816	−1.369	1.856	0.383	0.016	−2.144	−0.187	−1.561	1.441	−2.246
0.784	0.607	0.663	−0.764	−1.395	1.738	−2.055	2.962	−1.616	1.326
2.576	−3.024	0.191	1.084	−3.698	−3.031	−0.517	−0.179	0.681	−0.719
−1.232	1.234	−0.046	1.338	1.726	1.448	2.216	−1.662	2.188	2.308
2.129	−1.936	3.381	1.319	−3.131	−1.037	1.191	1.449	0.690	−0.251
−2.753	1.049	1.616	1.232	2.910	0.389	−3.766	2.044	1.459	−0.002
0.071	1.869	−5.827	0.866	−1.191	2.508	1.552	−1.052	1.914	−0.274
0.507	0.595	−0.202	−0.775	−1.732	−2.771	0.049	5.221	3.059	0.015
0.384	−1.574	1.414	−0.789	−1.263	−0.470	0.020	1.489	0.497	1.316
1.688	4.311	2.305	−5.632	1.776	1.540	0.208	0.611	0.810	−1.241
−0.045	−1.563	3.687	−0.160	−0.101	1.838	1.590	1.222	0.377	2.069
2.516	−1.339	0.956	−1.285	0.301	3.739	−3.320	0.183	0.993	−4.678
0.536	1.965	−0.580	−0.307	1.564	0.163	−2.239	−2.460	−2.003	−1.609
0.775	1.427	−0.626	−1.134	−3.109	1.652	2.331	−0.188	2.137	−1.316
0.964	−3.740	1.995	−1.349	−1.068	−0.172	1.907	5.515	0.863	−1.018
2.597	2.328	−0.722	3.057	1.632	0.655	0.972	1.401	1.840	4.508
−1.343	−2.859	0.903	−0.631	−2.810	3.345	1.997	0.356	1.215	0.501
−1.097	0.798	−1.057	3.880	2.321	−1.677	−3.746	−1.125	−1.090	−1.972
−0.977	0.225	−0.004	−0.513	3.613	1.030	2.349	−1.278	−1.301	−5.159
2.421	−1.732	2.170	0.451	1.013	−0.912	0.615	−0.532	1.453	−2.155
0.921	−0.932	−2.511	−0.164	0.154	−0.004	0.516	2.240	−0.020	4.432
−1.854	−3.192	−3.633	0.067	3.709	0.560	−0.156	0.964	−2.618	−0.718
2.457	−0.566	−1.439	0.194	1.440	−1.568	−2.407	−1.356	0.849	0.801
1.143	0.212	4.088	−0.832	−0.361	0.303	−2.984	1.378	−0.649	−2.399
1.184	1.622	−1.896	0.026	−2.163	−1.683	3.778	3.585	−3.853	2.352
3.842	1.179	−0.987	0.498	2.348	3.263	1.924	−4.421	−0.680	2.129
1.930	0.114	−6.145	0.737	−0.353	2.478	−2.104	0.020	−2.250	−1.096
−0.174	−0.403	−1.539	1.740	−1.293	−1.922	1.228	1.433	−2.659	2.923
3.017	2.409	1.876	4.534	−0.539	−1.534	−0.847	−0.107	0.796	−1.257
2.632	−2.417	0.136	−1.155	4.277	−1.035	−0.968	−0.400	1.393	−0.858
−1.589	−2.199	0.776	0.821	3.237	4.810	1.012	−4.102	1.088	1.958
−1.308	0.561	−0.882	4.041	1.923	−0.717	0.599	1.705	0.241	2.677
−1.881	−1.808	−2.767	0.426	0.234	−4.060	1.036	−1.657	0.471	1.753
2.869	4.397	1.986	−2.123	−0.065	−0.705	−0.968	−2.265	−1.979	−1.114
0.252	−1.324	0.302	2.426	0.710	−1.454	−0.319	2.277	−0.971	−3.217
−0.833	1.653	−2.738	2.856	−0.789	−0.873	−0.809	−1.538	−1.334	2.289
0.276	0.020	−0.162	−1.720	0.048	0.401	−2.073	2.430	2.776	1.174
0.742	3.058	1.994	3.090	0.170	−0.789	−2.526	−0.980	−1.331	−1.834
0.770	1.419	4.391	1.502	−2.856	−3.648	−1.179	1.556	3.176	2.613
−2.208	1.766	−0.282	3.051	−1.734	−0.032	1.234	−0.626	1.052	−3.146
−1.161	−0.803	5.530	2.219	−0.371	1.372	−1.649	−2.059	1.456	0.677
−4.276	−0.196	−1.456	0.139	0.094	2.367	−1.902	1.123	−1.222	0.323
−1.615	−0.140	0.697	−0.647	1.289	1.416	0.811	0.523	1.406	−1.022
−3.831	−0.105	−2.271	−3.207	0.539	−1.010	2.646	−1.985	0.347	0.712

RANDOM NORMAL NUMBERS, $\mu = 0$, $\sigma = 2$

11	12	13	14	15	16	17	18	19	20
−0.686	0.678	−0.150	−0.334	5.096	0.708	0.403	1.538	1.217	−2.456
0.106	−0.018	2.558	−0.049	−1.061	−0.574	−0.510	−1.036	−0.168	2.516
−0.638	3.191	−4.587	−0.499	−0.510	−1.521	1.325	−1.355	−1.036	−3.305
−3.088	−0.998	0.883	2.230	0.603	0.906	−2.303	0.152	1.423	2.706
1.017	−2.496	−4.981	1.769	−0.252	3.018	2.764	1.105	−1.527	−1.187
0.132	−1.520	−1.748	−3.513	0.878	−0.483	−0.354	−1.103	−2.178	2.192
1.217	−2.380	−0.017	−0.072	−2.066	0.251	0.035	1.641	−1.298	2.070
0.540	−3.950	1.287	−0.771	−2.946	−1.181	−2.286	−1.561	0.420	−0.746
−0.395	−1.421	−2.163	0.270	−1.257	5.610	0.287	−1.138	−0.979	−2.224
−3.279	−2.813	1.125	−3.982	−0.102	0.576	−0.531	−0.695	−3.385	−1.045
3.510	3.235	2.623	−2.582	1.274	2.440	0.824	1.983	−0.770	2.489
−0.408	1.922	2.351	−0.146	−0.039	−0.648	−3.041	0.522	−1.659	−0.515
−2.434	1.297	2.813	−0.651	3.409	0.108	1.716	−1.801	0.344	0.923
0.541	0.820	−0.254	2.851	−3.027	1.553	2.218	1.758	1.003	−1.148
−0.813	1.562	2.116	−4.375	−2.289	1.593	0.163	−1.991	0.355	1.364
−0.238	−0.450	0.364	0.677	−0.711	−1.661	1.071	0.682	0.347	0.113
−1.214	−5.369	3.300	0.461	3.197	−0.368	−3.190	2.868	−0.943	0.931
3.521	1.655	2.373	1.993	−1.096	1.875	−1.143	−3.658	2.664	0.378
−1.075	−3.475	−2.069	−0.971	−0.909	−1.796	−0.760	−1.794	−1.576	3.863
−1.213	−1.760	0.397	−0.323	2.659	0.666	−4.368	2.704	1.160	−1.377
0.408	2.865	3.666	−0.433	−1.798	−1.434	−3.688	2.261	−1.084	0.722
−1.809	−2.890	−3.537	−2.701	0.656	0.684	0.905	1.953	2.720	−0.263
−1.633	0.283	−3.937	−0.224	−0.549	0.016	−1.265	−1.650	−1.506	0.504
−1.181	2.578	0.568	0.286	1.152	−0.929	−3.335	0.020	1.171	1.366
0.374	1.225	−0.213	−1.951	0.126	−1.551	−0.147	0.605	2.450	−1.514
−1.828	−3.459	2.624	2.605	0.698	−0.984	−2.289	−3.389	1.647	−2.592
−3.073	1.381	6.111	0.458	−0.792	−0.785	−1.254	2.784	−0.248	−0.965
−0.817	−1.048	−0.603	−0.647	−2.140	1.970	1.612	−2.050	1.962	−3.520
−0.778	−2.697	2.431	−2.011	2.810	0.010	1.830	−1.425	1.425	−2.506
1.866	0.259	−1.360	2.165	1.845	−0.326	2.054	−0.825	5.348	−0.384
0.715	−0.981	−0.126	0.263	−0.692	−3.790	−3.119	−0.547	−1.450	−0.791
0.802	−0.906	−0.726	0.071	3.693	−0.409	1.536	−0.907	3.216	−3.096
−0.363	0.030	−2.423	−0.517	−4.567	1.092	−1.194	0.253	−2.816	0.766
2.878	−2.689	0.797	0.820	0.764	0.366	−0.891	−0.122	0.196	1.052
−2.245	1.324	0.101	0.431	−2.152	0.779	−0.708	0.028	1.317	−1.259
−0.286	0.390	1.204	−4.414	−0.164	−3.724	0.207	1.835	0.334	0.660
−1.434	−0.736	−0.040	0.213	0.215	−0.565	0.915	−0.022	0.487	−0.487
0.004	−1.773	−0.480	0.768	−0.837	−0.513	0.828	4.563	1.298	2.837
1.299	−1.915	0.346	1.037	−2.953	−1.968	−1.704	1.639	2.802	−2.965
−1.694	1.993	1.021	−2.152	0.679	−0.763	0.577	2.860	0.329	−2.702
−0.506	0.328	−2.091	−0.238	2.582	0.429	1.647	−1.048	−1.367	1.054
0.527	−3.033	−0.893	−0.776	−0.383	−0.708	−0.482	−2.686	1.369	1.040
3.815	−1.282	1.877	−1.177	0.000	−0.059	0.754	0.529	−0.522	2.073
1.838	−0.569	3.556	−0.956	−2.106	0.371	1.806	0.449	−0.867	2.664
0.810	3.394	1.224	−4.428	4.645	−0.644	−2.579	−2.198	2.683	1.338
4.048	−0.706	1.326	2.187	0.611	2.962	−2.137	−0.657	−3.539	−1.526
1.619	−1.214	−0.860	−0.625	−2.534	0.519	−2.539	0.737	−0.622	−0.146
1.732	−3.199	2.104	1.752	0.087	−0.333	3.943	0.037	0.135	1.756
−1.580	−3.456	2.934	0.580	1.665	2.331	−1.413	−1.558	2.144	1.876
1.176	−0.195	0.127	0.060	−3.145	−0.001	0.219	−1.803	−5.255	1.524

RANDOM NORMAL NUMBERS, $\mu = 0$, $\sigma = 2$

21	22	23	24	25	26	27	28	29	30
−0.625	−1.119	0.772	−1.479	0.164	3.051	0.297	1.904	2.864	3.093
1.375	1.994	1.004	−3.128	−1.517	−2.916	2.196	3.544	−1.858	−1.021
−1.835	0.393	−1.426	−0.469	−0.009	−2.366	0.408	−0.669	−0.266	−0.907
0.764	−2.796	−1.932	−1.144	−4.177	−2.150	4.163	1.003	−1.088	−0.346
−0.913	−4.834	2.310	−0.154	−2.007	−1.741	−3.570	1.361	−0.219	−1.424
−4.228	0.846	−0.794	−1.756	2.621	0.128	−1.369	2.090	−4.471	0.440
−2.724	2.694	−0.585	1.094	2.116	−1.176	0.180	1.438	1.260	−1.730
4.168	−0.764	−0.791	−2.517	−2.103	0.901	0.141	1.796	−4.435	1.711
3.286	2.374	1.605	−0.951	−1.308	−0.903	1.562	3.537	3.340	−1.417
0.197	0.212	1.303	−0.289	1.441	−2.913	−0.606	−1.302	1.281	0.147
0.713	−1.532	−4.409	−2.502	−1.488	1.696	−2.390	0.517	−2.406	−0.457
0.925	−2.267	2.010	−1.381	−2.057	0.988	−0.024	−2.096	0.116	1.383
−3.312	1.604	0.955	−0.184	0.074	−0.714	2.059	−2.293	0.899	−0.837
0.320	−2.893	−1.005	1.527	−0.990	1.930	−1.512	1.333	3.188	−1.555
0.619	−1.545	1.543	−0.207	−0.586	2.409	−2.454	−0.738	−0.060	−1.533
0.119	−0.542	−2.461	−2.475	−1.265	−3.598	0.983	−1.702	−1.735	−4.773
1.814	−0.053	−0.063	−2.921	2.076	−0.535	2.585	−3.066	−0.771	1.553
−2.068	0.648	2.066	0.610	−0.681	0.845	1.349	0.515	−1.106	−3.860
−1.881	−2.033	1.704	1.161	0.316	1.623	−3.370	−0.261	−3.559	−0.647
−2.125	0.620	−0.838	2.278	0.230	2.962	1.925	−2.209	−0.676	0.859
2.054	−2.290	2.264	1.598	2.064	−1.129	−1.381	−1.149	−0.488	0.568
−2.516	−2.190	−0.629	2.361	1.734	0.607	0.935	1.275	3.125	−0.224
−0.143	−1.222	1.061	−2.668	−4.419	0.569	0.259	−0.027	1.989	4.602
−0.007	0.017	−0.811	−0.166	0.850	0.565	0.184	−2.887	1.101	0.192
−1.749	0.231	−2.380	−3.177	−1.077	4.460	0.494	1.941	−0.106	0.015
1.300	−0.289	−2.657	−0.160	−0.490	−0.329	1.602	−1.110	4.204	2.552
0.588	−1.072	0.935	−0.164	0.113	1.139	−0.923	−0.953	0.001	−0.033
1.719	−1.183	−1.051	−0.944	0.734	1.965	2.121	2.213	3.826	−2.004
0.726	1.867	0.624	2.066	−2.792	−2.507	−0.816	−0.569	0.002	−1.934
2.369	−0.361	2.216	−1.500	−0.350	−1.063	−3.979	−3.626	−1.326	−0.488
1.790	−0.290	2.601	6.261	−0.622	−0.534	0.477	0.075	0.167	−2.351
1.801	−2.408	0.408	−2.039	0.175	3.839	3.096	−0.001	2.912	−0.560
0.392	1.600	−0.940	−0.160	−0.885	−1.083	−3.503	1.814	−0.563	−2.682
−4.113	−3.018	0.523	−1.915	−0.722	−2.769	0.210	−0.381	−0.724	−2.013
−0.393	−0.828	−0.102	−2.457	1.702	2.257	−2.473	−1.459	−1.385	−3.669
0.688	−0.214	2.741	2.906	−0.778	1.158	0.713	0.815	−0.670	0.144
1.957	1.104	3.540	2.726	−0.028	−0.181	−1.477	−4.434	0.457	0.057
1.823	−1.371	−4.951	3.333	0.248	1.691	2.311	−2.996	1.573	2.319
−0.277	0.346	−1.354	3.170	0.268	0.773	1.242	3.542	0.940	−0.535
−0.484	1.447	−0.512	−1.379	−0.808	1.014	2.103	0.005	−2.122	0.843
3.209	−1.924	−0.833	1.158	3.203	−0.040	−0.880	−2.217	0.007	0.022
1.834	2.064	−0.319	2.672	1.281	4.921	0.819	0.634	−4.961	−0.739
−1.618	0.705	0.220	−0.177	−0.117	−4.699	2.210	0.035	2.403	−0.816
2.553	1.710	−2.844	−4.619	−4.328	0.459	−2.373	−1.069	2.792	1.942
−1.665	1.627	1.072	−0.902	1.336	3.850	−0.804	1.254	−2.493	−1.101
−0.468	2.177	1.703	1.897	1.139	−1.606	−1.139	−1.435	5.162	−0.146
−1.296	−0.646	0.193	0.534	−0.863	−3.178	2.461	−1.275	0.731	2.983
−3.086	−0.115	2.325	0.088	4.652	2.833	−0.054	−0.670	−2.313	−1.956
−1.324	0.102	0.665	0.878	−1.760	−1.038	0.685	−1.034	0.380	−0.463
1.936	2.264	0.379	4.480	−3.841	−3.992	−3.565	2.558	−0.906	−0.432

RANDOM NORMAL NUMBERS, $\mu = 0$, $\sigma = 2$

31	32	33	34	35	36	37	38	39	40
−0.660	−0.996	−0.264	−1.823	0.818	−0.410	−1.786	2.399	1.986	0.242
1.785	−0.471	0.082	−3.006	−2.286	−0.222	0.388	−0.110	−0.358	−0.333
0.880	0.224	2.561	2.165	2.974	2.516	−4.148	−0.241	−1.318	−0.677
1.021	3.100	−1.783	−2.063	−2.176	1.959	0.248	0.597	1.394	0.612
−2.420	5.579	2.351	1.601	1.045	−2.857	1.400	3.411	−0.239	−2.323
−2.542	−3.145	−2.432	−0.444	−1.276	−3.342	3.479	2.630	−0.405	1.845
−2.437	0.104	1.110	0.008	−2.173	2.294	−0.529	1.723	−1.609	2.119
3.280	−1.213	−3.063	3.637	−0.038	0.217	−0.790	−1.412	−0.055	−0.612
0.502	−0.767	−1.569	0.386	−1.990	−0.062	3.319	−2.448	−0.445	0.059
−1.684	0.290	3.179	0.158	3.562	−1.929	−1.170	1.179	0.110	3.655
0.023	1.652	3.049	−1.410	−1.447	−0.638	−2.483	2.386	−0.331	1.215
−2.741	−2.313	−2.069	−1.305	−0.934	−7.769	2.654	−1.032	1.489	0.671
−0.746	2.099	−3.225	1.533	−1.741	−1.922	0.895	−2.974	−0.828	1.734
−0.934	−4.158	−3.297	−2.859	−4.026	2.722	−1.268	0.991	−1.196	−0.458
−1.574	0.097	2.122	−3.279	−0.820	0.483	2.196	0.642	−1.488	0.374
1.261	−0.663	0.616	−2.801	1.065	4.845	0.418	−0.226	1.897	3.554
2.030	1.692	0.265	0.511	−1.959	0.247	−1.381	−2.625	0.695	−2.248
−4.452	0.900	−1.646	0.573	0.973	−0.350	2.649	4.114	2.497	0.287
−0.075	−2.069	−0.574	0.001	−0.784	−1.235	−3.191	2.128	1.168	−0.742
0.369	0.919	−2.760	1.878	−5.001	−1.670	0.913	−2.853	0.002	1.885
1.360	−2.214	−2.175	0.193	3.298	−0.103	2.226	0.164	−2.429	−0.580
−3.271	2.845	−0.102	−0.822	−3.646	0.361	−3.188	−1.031	1.846	−1.622
−0.908	−3.907	1.407	0.078	1.324	0.276	−2.805	0.604	1.632	2.413
−1.323	2.717	−0.083	−1.645	1.103	−1.539	−0.173	2.429	−0.343	0.011
1.095	−0.871	1.636	2.345	−3.127	0.500	1.250	−0.072	−3.248	2.603
−1.907	−0.869	−4.388	−0.114	1.890	0.218	0.510	−0.768	−2.610	3.635
1.508	−0.333	−2.433	1.237	−1.733	−2.826	−3.761	−1.125	0.720	−0.832
2.937	1.887	−0.430	−5.194	4.716	−2.950	−0.393	−1.111	0.008	−0.186
−4.706	−1.302	−2.011	−0.124	−2.037	0.140	1.392	−1.869	−2.249	−0.075
5.019	−3.900	1.300	−0.034	−1.679	−0.621	0.285	1.197	−0.871	−1.240
−0.910	−0.495	0.074	3.144	−2.631	−3.152	0.192	−1.073	0.646	4.381
1.304	−1.010	−0.739	−1.028	2.886	−1.418	1.314	0.779	−2.139	0.173
0.371	−5.663	−0.017	−1.551	−3.508	1.305	−0.819	−0.199	−0.331	−0.358
−2.039	−3.961	0.679	2.451	−2.802	1.449	−0.964	−1.170	0.891	1.560
−0.911	1.904	0.062	−2.375	−1.548	−0.361	2.692	3.772	2.005	3.718
−1.720	0.871	3.594	0.889	0.162	0.112	−0.053	−2.597	−1.310	−2.234
−4.091	0.430	2.222	−0.141	0.506	2.751	−0.472	−1.141	1.671	−0.920
−1.797	−1.272	1.847	0.039	0.689	−0.080	1.457	−3.856	1.332	−2.898
−0.719	0.829	2.570	1.107	−0.314	−3.750	1.041	−1.657	−0.233	1.417
−1.890	3.240	1.877	2.552	3.389	0.215	1.979	−0.895	−1.996	0.611
−1.952	−1.276	−2.754	−0.049	−2.916	3.820	0.381	1.337	2.211	3.456
0.502	1.812	−0.577	0.551	−0.257	0.883	4.377	−4.180	−2.266	−0.100
1.971	2.333	−0.945	2.618	2.953	−1.997	1.491	−0.082	2.617	0.749
0.561	−1.506	4.127	0.933	−1.930	0.460	−0.008	0.352	−1.274	0.271
−1.409	−0.638	2.757	0.461	1.331	2.030	−0.846	−1.035	−1.580	−0.772
−2.066	0.218	0.070	−3.420	0.089	−0.084	4.944	−4.285	0.200	0.276
−2.734	3.622	−0.300	1.648	1.328	0.479	−0.498	1.997	2.203	2.792
−1.434	1.441	0.258	−1.893	−2.925	−1.753	0.272	0.747	−0.999	−0.155
−0.071	−4.344	−2.763	4.371	1.547	2.588	2.914	0.261	3.381	5.445
4.574	1.751	3.420	−1.383	0.966	−2.731	3.444	1.410	2.740	−2.011

RANDOM NORMAL NUMBERS, $\mu = 0$, $\sigma = 2$

41	42	43	44	45	46	47	48	49	50
−1.739	0.276	1.761	0.092	0.820	1.772	−3.258	0.707	−0.578	−1.611
−1.776	−1.482	1.399	1.031	−0.546	−0.204	2.591	2.129	1.615	0.919
−1.894	0.388	1.023	−1.493	1.513	1.003	2.547	−2.443	−1.855	2.898
−2.042	1.064	−2.399	−0.333	−2.141	−1.022	−2.976	−0.485	0.073	−0.891
0.287	0.120	−2.013	0.598	0.001	3.454	2.077	−1.966	−4.187	0.452
0.739	−4.324	0.088	1.124	0.610	0.368	0.953	−0.141	−0.441	3.163
0.749	0.597	2.194	−0.771	1.063	0.246	0.465	−3.122	−1.995	3.015
−1.111	−2.558	0.146	−0.590	−3.278	2.649	−1.299	−1.809	3.938	−1.766
−0.347	2.324	0.083	−0.152	−3.563	−1.062	0.901	0.882	0.865	0.581
−0.105	1.781	−0.775	−0.726	−3.211	−1.200	−2.688	1.639	−0.945	−1.022
1.968	2.056	−4.124	−1.126	−2.798	−1.150	−1.632	−3.405	1.182	1.985
1.614	−1.436	−4.649	−1.168	2.549	0.522	−0.616	2.009	−0.465	1.362
−1.671	−0.907	−0.459	2.880	2.640	−0.751	−2.414	−1.195	−2.334	−0.240
−1.328	0.335	−0.049	−1.903	0.225	−0.140	−1.121	0.820	0.282	0.635
−0.623	−0.823	1.655	1.997	−3.841	3.318	1.035	1.056	2.112	2.166
−2.292	−1.662	2.136	−0.223	1.372	−3.612	−0.276	−4.097	−0.419	−0.017
3.146	1.248	0.090	−1.069	−0.022	1.017	−1.157	1.803	−1.585	−1.526
1.553	−1.369	0.044	0.606	−1.734	−1.443	−3.016	−0.977	3.150	0.264
−3.179	3.510	−2.299	0.371	1.071	−1.044	−1.352	1.740	1.936	0.242
1.701	−0.455	2.119	−1.716	−2.857	−0.991	−1.621	2.934	3.487	0.754
−2.088	1.495	2.961	−2.029	−0.072	−0.664	0.992	1.659	0.834	−2.175
−3.757	0.316	0.763	−3.035	0.907	−3.804	−3.403	3.689	0.901	−2.386
−1.177	−1.422	−4.712	0.235	−1.048	−2.627	0.794	−1.473	2.598	−0.364
−1.380	−1.661	−1.714	−1.396	0.477	1.750	−2.458	−5.077	−0.194	1.093
−0.852	0.562	−0.199	0.802	0.494	−0.294	0.205	0.260	−2.616	4.117
2.591	1.323	0.458	4.020	−1.907	−0.065	−2.786	0.137	0.446	4.368
−2.240	2.744	0.551	−3.005	−2.677	4.492	2.928	0.061	−0.216	2.566
−1.488	−0.163	−0.187	2.081	−0.993	1.160	1.301	−2.236	1.586	0.011
0.622	−0.988	−0.956	−0.484	−0.648	−3.467	−3.778	1.181	1.740	0.092
−0.949	−2.527	−1.934	1.318	0.422	3.848	0.050	−1.448	0.278	3.041
−4.952	0.019	1.793	0.881	0.282	0.621	1.202	−0.373	3.665	3.386
−0.751	3.342	0.969	0.821	1.983	−0.533	−1.273	−2.214	−0.774	−1.210
0.618	−0.688	−2.960	−5.252	−0.543	0.104	−0.468	−3.139	0.594	−1.302
2.371	0.160	1.715	0.319	1.387	5.138	3.883	−1.869	−0.899	−1.019
−1.184	0.047	1.453	−0.889	−1.292	0.197	−0.302	−1.497	−1.838	−0.940
−0.287	2.329	2.028	−1.765	1.669	−1.024	1.600	0.454	3.098	2.275
1.764	−2.839	−1.942	0.008	4.001	0.083	−1.631	2.968	−0.146	−2.079
1.149	−1.571	1.296	1.510	−0.599	0.083	−0.688	6.017	0.012	−1.451
2.984	−1.432	−0.960	−2.124	1.353	0.934	0.666	3.096	2.905	−1.472
−1.701	−0.004	2.710	0.573	2.424	−0.119	−1.410	3.413	−3.588	0.047
−2.333	0.912	−0.773	−2.016	2.253	2.784	3.764	0.559	4.791	1.288
−0.214	2.787	0.095	−3.174	1.460	0.411	0.922	−0.474	3.113	−1.067
1.214	0.785	−2.686	1.909	−1.747	−4.551	0.589	−0.573	−1.364	−2.583
0.878	0.097	1.650	1.437	−1.643	−2.608	1.122	0.538	0.664	−0.323
−0.105	−0.297	3.821	2.105	2.021	−1.922	1.472	0.042	1.403	1.465
−0.593	0.136	0.910	−0.549	−1.472	3.214	−2.273	3.458	1.436	0.500
2.198	2.325	−1.229	−0.276	1.560	−0.482	−0.482	0.455	−0.181	1.417
1.160	0.139	0.997	−0.082	−0.689	0.995	−5.301	0.998	3.413	−1.797
3.024	−1.561	0.982	−1.244	1.407	−0.063	−1.176	2.355	2.006	−4.833
0.955	0.174	−0.401	2.472	0.584	3.811	1.115	0.951	−2.136	−2.324

XII.7 ORTHOGONAL POLYNOMIALS

In fitting a curvilinear model of the form

$$y_i = \beta_0 + \beta_1 x_i + \beta_2 x_i^2 + \cdots + \beta_p x_i^p + e_i \,,$$
$$i = 1, 2, \ldots, n,$$

it is convenient computationally to fit the model using orthogonal polynomials. Here one fits the model

$$y_i = \alpha_0 \xi_0(x) + \alpha_1 \xi_1(x) + \cdots + \alpha_p \xi_p(x) + e_i$$

where the $\xi_j(x)$ are orthogonal polynomials in x of the jth degree, namely, the Tchebycheff polynomials. The least-squares estimators $\hat{\alpha}_j$ of the α_j are given by

$$\hat{\alpha}_j = \frac{\sum_i y_i \xi_j(x_i)}{\sum_i [\xi_j(x_i)]^2} \,.$$

The estimators $\hat{\alpha}_j$ for any $j \leq n - 1$ are independent normal variates with means α_j for $j \leq p$ and 0 for $j > p$ and with variances $\dfrac{\sigma^2}{\sum_i [\xi_j(x_i)]^2}$. A mean-square estimate of σ^2 is provided by the error sum of squares

$$s^2 = \left\{ \sum_{i=1}^{n} y_i^2 - \sum_{j=0}^{p} \hat{\alpha}_j^2 \left(\sum_{i=1}^{n} \left[\xi_j(x_i) \right]^2 \right) \right\} \Big/ (n - p - 1) \,.$$

Thus the ratios $\dfrac{(\alpha_j - \hat{\alpha}_j) \sqrt{\sum_i [\xi_j(x_i)]^2}}{s}$ with $\hat{\alpha}_j = 0$ for $j > p$ is distributed as Student's t-distribution.

This table provides values of $\xi_j(x_i)$ for various values of n and j. To avoid fractional values and to reduce the size of the integers, the table is arranged so that the highest power of x_i in $\xi_j(x_i)$ has a coefficient λ_j. The two values at the bottom of each column are the values $D_j = \sum_{i=1}^{n} [\xi_j(x_i)]^2$ and λ_j.

ORTHOGONAL POLYNOMIALS

n = 3

	ξ'_1	ξ'_2
	−1	+1
	0	−2
	+1	+1
D	2	6
λ	1	3

n = 4

	ξ'_1	ξ'_2	ξ'_3
	−3	+1	−1
	−1	−1	+3
	+1	−1	−3
	+3	+1	+1
D	20	4	20
λ	2	1	$\frac{10}{3}$

n = 5

	ξ'_1	ξ'_2	ξ'_3	ξ'_4
	−2	+2	−1	+1
	−1	−1	+2	−4
	0	−2	0	+6
	+1	−1	−2	−4
	+2	+2	+1	+1
D	10	14	10	70
λ	1	1	$\frac{5}{6}$	$\frac{35}{12}$

n = 6

	ξ'_1	ξ'_2	ξ'_3	ξ'_4	ξ'_5
	−5	+5	−5	+1	−1
	−3	−1	+7	−3	+5
	−1	−4	+4	+2	−10
	+1	−4	−4	+2	+10
	+3	−1	−7	−3	−5
	+5	+5	+5	+1	+1
D	70	84	180	28	252
λ	2	$\frac{3}{2}$	$\frac{5}{3}$	$\frac{7}{12}$	$\frac{21}{10}$

n = 7

	ξ'_1	ξ'_2	ξ'_3	ξ'_4	ξ'_5
	−3	+5	−1	+3	−1
	−2	0	+1	−7	+4
	−1	−3	+1	+1	−5
	0	−4	0	+6	0
	+1	−3	−1	+1	+5
	+2	0	−1	−7	−4
	+3	+5	+1	+3	+1
D	28	84	6	154	84
λ	1	1	$\frac{1}{6}$	$\frac{7}{12}$	$\frac{7}{20}$

n = 8

	ξ'_1	ξ'_2	ξ'_3	ξ'_4	ξ'_5
	−7	+7	−7	+7	−7
	−5	+1	+5	−13	+23
	−3	−3	+7	−3	−17
	−1	−5	+3	+9	−15
	+1	−5	−3	+9	+15
	+3	−3	−7	−3	+17
	+5	+1	−5	−13	−23
	+7	+7	+7	+7	+7
D	168	168	264	616	2184
λ	2	1	$\frac{2}{3}$	$\frac{7}{12}$	$\frac{7}{10}$

n = 9

	ξ'_1	ξ'_2	ξ'_3	ξ'_4	ξ'_5
	0	−20	0	+18	0
	+1	−17	−9	+9	+9
	+2	−8	−13	−11	+4
	+3	+7	−7	−21	−11
	+4	+28	+14	+14	+4
D	60	2,772	990	2,002	468
λ	1	3	$\frac{5}{6}$	$\frac{7}{12}$	$\frac{3}{20}$

n = 10

	ξ'_1	ξ'_2	ξ'_3	ξ'_4	ξ'_5
	+1	−4	−12	+18	+6
	+3	−3	−31	+3	+11
	+5	−1	−35	−17	+1
	+7	+2	−14	−22	−14
	+9	+6	+42	+18	+6
D	330	132	8,580	2,860	780
λ	2	$\frac{1}{2}$	$\frac{5}{3}$	$\frac{5}{12}$	$\frac{1}{10}$

n = 11

	ξ'_1	ξ'_2	ξ'_3	ξ'_4	ξ'_5
	0	−10	0	+6	0
	+1	−9	−14	+4	+4
	+2	−6	−23	−1	+4
	+3	−1	−22	−6	−1
	+4	+6	−6	−6	−6
	+5	+15	+30	+6	+3
D	110	858	4,290	286	156
λ	1	1	$\frac{5}{6}$	$\frac{1}{12}$	$\frac{1}{40}$

n = 12

	ξ'_1	ξ'_2	ξ'_3	ξ'_4	ξ'_5
	+1	−35	−7	+28	+20
	+3	−29	−19	+12	+44
	+5	−17	−25	−13	+29
	+7	+1	−21	−33	−21
	+9	+25	−3	−27	−57
	+11	+55	+33	+33	+33
D	572	12,012	5,148	8,008	15,912
λ	2	3	$\frac{2}{3}$	$\frac{7}{24}$	$\frac{3}{20}$

n = 13

	ξ'_1	ξ'_2	ξ'_3	ξ'_4	ξ'_5
	0	−14	0	+84	0
	+1	−13	−4	+64	+20
	+2	−10	−7	+11	+26
	+3	−5	−8	−54	+11
	+4	+2	−6	−96	−18
	+5	+11	0	−66	−33
	+6	+22	+11	+99	+22
D	182	2,002	572	68,068	6,188
λ	1	1	$\frac{1}{6}$	$\frac{7}{12}$	$\frac{7}{120}$

n = 14

	ξ'_1	ξ'_2	ξ'_3	ξ'_4	ξ'_5
	+1	−8	−24	+108	+60
	+3	−7	−67	+63	+145
	+5	−5	−95	−13	+139
	+7	−2	−98	−92	+28
	+9	+2	−66	−132	−132
	+11	+7	+11	−77	−187
	+13	+13	+143	+143	+143
D	910	728	97,240	136,136	235,144
λ	2	$\frac{1}{2}$	$\frac{5}{3}$	$\frac{7}{12}$	$\frac{7}{30}$

n = 15

	ξ'_1	ξ'_2	ξ'_3	ξ'_4	ξ'_5
	0	−56	0	+756	0
	+1	−53	−27	+621	+675
	+2	−44	−49	+251	+1000
	+3	−29	−61	−249	+751
	+4	−8	−58	−704	−44
	+5	+19	−35	−869	−979
	+6	+52	+13	−429	−1144
	+7	+91	+91	+1001	+1001
D	280	37,128	39,780	6,466,460	10,581,480
λ	1	3	$\frac{5}{6}$	$\frac{35}{12}$	$\frac{21}{20}$

n = 16

	ξ'_1	ξ'_2	ξ'_3	ξ'_4	ξ'_5
	+1	−21	−63	+189	+45
	+3	−19	−179	+129	+115
	+5	−15	−265	+23	+131
	+7	−9	−301	−101	+77
	+9	−1	−267	−201	−33
	+11	+9	−143	−221	−143
	+13	+21	+91	−91	−143
	+15	+35	+455	+273	+143
D	1,360	5,712	1,007,760	470,288	201,552
λ	2	1	$\frac{10}{3}$	$\frac{7}{12}$	$\frac{1}{10}$

ORTHOGONAL POLYNOMIALS

17

	ξ'_1	ξ'_2	ξ'_3	ξ'_4	ξ'_5
	0	−24	0	+36	0
	+1	−23	−7	+31	+55
	+2	−20	−13	+17	+88
	+3	−15	−17	−3	+83
	+4	−8	−18	−24	+36
	+5	+1	−15	−39	−39
	+6	+12	−7	−39	−104
	+7	+25	+7	−13	−91
	+8	+40	+28	+52	+104
D	408	7,752	3,876	16,796	100,776
λ	1	1	$\frac{1}{6}$	$\frac{1}{12}$	$\frac{1}{20}$

18

	ξ'_1	ξ'_2	ξ'_3	ξ'_4	ξ'_5
	+1	−40	−8	+44	+220
	+3	−37	−23	+33	+583
	+5	−31	−35	+13	+733
	+7	−22	−42	−12	+588
	+9	−10	−42	−36	+156
	+11	+5	−33	−51	−429
	+13	+23	−13	−47	−871
	+15	+44	+20	−12	−676
	+17	+68	+68	+68	+884
D	1,938	23,256	23,256	28,424	6,953,544
λ	2	$\frac{3}{2}$	$\frac{1}{3}$	$\frac{1}{12}$	$\frac{3}{10}$

19

	ξ'_1	ξ'_2	ξ'_3	ξ'_4	ξ'_5
	0	−30	0	+396	0
	+1	−29	−44	+352	+44
	+2	−26	−83	+227	+74
	+3	−21	−112	+42	+79
	+4	−14	−126	−168	+54
	+5	−5	−120	−354	+3
	+6	+6	−89	−453	−58
	+7	+19	−28	−388	−98
	+8	+34	+68	−68	−68
	+9	+51	+204	+612	+102
D	570	13,566	213,180	2,288,132	89,148
λ	1	1	$\frac{5}{6}$	$\frac{7}{12}$	$\frac{1}{40}$

20

	ξ'_1	ξ'_2	ξ'_3	ξ'_4	ξ'_5
	+1	−33	−99	+1188	+396
	+3	−31	−287	+948	+1076
	+5	−27	−445	+503	+1441
	+7	−21	−553	−77	+1351
	+9	−13	−591	−687	+771
	+11	−3	−539	−1187	−187
	+13	+9	−377	−1402	−1222
	+15	+23	−85	−1122	−1802
	+17	+39	+357	−102	−1122
	+19	+57	+969	+1938	+1938
D	2,660	17,556	4,903,140	22,881,320	31,201,800
λ	2	1	$\frac{10}{3}$	$\frac{35}{24}$	$\frac{7}{20}$

21

	ξ'_1	ξ'_2	ξ'_3	ξ'_4	ξ'_5
	0	−110	0	+594	0
	+1	−107	−54	+540	+1404
	+2	−98	−103	+385	+2444
	+3	−83	−142	+150	+2819
	+4	−62	−166	−130	+2354
	+5	−35	−170	−406	+1063
	+6	−2	−149	−615	−788
	+7	+37	−98	−680	−2618
	+8	+82	−12	−510	−3468
	+9	+133	+114	0	−1938
	+10	+190	+285	+969	+3876
D	770	201,894	432,630	5,720,330	121,687,020
λ	1	3	$\frac{5}{6}$	$\frac{7}{12}$	$\frac{21}{40}$

22

	ξ'_1	ξ'_2	ξ'_3	ξ'_4	ξ'_5
	+1	−20	−12	+702	+390
	+3	−19	−35	+585	+1079
	+5	−17	−55	+365	+1509
	+7	−14	−70	+70	+1554
	+9	−10	−78	−258	+1158
	+11	−5	−77	−563	+363
	+13	+1	−65	−775	−663
	+15	+8	−40	−810	−1598
	+17	+16	0	−570	−1938
	+19	+25	+57	+57	−969
	+21	+35	+133	+1197	+2261
D	3,542	7,084	96,140	8,748,740	40,562,340
λ	2	$\frac{1}{2}$	$\frac{1}{3}$	$\frac{7}{12}$	$\frac{7}{30}$

ORTHOGONAL POLYNOMIALS

23

	ξ'_1	ξ'_2	ξ'_3	ξ'_4	ξ'_5
	0	−44	0	+858	0
	+1	−43	−13	+793	+65
	+2	−40	−25	+605	+116
	+3	−35	−35	+315	+141
	+4	−28	−42	−42	+132
	+5	−19	−45	−417	+87
	+6	−8	−43	−747	+12
	+7	+5	−35	−955	−77
	+8	+20	−20	−950	−152
	+9	+37	+3	−627	−171
	+10	+56	+35	+133	−76
	+11	+77	+77	+1463	+209
D	1,012	35,420	32,890	13,123,110	340,860
λ	1	1	$\frac{1}{6}$	$\frac{7}{12}$	$\frac{1}{60}$

24

	ξ'_1	ξ'_2	ξ'_3	ξ'_4	ξ'_5
	+1	−143	−143	+143	+715
	+3	−137	−419	+123	+2005
	+5	−125	−665	+85	+2893
	+7	−107	−861	+33	+3171
	+9	−83	−987	−27	+2721
	+11	−53	−1023	−87	+1551
	+13	−17	−949	−137	−169
	+15	+25	−745	−165	−2071
	+17	+73	−391	−157	−3553
	+19	+127	+133	−97	−3743
	+21	+187	+847	+33	−1463
	+23	+253	+1771	+253	+4807
D	4,600	394,680	17,760,600	394,680	177,928,920
λ	2	3	$\frac{10}{3}$	$\frac{1}{12}$	$\frac{3}{10}$

25

	ξ'_1	ξ'_2	ξ'_3	ξ'_4	ξ'_5
	0	−52	0	+858	0
	+1	−51	−77	+803	+275
	+2	−48	−149	+643	+500
	+3	−43	−211	+393	+631
	+4	−36	−258	+78	+636
	+5	−27	−285	−267	+501
	+6	−16	−287	−597	+236
	+7	−3	−259	−857	−119
	+8	+12	−196	−982	−488
	+9	+29	−93	−897	−753
	+10	+48	+55	−517	−748
	+11	+69	+253	+253	−253
	+12	+92	+506	+1518	+1012
D	1,300	53,820	1,480,050	14,307,150	7,803,900
λ	1	1	$\frac{5}{6}$	$\frac{5}{12}$	$\frac{1}{20}$

26

	ξ'_1	ξ'_2	ξ'_3	ξ'_4	ξ'_5
	+1	−28	−84	+1386	+330
	+3	−27	−247	+1221	+935
	+5	−25	−395	+905	+1381
	+7	−22	−518	+466	+1582
	+9	−18	−606	−54	+1482
	+11	−13	−649	−599	+1067
	+13	−7	−637	−1099	+377
	+15	0	−560	−1470	−482
	+17	+8	−408	−1614	−1326
	+19	+17	−171	−1419	−1881
	+21	+27	+161	−759	−1771
	+23	+38	+598	+506	−506
	+25	+50	+1150	+2530	+2530
D	5,850	16,380	7,803,900	40,060,020	48,384,180
λ	2	$\frac{1}{2}$	$\frac{5}{3}$	$\frac{7}{12}$	$\frac{1}{10}$

27

	ξ'_1	ξ'_2	ξ'_3	ξ'_4	ξ'_5
	0	−182	0	+1638	0
	+1	−179	−18	+1548	+3960
	+2	−170	−35	+1285	+7304
	+3	−155	−50	+870	+9479
	+4	−134	−62	+338	+10058
	+5	−107	−70	−262	+8803
	+6	−74	−73	−867	+5728
	+7	−35	−70	−1400	+1162
	+8	+10	−60	−1770	−4188
	+9	+61	−42	−1872	−9174
	+10	+118	−15	−1587	−12144
	+11	+181	+22	−782	−10879
	+12	+250	+70	+690	−2530
	+13	+325	+130	+2990	+16445
D	1,638	712,530	101,790	56,448,210	2,032,135,560
λ	1	3	$\frac{1}{6}$	$\frac{7}{12}$	$\frac{21}{40}$

28

	ξ'_1	ξ'_2	ξ'_3	ξ'_4	ξ'_5
	+1	−65	−39	+936	+1560
	+3	−63	−115	+840	+4456
	+5	−59	−185	+655	+6701
	+7	−53	−245	+395	+7931
	+9	−45	−291	+81	+7887
	+11	−35	−319	−259	+6457
	+13	−23	−325	−590	+3718
	+15	−9	−305	−870	−22
	+17	+7	−255	−1050	−4182
	+19	+25	−171	−1074	−7866
	+21	+45	−49	−879	−9821
	+23	+67	+115	−395	−8395
	+25	+91	+325	+455	−1495
	+27	+117	+585	+1755	+13455
D	7,308	95,004	2,103,660	19,634,160	1,354,757,040
λ	2	1	$\frac{2}{3}$	$\frac{7}{24}$	$\frac{7}{20}$

ORTHOGONAL POLYNOMIALS

	29				
	ξ'_1	ξ'_2	ξ'_3	ξ'_4	ξ'_5
	0	−70	0	+2184	0
	+1	−69	−104	+2080	+1768
	+2	−66	−203	+1775	+3298
	+3	−61	−292	+1290	+4373
	+4	−54	−366	+660	+4818
	+5	−45	−420	−66	+4521
	+6	−34	−449	−825	+3454
	+7	−21	−448	−1540	+1695
	+8	−6	−412	−2120	−556
	+9	+11	−336	+2460	−2946
	+10	+30	−215	−2441	−4958
	+11	+51	−44	−1930	−5885
	+12	+74	+182	−780	−4810
	+13	+99	+468	+1170	−585
	+14	+126	+819	+4095	+8190
D	2,030	113,274	4,207,320	107,987,880	500,671,080
λ	1	1	$\frac{5}{6}$	$\frac{7}{12}$	$\frac{7}{40}$

	30				
	ξ'_1	ξ'_2	ξ'_3	ξ'_4	ξ'_5
	+1	−112	−112	+12376	+1768
	+3	−109	−331	+11271	+5083
	+5	−103	−535	+9131	+7753
	+7	−94	−714	+6096	+9408
	+9	−82	−858	+2376	+9768
	+11	−67	−957	−1749	+8679
	+13	−49	−1001	−5929	+6149
	+15	−28	−980	−9744	+2384
	+17	−4	−884	−12704	−2176
	+19	+23	−703	−14249	−6821
	+21	+53	−427	−13749	−10535
	+23	+86	−46	−10504	−11960
	+25	+122	+450	−3744	−9360
	+27	+161	+1071	+7371	−585
	+29	+203	+1827	+23751	+16965
D	8,990	302,064	21,360,240	3,671,587,920	2,145,733,200
λ	2	$\frac{3}{2}$	$\frac{5}{3}$	$\frac{35}{12}$	$\frac{3}{10}$

	31				
	ξ'_1	ξ'_2	ξ'_3	ξ'_4	ξ'_5
	+0	−80	0	+408	0
	+1	−79	−119	+391	+221
	+2	−76	−233	+341	+416
	+3	−71	−337	+261	+561
	+4	−64	−426	+156	+636
	+5	−55	−495	+33	+627
	+6	−44	−539	−99	+528
	+7	−31	−553	−229	+343
	+8	−16	−532	−344	+88
	+9	+1	−471	−429	−207
	+10	+20	−365	−467	−496
	+11	+41	−209	−439	−715
	+12	+64	+2	−324	−780
	+13	+89	+273	−99	−585
	+14	+116	+609	+261	0
	+15	+145	+1015	+783	+1131
D	2,480	158,224	6,724,520	4,034,712	9,536,592
λ	1	1	$\frac{5}{6}$	$\frac{1}{12}$	$\frac{1}{60}$

	32				
	ξ'_1	ξ'_2	ξ'_3	ξ'_4	ξ'_5
	+1	−85	−51	+459	+255
	+3	−83	−151	+423	+737
	+5	−79	−245	+353	+1137
	+7	−73	−329	+253	+1407
	+9	−65	−399	+129	+1509
	+11	−55	−451	−11	+1419
	+13	−43	−481	−157	+1131
	+15	−29	−485	−297	+661
	+17	−13	−459	−417	+51
	+19	+5	−399	−501	−627
	+21	+25	−301	−531	−1267
	+23	+47	−161	−487	−1725
	+25	+71	+25	−347	−1815
	+27	+97	+261	−87	−1305
	+29	+125	+551	+319	+87
	+31	+155	+899	+899	+2697
D	10,912	185,504	5,379,616	5,379,616	54,285,216
λ	2	1	$\frac{2}{3}$	$\frac{1}{12}$	$\frac{1}{30}$

ORTHOGONAL POLYNOMIALS

	33					34				
	ξ'_1	ξ'_2	ξ'_3	ξ'_4	ξ'_5	ξ'_1	ξ'_2	ξ'_3	ξ'_4	ξ'_5
	0	−272	0	+3672	0	1	−48	−144	+4104	+6840
	+1	−269	−27	+3537	+2565	3	−47	−427	+3819	+19855
	+2	−260	−53	+3139	+4864	5	−45	−695	+3263	+30917
	+3	−245	−77	+2499	+6649	7	−42	−938	+2464	+38864
	+4	−224	−98	+1652	+7708	9	−38	−1146	+1464	+42744
	+5	−197	−115	+647	+7883	11	−33	−1309	+319	+41899
	+6	−164	−127	−453	+7088	13	−27	−1417	−901	+36049
	+7	−125	−133	−1571	+5327	15	−20	−1460	−2112	+25376
	+8	−80	−132	−2616	+2712	17	−12	−1428	−3216	+10608
	+9	−29	−123	−3483	−519	19	−3	−1311	−4101	−6897
	+10	+28	−105	−4053	−3984	21	+7	−1099	−4641	−25067
	+11	+91	−77	−4193	−7139	23	+18	−782	−4696	−41032
	+12	+160	−38	−3756	−9260	25	+30	−350	−4112	−51040
	+13	+235	+13	−2581	−9425	27	+43	+207	−2721	−50373
	+14	+316	+77	−493	−6496	29	+57	+899	−341	−33263
	+15	+403	+155	+2697	+899	31	+72	+1736	+3224	+7192
	+16	+496	+248	+7192	+14384	33	+88	+2728	+8184	+79112
D	2,992	1,947,792	417,384	348,330,136	1,547,128,656	13,090	62,832	51,477,360	456,432,592	46,929,569,232
λ	1	3	$\frac{1}{6}$	$\frac{7}{12}$	$\frac{3}{20}$	2	$\frac{1}{2}$	$\frac{5}{3}$	$\frac{7}{12}$	$\frac{7}{10}$

	35				
	ξ'_1	ξ'_2	ξ'_3	ξ'_4	ξ'_5
	0	−102	0	+23256	0
	1	−101	−152	+22496	+3800
	2	−98	−299	+20251	+7250
	3	−93	−436	+16626	+10021
	4	−86	−558	+11796	+11826
	5	−77	−660	+6006	+12441
	6	−66	−737	−429	+11726
	7	−53	−784	−7124	+9646
	8	−38	−796	−13624	+6292
	9	−21	−768	−19404	+1902
	10	−2	−695	−23869	−3118
	11	+19	−572	−26354	−8173
	12	+42	−394	−26124	−12458
	13	+67	−156	−22374	−14937
	14	+94	+147	−14229	−14322
	15	+123	+520	−744	−9052
	16	+154	+968	+19096	+2728
	17	+187	+1496	+46376	+23188
D	3,570	290,598	15,775,320	14,834,059,240	4,045,652,520
λ	1	1	$\frac{5}{6}$	$\frac{35}{12}$	$\frac{7}{40}$

ORTHOGONAL POLYNOMIALS

36

	ξ_1'	ξ_2'	ξ_3'	ξ_4'	ξ_5'
	1	−323	−323	+2584	+12920
	3	−317	−959	+2424	+37640
	5	−305	−1565	+2111	+59063
	7	−287	−2121	+1659	+75201
	9	−263	−2607	+1089	+84381
	11	−233	−3003	+429	+85371
	13	−197	−3289	−286	+77506
	15	−155	−3445	−1014	+60814
	17	−107	−3451	−1706	+36142
	19	−53	−3287	−2306	+5282
	21	+7	−2933	−2751	−28903
	23	+73	−2369	−2971	−62353
	25	+145	−1575	−2889	−89685
	27	+223	−531	−2421	−104067
	29	+307	+783	−1476	−97092
	31	+397	+2387	+44	−58652
	33	+493	+4301	+2244	+23188
	35	+595	+6545	+5236	+162316
D	15,540	3,011,652	307,618,740	191,407,216	199,046,103,984
λ	2	3	$\frac{10}{3}$	$\frac{7}{24}$	$\frac{21}{20}$

37

	ξ_1'	ξ_2'	ξ_3'	ξ_4'	ξ_5'
	0	−114	0	+5814	0
	1	−113	−34	+5644	+680
	2	−110	−67	+5141	+1304
	3	−105	−98	+4326	+1819
	4	−98	−126	+3234	+2178
	5	−89	−150	+1914	+2343
	6	−78	−169	+429	+2288
	7	−65	−182	−1144	+2002
	8	−50	−188	−2714	+1492
	9	−33	−186	−4176	+786
	10	−14	−175	−5411	−64
	11	+7	−154	−6286	−979
	12	+30	−122	−6654	−1850
	13	+55	−78	−6354	−2535
	14	+82	−21	−5211	−2856
	15	+111	+50	−3036	−2596
	16	+142	+136	+374	−1496
	17	+175	+238	+5236	+748
	18	+210	+357	+11781	+4488
D	4,218	383,838	932,178	980,961,982	152,877,192
λ	1	1	$\frac{1}{6}$	$\frac{7}{12}$	$\frac{1}{40}$

38

	ξ_1'	ξ_2'	ξ_3'	ξ_4'	ξ_5'
	1	−60	−36	+918	+1530
	3	−59	−107	+867	+4471
	5	−57	−175	+767	+7061
	7	−54	−238	+622	+9086
	9	−50	−294	+438	+10362
	11	−45	−341	+223	+10747
	13	−39	−377	−13	+10153
	15	−32	−400	−258	+8558
	17	−24	−408	−498	+6018
	19	−15	−399	−717	+2679
	21	−5	−371	−897	−1211
	23	+6	−322	−1018	−5290
	25	+18	−250	−1058	−9070
	27	+31	−153	−993	−11925
	29	+45	−29	−797	−13079
	31	+60	+124	−442	−11594
	33	+76	+308	+102	−6358
	35	+93	+525	+867	+3927
	37	+111	+777	+1887	+20757
D	18,278	109,668	4,496,388	25,479,532	3,286,859,628
λ	2	$\frac{1}{2}$	$\frac{1}{3}$	$\frac{1}{12}$	$\frac{1}{10}$

ORTHOGONAL POLYNOMIALS

	39			
ξ_1'	ξ_2'	ξ_3'	ξ_4'	ξ_5'
0	−380	0	+1026	0
1	−377	−189	+999	+5049
2	−368	−373	+919	+9724
3	−353	−547	+789	+13669
4	−332	−706	+614	+16564
5	−305	−845	+401	+18143
6	−272	−959	+159	+18212
7	−233	−1043	−101	+16667
8	−188	−1092	−366	+13512
9	−137	−1101	−621	+8877
10	−80	−1065	−849	+3036
11	−17	−979	−1031	−3575
12	+52	−838	−1146	−10340
13	+127	−637	−1171	−16445
14	+208	−371	−1081	−20860
15	+295	−35	−849	−22321
16	+388	+376	−446	−19312
17	+487	+867	+159	−10047
18	+592	+1443	+999	+7548
19	+703	+2109	+2109	+35853
D 4,940	4,496,388	33,722,910	32,224,114	9,860,578,884
λ 1	3	$\frac{5}{6}$	$\frac{1}{12}$	$\frac{3}{20}$

	40			
ξ_1'	ξ_2'	ξ_3'	ξ_4'	ξ_5'
1	−133	−399	+39501	+627
3	−131	−1187	+37521	+1837
5	−127	−1945	+33631	+2917
7	−121	−2653	+27971	+3787
9	−113	−3291	+20751	+4377
11	−103	−3839	+12251	+4631
13	−91	−4277	+2821	+4511
15	−77	−4585	−7119	+4001
17	−61	−4743	−17079	+3111
19	−43	−4731	−26499	+1881
21	−23	−4529	−34749	+385
23	−1	−4117	−41129	−1265
25	+23	−3475	−44869	−2915
27	+49	−2583	−45129	−4365
29	+77	−1421	−40999	−5365
31	+107	+31	−31499	−5611
33	+139	+1793	−15579	−4741
35	+173	+3885	+7881	−2331
37	+209	+6327	+40071	+2109
39	+247	+9139	+82251	+9139
D 21,320	567,112	644,482,280	49,625,135,560	644,482,280
λ 2	1	$\frac{10}{3}$	$\frac{35}{12}$	$\frac{1}{30}$

ORTHOGONAL POLYNOMIALS

41				
ξ_1'	ξ_2'	ξ_3'	ξ_4'	ξ_5'
0	−140	0	+8778	0
1	−139	−209	+8569	+4807
2	−136	−413	+7949	+9292
3	−131	−607	+6939	+13147
4	−124	−786	+5574	+16092
5	−115	−945	+3903	+17889
6	−104	−1079	+1989	+18356
7	−91	−1183	−91	+17381
8	−76	−1252	−2246	+14936
9	−59	−1281	−4371	+11091
10	−40	−1265	−6347	+6028
11	−19	−1199	−8041	+55
12	+4	−1078	−9306	−6380
13	+29	−897	−9981	−12675
14	+56	−651	−9891	−18060
15	+85	−335	−8847	−21583
16	+116	+56	−6646	−22096
17	+149	+527	−3071	−18241
18	+184	+1083	+2109	−8436
19	+221	+1729	+9139	+9139
20	+260	+2470	+18278	+36556
D 5,740	641,732	47,900,710	2,481,256,778	10,376,164,708
λ 1	1	$\frac{5}{6}$	$\frac{7}{12}$	$\frac{7}{60}$

42				
ξ_1'	ξ_2'	ξ_3'	ξ_4'	ξ_5'
1	−220	−44	+9614	+48070
3	−217	−131	+9177	+141151
5	−211	−215	+8317	+225181
7	−202	−294	+7062	+294546
9	−190	−366	+5454	+344262
11	−175	−429	+3549	+370227
13	−157	−481	+1417	+369473
15	−136	−520	−858	+340418
17	−112	−544	−3178	+283118
19	−85	−551	−5431	+199519
21	−55	−539	−7491	+93709
23	−22	−506	−9218	−27830
25	+14	−450	−10458	−155970
27	+53	−369	−11043	−278685
29	+95	−261	−10791	−380799
31	+140	−124	−9506	−443734
33	+188	+44	−6978	−445258
35	+239	+245	−2983	−359233
37	+293	+481	+2717	−155363
39	+350	+754	+10374	+201058
41	+410	+1066	+20254	+749398
D 24,682	1,629,012	9,075,924	3,084,805,724	4,389,117,671,484
λ 2	$\frac{3}{2}$	$\frac{1}{3}$	$\frac{7}{12}$	$\frac{21}{10}$

ORTHOGONAL POLYNOMIALS

	43				
	ξ_1'	ξ_2'	ξ_3'	ξ_4'	ξ_5'
	0	−154	0	+10626	0
	1	−153	−46	+10396	+8740
	2	−150	−91	+9713	+16948
	3	−145	−134	+8598	+24113
	4	−138	−174	+7086	+29766
	5	−129	−210	+5226	+33501
	6	−118	−241	+3081	+34996
	7	−105	−266	+728	+34034
	8	−90	−284	−1742	+30524
	9	−73	−294	−4224	+24522
	10	−54	−295	−6599	+16252
	11	−33	−286	−8734	+6127
	12	−10	−266	−10482	−5230
	13	+15	−234	−11682	−16965
	14	+42	−189	−12159	−27972
	15	+71	−130	−11724	−36872
	16	+102	−56	−10174	−41992
	17	+135	+34	−7292	−41344
	18	+170	+141	−2847	−32604
	19	+207	+266	+3406	−13091
	20	+246	+410	+11726	+20254
	21	+287	+574	+22386	+70889
D	6,622	814,506	2,676,234	3,815,417,606	39,541,600,644
λ	1	1	$\frac{1}{6}$	$\frac{7}{12}$	$\frac{7}{40}$

	44				
	ξ_1'	ξ_2'	ξ_3'	ξ_4'	ξ_5'
	1	−161	−483	+5796	+1380
	3	−159	−1439	+5556	+4060
	5	−155	−2365	+5083	+6503
	7	−149	−3241	+4391	+8561
	9	−141	−4047	+3501	+10101
	11	−131	−4763	+2441	+11011
	13	−119	−5369	+1246	+11206
	15	−105	−5845	−42	+10634
	17	−89	−6171	−1374	+9282
	19	−71	−6327	−2694	+7182
	21	−51	−6293	−3939	+4417
	23	−29	−6049	−5039	+1127
	25	−5	−5575	−5917	−2485
	27	+21	−4851	−6489	−6147
	29	+49	−3857	−6664	−9512
	31	+79	−2573	−6344	−12152
	33	+111	−979	−5424	−13552
	35	+145	+945	−3792	−13104
	37	+181	+3219	−1329	−10101
	39	+219	+5863	+2091	−3731
	41	+259	+8897	+6601	+6929
	43	+301	+12341	+12341	+22919
D	28,380	913,836	1,257,829,980	1,173,974,648	4,162,273,752
λ	2	1	$\frac{10}{3}$	$\frac{7}{24}$	$\frac{1}{20}$

ORTHOGONAL POLYNOMIALS

45

	ξ'_1	ξ'_2	ξ'_3	ξ'_4	ξ'_5
	0	−506	0	+9108	0
	1	−503	−252	+8928	+4500
	2	−494	−499	+8393	+8750
	3	−479	−736	+7518	+12509
	4	−458	−958	+6328	+15554
	5	−431	−1160	+4858	+17689
	6	−398	−1337	+3153	+18754
	7	−359	−1484	+1268	+18634
	8	−314	−1596	−732	+17268
	9	−263	−1668	−2772	+14658
	10	−206	−1695	−4767	+10878
	11	−143	−1672	−6622	+6083
	12	−74	−1594	−8232	+518
	13	+1	−1456	−9482	−5473
	14	+82	−1253	−10247	−11438
	15	+169	−980	−10392	−16808
	16	+262	−632	−9772	−20888
	17	+361	−204	−8232	−22848
	18	+466	+309	−5607	−21714
	19	+577	+912	−1722	−16359
	20	+694	+1610	+3608	−5494
	21	+817	+2408	+10578	−12341
	22	+946	+3311	+19393	+38786
D	7,590	9,203,634	92,036,340	2,934,936,620	12,006,558,900
λ	1	3	$\frac{5}{6}$	$\frac{5}{12}$	$\frac{3}{40}$

46

	ξ'_2	ξ'_3	ξ'_4	ξ'_5
	−88	−264	+1980	+3300
	−87	−787	+1905	+9725
	−85	−1295	+1757	+15631
	−82	−1778	+1540	+20692
	−78	−2226	+1260	+24612
	−73	−2629	+925	+27137
	−67	−2977	+545	+28067
	−60	−3260	+132	−27268
	−52	−3468	−300	+24684
	−43	−3591	−735	+20349
	−33	−3619	−1155	+14399
	−22	−3542	−1540	+7084
	−10	−3350	−1868	−1220
	+3	−3033	−2115	−9999
	+17	−2581	−2255	−18589
	+32	−1984	−2260	−26164
	+48	−1232	−2100	−31724
	+65	−315	−1743	−34083
	+83	+777	−1155	−31857
	+102	+2054	−300	−23452
	+122	+3526	+860	−7052
	+143	+5203	+2365	+19393
	+165	+7095	+4257	+58179
D	285,384	429,502,920	143,167,640	27,214,866,840
λ	$\frac{1}{2}$	$\frac{5}{3}$	$\frac{1}{12}$	$\frac{1}{10}$

ORTHOGONAL POLYNOMIALS

	47			
	ξ_2'	ξ_3'	ξ_4'	ξ_5'
	−184	0	+15180	0
	−183	−55	+14905	+3575
	−180	−109	+14087	+6968
	−175	−161	+12747	+10003
	−168	−210	+10920	+12516
	−159	−255	+8655	+14361
	−148	−295	+6015	+15416
	−135	−329	+3077	+15589
	−120	−356	−68	+14824
	−103	−375	−3315	+13107
	−84	−385	−6545	+10472
	−63	−385	−9625	+7007
	−40	−374	−12408	+2860
	−15	−351	−14733	−1755
	+12	−315	−16425	−6552
	+41	−265	−17295	−11167
	+72	−200	−17140	−15152
	+105	−119	−15743	−17969
	+140	−21	−12873	−18984
	+177	+95	−8285	−17461
	+216	+230	−1720	−12556
	+257	+385	+7095	−3311
	+300	+561	+18447	+11352
	+345	+759	+32637	+32637
D	1,271,256	4,994,220	8,518,474,580	8,629,104,120
λ	1	$\frac{1}{6}$	$\frac{7}{12}$	$\frac{1}{20}$

	48			
	ξ_2'	ξ_3'	ξ_4'	ξ_5'
	−575	−115	+16445	+82225
	−569	−343	+15873	+242671
	−557	−565	+14743	+391231
	−539	−777	+13083	+520401
	−515	−975	+10935	+623307
	−485	−1155	+8355	+693957
	−449	−1313	+5413	+727493
	−407	−1445	+2193	+720443
	−359	−1547	−1207	+670973
	−305	−1615	−4675	+579139
	−245	−1645	−8085	+447139
	−179	−1633	−11297	+279565
	−107	−1575	−14157	+83655
	−29	−1467	−16497	−130455
	+55	−1305	−18135	−349479
	+145	−1085	−18875	−556729
	+241	−803	−18507	−731863
	+343	−455	−16807	−850633
	+451	−37	−13537	−884633
	+565	+455	−8445	−801047
	+685	+1025	−1265	−562397
	+811	+1677	+8283	−126291
	+943	+2415	+20493	+554829
	+1081	+3243	+35673	+1533939
D	12,712,560	92,620,080	10,301,411,120	19,208,385,771,120
λ	3	$\frac{2}{3}$	$\frac{7}{12}$	$\frac{21}{10}$

ORTHOGONAL POLYNOMIALS

	49			
	ξ_2'	ξ_3'	ξ_4'	ξ_5'
	−200	0	+17940	0
	−199	−299	+17641	+9867
	−196	−593	+16751	+19272
	−191	−877	+15291	+27767
	−184	−1146	+13296	+34932
	−175	−1395	+10815	+40389
	−164	−1619	+7911	+43816
	−151	−1813	+4661	+44961
	−136	−1972	+1156	+43656
	−119	−2091	−2499	+39831
	−100	−2165	−6185	+33528
	−79	−2189	−9769	+24915
	−56	−2158	−13104	+14300
	−31	−2067	−16029	+2145
	−4	−1911	−18369	−10920
	+25	−1685	−19935	−24083
	+56	−1384	−20524	−36336
	+89	−1003	−19919	−46461
	+124	−537	−17889	−53016
	+161	+19	−14189	−54321
	+200	+670	−8560	−48444
	+241	+1421	−729	−33187
	+284	+2277	+9591	−6072
	+329	+3243	+22701	+35673
	+376	+4324	+38916	+95128
D	1,566,040	167,230,700	12,408,517,940	74,451,107,640
λ	1	$\frac{5}{6}$	$\frac{7}{12}$	$\frac{7}{60}$

ORTHOGONAL POLYNOMIALS

	50			
	ξ_2'	ξ_3'	ξ_4'	ξ_5'
	−104	−312	+96876	+10764
	−103	−931	+93771	+31809
	−101	−1535	+87631	+51419
	−98	−2114	+78596	+68684
	−94	−2658	+66876	+82764
	−89	−3157	+52751	+92917
	−83	−3601	+36571	−98527
	−76	−3980	+18756	−99132
	−68	−4284	−204	+94452
	−59	−4503	−19749	+84417
	−49	−4627	−39249	+69195
	−38	−4646	−58004	+49220
	−26	−4550	−75244	+25220
	−13	−4329	−90129	−1755
	+1	−3973	−101749	−30305
	+16	−3472	−109124	−58652
	+32	−2816	−111204	−84612
	+49	−1995	−106869	−105567
	+67	−999	−94929	−118437
	+86	+182	−74124	−119652
	+106	+1558	−43124	−105124
	+127	+3139	−529	−70219
	+149	+4935	+55131	−9729
	+172	+6956	+125396	+82156
	+196	+9212	+211876	+211876
D	433,160	770,715,400	372,255,538,200	372,255,538,200
λ	$\frac{1}{2}$	$\frac{5}{3}$	$\frac{35}{12}$	$\frac{7}{30}$

XIII. MISCELLANEOUS MATHEMATICAL TABLES

XIII.1 EXPONENTIAL FUNCTIONS

x	e^x	e^{-x}	x	e^x	e^{-x}
0.00	1.0000	1.000000	**0.50**	1.6487	0.606531
0.01	1.0101	0.990050	0.51	1.6653	.600496
0.02	1.0202	.980199	0.52	1.6820	.594521
0.03	1.0305	.970446	0.53	1.6989	.588605
0.04	1.0408	.960789	0.54	1.7160	.582748
0.05	1.0513	0.951229	**0.55**	1.7333	0.576950
0.06	1.0618	.941765	0.56	1.7507	.571209
0.07	1.0725	.932394	0.57	1.7683	.565525
0.08	1.0833	.923116	0.58	1.7860	.559898
0.09	1.0942	.913931	0.59	1.8040	.554327
0.10	1.1052	0.904837	**0.60**	1.8221	0.548812
0.11	1.1163	.895834	0.61	1.8404	.543351
0.12	1.1275	.886920	0.62	1.8589	.537944
0.13	1.1388	.878095	0.63	1.8776	.532592
0.14	1.1503	.869358	0.64	1.8965	.527292
0.15	1.1618	0.860708	**0.65**	1.9155	0.522046
0.16	1.1735	.852144	0.66	1.9348	.516851
0.17	1.1853	.843665	0.67	1.9542	.511709
0.18	1.1972	.835270	0.68	1.9739	.506617
0.19	1.2092	.826959	0.69	1.9937	.501576
0.20	1.2214	0.818731	**0.70**	2.0138	0.496585
0.21	1.2337	.810584	0.71	2.0340	.491644
0.22	1.2461	.802519	0.72	2.0544	.486752
0.23	1.2586	.794534	0.73	2.0751	.481909
0.24	1.2712	.786628	0.74	2.0959	.477114
0.25	1.2840	0.778801	**0.75**	2.1170	0.472367
0.26	1.2969	.771052	0.76	2.1383	.467666
0.27	1.3100	.763379	0.77	2.1598	.463013
0.28	1.3231	.755784	0.78	2.1815	.458406
0.29	1.3364	.748264	0.79	2.2034	.453845
0.30	1.3499	0.740818	**0.80**	2.2255	0.449329
0.31	1.3634	.733447	0.81	2.2479	.444858
0.32	1.3771	.726149	0.82	2.2705	.440432
0.33	1.3910	.718924	0.83	2.2933	.436049
0.34	1.4049	.711770	0.84	2.3164	.431711
0.35	1.4191	0.704688	**0.85**	2.3396	0.427415
0.36	1.4333	.697676	0.86	2.3632	.423162
0.37	1.4477	.690734	0.87	2.3869	.418952
0.38	1.4623	.683861	0.88	2.4109	.414783
0.39	1.4770	.677057	0.89	2.4351	.410656
0.40	1.4918	0.670320	**0.90**	2.4596	0.406570
0.41	1.5068	.663650	0.91	2.4843	.402524
0.42	1.5220	.657047	0.92	2.5093	.398519
0.43	1.5373	.650509	0.93	2.5345	.394554
0.44	1.5527	.644036	0.94	2.5600	.390628
0.45	1.5683	0.637628	**0.95**	2.5857	0.386741
0.46	1.5841	.631284	0.96	2.6117	.382893
0.47	1.6000	.625002	0.97	2.6379	.379083
0.48	1.6161	.618783	0.98	2.6645	.375311
0.49	1.6323	.612626	0.99	2.6912	.371577
0.50	1.6487	0.606531	**1.00**	2.7183	0.367879

EXPONENTIAL FUNCTIONS

x	e^x	e^{-x}	x	e^x	e^{-x}
1.00	2.7183	0.367879	**1.50**	4.4817	0.223130
1.01	2.7456	.364219	1.51	4.5267	.220910
1.02	2.7732	.360595	1.52	4.5722	.218712
1.03	2.8011	.357007	1.53	4.6182	.216536
1.04	2.8292	.353455	1.54	4.6646	.214381
1.05	2.8577	0.349938	**1.55**	4.7115	0.212248
1.06	2.8864	.346456	1.56	4.7588	.210136
1.07	2.9154	.343009	1.57	4.8066	.208045
1.08	2.9447	.339596	1.58	4.8550	.205975
1.09	2.9743	.336216	1.59	4.9037	.203926
1.10	3.0042	0.332871	**1.60**	4.9530	0.201897
1.11	3.0344	.329559	1.61	5.0028	.199888
1.12	3.0649	.326280	1.62	5.0531	.197899
1.13	3.0957	.323033	1.63	5.1039	.195930
1.14	3.1268	.319819	1.64	5.1552	.193980
1.15	3.1582	0.316637	**1.65**	5.2070	0.192050
1.16	3.1899	.313486	1.66	5.2593	.190139
1.17	3.2220	.310367	1.67	5.3122	.188247
1.18	3.2544	.307279	1.68	5.3656	.186374
1.19	3.2871	.304221	1.69	5.4195	.184520
1.20	3.3201	0.301194	**1.70**	5.4739	0.182684
1.21	3.3535	.298197	1.71	5.5290	.180866
1.22	3.3872	.295230	1.72	5.5845	.179066
1.23	3.4212	.292293	1.73	5.6407	.177284
1.24	3.4556	.289384	1 74	5.6973	175520
1.25	3.4903	0.286505	**1.75**	5.7546	0.173774
1.26	3.5254	.283654	1.76	5.8124	.172045
1.27	3.5609	.280832	1.77	5.8709	170333
1.28	3.5966	.278037	1.78	5.9299	168638
1.29	3.6328	.275271	1.79	5.9895	.166960
1.30	3.6693	0.272532	**1.80**	6.0496	0.165299
1.31	3.7062	.269820	1.81	6.1104	.163654
1.32	3.7434	.267135	1.82	6.1719	.162026
1.33	3.7810	.264477	1.83	6.2339	.160414
1.34	3.8190	.261846	1.84	6.2965	.158817
1.35	3.8574	0.259240	**1.85**	6.3598	0.157237
1.36	3.8962	.256661	1.86	6.4237	.155673
1.37	3.9354	.254107	1.87	6.4883	.154124
1.38	3.9749	.251579	1.88	6.5535	.152590
1.39	4.0149	.249075	1.89	6.6194	.151072
1.40	4.0552	0.246597	**1.90**	6.6859	0.149569
1.41	4.0960	.244143	1.91	6.7531	.148080
1.42	4.1371	.241714	1.92	6.8210	.146607
1.43	4.1787	.239309	1.93	6.8895	.145148
1.44	4.2207	.236928	1.94	6.9588	.143704
1.45	4.2631	0.234570	**1.95**	7.0287	0.142274
1.46	4.3060	.232236	1.96	7.0993	.140858
1.47	4.3492	.229925	1.97	7.1707	.139457
1.48	4.3929	.227638	1.98	7.2427	.138069
1.49	4.4371	.225373	1.99	7.3155	.136695
1.50	4.4817	0.223130	**2.00**	7.3891	0.135335

EXPONENTIAL FUNCTIONS

x	e^x	e^{-x}	x	e^x	e^{-x}
2.00	7.3891	0.135335	**2.50**	12.182	0.082085
2.01	7.4633	.133989	2.51	12.305	.081268
2.02	7.5383	.132655	2.52	12.429	.080460
2.03	7.6141	.131336	2.53	12.554	.079659
2.04	7.6906	.130029	2.54	12.680	.078866
2.05	7.7679	0.128735	**2.55**	12.807	0.078082
2.06	7.8460	.127454	2.56	12.936	.077305
2.07	7.9248	.126186	2.57	13.066	.076536
2.08	8.0045	.124930	2.58	13.197	.075774
2.09	8.0849	.123687	2.59	13.330	.075020
2.10	8.1662	0.122456	**2.60**	13.464	0.074274
2.11	8.2482	.121238	2.61	13.599	.073535
2.12	8.3311	.120032	2.62	13.736	.072803
2.13	8.4149	.118837	2.63	13.874	.072078
2.14	8.4994	.117655	2.64	14.013	.071361
2.15	8.5849	0.116484	**2.65**	14.154	0.070651
2.16	8.6711	.115325	2.66	14.296	.069948
2.17	8.7583	.114178	2.67	14.440	.069252
2.18	8.8463	.113042	2.68	14.585	.068563
2.19	8.9352	.111917	2.69	14.732	.067881
2.20	9.0250	0.110803	**2.70**	14.880	0.067206
2.21	9.1157	.109701	2.71	15.029	.066537
2.22	9.2073	.108609	2.72	15.180	.065875
2.23	9.2999	.107528	2.73	15.333	.065219
2.24	9.3933	.106459	2.74	15.487	.064570
2.25	9.4877	0.105399	**2.75**	15.643	0.063928
2.26	9.5831	.104350	2.76	15.800	.063292
2.27	9.6794	.103312	2.77	15.959	.062662
2.28	9.7767	.102284	2.78	16.119	.062039
2.29	9.8749	.101266	2.79	16.281	.061421
2.30	9.9742	0.100259	**2.80**	16.445	0.060810
2.31	10.074	.099261	2.81	16.610	.060205
2.32	10.176	.098274	2.82	16.777	.059606
2.33	10.278	.097296	2.83	16.945	.059013
2.34	10.381	.096328	2.84	17.116	.058426
2.35	10.486	0.095369	**2.85**	17.288	0.057844
2.36	10.591	.094420	2.86	17.462	.057269
2.37	10.697	.093481	2.87	17.637	.056699
2.38	10.805	.092551	2.88	17.814	.056135
2.39	10.913	.091630	2.89	17.993	.055576
2.40	11.023	0.090718	**2.90**	18.174	0.055023
2.41	11.134	.089815	2.91	18.357	.054476
2.42	11.246	.088922	2.92	18.541	.053934
2.43	11.359	.088037	2.93	18.728	.053397
2.44	11.473	.087161	2.94	18.916	.052866
2.45	11.588	0.086294	**2.95**	19.106	0.052340
2.46	11.705	.085435	2.96	19.298	.051819
2.47	11.822	.084585	2.97	19.492	.051303
2.48	11.941	.083743	2.98	19.688	.050793
2.49	12.061	.082910	2.99	19.886	.050287
2.50	12.182	0.082085	**3.00**	20.086	0.049787

EXPONENTIAL FUNCTIONS

x	e^x	e^{-x}	x	e^x	e^{-x}
3.00	20.086	0.049787	**3.50**	33.115	0.030197
3.01	20.287	.049292	3.51	33.448	.029897
3.02	20.491	.048801	3.52	33.784	.029599
3.03	20.697	.048316	3.53	34.124	.029305
3.04	20.905	.047835	3.54	34.467	.029013
3.05	21.115	0.047359	**3.55**	34.813	0.028725
3.06	21.328	.046888	3.56	35.163	.028439
3.07	21.542	.046421	3.57	35.517	.028156
3.08	21.758	.045959	3.58	35.874	.027876
3.09	21.977	.045502	3.59	36.234	.027598
3.10	22.198	0.045049	**3.60**	36.598	0.027324
3.11	22.421	.044601	3.61	36.966	.027052
3.12	22.646	.044157	3.62	37.338	.026783
3.13	22.874	.043718	3.63	37.713	.026516
3.14	23.104	.043283	3.64	38.092	.026252
3.15	23.336	0.042852	**3.65**	38.475	0.025991
3.16	23.571	.042426	3.66	38.861	.025733
3.17	23.807	.042004	3.67	39.252	.025476
3.18	24.047	.041586	3.68	39.646	.025223
3.19	24.288	.041172	3.69	40.045	.024972
3.20	24.533	0.040762	**3.70**	40.447	0.024724
3.21	24.779	.040357	3.71	40.854	.024478
3.22	25.028	.039955	3.72	41.264	.024234
3.23	25.280	.039557	3.73	41.679	.023993
3.24	25.534	.039164	3.74	42.098	.023754
3.25	25.790	0.038774	**3.75**	42.521	0.023518
3.26	26.050	.038388	3.76	42.948	.023284
3.27	26.311	.038006	3.77	43.380	.023052
3.28	26.576	.037628	3.78	43.816	.022823
3.29	26.843	.037254	3.79	44.256	.022596
3.30	27.113	0.036883	**3.80**	44.701	0.022371
3.31	27.385	.036516	3.81	45.150	.022148
3.32	27.660	.036153	3.82	45.604	.021928
3.33	27.938	.035793	3.83	46.063	.021710
3.34	28.219	.035437	3.84	46.525	.021494
3.35	28.503	0.035084	**3.85**	46.993	0.021280
3.36	28.789	.034735	3.86	47.465	.021068
3.37	29.079	.034390	3.87	47.942	.020858
3.38	29.371	.034047	3.88	48.424	.020651
3.39	29.666	.033709	3.89	48.911	.020445
3.40	29.964	0.033373	**3.90**	49.402	0.020242
3.41	30.265	.033041	3.91	49.899	.020041
3.42	30.569	.032712	3.92	50.400	.019841
3.43	30.877	.032387	3.93	50.907	.019644
3.44	31.187	.032065	3.94	51.419	.019448
3.45	31.500	0.031746	**3.95**	51.935	0.019255
3.46	31.817	.031430	3.96	52.457	.019063
3.47	32.137	.031117	3.97	52.985	.018873
3.48	32.460	.030807	3.98	53.517	.018686
3.49	32.786	.030501	3.99	54.055	.018500
3.50	33.115	0.030197	**4.00**	54.598	0.018316

EXPONENTIAL FUNCTIONS

x	e^x	e^{-x}	x	e^x	e^{-x}
4.00	54.598	0.018316	**4.50**	90.017	0.011109
4.01	55.147	.018133	4.51	90.922	.010998
4.02	55.701	.017953	4.52	91.836	.010889
4.03	56.261	.017774	4.53	92.759	.010781
4.04	56.826	.017597	4.54	93.691	.010673
4.05	57.397	0.017422	**4.55**	94.632	0.010567
4.06	57.974	.017249	4.56	95.583	.010462
4.07	58.557	.017077	4.57	96.544	.010358
4.08	59.145	.016907	4.58	97.514	.010255
4.09	59.740	.016739	4.59	98.494	.010153
4.10	60.340	0.016573	**4.60**	99.484	0.010052
4.11	60.947	.016408	4.61	100.48	.009952
4.12	61.559	.016245	4.62	101.49	.009853
4.13	62.178	.016083	4.63	102.51	.009755
4.14	62.803	.015923	4.64	103.54	.009658
4.15	63.434	0.015764	**4.65**	104.58	0.009562
4.16	64.072	.015608	4.66	105.64	.009466
4.17	64.715	.015452	4.67	106.70	.009372
4.18	65.366	.015299	4.68	107.77	.009279
4.19	66.023	.015146	4.69	108.85	.009187
4.20	66.686	0.014996	**4.70**	109.95	0.009095
4.21	67.357	.014846	4.71	111.05	.009005
4.22	68.033	.014699	4.72	112.17	.008915
4.23	68.717	.014552	4.73	113.30	.008826
4.24	69.408	.014408	4.74	114.43	.008739
4.25	70.105	0.014264	**4.75**	115.58	0.008652
4.26	70.810	.014122	4.76	116.75	.008566
4.27	71.522	.013982	4.77	117.92	.008480
4.28	72.240	.013843	4.78	119.10	.008396
4.29	72.966	.013705	4.79	120.30	.008312
4.30	73.700	0.013569	**4.80**	121.51	0.008230
4.31	74.440	.013434	4.81	122.73	.008148
4.32	75.189	.013300	4.82	123.97	.008067
4.33	75.944	.013168	4.83	125.21	.007987
4.34	76.708	.013037	4.84	126.47	.007907
4.35	77.478	0.012907	**4.85**	127.74	0.007828
4.36	78.257	.012778	4.86	129.02	.007750
4.37	79.044	.012651	4.87	130.32	.007673
4.38	79.838	.012525	4.88	131.63	.007597
4.39	80.640	.012401	4.89	132.95	.007521
4.40	81.451	0.012277	**4.90**	134.29	0.007447
4.41	82.269	.012155	4.91	135.64	.007372
4.42	83.096	.012034	4.92	137.00	.007299
4.43	83.931	.011914	4.93	138.38	.007227
4.44	84.775	.011796	4.94	139.77	.007155
4.45	85.627	0.011679	**4.95**	141.17	0.007083
4.46	86.488	.011562	4.96	142.59	.007013
4.47	87.357	.011447	4.97	144.03	.006943
4.48	88.235	.011333	4.98	145.47	.006874
4.49	89.121	.011221	4.99	146.94	.006806
4.50	90.017	0.011109	**5.00**	148.41	0.006738

EXPONENTIAL FUNCTIONS

x	e^x	e^{-x}	x	e^x	e^{-x}
5.00	148.41	0.006738	**5.50**	244.69	0.0040868
5.01	149.90	.006671	5.55	257.24	.0038875
5.02	151.41	.006605	5.60	270.43	.0036979
5.03	152.93	.006539	5.65	284.29	.0035175
5.04	154.47	.006474	5.70	298.87	.0033460
5.05	156.02	0.006409	**5.75**	314.19	0.0031828
5.06	157.59	.006346	5.80	330.30	.0030276
5.07	159.17	.006282	5.85	347.23	.0028799
5.08	160.77	.006220	5.90	365.04	.0027394
5.09	162.39	.006158	5.95	383.75	.0026058
5.10	164.02	0.006097	**6.00**	403.43	0.0024788
5.11	165.67	.006036	6.05	424.11	.0023579
5.12	167.34	.005976	6.10	445.86	.0022429
5.13	169.02	.005917	6.15	468.72	.0021335
5.14	170.72	.005858	6.20	492.75	.0020294
5.15	172.43	0.005799	**6.25**	518.01	0.0019305
5.16	174.16	.005742	6.30	544.57	.0018363
5.17	175.91	.005685	6.35	572.49	.0017467
5.18	177.68	.005628	6.40	601.85	.0016616
5.19	179.47	.005572	6.45	632.70	.0015805
5.20	181.27	0.005517	**6.50**	665.14	0.0015034
5.21	183.09	.005462	6.55	699.24	.0014301
5.22	184.93	.005407	6.60	735.10	.0013604
5.23	186.79	.005354	6.65	772.78	.0012940
5.24	188.67	.005300	6.70	812.41	.0012309
5.25	190.57	0.005248	**6.75**	854.06	0.0011709
5.26	192.48	.005195	6.80	897.85	.0011138
5.27	194.42	.005144	6.85	943.88	.0010595
5.28	196.37	.005092	6.90	992.27	.0010078
5.29	198.34	.005042	6.95	1043.1	.0009586
5.30	200.34	0.004992	**7.00**	1096.6	0.0009119
5.31	202.35	.004942	7.05	1152.9	.0008674
5.32	204.38	.004893	7.10	1212.0	.0008251
5.33	206.44	.004844	7.15	1274.1	.0007849
5.34	208.51	.004796	7.20	1339.4	.0007466
5.35	210.61	0.004748	**7.25**	1408.1	0.0007102
5.36	212.72	.004701	7.30	1480.3	.0006755
5.37	214.86	.004654	7.35	1556.2	.0006426
5.38	217.02	.004608	7.40	1636.0	.0006113
5.39	219.20	.004562	7.45	1719.9	.0005814
5.40	221.41	0.004517	**7.50**	1808.0	0.0005531
5.41	223.63	.004472	7.55	1900.7	.0005261
5.42	225.88	.004427	7.60	1998.2	.0005005
5.43	228.15	.004383	7.65	2100.6	.0004760
5.44	230.44	.004339	7.70	2208.3	.0004528
5.45	232.76	0.004296	**7.75**	2321.6	0.0004307
5.46	235.10	.004254	7.80	2440.6	.0004097
5.47	237.46	.004211	7.85	2565.7	.0003898
5.48	239.85	.004169	7.90	2697.3	.0003707
5.49	242.26	.004128	7.95	2835.6	.0003527
5.50	244.69	0.004087	**8.00**	2981.0	0.0003355

EXPONENTIAL FUNCTIONS

x	e^x	e^{-x}	x	e^x	e^{-x}
8.00	2981.0	0.0003355	**9.00**	8103.1	0.0001234
8.05	3133.8	.0003191	9.05	8518.5	.0001174
8.10	3294.5	.0003035	9.10	8955.3	.0001117
8.15	3463.4	.0002887	9.15	9414.4	.0001062
8.20	3641.0	.0002747	9.20	9897.1	.0001010
8.25	3827.6	0.0002613	**9.25**	10405	0.0000961
8.30	4023.9	.0002485	9.30	10938	.0000914
8.35	4230.2	.0002364	9.35	11499	.0000870
8.40	4447.1	.0002249	9.40	12088	.0000827
8.45	4675.1	.0002139	9.45	12708	.0000787
8.50	4914.8	0.0002035	**9.50**	13360	0.0000749
8.55	5166.8	.0001935	9.55	14045	.0000712
8.60	5431.7	.0001841	9.60	14765	.0000677
8.65	5710.1	.0001751	9.65	15522	.0000644
8.70	6002.9	.0001666	9.70	16318	.0000613
8.75	6310.7	0.0001585	**9.75**	17154	0.0000583
8.80	6634.2	.0001507	9.80	18034	.0000555
8.85	6974.4	.0001434	9.85	18958	.0000527
8.90	7332.0	.0001364	9.90	19930	.0000502
8.95	7707.9	.0001297	9.95	20952	0.0000477
9.00	8103.1	0.0001234	10.00	22026	0.0000454

XIII.2 SUMS OF POWERS OF INTEGERS $\sum_{k=1}^{n} k^m$

$(m = 1, 2, 3, 4);\ 1 \leq n \leq 40$

n	Σk	Σk^2	Σk^3	Σk^4
1	1	1	1	1
2	3	5	9	17
3	6	14	36	98
4	10	30	100	354
5	15	55	225	979
6	21	91	441	2275
7	28	140	784	4676
8	36	204	1296	8772
9	45	285	2025	15333
10	55	385	3025	25333
11	66	506	4356	39974
12	78	650	6084	60710
13	91	819	8281	89271
14	105	1015	11025	127687
15	120	1240	14400	178312
16	136	1496	18496	243848
17	153	1785	23409	327369
18	171	2109	29241	432345
19	190	2470	36100	562666
20	210	2870	44100	722666
21	231	3311	53361	917147
22	253	3795	64009	1151403
23	276	4324	76176	1431244
24	300	4900	90000	1763020
25	325	5525	105625	2153645
26	351	6201	123201	2610621
27	378	6930	142884	3142062
28	406	7714	164836	3756718
29	435	8555	189225	4463999
30	465	9455	216225	5273999
31	496	10416	246016	6197520
32	528	11440	278784	7246096
33	561	12529	314721	8432017
34	595	13685	354025	9768353
35	630	14910	396900	11268978
36	666	16206	443556	12948594
37	703	17575	494209	14822755
38	741	19019	549081	16907891
39	780	20540	608400	19221332
40	820	22140	672400	21781332

SUMS OF POWERS OF THE FIRST n INTEGERS

$$\sum_{k=1}^{n} k = 1 + 2 + 3 + \cdots + n = \frac{n(n+1)}{2}$$

$$\sum_{k=1}^{n} k^2 = 1^2 + 2^2 + 3^2 + \cdots + n^2 = \frac{n(n+1)(2n+1)}{6}$$

$$\sum_{k=1}^{n} k^3 = \frac{n^2(n+1)^2}{4}$$

$$\sum_{k=1}^{n} k^4 = \frac{n}{30}(n+1)(2n+1)(3n^2+3n-1).$$

$$\sum_{k=1}^{n} k^5 = \frac{n^2}{12}(n+1)^2(2n^2+2n-1).$$

$$\sum_{k=1}^{n} k^6 = \frac{n}{42}(n+1)(2n+1)(3n^4+6n^3-3n+1).$$

$$\sum_{k=1}^{n} k^7 = \frac{n^2}{24}(n+1)^2(3n^4+6n^3-n^2-4n+2).$$

$$\sum_{k=1}^{n} k^8 = \frac{n}{90}(n+1)(2n+1)(5n^6+15n^5+5n^4-15n^3-n^2+9n-3).$$

$$\sum_{k=1}^{n} k^9 = \frac{n^2}{20}(n+1)^2(2n^6+6n^5+n^4-8n^3+n^2+6n-3).$$

$$\sum_{k=1}^{n} k^{10} = \frac{n}{66}(n+1)(2n+1)(3n^8+12n^7+8n^6-18n^5 - 10n^4+24n^3+2n^2-15n+5).$$

Note that

$\sum_{k=1}^{n} k^p = 1^p + 2^p + 3^p + \cdots + n^p$ is a function of n which can be conveniently generated by use of the *following proposition*

If
$$\sum_{k=1}^{n} k^p = a_1 n^{p+1} + a_2 n^p + a_3 n^{p-1} + \cdots + a_{p+1} n$$

then

$$\sum_{k=1}^{n} k^{p+1} = \frac{p+1}{p+2} a_1 n^{p+2} + \frac{p+1}{p+1} a_2 n^{p+1} + \frac{p+1}{p} a_3 n^p + \cdots + \frac{p+1}{2} a_{p+1} n^2 + \left[1 - (p+1)\sum_{k=1}^{p+1} \frac{a_k}{(p+3-k)}\right] n$$

Example *Since* $\sum_{k=1}^{n} k = \frac{1}{2}n^2 + \frac{1}{2}n$, then

$$\sum_{k=1}^{n} k^2 = \frac{1}{3}n^3 + \frac{1}{2}n^2 + \frac{1}{6}n$$ and from this result

$$\sum_{k=1}^{n} k^3 = \frac{1}{4}n^4 + \frac{1}{2}n^3 + \frac{1}{4}n^2 \quad \text{etc.}$$

This proposition is extracted from a paper written by Michael A. Budin and Arnold J. Cantor entitled "Simplified Computation of Sums of Powers of Integers."

XIII.3 FACTORIALS, EXACT VALUES

n	$n!$
0	1 (by definition)
1	1
2	2
3	6
4	24
5	120
6	720
7	5040
8	40,320
9	362,880
10	3,628,800
11	39,916,800
12	479,001,600
13	6,227,020,800
14	87,178,291,200
15	1,307,674,368,000
16	20,922,789,888,000
17	355,687,428,096,000
18	6,402,373,705,728,000
19	121,645,100,408,832,000
20	2,432,902,008,176,640,000
21	51,090,942,171,709,440,000
22	1,124,000,727,777,607,680,000
23	25,852,016,738,884,976,640,000
24	620,448,401,733,239,439,360,000
25	15,511,210,043,330,985,984,000,000
26	403,291,461,126,605,635,584,000,000
27	10,888,869,450,418,352,160,768,000,000
28	304,888,344,611,713,860,501,504,000,000
29	8,841,761,993,739,701,954,543,616,000,000
30	265,252,859,812,191,058,636,308,480,000,000
31	8.22284×10^{33}
32	2.63131×10^{35}
33	8.68332×10^{36}
34	2.95233×10^{38}
35	1.03331×10^{40}
36	3.71993×10^{41}
37	1.37638×10^{43}
38	5.23023×10^{44}
39	2.03979×10^{46}

$\underline{|n} = n! = e^{-n} n^n \sqrt{2\pi n}$. approximately, known as Stirling's formula

$\log_e n! = n \log_e n - n$, approximately.

XIII.4 SPECIAL FUNCTIONS

The Gamma Function

Definition: $\Gamma(n) = \int_0^\infty t^{n-1} e^{-t} dt \quad n > 0$

Recursion Formula: $\Gamma(n+1) = n\Gamma(n)$

$\Gamma(n+1) = n!$ if $n = 0,1,2,\ldots$ where $0! = 1$

For $n < 0$ the gamma function can be defined by using

$$\Gamma(n) = \frac{\Gamma(n+1)}{n}$$

Graph:

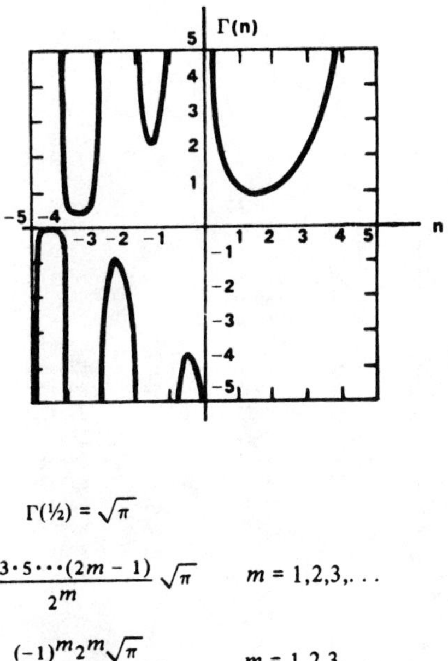

Special Values: $\Gamma(\tfrac{1}{2}) = \sqrt{\pi}$

$$\Gamma(m + \tfrac{1}{2}) = \frac{1 \cdot 3 \cdot 5 \cdots (2m-1)}{2^m}\sqrt{\pi} \qquad m = 1,2,3,\ldots$$

$$\Gamma(-m + \tfrac{1}{2}) = \frac{(-1)^m 2^m \sqrt{\pi}}{1 \cdot 3 \cdot 5 \cdots (2m-1)} \qquad m = 1,2,3,\ldots$$

Definition: $$\Gamma(x+1) = \lim_{k \to \infty} \frac{1 \cdot 2 \cdot 3 \cdots k}{(x+1)(x+2)\cdots(x+k)} k^x$$

$$\frac{1}{\Gamma(x)} = x e^{\gamma x} \prod_{m=1}^{\infty} \left\{ \left(1 + \frac{x}{m}\right) e^{-x/m} \right\}$$

This is an infinite product representation for the gamma function where γ is Euler's constant.

Properties:

$$\Gamma'(1) = \int_0^\infty e^{-x} \ln x \, dx = -\gamma$$

$$\frac{\Gamma'(x)}{\Gamma(x)} = -\gamma + \left(\frac{1}{1} - \frac{1}{x}\right) + \left(\frac{1}{2} - \frac{1}{x+1}\right) + \ldots + \left(\frac{1}{n} - \frac{1}{x+n-1}\right) + \ldots$$

$$\Gamma(x+1) = \sqrt{2\pi x}\, x^x e^{-x} \left\{1 + \frac{1}{12x} + \frac{1}{288x^2} - \frac{139}{51{,}840x^3} + \ldots\right\}$$

This is called *Stirling's asymptotic series.*

If we let $x = n$ a positive integer, then a useful approximation for $n!$ where n is large [e.g. $n > 10$] is given by *Stirling's formula*

$$n! \approx \sqrt{2\pi n}\, n^n e^{-n}$$

GAMMA FUNCTION*

Values of $\Gamma(n) = \int_0^\infty e^{-x} x^{n-1} dx; \Gamma(n+1) = n\Gamma(n)$

n	$\Gamma(n)$	n	$\Gamma(n)$	n	$\Gamma(n)$	n	$\Gamma(n)$
1.00	1.00000	1.25	.90640	1.50	.88623	1.75	.91906
1.01	.99433	1.26	.90440	1.51	.88659	1.76	.92137
1.02	.98884	1.27	.90250	1.52	.88704	1.77	.92376
1.03	.98355	1.28	.90072	1.53	.88757	1.78	.92623
1.04	.97844	1.29	.89904	1.54	.88818	1.79	.92877
1.05	.97350	1.30	.89747	1.55	.88887	1.80	.93138
1.06	.96874	1.31	.89600	1.56	.88964	1.81	.93408
1.07	.96415	1.32	.89464	1.57	.89049	1.82	.93685
1.08	.95973	1.33	.89338	1.58	.89142	1.83	.93969
1.09	.95546	1.34	.89222	1.59	.89243	1.84	.94261
1.10	.95135	1.35	.89115	1.60	.89352	1.85	.94561
1.11	.94740	1.36	.89018	1.61	.89468	1.86	.94869
1.12	.94359	1.37	.88931	1.62	.89592	1.87	.95184
1.13	.93993	1.38	.88854	1.63	.89724	1.88	.95507
1.14	.93642	1.39	.88785	1.64	.89864	1.89	.95838
1.15	.93304	1.40	.88726	1.65	.90012	1.90	.96177
1.16	.92980	1.41	.88676	1.66	.90167	1.91	.96523
1.17	.92670	1.42	.88636	1.67	.90330	1.92	.96877
1.18	.92373	1.43	.88604	1.68	.90500	1.93	.97240
1.19	.92089	1.44	.88581	1.69	.90678	1.94	.97610
1.20	.91817	1.45	.88566	1.70	.90864	1.95	.97988
1.21	.91558	1.46	.88560	1.71	.91057	1.96	.98374
1.22	.91311	1.47	.88563	1.72	.91258	1.97	.98768
1.23	.91075	1.48	.88575	1.73	.91466	1.98	.99171
1.24	.90852	1.49	.88595	1.74	.91683	1.99	.99581
						2.00	1.00000

* For large positive values of x, $\Gamma(x)$ approximates Stirling's asymptotic series

$$x^x e^{-x} \sqrt{\frac{2\pi}{x}} \left[1 + \frac{1}{12x} + \frac{1}{288x^2} - \frac{139}{51840x^3} - \frac{571}{2488320x^4} + \cdots\right]$$

The Beta Function

Definition: $B(m,n) = \int_0^1 t^{m-1}(1-t)^{n-1}dt \quad m > 0, n > 0$

Relationship with Gamma Function $B(m,n) = \dfrac{\Gamma(m)\Gamma(n)}{\Gamma(m+n)}$

Properties:

$$B(m,n) = B(n,m)$$

$$B(m,n) = 2\int_0^{\pi/2} \sin^{2m-1}\theta \cos^{2n-1}\theta \, d\theta$$

$$B(m,n) = \int_0^{\infty} \frac{t^{m-1}}{(1+t)^{m+n}} dt$$

$$B(m,n) = r^n(r+1)^m \int_0^1 \frac{t^{m-1}(1-t)^{n-1}}{(r+t)^{m+n}} dt$$

The Error Function

Definition: $\operatorname{erf} x = \dfrac{2}{\sqrt{\pi}} \int_0^x e^{-t^2} dt$

Series: $\operatorname{erf} x = \dfrac{2}{\sqrt{\pi}} \left(x - \dfrac{x^3}{3} + \dfrac{1}{2!}\dfrac{x^5}{5} - \dfrac{1}{3!}\dfrac{x^7}{7} + \ldots\right)$

Property: $\operatorname{erf} x = -\operatorname{erf}(-x)$

Relationship with Normal Probability Function f(t): $\int_0^x f(t)\,dt = \dfrac{1}{2}\operatorname{erf}\left(\dfrac{x}{\sqrt{2}}\right)$

To evaluate *erf* (2.3), one proceeds as follows: Since $\dfrac{x}{\sqrt{2}} = 2.3$, one finds $x = (2.3)(\sqrt{2}) = 3.25$. In the normal probability function table (pg. 106), one finds the entry 0.4994 opposite the value 3.25. Thus *erf* (2.3) = 2(0.4994) = 0.9988.

$$\operatorname{erfc} z = 1 - \operatorname{erf} z = \frac{2}{\sqrt{\pi}} \int_z^{\infty} e^{-t^2} dt$$

is known as the complementary error function.

XIII.5 COEFFICIENTS FOR ORTHOGONAL POLYNOMIALS, AND FOR x^m IN TERMS OF ORTHOGONAL POLYNOMIALS[a]

I. Legendre Polynomials: $P_n(x) = a_n^{-1} \sum_{m=0}^{n} c_m x^m \qquad x^n = b_n^{-1} \sum_{m=0}^{n} d_m P_m(x)$

	a_n \ b_n	x^0	x^1	x^2	x^3	x^4	x^5	x^6	x^7
b_n		1	1	3	5	35	63	231	429
P_0	1	1 1		1		7		33	
P_1	1		1 1		3		27		143
P_2	2	−1		3 2		20		110	
P_3	2		−3		5 2		28		182
P_4	8	3		−30		35 8		72	
P_5	8		15		−70		63 8		88
P_6	16	−5		105		−315		231 16	
P_7	16		−35		315		−693		429 16

$P_6(x) = \frac{1}{16}[231x^6 - 315x^4 + 105x^2 - 5] \qquad x^6 = \frac{1}{231}[33P_0 + 110P_2 + 72P_4 + 16P_6]$

II. Tschebysheff Polynomials: $T_n(x) = \sum_{m=0}^{n} c_m x^m \qquad x^n = b_n^{-1} \sum_{m=0}^{n} d_m T_m(x)$

	x^0	x^1	x^2	x^3	x^4	x^5	x^6	x^7
b_n	1	1	2	4	8	16	32	64
T_0	1 1		1		3		10	
T_1		1 1		3		10		35
T_2	−1		2 1		4		15	
T_3		−3		4 1		5		21
T_4	1		−8		8 1		6	
T_5		5		−20		16 1		7
T_6	−1		18		−48		32 1	
T_7		−7		56		−112		64 1

$T_6(x) = 32x^6 - 48x^4 + 18x^2 - 1 \qquad x^6 = \frac{1}{32}[10T_0 + 15T_2 + 6T_4 + T_6]$

III. Tschebysheff Polynomials: $U_n(x) = \sum_{m=0}^{n} c_m x^m \qquad x^n = b_n^{-1} \sum_{m=0}^{n} d_m U_m(x)$

	x^0	x^1	x^2	x^3	x^4	x^5	x^6	x^7
b_n	1	2	4	8	16	32	64	128
U_0	1 1		1		2		5	
U_1		2 1		2		5		14
U_2	−1		4 1		3		9	
U_3		−4		8 1		4		14
U_4	1		−12		16 1		5	
U_5		6		−32		32 1		6
U_6	−1		24		−80		64 1	
U_7		−8		80		−192		128 1

$U_6(x) = 64x^6 - 80x^4 + 24x^2 - 1 \qquad x^6 = \frac{1}{64}[5U_0 + 9U_2 + 5U_4 + U_6]$

Coefficients for Orthogonal Polynomials, and for x^n in Terms of Orthogonal Polynomials[a] (continued)

IV. Jacobi Polynomials $P_n^{(\alpha,\beta)}(x) = a_n^{-1} \sum_{m=0}^{n} c_m (x-1)^m$

	α_n	$(x-1)^0$	$(x-1)^1$	$(x-1)^2$	$(x-1)^3$	$(x-1)^4$	$(x-1)^5$	$(x-1)^6$
$P_0\ (\alpha,\beta)$	1	1						
$P_1\ (\alpha,\beta)$	2	$2(\alpha+1)$	$\alpha+\beta+2$					
$P_2\ (\alpha,\beta)$	8	$4(\alpha+1)_2$	$4(\alpha+\beta+3)(\alpha+2)$	$(\alpha+\beta+3)_2$				
$P_3\ (\alpha,\beta)$	48	$8(\alpha+1)_3$	$12(\alpha+\beta+4)(\alpha+2)_2$	$6(\alpha+\beta+4)_2(\alpha+3)$	$(\alpha+\beta+4)_3$			
$P_4\ (\alpha,\beta)$	384	$16(\alpha+1)_4$	$32(\alpha+\beta+5)(\alpha+2)_3$	$24(\alpha+\beta+5)_2(\alpha+3)_2$	$8(\alpha+\beta+5)_3(\alpha+4)$	$(\alpha+\beta+5)_4$		
$P_5\ (\alpha,\beta)$	3840	$32(\alpha+1)_5$	$80(\alpha+\beta+6)(\alpha+2)_4$	$80(\alpha+\beta+6)_2(\alpha+3)_3$	$40(\alpha+\beta+6)_3(\alpha+4)_2$	$10(\alpha+\beta+6)_4(\alpha+5)$	$(\alpha+\beta+6)_5$	
$P_6\ (\alpha,\beta)$	46080	$64(\alpha+1)_6$	$192(\alpha+\beta+7)(\alpha+2)_5$	$240(\alpha+\beta+7)_2(\alpha+3)_4$	$160(\alpha+\beta+7)_3(\alpha+4)_3$	$60(\alpha+\beta+7)_4(\alpha+5)_2$	$12(\alpha+\beta+7)_5(\alpha+6)$	$(\alpha+\beta+7)_6$

$$(m)_n = m(m+1)(m+2)\ldots(m+n-1)$$

$$P_5^{(1,1)}(x) = \frac{1}{3840}\left[(8)_5(x-1)^5+10(8)_4(6)(x-1)^4+40(8)_2(5)_2(x-1)^3+80(8)_2(4)_3(x-1)^2+80(8)(3)_4(x-1)+32(2)_5\right]$$

$$P_5^{(1,1)}(x) = \frac{1}{3840}\left[95040(x-1)^5+475200(x-1)^4+864000(x-1)^3+691200(x-1)^2+230400(x-1)+23040\right]$$

Coefficients for Orthogonal Polynomials, and for x^n in Terms of Orthogonal Polynomials* (continued)

V. Laguerre Polynomials: $L_n(x) = \sum_{m=0}^{n} c_m x^m \qquad x^n = b_n^{-1} \sum_{m=0}^{n} d_m L_m(x)$

	x^0	x^1	x^2	x^3	x^4	x^5	x^6	x^7
b_m	1	1	2	6	24	120	720	5040
L_0	1 1	1	2	6	24	120	720	5040
L_1	1	−1 −1	−4	−18	−96	−600	−4320	−35280
L_2	2	−4	1 2	18	144	1200	10800	105840
L_3	6	−18	9	−1 −6	−96	−1200	−14400	−176400
L_4	24	−96	72	−16	1 24	600	10800	17640
L_5	120	−600	600	−200	25	−1 −120	−4320	−105840
L_6	720	−4320	5400	−2400	450	−36	1 720	35280
L_7	5040	−35280	52920	−29400	7350	−882	49	−1 −5040

$$L_6(x) = x^6 - 36x^5 + 450x^4 - 2400x^3 + 5400x^2 - 4320x + 720$$

$$x^6 = \frac{1}{720}[720L_0 - 4320L_1 + 10800L_2 - 14400L_3 + 10800L_4 - 4320L_5 + 720L_6]$$

VI. Hermite polynomials: $H_n(x) = \sum_{m=0}^{n} c_m x^m \qquad x^n = b_n^{-1} \sum_{m=0}^{n} d_m H_m(x)$

	x^0	x^1	x^2	x^3	x^4	x^5	x^6	x^7
b_n	1	2	4	8	16	32	64	128
H_0	1 1		2		12		120	
H_1		2 1		6		60		840
H_2	−2		4 1		12		180	
H_3		−12		8 1		20		420
H_4	12		−48		16 1		30	
H_5		120		−160		32 1		42
H_6	−120		720		−480		64 1	
H_7		−1680		3360		−1344		128 1

$$H_6(x) = 64x^6 - 480x^4 + 720x^2 - 120 \qquad x^6 = \frac{1}{64}[120H_0 + 180H_2 + 30H_4 + H_6]$$

Abridged from Abramowitz, M. and Stegun, I. A., Eds., *Handbook of Mathematical Functions*, National Bureau of Standards, Washington, D. C., 1964.

XIII.6 DERIVATIVES*

In the following formulas u, v, w represent functions of x, while a, c, n represent fixed real numbers. All arguments in the trigonometric functions are measured in radians, and all inverse trigonometric and hyperbolic functions represent principal values.

1. $\frac{d}{dx}(a) = 0$

2. $\frac{d}{dx}(x) = 1$

3. $\frac{d}{dx}(au) = a\frac{du}{dx}$

4. $\frac{d}{dx}(u + v - w) = \frac{du}{dx} + \frac{dv}{dx} - \frac{dw}{dx}$

5. $\frac{d}{dx}(uv) = u\frac{dv}{dx} + v\frac{du}{dx}$

6. $\frac{d}{dx}(uvw) = uv\frac{dw}{dx} + vw\frac{du}{dx} + uw\frac{dv}{dx}$ and so on to n factors

7. $\frac{d}{dx}\left(\frac{u}{v}\right) = \frac{v\frac{du}{dx} - u\frac{dv}{dx}}{v^2} = \frac{1}{v}\frac{du}{dx} - \frac{u}{v^2}\frac{dv}{dx}$

8. $\frac{d}{dx}(u^n) = nu^{n-1}\frac{du}{dx}$

9. $\frac{d}{dx}(\sqrt{u}) = \frac{1}{2\sqrt{u}}\frac{du}{dx}$

10. $\frac{d}{dx}\left(\frac{1}{u}\right) = -\frac{1}{u^2}\frac{du}{dx}$

11. $\frac{d}{dx}\left(\frac{1}{u^n}\right) = -\frac{n}{u^{n+1}}\frac{du}{dx}$

12. $\frac{d}{dx}\left(\frac{u^n}{v^m}\right) = \frac{u^{n-1}}{v^{m+1}}\left(nv\frac{du}{dx} - mu\frac{dv}{dx}\right)$

13. $\frac{d}{dx}(u^n v^m) = u^{n-1}v^{m-1}\left(nv\frac{du}{dx} + mu\frac{dv}{dx}\right)$

*Let $y = f(x)$ and $\frac{dy}{dx} = \frac{d[f(x)]}{dx} = f'(x)$ define respectively a function and its derivative for any value x in their common domain. The differential for the function at such a value x is accordingly defined as

$$dy = d[f(x)] = \frac{dy}{dx}dx = \frac{d[f(x)]}{dx}dx = f'(x)dx$$

Each derivative formula has an associated differential formula. For example, formula 6 above has the differential formula

$$d(uvw) = uv\,dw + vw\,du + uw\,dv$$

DERIVATIVES (Continued)

14. $\frac{d}{dx}[f(u)] = \frac{d}{du}[f(u)] \cdot \frac{du}{dx}$

15. $\frac{d^2}{dx^2}[f(u)] = \frac{df(u)}{du} \cdot \frac{d^2u}{dx^2} + \frac{d^2f(u)}{du^2} \cdot \left(\frac{du}{dx}\right)^2$

16. $\frac{d^n}{dx^n}[uv] = \binom{n}{0} v \frac{d^n u}{dx^n} + \binom{n}{1} \frac{dv}{dx} \frac{d^{n-1}u}{dx^{n-1}} + \binom{n}{2} \frac{d^2v}{dx^2} \frac{d^{n-2}u}{dx^{n-2}} + \cdots + \binom{n}{k} \frac{d^kv}{dx^k} \frac{d^{n-k}u}{dx^{n-k}} + \cdots + \binom{n}{n} u \frac{d^nv}{dx^n}$

where $\binom{n}{r} = \frac{n!}{r!(n-r)!}$ the binomial coefficient, n non-negative integer and $\binom{n}{0} = 1$

17. $\frac{du}{dx} = \frac{1}{\frac{dx}{du}}$ if $\frac{dx}{du} \neq 0$

18. $\frac{d}{dx}(\log_a u) = (\log_a e)\frac{1}{u}\frac{du}{dx}$

19. $\frac{d}{dx}(\log_e u) = \frac{1}{u}\frac{du}{dx}$

20. $\frac{d}{dx}(a^u) = a^u(\log_e a)\frac{du}{dx}$

21. $\frac{d}{dx}(e^u) = e^u\frac{du}{dx}$

22. $\frac{d}{dx}(u^v) = vu^{v-1}\frac{du}{dx} + (\log_e u)u^v\frac{dv}{dx}$

23. $\frac{d}{dx}(\sin u) = \frac{du}{dx}(\cos u)$

24. $\frac{d}{dx}(\cos u) = -\frac{du}{dx}(\sin u)$

25. $\frac{d}{dx}(\tan u) = \frac{du}{dx}(\sec^2 u)$

26. $\frac{d}{dx}(\cot u) = -\frac{du}{dx}(\csc^2 u)$

27. $\frac{d}{dx}(\sec u) = \frac{du}{dx}\sec u \cdot \tan u$

28. $\frac{d}{dx}(\csc u) = -\frac{du}{dx}\csc u \cdot \cot u$

29. $\frac{d}{dx}(\text{vers } u) = \frac{du}{dx}\sin u$

DERIVATIVES (Continued)

30. $\frac{d}{dx}(\text{arc sin } u) = \frac{1}{\sqrt{1-u^2}}\frac{du}{dx}, \quad \left(-\frac{\pi}{2} \le \text{arc sin } u \le \frac{\pi}{2}\right)$

31. $\frac{d}{dx}(\text{arc cos } u) = -\frac{1}{\sqrt{1-u^2}}\frac{du}{dx}, \quad (0 \le \text{arc cos } u \le \pi)$

32. $\frac{d}{dx}(\text{arc tan } u) = \frac{1}{1+u^2}\frac{du}{dx}, \quad \left(-\frac{\pi}{2} < \text{arc tan } u < \frac{\pi}{2}\right)$

33. $\frac{d}{dx}(\text{arc cot } u) = -\frac{1}{1+u^2}\frac{du}{dx}, \quad (0 \le \text{arc cot } u \le \pi)$

34. $\frac{d}{dx}(\text{arc sec } u) = \frac{1}{u\sqrt{u^2-1}}\frac{du}{dx}, \quad \left(0 \le \text{arc sec } u < \frac{\pi}{2}, -\pi \le \text{arc sec } u < -\frac{\pi}{2}\right)$

35. $\frac{d}{dx}(\text{arc csc } u) = -\frac{1}{u\sqrt{u^2-1}}\frac{du}{dx}, \quad \left(0 < \text{arc csc } u \le \frac{\pi}{2}, -\pi < \text{arc csc } u \le -\frac{\pi}{2}\right)$

36. $\frac{d}{dx}(\text{arc vers } u) = \frac{1}{\sqrt{2u-u^2}}\frac{du}{dx}, \quad (0 \le \text{arc vers } u \le \pi)$

37. $\frac{d}{dx}(\sinh u) = \frac{du}{dx}(\cosh u)$

38. $\frac{d}{dx}(\cosh u) = \frac{du}{dx}(\sinh u)$

39. $\frac{d}{dx}(\tanh u) = \frac{du}{dx}(\text{sech}^2\, u)$

40. $\frac{d}{dx}(\coth u) = -\frac{du}{dx}(\text{csch}^2\, u)$

41. $\frac{d}{dx}(\text{sech } u) = -\frac{du}{dx}(\text{sech } u \cdot \tanh u)$

42. $\frac{d}{dx}(\text{csch } u) = -\frac{du}{dx}(\text{csch } u \cdot \coth u)$

43. $\frac{d}{dx}(\sinh^{-1} u) = \frac{d}{dx}[\log(u + \sqrt{u^2+1})] = \frac{1}{\sqrt{u^2+1}}\frac{du}{dx}$

44. $\frac{d}{dx}(\cosh^{-1} u) = \frac{d}{dx}[\log(u + \sqrt{u^2-1})] = \frac{1}{\sqrt{u^2-1}}\frac{du}{dx}, \quad (u > 1, \cosh^{-1} u > 0)$

45. $\frac{d}{dx}(\tanh^{-1} u) = \frac{d}{dx}\left[\frac{1}{2}\log\frac{1+u}{1-u}\right] = \frac{1}{1-u^2}\frac{du}{dx}, \quad (u^2 < 1)$

46. $\frac{d}{dx}(\coth^{-1} u) = \frac{d}{dx}\left[\frac{1}{2}\log\frac{u+1}{u-1}\right] = \frac{1}{1-u^2}\frac{du}{dx}, \quad (u^2 > 1)$

47. $\frac{d}{dx}(\text{sech}^{-1} u) = \frac{d}{dx}\left[\log\frac{1+\sqrt{1-u^2}}{u}\right] = -\frac{1}{u\sqrt{1-u^2}}\frac{du}{dx}, \quad (0 < u < 1, \text{sech}^{-1} u > 0)$

DERIVATIVES (Continued)

48. $\frac{d}{dx}(\operatorname{csch}^{-1} u) = \frac{d}{dx}\left[\log \frac{1 + \sqrt{1 + u^2}}{u}\right] = -\frac{1}{|u|\sqrt{1 + u^2}}\frac{du}{dx}$

49. $\frac{d}{dq}\int_p^q f(x)\,dx = f(q),$ [p constant]

50. $\frac{d}{dp}\int_p^q f(x)\,dx = -f(p),$ [q constant]

51. $\frac{d}{da}\int_p^q f(x, a)\,dx = \int_p^q \frac{\partial}{\partial a}[f(x, a)]\,dx + f(q, a)\frac{dq}{da} - f(p, a)\frac{dp}{da}$

XIII.7 INTEGRATION

The following is a brief discussion of some integration techniques. A more complete discussion can be found in a number of good text books. However, the purpose of this introduction is simply to discuss a few of the important techniques which may be used, in conjunction with the integral table which follows, to integrate particular functions.

No matter how extensive the integral table, it is a fairly uncommon occurrence to find in the table the exact integral desired. Usually some form of transformation will have to be made. The simplest type of transformation, and yet the most general, is substitution. Simple forms of substitution, such as $y = ax$, are employed almost unconsciously by experienced users of integral tables. Other substitutions may require more thought. In some sections of the tables, appropriate substitutions are suggested for integrals which are similar to, but not exactly like, integrals in the table. Finding the right substitution is largely a matter of intuition and experience.

Several precautions must be observed when using substitutions:

1. Be sure to make the substitution in the dx term, as well as everywhere else in the integral.
2. Be sure that the function substituted is one-to-one and continuous. If this is not the case, the integral must be restricted in such a way as to make it true. See the example following.
3. With definite integrals, the limits should also be expressed in terms of the new dependent variable. With indefinite integrals, it is necessary to perform the reverse substitution to obtain the answer in terms of the original independent variable. This may also be done for definite integrals, but it is usually easier to change the limits.

Example:

$$\int \frac{x^4}{\sqrt{a^2 - x^2}}\, dx$$

Here we make the substitution $x = |a| \sin\theta$. Then $dx = |a| \cos\theta\, d\theta$, and

$$\sqrt{a^2 - x^2} = \sqrt{a^2 - a^2 \sin^2\theta} = |a|\sqrt{1 - \sin^2\theta} = |a \cos\theta|$$

Notice the absolute value signs. It is very important to keep in mind that a square root radical always denotes the positive square root, and to assure the sign is always kept positive. Thus $\sqrt{x^2} = |x|$. Failure to observe this is a common cause of errors in integration.

Notice also that the indicated substitution is not a one-to-one function, that is, it does not have a unique inverse. Thus we must restrict the range of θ in such a way as to make the function one-to-one. Fortunately, this is easily done by solving for θ

$$\theta = \sin^{-1} \frac{x}{|a|}$$

and restricting the inverse sine to the principal values, $-\frac{\pi}{2} \le \theta \le \frac{\pi}{2}$.

Thus the integral becomes

$$\int \frac{a^4 \sin^4\theta |a| \cos\theta\, d\theta}{|a|\,|\cos\theta|}$$

Now, however, in the range of values chosen for θ, $\cos\theta$ is always positive. Thus we may remove the absolute value signs from $\cos\theta$ in the denominator. (This is one of the reasons that the principal values of the inverse trigonometric functions are defined as they are.)

Then the $\cos\theta$ terms cancel, and the integral becomes

$$a^4 \int \sin^4\theta \, d\theta$$

By application of integral formulas 299 and 296, we integrate this to

$$-a^4 \frac{\sin^3\theta\cos\theta}{4} - \frac{3a^4}{8}\cos\theta\sin\theta + \frac{3a^4}{8}\theta + C$$

We now must perform the inverse substitution to get the result in terms of x. We have

$$\theta = \sin^{-1}\frac{x}{|a|}$$

$$\sin\theta = \frac{x}{|a|}$$

Then

$$\cos\theta = \pm\sqrt{1 - \sin^2\theta} = \pm\sqrt{1 - \frac{x^2}{a^2}} = \pm\frac{\sqrt{a^2 - x^2}}{|a|}.$$

Because of the previously mentioned fact that $\cos\theta$ is positive, we may omit the $\pm$ sign. The reverse substitution then produces the final answer

$$\int \frac{x^4}{\sqrt{a^2 - x^2}} dx = -\tfrac{1}{4}x^3\sqrt{a^2 - x^2} - \tfrac{3}{8}a^2 x\sqrt{a^2 - x^2} + \frac{3a^4}{8}\sin^{-1}\frac{x}{|a|} + C.$$

Any rational function of x may be integrated, if the denominator is factored into linear and irreducible quadratic factors. The function may then be broken into partial fractions, and the individual partial fractions integrated by use of the appropriate formula from the integral table. See the section on partial fractions for further information.

Many integrals may be reduced to rational functions by proper substitutions. For example,

$$z = \tan\frac{x}{2}$$

will reduce any rational function of the six trigonometric functions of x to a rational function of z. (Frequently there are other substitutions which are simpler to use, but this one will always work. See integral formula number 484.)

Any rational function of x and $\sqrt{ax + b}$ may be reduced to a rational function of z by making the substitution

$$z = \sqrt{ax + b}.$$

Other likely substitutions will be suggested by looking at the form of the integrand.

The other main method of transforming integrals is integration by parts. This involves applying formula number 5 or 6 in the accompanying integral table. The critical factor in this method is the choice of the functions u and v. In order for the method to be successful, $v = \int dv$ and $\int v\,du$ must be easier to integrate than the original integral. Again, this choice is largely a matter of intuition and experience.

Example:

$$\int x \sin x \, dx$$

Two obvious choices are $u = x$, $dv = \sin x\,dx$, or $u = \sin x$, $dv = x\,dx$. Since a preliminary mental calculation indicates that $\int v\,du$ in the second choice would be more, rather than less, complicated than the original integral (it would contain x^2), we use the first choice.

$$u = x \qquad du = dx$$

$$dv = \sin x\,dx \qquad v = -\cos x$$

$$\int x \sin x\,dx = \int u\,dv = uv - \int v\,du = -x\cos x + \int \cos x\,dx$$

$$= \sin x - x\cos x$$

Of course, this result could have been obtained directly from the integral table, but it provides a simple example of the method. In more complicated examples the choice of u and v may not be so obvious, and several different choices may have to be tried Of course, there is no guarantee that any of them will work.

Integration by parts may be applied more than once, or combined with substitution. A fairly common case is illustrated by the following example.

Example:

$$\int e^x \sin x\,dx$$

Let

$$u = e^x \qquad \text{Then} \quad du = e^x\,dx$$

$$dv = \sin x\,dx \qquad v = -\cos x$$

$$\int e^x \sin x\,dx = \int u\,dv = uv - \int v\,du = -e^x\cos x + \int e^x \cos x\,dx$$

In this latter integral,

$$\text{let} \quad u = e^x \qquad \text{Then} \quad du = e^x\,dx$$

$$dv = \cos x\,dx \qquad v = \sin x$$

$$\int e^x \sin x\,dx = -e^x\cos x + \int e^x\cos x\,dx = -e^x\cos x + \int u\,dv$$

$$= -e^x\cos x + uv - \int v\,du$$

$$= -e^x\cos x + e^x\sin x - \int e^x\sin x\,dx$$

This looks as if a circular transformation has taken place, since we are back at the same integral we started from. However, the above equation can be solved algebraically for the required integral:

$$\int e^x \sin x\,dx = \tfrac{1}{2}(e^x\sin x - e^x\cos x)$$

In the second integration by parts, if the parts had been chosen as $u = \cos x$, $dv = e^x\,dx$, we would indeed have made a circular transformation, and returned to the starting place. In general, when doing repeated integration by parts, one should never choose the function u at any stage to be the same as the function v at the previous stage, or a constant times the previous v.

The following rule is called the extended rule for integration by parts. It is the result of $n + 1$ successive applications of integration by parts.

If

$$g_1(x) = \int g(x)\,dx, \qquad g_2(x) = \int g_1(x)\,dx,$$

$$g_3(x) = \int g_2(x)\,dx, \ldots, g_m(x) = \int g_{m-1}(x)\,dx, \ldots,$$

then

$$\int f(x)\cdot g(x)\,dx = f(x)\cdot g_1(x) - f'(x)\cdot g_2(x) + f''(x)\cdot g_3(x) - + \cdots$$
$$+ (-1)^n f^{(n)}(x) g_{n+1}(x) + (-1)^{n+1} \int f^{(n+1)}(x) g_{n+1}(x)\,dx.$$

A useful special case of the above rule is when $f(x)$ is a polynomial of degree n. Then $f^{(n+1)}(x) = 0$, and

$$\int f(x)\cdot g(x)\,dx = f(x)\cdot g_1(x) - f'(x)\cdot g_2(x) + f''(x)\cdot g_3(x) - + \cdots + (-1)^n f^{(n)}(x) g_{n+1}(x) + C$$

Example:
If $f(x) = x^2$, $g(x) = \sin x$

$$\int x^2 \sin x\,dx = -x^2 \cos x + 2x \sin x + 2 \cos x + C$$

Another application of this formula occurs if

$$f''(x) = af(x) \quad \text{and} \quad g''(x) = bg(x),$$

where a and b are unequal constants. In this case, by a process similar to that used in the above example for $\int e^x \sin x\,dx$, we get the formula

$$\int f(x)g(x)\,dx = \frac{f(x)\cdot g'(x) - f'(x)\cdot g(x)}{b - a} + C$$

This formula could have been used in the example mentioned. Here is another example.

Example:
If $f(x) = e^{2x}$, $g(x) = \sin 3x$, then $a = 4$, $b = -9$, and

$$\int e^{2x} \sin 3x\,dx = \frac{3\,e^{2x}\cos 3x - 2\,e^{2x}\sin 3x}{-9 - 4} + C = \frac{e^{2x}}{13}(2 \sin 3x - 3 \cos 3x) + C$$

The following additional points should be observed when using this table.

1. A constant of integration is to be supplied with the answers for indefinite integrals.
2. Logarithmic expressions are to base $e = 2.71828\ldots$, unless otherwise specified, and are to be evaluated for the absolute value of the arguments involved therein.
3. All angles are measured in radians, and inverse trigonometric and hyperbolic functions represent principal values, unless otherwise indicated.
4. If the application of a formula produces either a zero denominator or the square root of a negative number in the result, there is usually available another form of the answer which avoids this difficulty. In many of the results, the excluded values are specified, but when such are omitted it is presumed that one can tell what these should be, especially when difficulties of the type herein mentioned are obtained.
5. When inverse trigonometric functions occur in the integrals, be sure that any replacements made for them are strictly in accordance with the rules for such functions. This causes

little difficulty when the argument of the inverse trigonometric function is positive, since then all angles involved are in the first quadrant. However, if the argument is negative, special care must be used. Thus if $u > 0$,

$$\sin^{-1} u = \cos^{-1}\sqrt{1 - u^2} = \csc^{-1}\frac{1}{u}, \text{ etc.}$$

However, if $u < 0$,

$$\sin^{-1} u = -\cos^{-1}\sqrt{1 - u^2} = -\pi - \csc^{-1}\frac{1}{u}, \text{ etc.}$$

See the section on inverse trigonometric functions for a full treatment of the allowable substitutions.

6. In integrals 340–345 and some others, the right side includes expressions of the form

$$A \tan^{-1} [B + C \tan f(x)].$$

In these formulas, the $\tan^{-1}$ does not necessarily represent the principal value. Instead of always employing the principal branch of the inverse tangent function, one must instead use that branch of the inverse tangent function upon which $f(x)$ lies for any particular choice of x.

Example:

$$\int_0^{4\pi} \frac{dx}{2 + \sin x} = \frac{2}{\sqrt{3}}\tan^{-1}\left.\frac{2\tan\frac{x}{2} + 1}{\sqrt{3}}\right]_0^{4\pi}$$

$$= \frac{2}{\sqrt{3}}\left[\tan^{-1}\frac{2\tan 2\pi + 1}{\sqrt{3}} - \tan^{-1}\frac{2\tan 0 + 1}{\sqrt{3}}\right]$$

$$= \frac{2}{\sqrt{3}}\left[\frac{13\pi}{6} - \frac{\pi}{6}\right] = \frac{4\pi}{\sqrt{3}} = \frac{4\sqrt{3}\pi}{3}$$

Here

$$\tan^{-1}\frac{2\tan 2\pi + 1}{\sqrt{3}} = \tan^{-1}\frac{1}{\sqrt{3}} = \frac{13\pi}{6},$$

since $f(x) = 2\pi$; and

$$\tan^{-1}\frac{2\tan 0 + 1}{\sqrt{3}} = \tan^{-1}\frac{1}{\sqrt{3}} = \frac{\pi}{6},$$

since $f(x) = 0$.

7. B_n and E_n where used in Integrals represents the Bernoulli and Euler numbers

INTEGRALS

ELEMENTARY FORMS

1. $\int a\,dx = ax$

2. $\int a \cdot f(x)\,dx = a \int f(x)\,dx$

3. $\int \phi(y)\,dx = \int \frac{\phi(y)}{y'}\,dy, \qquad \text{where } y' = \frac{dy}{dx}$

4. $\int (u + v)\,dx = \int u\,dx + \int v\,dx, \qquad \text{where } u \text{ and } v \text{ are any functions of } x$

5. $\int u\,dv = u \int dv - \int v\,du = uv - \int v\,du$

6. $\int u \frac{dv}{dx}\,dx = uv - \int v \frac{du}{dx}\,dx$

7. $\int x^n\,dx = \frac{x^{n+1}}{n+1}, \qquad \text{except } n = -1$

8. $\int \frac{f'(x)\,dx}{f(x)} = \log f(x), \qquad (df(x) = f'(x)\,dx)$

9. $\int \frac{dx}{x} = \log x$

10. $\int \frac{f'(x)\,dx}{2\sqrt{f(x)}} = \sqrt{f(x)}, \qquad (df(x) = f'(x)\,dx)$

11. $\int e^x\,dx = e^x$

12. $\int e^{ax}\,dx = e^{ax}/a$

13. $\int b^{ax}\,dx = \frac{b^{ax}}{a \log b}, \qquad (b > 0)$

14. $\int \log x\,dx = x \log x - x$

15. $\int a^x \log a\,dx = a^x, \qquad (a > 0)$

16. $\int \frac{dx}{a^2 + x^2} = \frac{1}{a} \tan^{-1} \frac{x}{a}$

INTEGRALS (Continued)

17. $$\int \frac{dx}{a^2 - x^2} = \begin{cases} \frac{1}{a}\tanh^{-1}\frac{x}{a} \\ \text{or} \\ \frac{1}{2a}\log\frac{a+x}{a-x}, & (a^2 > x^2) \end{cases}$$

18. $$\int \frac{dx}{x^2 - a^2} = \begin{cases} -\frac{1}{a}\coth^{-1}\frac{x}{a} \\ \text{or} \\ \frac{1}{2a}\log\frac{x-a}{x+a}, & (x^2 > a^2) \end{cases}$$

19. $$\int \frac{dx}{\sqrt{a^2 - x^2}} = \begin{cases} \sin^{-1}\frac{x}{|a|} \\ \text{or} \\ -\cos^{-1}\frac{x}{|a|}, & (a^2 > x^2) \end{cases}$$

20. $$\int \frac{dx}{\sqrt{x^2 \pm a^2}} = \log(x + \sqrt{x^2 \pm a^2})$$

21. $$\int \frac{dx}{x\sqrt{x^2 - a^2}} = \frac{1}{|a|}\sec^{-1}\frac{x}{a}$$

22. $$\int \frac{dx}{x\sqrt{a^2 \pm x^2}} = -\frac{1}{a}\log\left(\frac{a + \sqrt{a^2 \pm x^2}}{x}\right)$$

FORMS CONTAINING $(a + bx)$

For forms containing $a + bx$, but not listed in the table, the substitution $u = \frac{a + bx}{x}$ may prove helpful.

23. $$\int (a + bx)^n\,dx = \frac{(a + bx)^{n+1}}{(n+1)b}, \qquad (n \neq -1)$$

24. $$\int x(a + bx)^n\,dx$$

$$= \frac{1}{b^2(n+2)}(a + bx)^{n+2} - \frac{a}{b^2(n+1)}(a + bx)^{n+1}, \qquad (n \neq -1, -2)$$

25. $$\int x^2(a + bx)^n\,dx = \frac{1}{b^3}\left[\frac{(a + bx)^{n+3}}{n+3} - 2a\frac{(a + bx)^{n+2}}{n+2} + a^2\frac{(a + bx)^{n+1}}{n+1}\right]$$

INTEGRALS (Continued)

26. $$\int x^m(a+bx)^n\,dx = \begin{cases} \dfrac{x^{m+1}(a+bx)^n}{m+n+1} + \dfrac{an}{m+n+1}\displaystyle\int x^m(a+bx)^{n-1}\,dx \\ \text{or} \\ \dfrac{1}{a(n+1)}\Big[-x^{m+1}(a+bx)^{n+1} \\ \qquad + (m+n+2)\displaystyle\int x^m(a+bx)^{n+1}\,dx\Big] \\ \text{or} \\ \dfrac{1}{b(m+n+1)}\Big[x^m(a+bx)^{n+1} - ma\displaystyle\int x^{m-1}(a+bx)^n\,dx\Big] \end{cases}$$

27. $$\int \frac{dx}{a+bx} = \frac{1}{b}\log(a+bx)$$

28. $$\int \frac{dx}{(a+bx)^2} = -\frac{1}{b(a+bx)}$$

29. $$\int \frac{dx}{(a+bx)^3} = -\frac{1}{2b(a+bx)^2}$$

30. $$\int \frac{x\,dx}{a+bx} = \begin{cases} \dfrac{1}{b^2}[a+bx-a\log(a+bx)] \\ \text{or} \\ \dfrac{x}{b} - \dfrac{a}{b^2}\log(a+bx) \end{cases}$$

31. $$\int \frac{x\,dx}{(a+bx)^2} = \frac{1}{b^2}\left[\log(a+bx) + \frac{a}{a+bx}\right]$$

32. $$\int \frac{x\,dx}{(a+bx)^n} = \frac{1}{b^2}\left[\frac{-1}{(n-2)(a+bx)^{n-2}} + \frac{a}{(n-1)(a+bx)^{n-1}}\right], \qquad n \neq 1, 2$$

33. $$\int \frac{x^2\,dx}{a+bx} = \frac{1}{b^3}\left[\frac{1}{2}(a+bx)^2 - 2a(a+bx) + a^2\log(a+bx)\right]$$

34. $$\int \frac{x^2\,dx}{(a+bx)^2} = \frac{1}{b^3}\left[a+bx-2a\log(a+bx) - \frac{a^2}{a+bx}\right]$$

35. $$\int \frac{x^2\,dx}{(a+bx)^3} = \frac{1}{b^3}\left[\log(a+bx) + \frac{2a}{a+bx} - \frac{a^2}{2(a+bx)^2}\right]$$

36. $$\int \frac{x^2\,dx}{(a+bx)^n} = \frac{1}{b^3}\Big[\frac{-1}{(n-3)(a+bx)^{n-3}} + \frac{2a}{(n-2)(a+bx)^{n-2}} - \frac{a^2}{(n-1)(a+bx)^{n-1}}\Big], \qquad n \neq 1, 2, 3$$

INTEGRALS (Continued)

37. $\int \frac{dx}{x(a + bx)} = -\frac{1}{a} \log \frac{a + bx}{x}$

38. $\int \frac{dx}{x(a + bx)^2} = \frac{1}{a(a + bx)} - \frac{1}{a^2} \log \frac{a + bx}{x}$

39. $\int \frac{dx}{x(a + bx)^3} = \frac{1}{a^3}\left[\frac{1}{2}\left(\frac{2a + bx}{a + bx}\right)^2 + \log \frac{x}{a + bx}\right]$

40. $\int \frac{dx}{x^2(a + bx)} = -\frac{1}{ax} + \frac{b}{a^2} \log \frac{a + bx}{x}$

41. $\int \frac{dx}{x^3(a + bx)} = \frac{2bx - a}{2a^2x^2} + \frac{b^2}{a^3} \log \frac{x}{a + bx}$

42. $\int \frac{dx}{x^2(a + bx)^2} = -\frac{a + 2bx}{a^2x(a + bx)} + \frac{2b}{a^3} \log \frac{a + bx}{x}$

FORMS CONTAINING $c^2 \pm x^2$, $x^2 - c^2$

43. $\int \frac{dx}{c^2 + x^2} = \frac{1}{c} \tan^{-1} \frac{x}{c}$

44. $\int \frac{dx}{c^2 - x^2} = \frac{1}{2c} \log \frac{c + x}{c - x}, \qquad (c^2 > x^2)$

45. $\int \frac{dx}{x^2 - c^2} = \frac{1}{2c} \log \frac{x - c}{x + c}, \qquad (x^2 > c^2)$

46. $\int \frac{x\,dx}{c^2 \pm x^2} = \pm\frac{1}{2} \log (c^2 \pm x^2)$

47. $\int \frac{x\,dx}{(c^2 \pm x^2)^{n+1}} = \mp \frac{1}{2n(c^2 \pm x^2)^n}$

48. $\int \frac{dx}{(c^2 \pm x^2)^n} = \frac{1}{2c^2(n - 1)}\left[\frac{x}{(c^2 \pm x^2)^{n-1}} + (2n - 3) \int \frac{dx}{(c^2 \pm x^2)^{n-1}}\right]$

49. $\int \frac{dx}{(x^2 - c^2)^n} = \frac{1}{2c^2(n - 1)}\left[-\frac{x}{(x^2 - c^2)^{n-1}} - (2n - 3) \int \frac{dx}{(x^2 - c^2)^{n-1}}\right]$

50. $\int \frac{x\,dx}{x^2 - c^2} = \frac{1}{2} \log (x^2 - c^2)$

51. $\int \frac{x\,dx}{(x^2 - c^2)^{n+1}} = -\frac{1}{2n(x^2 - c^2)^n}$

INTEGRALS (Continued)

FORMS CONTAINING $a + bx$ and $c + dx$

$$u = a + bx, \qquad v = c + dx, \qquad k = ad - bc$$

If $k = 0$, then $v = \frac{c}{a}u$

52. $$\int \frac{dx}{u \cdot v} = \frac{1}{k} \cdot \log\left(\frac{v}{u}\right)$$

53. $$\int \frac{x\,dx}{u \cdot v} = \frac{1}{k}\left[\frac{a}{b}\log(u) - \frac{c}{d}\log(v)\right]$$

54. $$\int \frac{dx}{u^2 \cdot v} = \frac{1}{k}\left(\frac{1}{u} + \frac{d}{k}\log\frac{v}{u}\right)$$

55. $$\int \frac{x\,dx}{u^2 \cdot v} = \frac{-a}{bku} - \frac{c}{k^2}\log\frac{v}{u}$$

56. $$\int \frac{x^2\,dx}{u^2 \cdot v} = \frac{a^2}{b^2ku} + \frac{1}{k^2}\left[\frac{c^2}{d}\log(v) + \frac{a(k - bc)}{b^2}\log(u)\right]$$

57. $$\int \frac{dx}{u^n \cdot v^m} = \frac{1}{k(m-1)}\left[\frac{-1}{u^{n-1} \cdot v^{m-1}} - (m + n - 2)b\int \frac{dx}{u^n \cdot v^{m-1}}\right]$$

58. $$\int \frac{u}{v}\,dx = \frac{bx}{d} + \frac{k}{d^2}\log(v)$$

59. $$\int \frac{u^m\,dx}{v^n} = \begin{cases} \dfrac{-1}{k(n-1)}\left[\dfrac{u^{m+1}}{v^{n-1}} + b(n - m - 2)\displaystyle\int \frac{u^m}{v^{n-1}}\,dx\right] \\ \text{or} \\ \dfrac{-1}{d(n - m - 1)}\left[\dfrac{u^m}{v^{n-1}} + mk\displaystyle\int \frac{u^{m-1}}{v^n}\,dx\right] \\ \text{or} \\ \dfrac{-1}{d(n-1)}\left[\dfrac{u^m}{v^{n-1}} - mb\displaystyle\int \frac{u^{m-1}}{v^{n-1}}\,dx\right] \end{cases}$$

FORMS CONTAINING $(a + bx^n)$

60. $$\int \frac{dx}{a + bx^2} = \frac{1}{\sqrt{ab}}\tan^{-1}\frac{x\sqrt{ab}}{a}, \qquad (ab > 0)$$

61. $$\int \frac{dx}{a + bx^2} = \begin{cases} \dfrac{1}{2\sqrt{-ab}}\log\dfrac{a + x\sqrt{-ab}}{a - x\sqrt{-ab}}, & (ab < 0) \\ \text{or} \\ \dfrac{1}{\sqrt{-ab}}\tanh^{-1}\dfrac{x\sqrt{-ab}}{a}, & (ab < 0) \end{cases}$$

INTEGRALS (Continued)

62. $$\int \frac{dx}{a^2 + b^2x^2} = \frac{1}{ab}\tan^{-1}\frac{bx}{a}$$

63. $$\int \frac{x\,dx}{a + bx^2} = \frac{1}{2b}\log(a + bx^2)$$

64. $$\int \frac{x^2\,dx}{a + bx^2} = \frac{x}{b} - \frac{a}{b}\int \frac{dx}{a + bx^2}$$

65. $$\int \frac{dx}{(a + bx^2)^2} = \frac{x}{2a(a + bx^2)} + \frac{1}{2a}\int \frac{dx}{a + bx^2}$$

66. $$\int \frac{dx}{a^2 - b^2x^2} = \frac{1}{2ab}\log\frac{a + bx}{a - bx}$$

67. $$\int \frac{dx}{(a + bx^2)^{m+1}} = \begin{cases} \dfrac{1}{2ma}\dfrac{x}{(a + bx^2)^m} + \dfrac{2m - 1}{2ma}\displaystyle\int \frac{dx}{(a + bx^2)^m} \\ \text{or} \\ \dfrac{(2m)!}{(m!)^2}\left[\dfrac{x}{2a}\displaystyle\sum_{r=1}^{m}\frac{r!(r - 1)!}{(4a)^{m-r}(2r)!(a + bx^2)^r} + \dfrac{1}{(4a)^m}\displaystyle\int \frac{dx}{a + bx^2}\right] \end{cases}$$

68. $$\int \frac{x\,dx}{(a + bx^2)^{m+1}} = -\frac{1}{2bm(a + bx^2)^m}$$

69. $$\int \frac{x^2\,dx}{(a + bx^2)^{m+1}} = \frac{-x}{2mb(a + bx^2)^m} + \frac{1}{2mb}\int \frac{dx}{(a + bx^2)^m}$$

70. $$\int \frac{dx}{x(a + bx^2)} = \frac{1}{2a}\log\frac{x^2}{a + bx^2}$$

71. $$\int \frac{dx}{x^2(a + bx^2)} = -\frac{1}{ax} - \frac{b}{a}\int \frac{dx}{a + bx^2}$$

72. $$\int \frac{dx}{x(a + bx^2)^{m+1}} = \begin{cases} \dfrac{1}{2am(a + bx^2)^m} + \dfrac{1}{a}\displaystyle\int \frac{dx}{x(a + bx^2)^m} \\ \text{or} \\ \dfrac{1}{2a^{m+1}}\left[\displaystyle\sum_{r=1}^{m}\frac{a^r}{r(a + bx^2)^r} + \log\frac{x^2}{a + bx^2}\right] \end{cases}$$

73. $$\int \frac{dx}{x^2(a + bx^2)^{m+1}} = \frac{1}{a}\int \frac{dx}{x^2(a + bx^2)^m} - \frac{b}{a}\int \frac{dx}{(a + bx^2)^{m+1}}$$

74. $$\int \frac{dx}{a + bx^3} = \frac{k}{3a}\left[\frac{1}{2}\log\frac{(k + x)^3}{a + bx^3} + \sqrt{3}\tan^{-1}\frac{2x - k}{k\sqrt{3}}\right], \qquad \left(k = \sqrt[3]{\frac{a}{b}}\right)$$

75. $$\int \frac{x\,dx}{a + bx^3} = \frac{1}{3bk}\left[\frac{1}{2}\log\frac{a + bx^3}{(k + x)^3} + \sqrt{3}\tan^{-1}\frac{2x - k}{k\sqrt{3}}\right], \qquad \left(k = \sqrt[3]{\frac{a}{b}}\right)$$

INTEGRALS (Continued)

76. $$\int \frac{x^2\,dx}{a+bx^3} = \frac{1}{3b}\log(a+bx^3)$$

77. $$\int \frac{dx}{a+bx^4} = \frac{k}{2a}\left[\frac{1}{2}\log\frac{x^2+2kx+2k^2}{x^2-2kx+2k^2} + \tan^{-1}\frac{2kx}{2k^2-x^2}\right], \qquad \left(ab>0,\ k=\sqrt[4]{\frac{a}{4b}}\right)$$

78. $$\int \frac{dx}{a+bx^4} = \frac{k}{2a}\left[\frac{1}{2}\log\frac{x+k}{x-k} + \tan^{-1}\frac{x}{k}\right], \qquad \left(ab<0,\ k=\sqrt[4]{-\frac{a}{b}}\right)$$

79. $$\int \frac{x\,dx}{a+bx^4} = \frac{1}{2bk}\tan^{-1}\frac{x^2}{k}, \qquad \left(ab>0,\ k=\sqrt{\frac{a}{b}}\right)$$

80. $$\int \frac{x\,dx}{a+bx^4} = \frac{1}{4bk}\log\frac{x^2-k}{x^2+k}, \qquad \left(ab<0,\ k=\sqrt{-\frac{a}{b}}\right)$$

81. $$\int \frac{x^2\,dx}{a+bx^4} = \frac{1}{4bk}\left[\frac{1}{2}\log\frac{x^2-2kx+2k^2}{x^2+2kx+2k^2} + \tan^{-1}\frac{2kx}{2k^2-x^2}\right], \qquad \left(ab>0,\ k=\sqrt[4]{\frac{a}{4b}}\right)$$

82. $$\int \frac{x^2\,dx}{a+bx^4} = \frac{1}{4bk}\left[\log\frac{x-k}{x+k} + 2\tan^{-1}\frac{x}{k}\right], \qquad \left(ab<0,\ k=\sqrt[4]{-\frac{a}{b}}\right)$$

83. $$\int \frac{x^3\,dx}{a+bx^4} = \frac{1}{4b}\log(a+bx^4)$$

84. $$\int \frac{dx}{x(a+bx^n)} = \frac{1}{an}\log\frac{x^n}{a+bx^n}$$

85. $$\int \frac{dx}{(a+bx^n)^{m+1}} = \frac{1}{a}\int\frac{dx}{(a+bx^n)^m} - \frac{b}{a}\int\frac{x^n\,dx}{(a+bx^n)^{m+1}}$$

86. $$\int \frac{x^m\,dx}{(a+bx^n)^{p+1}} = \frac{1}{b}\int\frac{x^{m-n}\,dx}{(a+bx^n)^p} - \frac{a}{b}\int\frac{x^{m-n}\,dx}{(a+bx^n)^{p+1}}$$

87. $$\int \frac{dx}{x^m(a+bx^n)^{p+1}} = \frac{1}{a}\int\frac{dx}{x^m(a+bx^n)^p} - \frac{b}{a}\int\frac{dx}{x^{m-n}(a+bx^n)^{p+1}}$$

INTEGRALS (Continued)

88. $$\int x^m(a+bx^n)^p\,dx = \begin{cases} \dfrac{1}{b(np+m+1)}\left[x^{m-n+1}(a+bx^n)^{p+1} - a(m-n+1)\displaystyle\int x^{m-n}(a+bx^n)^p\,dx\right] \\ \text{or} \\ \dfrac{1}{np+m+1}\left[x^{m+1}(a+bx^n)^p + anp\displaystyle\int x^m(a+bx^n)^{p-1}\,dx\right] \\ \text{or} \\ \dfrac{1}{a(m+1)}\left[x^{m+1}(a+bx^n)^{p+1} - (m+1+np+n)b\displaystyle\int x^{m+n}(a+bx^n)^p\,dx\right] \\ \text{or} \\ \dfrac{1}{an(p+1)}\left[-x^{m+1}(a+bx^n)^{p+1} + (m+1+np+n)\displaystyle\int x^m(a+bx^n)^{p+1}\,dx\right] \end{cases}$$

FORMS CONTAINING $c^3 \pm x^3$

89. $$\int \frac{dx}{c^3 \pm x^3} = \pm\frac{1}{6c^2}\log\frac{(c\pm x)^3}{c^3 \pm x^3} + \frac{1}{c^2\sqrt{3}}\tan^{-1}\frac{2x \mp c}{c\sqrt{3}}$$

90. $$\int \frac{dx}{(c^3 \pm x^3)^2} = \frac{x}{3c^3(c^3 \pm x^3)} + \frac{2}{3c^3}\int\frac{dx}{c^3 \pm x^3}$$

91. $$\int \frac{dx}{(c^3 \pm x^3)^{n+1}} = \frac{1}{3nc^3}\left[\frac{x}{(c^3 \pm x^3)^n} + (3n-1)\int\frac{dx}{(c^3 \pm x^3)^n}\right]$$

92. $$\int \frac{x\,dx}{c^3 \pm x^3} = \frac{1}{6c}\log\frac{c^3 \pm x^3}{(c\pm x)^3} \pm \frac{1}{c\sqrt{3}}\tan^{-1}\frac{2x \mp c}{c\sqrt{3}}$$

93. $$\int \frac{x\,dx}{(c^3 \pm x^3)^2} = \frac{x^2}{3c^3(c^3 \pm x^3)} + \frac{1}{3c^3}\int\frac{x\,dx}{c^3 \pm x^3}$$

94. $$\int \frac{x\,dx}{(c^3 \pm x^3)^{n+1}} = \frac{1}{3nc^3}\left[\frac{x^2}{(c^3 \pm x^3)^n} + (3n-2)\int\frac{x\,dx}{(c^3 \pm x^3)^n}\right]$$

95. $$\int \frac{x^2\,dx}{c^3 \pm x^3} = \pm\frac{1}{3}\log(c^3 \pm x^3)$$

INTEGRALS (Continued)

96. $$\int \frac{x^2\,dx}{(c^3 \pm x^3)^{n+1}} = \mp \frac{1}{3n(c^3 \pm x^3)^n}$$

97. $$\int \frac{dx}{x(c^3 \pm x^3)} = \frac{1}{3c^3} \log \frac{x^3}{c^3 \pm x^3}$$

98. $$\int \frac{dx}{x(c^3 \pm x^3)^2} = \frac{1}{3c^3(c^3 \pm x^3)} + \frac{1}{3c^6} \log \frac{x^3}{c^3 \pm x^3}$$

99. $$\int \frac{dx}{x(c^3 \pm x^3)^{n+1}} = \frac{1}{3nc^3(c^3 \pm x^3)^n} + \frac{1}{c^3} \int \frac{dx}{x(c^3 \pm x^3)^n}$$

100. $$\int \frac{dx}{x^2(c^3 \pm x^3)} = -\frac{1}{c^3 x} \mp \frac{1}{c^3} \int \frac{x\,dx}{c^3 \pm x^3}$$

101. $$\int \frac{dx}{x^2(c^3 \pm x^3)^{n+1}} = \frac{1}{c^3} \int \frac{dx}{x^2(c^3 \pm x^3)^n} \mp \frac{1}{c^3} \int \frac{x\,dx}{(c^3 \pm x^3)^{n+1}}$$

FORMS CONTAINING $c^4 \pm x^4$

102. $$\int \frac{dx}{c^4 + x^4} = \frac{1}{2c^3\sqrt{2}} \left[\frac{1}{2} \log \frac{x^2 + cx\sqrt{2} + c^2}{x^2 - cx\sqrt{2} + c^2} + \tan^{-1} \frac{cx\sqrt{2}}{c^2 - x^2} \right]$$

103. $$\int \frac{dx}{c^4 - x^4} = \frac{1}{2c^3} \left[\frac{1}{2} \log \frac{c + x}{c - x} + \tan^{-1} \frac{x}{c} \right]$$

104. $$\int \frac{x\,dx}{c^4 + x^4} = \frac{1}{2c^2} \tan^{-1} \frac{x^2}{c^2}$$

105. $$\int \frac{x\,dx}{c^4 - x^4} = \frac{1}{4c^2} \log \frac{c^2 + x^2}{c^2 - x^2}$$

106. $$\int \frac{x^2\,dx}{c^4 + x^4} = \frac{1}{2c\sqrt{2}} \left[\frac{1}{2} \log \frac{x^2 - cx\sqrt{2} + c^2}{x^2 + cx\sqrt{2} + c^2} + \tan^{-1} \frac{cx\sqrt{2}}{c^2 - x^2} \right]$$

107. $$\int \frac{x^2\,dx}{c^4 - x^4} = \frac{1}{2c} \left[\frac{1}{2} \log \frac{c + x}{c - x} - \tan^{-1} \frac{x}{c} \right]$$

108. $$\int \frac{x^3\,dx}{c^4 \pm x^4} = \pm \frac{1}{4} \log (c^4 \pm x^4)$$

FORMS CONTAINING $(a + bx + cx^2)$

$$X = a + bx + cx^2 \text{ and } q = 4ac - b^2$$

If $q = 0$, then $X = c\left(x + \frac{b}{2c}\right)^2$, and formulas starting with 23 should be used in place of these.

109. $$\int \frac{dx}{X} = \frac{2}{\sqrt{q}} \tan^{-1} \frac{2cx + b}{\sqrt{q}}, \qquad (q > 0)$$

INTEGRALS (Continued)

110. $$\int \frac{dx}{X} = \begin{cases} \dfrac{-2}{\sqrt{-q}} \tanh^{-1} \dfrac{2cx+b}{\sqrt{-q}} \\ \text{or} \\ \dfrac{1}{\sqrt{-q}} \log \dfrac{2cx+b-\sqrt{-q}}{2cx+b+\sqrt{-q}}, \qquad (q<0) \end{cases}$$

111. $$\int \frac{dx}{X^2} = \frac{2cx+b}{qX} + \frac{2c}{q} \int \frac{dx}{X}$$

112. $$\int \frac{dx}{X^3} = \frac{2cx+b}{q}\left(\frac{1}{2X^2} + \frac{3c}{qX}\right) + \frac{6c^2}{q^2} \int \frac{dx}{X}$$

113. $$\int \frac{dx}{X^{n+1}} = \begin{cases} \dfrac{2cx+b}{nqX^n} + \dfrac{2(2n-1)c}{qn} \displaystyle\int \frac{dx}{X^n} \\ \text{or} \\ \dfrac{(2n)!}{(n!)^2}\left(\dfrac{c}{q}\right)^n \left[\dfrac{2cx+b}{q} \displaystyle\sum_{r=1}^{n} \left(\frac{q}{cX}\right)^r \left(\frac{(r-1)!r!}{(2r)!}\right) + \int \frac{dx}{X}\right] \end{cases}$$

114. $$\int \frac{x\,dx}{X} = \frac{1}{2c} \log X - \frac{b}{2c} \int \frac{dx}{X}$$

115. $$\int \frac{x\,dx}{X^2} = -\frac{bx+2a}{qX} - \frac{b}{q} \int \frac{dx}{X}$$

116. $$\int \frac{x\,dx}{X^{n+1}} = -\frac{2a+bx}{nqX^n} - \frac{b(2n-1)}{nq} \int \frac{dx}{X^n}$$

117. $$\int \frac{x^2}{X}\,dx = \frac{x}{c} - \frac{b}{2c^2} \log X + \frac{b^2-2ac}{2c^2} \int \frac{dx}{X}$$

118. $$\int \frac{x^2}{X^2}\,dx = \frac{(b^2-2ac)x+ab}{cqX} + \frac{2a}{q} \int \frac{dx}{X}$$

119. $$\int \frac{x^m\,dx}{X^{n+1}} = -\frac{x^{m-1}}{(2n-m+1)cX^n} - \frac{n-m+1}{2n-m+1} \cdot \frac{b}{c} \int \frac{x^{m-1}\,dx}{X^{n+1}} + \frac{m-1}{2n-m+1} \cdot \frac{a}{c} \int \frac{x^{m-2}\,dx}{X^{n+1}}$$

120. $$\int \frac{dx}{xX} = \frac{1}{2a} \log \frac{x^2}{X} - \frac{b}{2a} \int \frac{dx}{X}$$

121. $$\int \frac{dx}{x^2X} = \frac{b}{2a^2} \log \frac{X}{x^2} - \frac{1}{ax} + \left(\frac{b^2}{2a^2} - \frac{c}{a}\right) \int \frac{dx}{X}$$

122. $$\int \frac{dx}{xX^n} = \frac{1}{2a(n-1)X^{n-1}} - \frac{b}{2a} \int \frac{dx}{X^n} + \frac{1}{a} \int \frac{dx}{xX^{n-1}}$$

INTEGRALS (Continued)

123. $$\int \frac{dx}{x^m X^{n+1}} = -\frac{1}{(m-1)ax^{m-1}X^n} - \frac{n+m-1}{m-1}\cdot\frac{b}{a}\int \frac{dx}{x^{m-1}X^{n+1}} - \frac{2n+m-1}{m-1}\cdot\frac{c}{a}\int\frac{dx}{x^{m-2}X^{n+1}}$$

FORMS CONTAINING $\sqrt{a+bx}$

124. $$\int \sqrt{a+bx}\,dx = \frac{2}{3b}\sqrt{(a+bx)^3}$$

125. $$\int x\sqrt{a+bx}\,dx = -\frac{2(2a-3bx)\sqrt{(a+bx)^3}}{15b^2}$$

126. $$\int x^2\sqrt{a+bx}\,dx = \frac{2(8a^2-12abx+15b^2x^2)\sqrt{(a+bx)^3}}{105b^3}$$

127. $$\int x^m\sqrt{a+bx}\,dx = \begin{cases} \dfrac{2}{b(2m+3)}\left[x^m\sqrt{(a+bx)^3} - ma\displaystyle\int x^{m-1}\sqrt{a+bx}\,dx\right] \\ \text{or} \\ \dfrac{2}{b^{m+1}}\sqrt{a+bx}\displaystyle\sum_{r=0}^{m}\frac{m!(-a)^{m-r}}{r!(m-r)!(2r+3)}(a+bx)^{r+1} \end{cases}$$

128. $$\int \frac{\sqrt{a+bx}}{x}dx = 2\sqrt{a+bx} + a\int\frac{dx}{x\sqrt{a+bx}}$$

129. $$\int \frac{\sqrt{a+bx}}{x^2}dx = -\frac{\sqrt{a+bx}}{x} + \frac{b}{2}\int\frac{dx}{x\sqrt{a+bx}}$$

130. $$\int \frac{\sqrt{a+bx}}{x^m}dx = -\frac{1}{(m-1)a}\left[\frac{\sqrt{(a+bx)^3}}{x^{m-1}} + \frac{(2m-5)b}{2}\int\frac{\sqrt{a+bx}}{x^{m-1}}dx\right]$$

131. $$\int \frac{dx}{\sqrt{a+bx}} = \frac{2\sqrt{a+bx}}{b}$$

132. $$\int \frac{x\,dx}{\sqrt{a+bx}} = -\frac{2(2a-bx)}{3b^2}\sqrt{a+bx}$$

133. $$\int \frac{x^2\,dx}{\sqrt{a+bx}} = \frac{2(8a^2-4abx+3b^2x^2)}{15b^3}\sqrt{a+bx}$$

INTEGRALS (Continued)

134. $$\int \frac{x^m\,dx}{\sqrt{a+bx}} = \begin{cases} \dfrac{2}{(2m+1)b}\left[x^m\sqrt{a+bx} - ma\displaystyle\int \frac{x^{m-1}\,dx}{\sqrt{a+bx}}\right] \\ \text{or} \\ \dfrac{2(-a)^m\sqrt{a+bx}}{b^{m+1}} \displaystyle\sum_{r=0}^{m} \frac{(-1)^r m!(a+bx)^r}{(2r+1)r!(m-r)!a^r} \end{cases}$$

135. $$\int \frac{dx}{x\sqrt{a+bx}} = \frac{1}{\sqrt{a}}\log\left(\frac{\sqrt{a+bx}-\sqrt{a}}{\sqrt{a+bx}+\sqrt{a}}\right), \qquad (a>0)$$

136. $$\int \frac{dx}{x\sqrt{a+bx}} = \frac{2}{\sqrt{-a}}\tan^{-1}\sqrt{\frac{a+bx}{-a}}, \qquad (a<0)$$

137. $$\int \frac{dx}{x^2\sqrt{a+bx}} = -\frac{\sqrt{a+bx}}{ax} - \frac{b}{2a}\int \frac{dx}{x\sqrt{a+bx}}$$

138. $$\int \frac{dx}{x^n\sqrt{a+bx}} = \begin{cases} -\dfrac{\sqrt{a+bx}}{(n-1)ax^{n-1}} - \dfrac{(2n-3)b}{(2n-2)a}\displaystyle\int \frac{dx}{x^{n-1}\sqrt{a+bx}} \\ \text{or} \\ \dfrac{(2n-2)!}{[(n-1)!]^2}\left[-\dfrac{\sqrt{a+bx}}{a}\displaystyle\sum_{r=1}^{n-1}\frac{r!(r-1)!}{x^r(2r)!}\left(-\frac{b}{4a}\right)^{n-r-1} \right. \\ \qquad \left. + \left(-\dfrac{b}{4a}\right)^{n-1}\displaystyle\int \frac{dx}{x\sqrt{a+bx}}\right] \end{cases}$$

139. $$\int (a+bx)^{\pm\frac{n}{2}}\,dx = \frac{2(a+bx)^{\frac{2\pm n}{2}}}{b(2\pm n)}$$

140. $$\int x(a+bx)^{\pm\frac{n}{2}}\,dx = \frac{2}{b^2}\left[\frac{(a+bx)^{\frac{4\pm n}{2}}}{4\pm n} - \frac{a(a+bx)^{\frac{2\pm n}{2}}}{2\pm n}\right]$$

141. $$\int \frac{dx}{x(a+bx)^{\frac{m}{2}}} = \frac{1}{a}\int \frac{dx}{x(a+bx)^{\frac{m-2}{2}}} - \frac{b}{a}\int \frac{dx}{(a+bx)^{\frac{m}{2}}}$$

142. $$\int \frac{(a+bx)^{\frac{n}{2}}\,dx}{x} = b\int (a+bx)^{\frac{n-2}{2}}\,dx + a\int \frac{(a+bx)^{\frac{n-2}{2}}}{x}\,dx$$

143. $$\int f(x, \sqrt{a+bx})\,dx = \frac{2}{b}\int f\left(\frac{z^2-a}{b}, z\right)z\,dz, \qquad (z=\sqrt{a+bx})$$

INTEGRALS (Continued)

FORMS CONTAINING $\sqrt{a+bx}$ and $\sqrt{c+dx}$

$$u = a + bx \qquad v = c + dx \qquad k = ad - bc$$

If $k = 0$, then $v = \frac{c}{a}u$, and formulas starting with 124 should be used in place of these.

144. $$\int \frac{dx}{\sqrt{uv}} = \begin{cases} \dfrac{2}{\sqrt{bd}} \tanh^{-1} \dfrac{\sqrt{bduv}}{bv}, \ bd > o, \ k < o \\ \text{or} \\ \dfrac{2}{\sqrt{bd}} \tanh^{-1} \dfrac{\sqrt{bduv}}{du}, \ bd > o, \ k > o. \\ \text{or} \\ \dfrac{1}{\sqrt{bd}} \log \dfrac{(bv + \sqrt{bduv})^2}{v}, \qquad (bd > 0) \end{cases}$$

145. $$\int \frac{dx}{\sqrt{uv}} = \begin{cases} \dfrac{2}{\sqrt{-bd}} \tan^{-1} \dfrac{\sqrt{-bduv}}{bv} \\ \text{or} \\ -\dfrac{1}{\sqrt{-bd}} \sin^{-1}\left(\dfrac{2bdx + ad + bc}{|k|}\right), \qquad (bd < 0) \end{cases}$$

146. $$\int \sqrt{uv}\, dx = \frac{k + 2bv}{4bd}\sqrt{uv} - \frac{k^2}{8bd}\int \frac{dx}{\sqrt{uv}}$$

147. $$\int \frac{dx}{v\sqrt{u}} = \begin{cases} \dfrac{1}{\sqrt{kd}} \log \dfrac{d\sqrt{u} - \sqrt{kd}}{d\sqrt{u} + \sqrt{kd}} \\ \text{or} \\ \dfrac{1}{\sqrt{kd}} \log \dfrac{(d\sqrt{u} - \sqrt{kd})^2}{v}, \qquad (kd > 0) \end{cases}$$

148. $$\int \frac{dx}{v\sqrt{u}} = \frac{2}{\sqrt{-kd}} \tan^{-1} \frac{d\sqrt{u}}{\sqrt{-kd}}, \qquad (kd < 0)$$

149. $$\int \frac{x\, dx}{\sqrt{uv}} = \frac{\sqrt{uv}}{bd} - \frac{ad + bc}{2bd}\int \frac{dx}{\sqrt{uv}}$$

150. $$\int \frac{dx}{v\sqrt{uv}} = \frac{-2\sqrt{uv}}{kv}$$

INTEGRALS (Continued)

151. $\int \frac{v\,dx}{\sqrt{uv}} = \frac{\sqrt{uv}}{b} - \frac{k}{2b}\int \frac{dx}{\sqrt{uv}}$

152. $\int \sqrt{\frac{v}{u}}\,dx = \frac{v}{|v|}\int \frac{v\,dx}{\sqrt{uv}}$

153. $\int v^m\sqrt{u}\,dx = \frac{1}{(2m+3)d}\left(2v^{m+1}\sqrt{u} + k\int \frac{v^m\,dx}{\sqrt{u}}\right)$

154. $\int \frac{dx}{v^m\sqrt{u}} = -\frac{1}{(m-1)k}\left(\frac{\sqrt{u}}{v^{m-1}} + \left(m - \frac{3}{2}\right)b\int \frac{dx}{v^{m-1}\sqrt{u}}\right)$

155. $\int \frac{v^m\,dx}{\sqrt{u}} = \begin{cases} \frac{2}{b(2m+1)}\left[v^m\sqrt{u} - mk\int \frac{v^{m-1}}{\sqrt{u}}\,dx\right] \\ \text{or} \\ \frac{2(m!)^2\sqrt{u}}{b(2m+1)!}\sum_{r=0}^{m}\left(-\frac{4k}{b}\right)^{m-r}\frac{(2r)!}{(r!)^2}v^r \end{cases}$

FORMS CONTAINING $\sqrt{x^2 \pm a^2}$

156. $\int \sqrt{x^2 \pm a^2}\,dx = \frac{1}{2}[x\sqrt{x^2 \pm a^2} \pm a^2 \log(x + \sqrt{x^2 \pm a^2})]$

157. $\int \frac{dx}{\sqrt{x^2 \pm a^2}} = \log(x + \sqrt{x^2 \pm a^2})$

158. $\int \frac{dx}{x\sqrt{x^2 - a^2}} = \frac{1}{|a|}\sec^{-1}\frac{x}{a}$

159. $\int \frac{dx}{x\sqrt{x^2 + a^2}} = -\frac{1}{a}\log\left(\frac{a + \sqrt{x^2 + a^2}}{x}\right)$

160. $\int \frac{\sqrt{x^2 + a^2}}{x}\,dx = \sqrt{x^2 + a^2} - a\log\left(\frac{a + \sqrt{x^2 + a^2}}{x}\right)$

161. $\int \frac{\sqrt{x^2 - a^2}}{x}\,dx = \sqrt{x^2 - a^2} - |a|\sec^{-1}\frac{x}{a}$

162. $\int \frac{x\,dx}{\sqrt{x^2 \pm a^2}} = \sqrt{x^2 \pm a^2}$

163. $\int x\sqrt{x^2 \pm a^2}\,dx = \frac{1}{3}\sqrt{(x^2 \pm a^2)^3}$

INTEGRALS (Continued)

164. $$\int \sqrt{(x^2 \pm a^2)^3}\,dx = \frac{1}{4}\left[x\sqrt{(x^2 \pm a^2)^3} \pm \frac{3a^2x}{2}\sqrt{x^2 \pm a^2} + \frac{3a^4}{2}\log\left(x + \sqrt{x^2 \pm a^2}\right)\right]$$

165. $$\int \frac{dx}{\sqrt{(x^2 \pm a^2)^3}} = \frac{\pm x}{a^2\sqrt{x^2 \pm a^2}}$$

166. $$\int \frac{x\,dx}{\sqrt{(x^2 \pm a^2)^3}} = \frac{-1}{\sqrt{x^2 \pm a^2}}$$

167. $$\int x\sqrt{(x^2 \pm a^2)^3}\,dx = \tfrac{1}{5}\sqrt{(x^2 \pm a^2)^5}$$

168. $$\int x^2\sqrt{x^2 \pm a^2}\,dx = \frac{x}{4}\sqrt{(x^2 \pm a^2)^3} \mp \frac{a^2}{8}x\sqrt{x^2 \pm a^2} - \frac{a^4}{8}\log\left(x + \sqrt{x^2 \pm a^2}\right)$$

169. $$\int x^3\sqrt{x^2 + a^2}\,dx = \left(\tfrac{1}{5}x^2 - \tfrac{2}{15}a^2\right)\sqrt{(a^2 + x^2)^3}$$

170. $$\int x^3\sqrt{x^2 - a^2}\,dx = \frac{1}{5}\sqrt{(x^2 - a^2)^5} + \frac{a^2}{3}\sqrt{(x^2 - a^2)^3}$$

171. $$\int \frac{x^2\,dx}{\sqrt{x^2 \pm a^2}} = \frac{x}{2}\sqrt{x^2 \pm a^2} \mp \frac{a^2}{2}\log\left(x + \sqrt{x^2 \pm a^2}\right)$$

172. $$\int \frac{x^3\,dx}{\sqrt{x^2 \pm a^2}} = \frac{1}{3}\sqrt{(x^2 \pm a^2)^3} \mp a^2\sqrt{x^2 \pm a^2}$$

173. $$\int \frac{dx}{x^2\sqrt{x^2 \pm a^2}} = \mp\frac{\sqrt{x^2 \pm a^2}}{a^2x}$$

174. $$\int \frac{dx}{x^3\sqrt{x^2 + a^2}} = -\frac{\sqrt{x^2 + a^2}}{2a^2x^2} + \frac{1}{2a^3}\log\frac{a + \sqrt{x^2 + a^2}}{x}$$

175. $$\int \frac{dx}{x^3\sqrt{x^2 - a^2}} = \frac{\sqrt{x^2 - a^2}}{2a^2x^2} + \frac{1}{2|a^3|}\sec^{-1}\frac{x}{a}$$

176. $$\int x^2\sqrt{(x^2 \pm a^2)^3}\,dx = \frac{x}{6}\sqrt{(x^2 \pm a^2)^5} \mp \frac{a^2x}{24}\sqrt{(x^2 \pm a^2)^3} - \frac{a^4x}{16}\sqrt{x^2 \pm a^2} \mp \frac{a^6}{16}\log\left(x + \sqrt{x^2 \pm a^2}\right)$$

177. $$\int x^3\sqrt{(x^2 \pm a^2)^3}\,dx = \frac{1}{7}\sqrt{(x^2 \pm a^2)^7} \mp \frac{a^2}{5}\sqrt{(x^2 \pm a^2)^5}$$

INTEGRALS (Continued)

178. $\int \frac{\sqrt{x^2 \pm a^2}\,dx}{x^2} = -\frac{\sqrt{x^2 \pm a^2}}{x} + \log(x + \sqrt{x^2 \pm a^2})$

179. $\int \frac{\sqrt{x^2 + a^2}}{x^3}\,dx = -\frac{\sqrt{x^2 + a^2}}{2x^2} - \frac{1}{2a}\log\frac{a + \sqrt{x^2 + a^2}}{x}$

180. $\int \frac{\sqrt{x^2 - a^2}}{x^3}\,dx = -\frac{\sqrt{x^2 - a^2}}{2x^2} + \frac{1}{2|a|}\sec^{-1}\frac{x}{a}$

181. $\int \frac{\sqrt{x^2 \pm a^2}}{x^4}\,dx = \mp\frac{\sqrt{(x^2 \pm a^2)^3}}{3a^2x^3}$

182. $\int \frac{x^2\,dx}{\sqrt{(x^2 \pm a^2)^3}} = \frac{-x}{\sqrt{x^2 \pm a^2}} + \log(x + \sqrt{x^2 \pm a^2})$

183. $\int \frac{x^3\,dx}{\sqrt{(x^2 \pm a^2)^3}} = \sqrt{x^2 \pm a^2} \pm \frac{a^2}{\sqrt{x^2 \pm a^2}}$

184. $\int \frac{dx}{x\sqrt{(x^2 + a^2)^3}} = \frac{1}{a^2\sqrt{x^2 + a^2}} - \frac{1}{a^3}\log\frac{a + \sqrt{x^2 + a^2}}{x}$

185. $\int \frac{dx}{x\sqrt{(x^2 - a^2)^3}} = -\frac{1}{a^2\sqrt{x^2 - a^2}} - \frac{1}{|a^3|}\sec^{-1}\frac{x}{a}$

186. $\int \frac{dx}{x^2\sqrt{(x^2 \pm a^2)^3}} = -\frac{1}{a^4}\left[\frac{\sqrt{x^2 \pm a^2}}{x} + \frac{x}{\sqrt{x^2 \pm a^2}}\right]$

187. $\int \frac{dx}{x^3\sqrt{(x^2 + a^2)^3}} = -\frac{1}{2a^2x^2\sqrt{x^2 + a^2}} - \frac{3}{2a^4\sqrt{x^2 + a^2}}$

$$+ \frac{3}{2a^5}\log\frac{a + \sqrt{x^2 + a^2}}{x}$$

188. $\int \frac{dx}{x^3\sqrt{(x^2 - a^2)^3}} = \frac{1}{2a^2x^2\sqrt{x^2 - a^2}} - \frac{3}{2a^4\sqrt{x^2 - a^2}} - \frac{3}{2|a^5|}\sec^{-1}\frac{x}{a}$

189. $\int \frac{x^m}{\sqrt{x^2 \pm a^2}}\,dx = \frac{1}{m}x^{m-1}\sqrt{x^2 \pm a^2} \mp \frac{m-1}{m}a^2\int \frac{x^{m-2}}{\sqrt{x^2 \pm a^2}}\,dx$

190. $\int \frac{x^{2m}}{\sqrt{x^2 \pm a^2}}\,dx = \frac{(2m)!}{2^{2m}(m!)^2}\left[\sqrt{x^2 \pm a^2}\sum_{r=1}^{m}\frac{r!(r-1)!}{(2r)!}(\mp a^2)^{m-r}(2x)^{2r-1}\right.$

$$\left. + (\mp a^2)^m \log(x + \sqrt{x^2 \pm a^2})\right]$$

191. $\int \frac{x^{2m+1}}{\sqrt{x^2 \pm a^2}}\,dx = \sqrt{x^2 \pm a^2}\sum_{r=0}^{m}\frac{(2r)!(m!)^2}{(2m+1)!(r!)^2}(\mp 4a^2)^{m-r}x^{2r}$

INTEGRALS (Continued)

192. $$\int \frac{dx}{x^m\sqrt{x^2 \pm a^2}} = \mp \frac{\sqrt{x^2 \pm a^2}}{(m-1)a^2x^{m-1}} \mp \frac{(m-2)}{(m-1)a^2}\int \frac{dx}{x^{m-2}\sqrt{x^2 \pm a^2}}$$

193. $$\int \frac{dx}{x^{2m}\sqrt{x^2 \pm a^2}} = \sqrt{x^2 \pm a^2}\sum_{r=0}^{m-1} \frac{(m-1)!m!(2r)!2^{2m-2r-1}}{(r!)^2(2m)!(\mp a^2)^{m-r}x^{2r+1}}$$

194. $$\int \frac{dx}{x^{2m+1}\sqrt{x^2 + a^2}} = \frac{(2m)!}{(m!)^2}\left[\frac{\sqrt{x^2 + a^2}}{a^2}\sum_{r=1}^{m} (-1)^{m-r+1} \frac{r!(r-1)!}{2(2r)!(4a^2)^{m-r}x^{2r}} + \frac{(-1)^{m+1}}{2^{2m}a^{2m+1}}\log \frac{\sqrt{x^2+a^2}+a}{x}\right]$$

195. $$\int \frac{dx}{x^{2m+1}\sqrt{x^2 - a^2}} = \frac{(2m)!}{(m!)^2}\left[\frac{\sqrt{x^2 - a^2}}{a^2}\sum_{r=1}^{m} \frac{r!(r-1)!}{2(2r)!(4a^2)^{m-r}x^{2r}} + \frac{1}{2^{2m}|a|^{2m+1}}\sec^{-1}\frac{x}{a}\right]$$

196. $$\int \frac{dx}{(x-a)\sqrt{x^2 - a^2}} = -\frac{\sqrt{x^2 - a^2}}{a(x-a)}$$

197. $$\int \frac{dx}{(x+a)\sqrt{x^2 - a^2}} = \frac{\sqrt{x^2 - a^2}}{a(x+a)}$$

198. $$\int f(x, \sqrt{x^2 + a^2})\, dx = a\int f(a \tan u, a \sec u)\sec^2 u\, du, \qquad \left(u = \tan^{-1}\frac{x}{a}, a > 0\right)$$

199. $$\int f(x, \sqrt{x^2 - a^2})\, dx = a\int f(a \sec u, a \tan u)\sec u \tan u\, du, \qquad \left(u = \sec^{-1}\frac{x}{a}, a > 0\right)$$

FORMS CONTAINING $\sqrt{a^2 - x^2}$

200. $$\int \sqrt{a^2 - x^2}\, dx = \frac{1}{2}\left[x\sqrt{a^2 - x^2} + a^2 \sin^{-1}\frac{x}{|a|}\right]$$

201. $$\int \frac{dx}{\sqrt{a^2 - x^2}} = \begin{cases} \sin^{-1}\dfrac{x}{|a|} \\ \text{or} \\ -\cos^{-1}\dfrac{x}{|a|} \end{cases}$$

202. $$\int \frac{dx}{x\sqrt{a^2 - x^2}} = -\frac{1}{a}\log\left(\frac{a + \sqrt{a^2 - x^2}}{x}\right)$$

INTEGRALS (Continued)

203. $\int \frac{\sqrt{a^2 - x^2}}{x} dx = \sqrt{a^2 - x^2} - a \log\left(\frac{a + \sqrt{a^2 - x^2}}{x}\right)$

204. $\int \frac{x\,dx}{\sqrt{a^2 - x^2}} = -\sqrt{a^2 - x^2}$

205. $\int x\sqrt{a^2 - x^2}\,dx = -\frac{1}{3}\sqrt{(a^2 - x^2)^3}$

206. $\int \sqrt{(a^2 - x^2)^3}\,dx = \frac{1}{4}\left[x\sqrt{(a^2 - x^2)^3} + \frac{3a^2x}{2}\sqrt{a^2 - x^2} + \frac{3a^4}{2}\sin^{-1}\frac{x}{|a|}\right]$

207. $\int \frac{dx}{\sqrt{(a^2 - x^2)^3}} = \frac{x}{a^2\sqrt{a^2 - x^2}}$

208. $\int \frac{x\,dx}{\sqrt{(a^2 - x^2)^3}} = \frac{1}{\sqrt{a^2 - x^2}}$

209. $\int x\sqrt{(a^2 - x^2)^3}\,dx = -\frac{1}{5}\sqrt{(a^2 - x^2)^5}$

210. $\int x^2\sqrt{a^2 - x^2}\,dx = -\frac{x}{4}\sqrt{(a^2 - x^2)^3} + \frac{a^2}{8}\left(x\sqrt{a^2 - x^2} + a^2\sin^{-1}\frac{x}{|a|}\right)$

211. $\int x^3\sqrt{a^2 - x^2}\,dx = (-\frac{1}{5}x^2 - \frac{2}{15}a^2)\sqrt{(a^2 - x^2)^3}$

212. $\int x^2\sqrt{(a^2 - x^2)^3}\,dx = -\frac{1}{6}x\sqrt{(a^2 - x^2)^5} + \frac{a^2x}{24}\sqrt{(a^2 - x^2)^3}$

$+ \frac{a^4x}{16}\sqrt{a^2 - x^2} + \frac{a^6}{16}\sin^{-1}\frac{x}{|a|}$

213. $\int x^3\sqrt{(a^2 - x^2)^3}\,dx = \frac{1}{7}\sqrt{(a^2 - x^2)^7} - \frac{a^2}{5}\sqrt{(a^2 - x^2)^5}$

214. $\int \frac{x^2\,dx}{\sqrt{a^2 - x^2}} = -\frac{x}{2}\sqrt{a^2 - x^2} + \frac{a^2}{2}\sin^{-1}\frac{x}{|a|}$

215. $\int \frac{dx}{x^2\sqrt{a^2 - x^2}} = -\frac{\sqrt{a^2 - x^2}}{a^2x}$

216. $\int \frac{\sqrt{a^2 - x^2}}{x^2} dx = -\frac{\sqrt{a^2 - x^2}}{x} - \sin^{-1}\frac{x}{|a|}$

217. $\int \frac{\sqrt{a^2 - x^2}}{x^3} dx = -\frac{\sqrt{a^2 - x^2}}{2x^2} + \frac{1}{2a}\log\frac{a + \sqrt{a^2 - x^2}}{x}$

218. $\int \frac{\sqrt{a^2 - x^2}}{x^4} dx = -\frac{\sqrt{(a^2 - x^2)^3}}{3a^2x^3}$

INTEGRALS (Continued)

219. $$\int \frac{x^2\,dx}{\sqrt{(a^2-x^2)^3}} = \frac{x}{\sqrt{a^2-x^2}} - \sin^{-1}\frac{x}{|a|}$$

220. $$\int \frac{x^3\,dx}{\sqrt{a^2-x^2}} = -\frac{2}{3}(a^2-x^2)^{3/2} - x^2(a^2-x^2)^{1/2} = -\frac{1}{3}\sqrt{a^2-x^2}(x^2+2a^2)$$

221. $$\int \frac{x^3\,dx}{\sqrt{(a^2-x^2)^3}} = 2(a^2-x^2)^{1/2} + \frac{x^2}{(a^2-x^2)^{1/2}} = -\frac{a^2}{\sqrt{a^2-x^2}} + \sqrt{a^2-x^2}$$

222. $$\int \frac{dx}{x^3\sqrt{a^2-x^2}} = -\frac{\sqrt{a^2-x^2}}{2a^2x^2} - \frac{1}{2a^3}\log\frac{a+\sqrt{a^2-x^2}}{x}$$

223. $$\int \frac{dx}{x\sqrt{(a^2-x^2)^3}} = \frac{1}{a^2\sqrt{a^2-x^2}} - \frac{1}{a^3}\log\frac{a+\sqrt{a^2-x^2}}{x}$$

224. $$\int \frac{dx}{x^2\sqrt{(a^2-x^2)^3}} = \frac{1}{a^4}\left[-\frac{\sqrt{a^2-x^2}}{x} + \frac{x}{\sqrt{a^2-x^2}}\right]$$

225. $$\int \frac{dx}{x^3\sqrt{(a^2-x^2)^3}} = -\frac{1}{2a^2x^2\sqrt{a^2-x^2}} + \frac{3}{2a^4\sqrt{a^2-x^2}} - \frac{3}{2a^5}\log\frac{a+\sqrt{a^2-x^2}}{x}$$

226. $$\int \frac{x^m}{\sqrt{a^2-x^2}}\,dx = -\frac{x^{m-1}\sqrt{a^2-x^2}}{m} + \frac{(m-1)a^2}{m}\int \frac{x^{m-2}}{\sqrt{a^2-x^2}}\,dx$$

227. $$\int \frac{x^{2m}}{\sqrt{a^2-x^2}}\,dx = \frac{(2m)!}{(m!)^2}\left[-\sqrt{a^2-x^2}\sum_{r=1}^{m}\frac{r!(r-1)!}{2^{2m-2r+1}(2r)!}a^{2m-2r}x^{2r-1} + \frac{a^{2m}}{2^{2m}}\sin^{-1}\frac{x}{|a|}\right]$$

228. $$\int \frac{x^{2m+1}}{\sqrt{a^2-x^2}}\,dx = -\sqrt{a^2-x^2}\sum_{r=0}^{m}\frac{(2r)!(m!)^2}{(2m+1)!(r!)^2}(4a^2)^{m-r}x^{2r}$$

229. $$\int \frac{dx}{x^m\sqrt{a^2-x^2}} = -\frac{\sqrt{a^2-x^2}}{(m-1)a^2x^{m-1}} + \frac{m-2}{(m-1)a^2}\int \frac{dx}{x^{m-2}\sqrt{a^2-x^2}}$$

230. $$\int \frac{dx}{x^{2m}\sqrt{a^2-x^2}} = -\sqrt{a^2-x^2}\sum_{r=0}^{m-1}\frac{(m-1)!m!(2r)!2^{2m-2r-1}}{(r!)^2(2m)!a^{2m-2r}x^{2r+1}}$$

231. $$\int \frac{dx}{x^{2m+1}\sqrt{a^2-x^2}} = \frac{(2m)!}{(m!)^2}\left[-\frac{\sqrt{a^2-x^2}}{a^2}\sum_{r=1}^{m}\frac{r!(r-1)!}{2(2r)!(4a^2)^{m-r}x^{2r}} + \frac{1}{2^{2m}a^{2m+1}}\log\frac{a-\sqrt{a^2-x^2}}{x}\right]$$

INTEGRALS (Continued)

232. $$\int \frac{dx}{(b^2 - x^2)\sqrt{a^2 - x^2}} = \frac{1}{2b\sqrt{a^2 - b^2}} \log \frac{(b\sqrt{a^2 - x^2} + x\sqrt{a^2 - b^2})^2}{b^2 - x^2}, \quad (a^2 > b^2)$$

233. $$\int \frac{dx}{(b^2 - x^2)\sqrt{a^2 - x^2}} = \frac{1}{b\sqrt{b^2 - a^2}} \tan^{-1} \frac{x\sqrt{b^2 - a^2}}{b\sqrt{a^2 - x^2}}, \quad (b^2 > a^2)$$

234. $$\int \frac{dx}{(b^2 + x^2)\sqrt{a^2 - x^2}} = \frac{1}{b\sqrt{a^2 + b^2}} \tan^{-1} \frac{x\sqrt{a^2 + b^2}}{b\sqrt{a^2 - x^2}}$$

235. $$\int \frac{\sqrt{a^2 - x^2}}{b^2 + x^2}\, dx = \frac{\sqrt{a^2 + b^2}}{|b|} \sin^{-1} \frac{x\sqrt{a^2 + b^2}}{|a|\sqrt{x^2 + b^2}} - \sin^{-1} \frac{x}{|a|}$$

236. $$\int f(x, \sqrt{a^2 - x^2})\, dx = a \int f(a \sin u, a \cos u) \cos u\, du, \quad \left(u = \sin^{-1} \frac{x}{a},\ a > 0\right)$$

FORMS CONTAINING $\sqrt{a + bx + cx^2}$

$$X = a + bx + cx^2,\ q = 4ac - b^2, \text{ and } k = \frac{4c}{q}$$

If $q = 0$, then $\sqrt{X} = \sqrt{c}\left|x + \frac{b}{2c}\right|$

237. $$\int \frac{dx}{\sqrt{X}} = \begin{cases} \dfrac{1}{\sqrt{c}} \log \dfrac{2\sqrt{cX} + 2cx + b}{\sqrt{q}} \\ \text{or} \\ \dfrac{1}{\sqrt{c}} \sinh^{-1} \dfrac{2cx + b}{\sqrt{q}}, \quad (c > 0) \end{cases}$$

238. $$\int \frac{dx}{\sqrt{X}} = -\frac{1}{\sqrt{-c}} \sin^{-1} \frac{2cx + b}{\sqrt{-q}}, \quad (c < 0)$$

239. $$\int \frac{dx}{X\sqrt{X}} = \frac{2(2cx + b)}{q\sqrt{X}}$$

240. $$\int \frac{dx}{X^2\sqrt{X}} = \frac{2(2cx + b)}{3q\sqrt{X}}\left(\frac{1}{X} + 2k\right)$$

241. $$\int \frac{dx}{X^n\sqrt{X}} = \begin{cases} \dfrac{2(2cx + b)\sqrt{X}}{(2n - 1)qX^n} + \dfrac{2k(n - 1)}{2n - 1} \displaystyle\int \frac{dx}{X^{n-1}\sqrt{X}} \\ \text{or} \\ \dfrac{(2cx + b)(n!)(n - 1)!4^n k^{n-1}}{q[(2n)!]\sqrt{X}} \displaystyle\sum_{r=0}^{n-1} \frac{(2r)!}{(4kX)^r (r!)^2} \end{cases}$$

INTEGRALS (Continued)

242. $$\int \sqrt{X}\,dx = \frac{(2cx+b)\sqrt{X}}{4c} + \frac{1}{2k}\int \frac{dx}{\sqrt{X}}$$

243. $$\int X\sqrt{X}\,dx = \frac{(2cx+b)\sqrt{X}}{8c}\left(X + \frac{3}{2k}\right) + \frac{3}{8k^2}\int \frac{dx}{\sqrt{X}}$$

244. $$\int X^2\sqrt{X}\,dx = \frac{(2cx+b)\sqrt{X}}{12c}\left(X^2 + \frac{5X}{4k} + \frac{15}{8k^2}\right) + \frac{5}{16k^3}\int \frac{dx}{\sqrt{X}}$$

245. $$\int X^n\sqrt{X}\,dx = \begin{cases} \dfrac{(2cx+b)X^n\sqrt{X}}{4(n+1)c} + \dfrac{2n+1}{2(n+1)k}\displaystyle\int X^{n-1}\sqrt{X}\,dx \\ \text{or} \\ \dfrac{(2n+2)!}{[(n+1)!]^2(4k)^{n+1}}\left[\dfrac{k(2cx+b)\sqrt{X}}{c}\displaystyle\sum_{r=0}^{n}\dfrac{r!(r+1)!(4kX)^r}{(2r+2)!} + \displaystyle\int\dfrac{dx}{\sqrt{X}}\right] \end{cases}$$

246. $$\int \frac{x\,dx}{\sqrt{X}} = \frac{\sqrt{X}}{c} - \frac{b}{2c}\int \frac{dx}{\sqrt{X}}$$

247. $$\int \frac{x\,dx}{X\sqrt{X}} = -\frac{2(bx+2a)}{q\sqrt{X}}$$

248. $$\int \frac{x\,dx}{X^n\sqrt{X}} = -\frac{\sqrt{X}}{(2n-1)cX^n} - \frac{b}{2c}\int \frac{dx}{X^n\sqrt{X}}$$

249. $$\int \frac{x^2\,dx}{\sqrt{X}} = \left(\frac{x}{2c} - \frac{3b}{4c^2}\right)\sqrt{X} + \frac{3b^2-4ac}{8c^2}\int \frac{dx}{\sqrt{X}}$$

250. $$\int \frac{x^2\,dx}{X\sqrt{X}} = \frac{(2b^2-4ac)x+2ab}{cq\sqrt{X}} + \frac{1}{c}\int \frac{dx}{\sqrt{X}}$$

251. $$\int \frac{x^2\,dx}{X^n\sqrt{X}} = \frac{(2b^2-4ac)x+2ab}{(2n-1)cqX^{n-1}\sqrt{X}} + \frac{4ac+(2n-3)b^2}{(2n-1)cq}\int \frac{dx}{X^{n-1}\sqrt{X}}$$

252. $$\int \frac{x^3\,dx}{\sqrt{X}} = \left(\frac{x^2}{3c} - \frac{5bx}{12c^2} + \frac{5b^2}{8c^3} - \frac{2a}{3c^2}\right)\sqrt{X} + \left(\frac{3ab}{4c^2} - \frac{5b^3}{16c^3}\right)\int \frac{dx}{\sqrt{X}}$$

253. $$\int \frac{x^n\,dx}{\sqrt{X}} = \frac{1}{nc}x^{n-1}\sqrt{X} - \frac{(2n-1)b}{2nc}\int \frac{x^{n-1}\,dx}{\sqrt{X}} - \frac{(n-1)a}{nc}\int \frac{x^{n-2}\,dx}{\sqrt{X}}$$

INTEGRALS (Continued)

254. $$\int x\sqrt{X}\,dx = \frac{X\sqrt{X}}{3c} - \frac{b(2cx+b)}{8c^2}\sqrt{X} - \frac{b}{4ck}\int\frac{dx}{\sqrt{X}}$$

255. $$\int xX\sqrt{X}\,dx = \frac{X^2\sqrt{X}}{5c} - \frac{b}{2c}\int X\sqrt{X}\,dx$$

256. $$\int xX^n\sqrt{X}\,dx = \frac{X^{n+1}\sqrt{X}}{(2n+3)c} - \frac{b}{2c}\int X^n\sqrt{X}\,dx$$

257. $$\int x^2\sqrt{X}\,dx = \left(x - \frac{5b}{6c}\right)\frac{X\sqrt{X}}{4c} + \frac{5b^2-4ac}{16c^2}\int\sqrt{X}\,dx$$

258. $$\int\frac{dx}{x\sqrt{X}} = -\frac{1}{\sqrt{a}}\log\frac{2\sqrt{aX}+bx+2a}{x}, \qquad (a > 0)$$

259. $$\int\frac{dx}{x\sqrt{X}} = \frac{1}{\sqrt{-a}}\sin^{-1}\left(\frac{bx+2a}{|x|\sqrt{-q}}\right), \qquad (a < 0)$$

260. $$\int\frac{dx}{x\sqrt{X}} = -\frac{2\sqrt{X}}{bx}, \qquad (a = 0)$$

261. $$\int\frac{dx}{x^2\sqrt{X}} = -\frac{\sqrt{X}}{ax} - \frac{b}{2a}\int\frac{dx}{x\sqrt{X}}$$

262. $$\int\frac{\sqrt{X}\,dx}{x} = \sqrt{X} + \frac{b}{2}\int\frac{dx}{\sqrt{X}} + a\int\frac{dx}{x\sqrt{X}}$$

263. $$\int\frac{\sqrt{X}\,dx}{x^2} = -\frac{\sqrt{X}}{x} + \frac{b}{2}\int\frac{dx}{x\sqrt{X}} + c\int\frac{dx}{\sqrt{X}}$$

FORMS INVOLVING $\sqrt{2ax - x^2}$

264. $$\int\sqrt{2ax-x^2}\,dx = \frac{1}{2}\left[(x-a)\sqrt{2ax-x^2} + a^2\sin^{-1}\frac{x-a}{|a|}\right]$$

265. $$\int\frac{dx}{\sqrt{2ax-x^2}} = \begin{cases}\cos^{-1}\dfrac{a-x}{|a|} \\ \text{or} \\ \sin^{-1}\dfrac{x-a}{|a|}\end{cases}$$

INTEGRALS (Continued)

266. $$\int x^n\sqrt{2ax - x^2}\,dx = \begin{cases} -\dfrac{x^{n-1}(2ax - x^2)^{3/2}}{n+2} + \dfrac{(2n+1)a}{n+2}\displaystyle\int x^{n-1}\sqrt{2ax - x^2}\,dx \\ \text{or} \\ \sqrt{2ax - x^2}\left[\dfrac{x^{n+1}}{n+2} - \displaystyle\sum_{r=0}^{n} \dfrac{(2n+1)!(r!)^2 a^{n-r+1}}{2^{n-r}(2r+1)!(n+2)!n!}x^r\right] \\ \qquad + \dfrac{(2n+1)!a^{n+2}}{2^n n!(n+2)!}\sin^{-1}\dfrac{x-a}{|a|} \end{cases}$$

267. $$\int \frac{\sqrt{2ax - x^2}}{x^n}\,dx = \frac{(2ax - x^2)^{3/2}}{(3-2n)ax^n} + \frac{n-3}{(2n-3)a}\int \frac{\sqrt{2ax - x^2}}{x^{n-1}}\,dx$$

268. $$\int \frac{x^n\,dx}{\sqrt{2ax - x^2}} = \begin{cases} \dfrac{-x^{n-1}\sqrt{2ax - x^2}}{n} + \dfrac{a(2n-1)}{n}\displaystyle\int \dfrac{x^{n-1}}{\sqrt{2ax - x^2}}\,dx \\ \text{or} \\ -\sqrt{2ax - x^2}\displaystyle\sum_{r=1}^{n} \dfrac{(2n)!r!(r-1)!a^{n-r}}{2^{n-r}(2r)!(n!)^2}x^{r-1} \\ \qquad + \dfrac{(2n)!a^n}{2^n(n!)^2}\sin^{-1}\dfrac{x-a}{|a|} \end{cases}$$

269. $$\int \frac{dx}{x^n\sqrt{2ax - x^2}} = \begin{cases} \dfrac{\sqrt{2ax - x^2}}{a(1-2n)x^n} + \dfrac{n-1}{(2n-1)a}\displaystyle\int \dfrac{dx}{x^{n-1}\sqrt{2ax - x^2}} \\ \text{or} \\ -\sqrt{2ax - x^2}\displaystyle\sum_{r=0}^{n-1} \dfrac{2^{n-r}(n-1)!n!(2r)!}{(2n)!(r!)^2 a^{n-r}x^{r+1}} \end{cases}$$

270. $$\int \frac{dx}{(2ax - x^2)^{3/2}} = \frac{x-a}{a^2\sqrt{2ax - x^2}}$$

271. $$\int \frac{x\,dx}{(2ax - x^2)^{3/2}} = \frac{x}{a\sqrt{2ax - x^2}}$$

MISCELLANEOUS ALGEBRAIC FORMS

272. $$\int \frac{dx}{\sqrt{2ax + x^2}} = \log(x + a + \sqrt{2ax + x^2})$$

273. $$\int \sqrt{ax^2 + c}\,dx = \frac{x}{2}\sqrt{ax^2 + c} + \frac{c}{2\sqrt{a}}\log(x\sqrt{a} + \sqrt{ax^2 + c}), \qquad (a > 0)$$

274. $$\int \sqrt{ax^2 + c}\,dx = \frac{x}{2}\sqrt{ax^2 + c} + \frac{c}{2\sqrt{-a}}\sin^{-1}\left(x\sqrt{-\frac{a}{c}}\right), \qquad (a < 0)$$

INTEGRALS (Continued)

275. $\int \sqrt{\frac{1+x}{1-x}}\,dx = \sin^{-1} x - \sqrt{1-x^2}$

276. $$\int \frac{dx}{x\sqrt{ax^n + c}} = \begin{cases} \dfrac{1}{n\sqrt{c}} \log \dfrac{\sqrt{ax^n + c} - \sqrt{c}}{\sqrt{ax^n + c} + \sqrt{c}} \\ \text{or} \\ \dfrac{2}{n\sqrt{c}} \log \dfrac{\sqrt{ax^n + c} - \sqrt{c}}{\sqrt{x^n}}, \qquad (c > 0) \end{cases}$$

277. $\int \frac{dx}{x\sqrt{ax^n + c}} = \frac{2}{n\sqrt{-c}} \sec^{-1} \sqrt{-\frac{ax^n}{c}}, \qquad (c < 0)$

278. $\int \frac{dx}{\sqrt{ax^2 + c}} = \frac{1}{\sqrt{a}} \log (x\sqrt{a} + \sqrt{ax^2 + c}), \qquad (a > 0)$

279. $\int \frac{dx}{\sqrt{ax^2 + c}} = \frac{1}{\sqrt{-a}} \sin^{-1}\left(x\sqrt{-\frac{a}{c}}\right), \qquad (a < 0)$

280. $$\int (ax^2 + c)^{m+\frac{1}{2}}\,dx = \begin{cases} \dfrac{x(ax^2 + c)^{m+\frac{1}{2}}}{2(m+1)} + \dfrac{(2m+1)c}{2(m+1)} \displaystyle\int (ax^2 + c)^{m-\frac{1}{2}}\,dx \\ \text{or} \\ x\sqrt{ax^2 + c} \displaystyle\sum_{r=0}^{m} \dfrac{(2m+1)!(r!)^2 c^{m-r}}{2^{2m-2r+1} m!(m+1)!(2r+1)!}(ax^2 + c)^r \\ \quad + \dfrac{(2m+1)!c^{m+1}}{2^{2m+1} m!(m+1)!} \displaystyle\int \dfrac{dx}{\sqrt{ax^2 + c}} \end{cases}$$

281. $\int x(ax^2 + c)^{m+\frac{1}{2}}\,dx = \frac{(ax^2 + c)^{m+\frac{3}{2}}}{(2m+3)a}$

282. $$\int \frac{(ax^2 + c)^{m+\frac{1}{2}}}{x}\,dx = \begin{cases} \dfrac{(ax^2 + c)^{m+\frac{1}{2}}}{2m+1} + c \displaystyle\int \dfrac{(ax^2 + c)^{m-\frac{1}{2}}}{x}\,dx \\ \text{or} \\ \sqrt{ax^2 + c} \displaystyle\sum_{r=0}^{m} \dfrac{c^{m-r}(ax^2 + c)^r}{2r+1} + c^{m+1} \displaystyle\int \dfrac{dx}{x\sqrt{ax^2 + c}} \end{cases}$$

283. $$\int \frac{dx}{(ax^2 + c)^{m+\frac{1}{2}}} = \begin{cases} \dfrac{x}{(2m-1)c(ax^2 + c)^{m-\frac{1}{2}}} + \dfrac{2m-2}{(2m-1)c} \displaystyle\int \dfrac{dx}{(ax^2 + c)^{m-\frac{1}{2}}} \\ \text{or} \\ \dfrac{x}{\sqrt{ax^2 + c}} \displaystyle\sum_{r=0}^{m-1} \dfrac{2^{2m-2r-1}(m-1)!m!(2r)!}{(2m)!(r!)^2 c^{m-r}(ax^2 + c)^r} \end{cases}$$

INTEGRALS (Continued)

284. $$\int \frac{dx}{x^m\sqrt{ax^2+c}} = -\frac{\sqrt{ax^2+c}}{(m-1)cx^{m-1}} - \frac{(m-2)a}{(m-1)c}\int \frac{dx}{x^{m-2}\sqrt{ax^2+c}}$$

285. $$\int \frac{1+x^2}{(1-x^2)\sqrt{1+x^4}}\,dx = \frac{1}{\sqrt{2}}\log\frac{x\sqrt{2}+\sqrt{1+x^4}}{1-x^2}$$

286. $$\int \frac{1-x^2}{(1+x^2)\sqrt{1+x^4}}\,dx = \frac{1}{\sqrt{2}}\tan^{-1}\frac{x\sqrt{2}}{\sqrt{1+x^4}}$$

287. $$\int \frac{dx}{x\sqrt{x^n+a^2}} = -\frac{2}{na}\log\frac{a+\sqrt{x^n+a^2}}{\sqrt{x^n}}$$

288. $$\int \frac{dx}{x\sqrt{x^n-a^2}} = -\frac{2}{na}\sin^{-1}\frac{a}{\sqrt{x^n}}$$

289. $$\int \sqrt{\frac{x}{a^3-x^3}}\,dx = \frac{2}{3}\sin^{-1}\left(\frac{x}{a}\right)^{\frac{3}{2}}$$

FORMS INVOLVING TRIGONOMETRIC FUNCTIONS

290. $$\int (\sin ax)\,dx = -\frac{1}{a}\cos ax$$

291. $$\int (\cos ax)\,dx = \frac{1}{a}\sin ax$$

292. $$\int (\tan ax)\,dx = -\frac{1}{a}\log\cos ax = \frac{1}{a}\log\sec ax$$

293. $$\int (\cot ax)\,dx = \frac{1}{a}\log\sin ax = -\frac{1}{a}\log\csc ax$$

294. $$\int (\sec ax)\,dx = \frac{1}{a}\log(\sec ax + \tan ax) = \frac{1}{a}\log\tan\left(\frac{\pi}{4}+\frac{ax}{2}\right)$$

295. $$\int (\csc ax)\,dx = \frac{1}{a}\log(\csc ax - \cot ax) = \frac{1}{a}\log\tan\frac{ax}{2}$$

296. $$\int (\sin^2 ax)\,dx = -\frac{1}{2a}\cos ax\sin ax + \frac{1}{2}x = \frac{1}{2}x - \frac{1}{4a}\sin 2ax$$

297. $$\int (\sin^3 ax)\,dx = -\frac{1}{3a}(\cos ax)(\sin^2 ax + 2)$$

298. $$\int (\sin^4 ax)\,dx = \frac{3x}{8} - \frac{\sin 2ax}{4a} + \frac{\sin 4ax}{32a}$$

299. $$\int (\sin^n ax)\,dx = -\frac{\sin^{n-1} ax\cos ax}{na} + \frac{n-1}{n}\int (\sin^{n-2} ax)\,dx$$

INTEGRALS (Continued)

300. $$\int (\sin^{2m} ax)\,dx = -\frac{\cos ax}{a}\sum_{r=0}^{m-1}\frac{(2m)!(r!)^2}{2^{2m-2r}(2r+1)!(m!)^2}\sin^{2r+1} ax + \frac{(2m)!}{2^{2m}(m!)^2}x$$

301. $$\int (\sin^{2m+1} ax)\,dx = -\frac{\cos ax}{a}\sum_{r=0}^{m}\frac{2^{2m-2r}(m!)^2(2r)!}{(2m+1)!(r!)^2}\sin^{2r} ax$$

302. $$\int (\cos^2 ax)\,dx = \frac{1}{2a}\sin ax \cos ax + \frac{1}{2}x = \frac{1}{2}x + \frac{1}{4a}\sin 2ax$$

303. $$\int (\cos^3 ax)\,dx = \frac{1}{3a}(\sin ax)(\cos^2 ax + 2)$$

304. $$\int (\cos^4 ax)\,dx = \frac{3x}{8} + \frac{\sin 2ax}{4a} + \frac{\sin 4ax}{32a}$$

305. $$\int (\cos^n ax)\,dx = \frac{1}{na}\cos^{n-1} ax \sin ax + \frac{n-1}{n}\int (\cos^{n-2} ax)\,dx$$

306. $$\int (\cos^{2m} ax)\,dx = \frac{\sin ax}{a}\sum_{r=0}^{m-1}\frac{(2m)!(r!)^2}{2^{2m-2r}(2r+1)!(m!)^2}\cos^{2r+1} ax + \frac{(2m)!}{2^{2m}(m!)^2}x$$

307. $$\int (\cos^{2m+1} ax)\,dx = \frac{\sin ax}{a}\sum_{r=0}^{m}\frac{2^{2m-2r}(m!)^2(2r)!}{(2m+1)!(r!)^2}\cos^{2r} ax$$

308. $$\int \frac{dx}{\sin^2 ax} = \int (\csc^2 ax)\,dx = -\frac{1}{a}\cot ax$$

309. $$\int \frac{dx}{\sin^m ax} = \int (\csc^m ax)\,dx = -\frac{1}{(m-1)a}\cdot\frac{\cos ax}{\sin^{m-1} ax} + \frac{m-2}{m-1}\int \frac{dx}{\sin^{m-2} ax}$$

310. $$\int \frac{dx}{\sin^{2m} ax} = \int (\csc^{2m} ax)\,dx = -\frac{1}{a}\cos ax \sum_{r=0}^{m-1}\frac{2^{2m-2r-1}(m-1)!m!(2r)!}{(2m)!(r!)^2\sin^{2r+1} ax}$$

311. $$\int \frac{dx}{\sin^{2m+1} ax} = \int (\csc^{2m+1} ax)\,dx =$$
$$-\frac{1}{a}\cos ax \sum_{r=0}^{m-1}\frac{(2m)!(r!)^2}{2^{2m-2r}(m!)^2(2r+1)!\sin^{2r+2} ax} + \frac{1}{a}\cdot\frac{(2m)!}{2^{2m}(m!)^2}\log\tan\frac{ax}{2}$$

312. $$\int \frac{dx}{\cos^2 ax} = \int (\sec^2 ax)\,dx = \frac{1}{a}\tan ax$$

313. $$\int \frac{dx}{\cos^n ax} = \int (\sec^n ax)\,dx = \frac{1}{(n-1)a}\cdot\frac{\sin ax}{\cos^{n-1} ax} + \frac{n-2}{n-1}\int \frac{dx}{\cos^{n-2} ax}$$

314. $$\int \frac{dx}{\cos^{2m} ax} = \int (\sec^{2m} ax)\,dx = \frac{1}{a}\sin ax \sum_{r=0}^{m-1}\frac{2^{2m-2r-1}(m-1)!m!(2r)!}{(2m)!(r!)^2\cos^{2r+1} ax}$$

INTEGRALS (Continued)

315. $$\int \frac{dx}{\cos^{2m+1} ax} = \int (\sec^{2m+1} ax)\, dx = \frac{1}{a} \sin ax \sum_{r=0}^{m-1} \frac{(2m)!(r!)^2}{2^{2m-2r}(m!)^2(2r+1)! \cos^{2r+2} ax} + \frac{1}{a} \cdot \frac{(2m)!}{2^{2m}(m!)^2} \log(\sec ax + \tan ax)$$

316. $$\int (\sin mx)(\sin nx)\, dx = \frac{\sin(m-n)x}{2(m-n)} - \frac{\sin(m+n)x}{2(m+n)}, \qquad (m^2 \neq n^2)$$

317. $$\int (\cos mx)(\cos nx)\, dx = \frac{\sin(m-n)x}{2(m-n)} + \frac{\sin(m+n)x}{2(m+n)}, \qquad (m^2 \neq n^2)$$

318. $$\int (\sin ax)(\cos ax)\, dx = \frac{1}{2a} \sin^2 ax$$

319. $$\int (\sin mx)(\cos nx)\, dx = -\frac{\cos(m-n)x}{2(m-n)} - \frac{\cos(m+n)x}{2(m+n)}, \qquad (m^2 \neq n^2)$$

320. $$\int (\sin^2 ax)(\cos^2 ax)\, dx = -\frac{1}{32a} \sin 4ax + \frac{x}{8}$$

321. $$\int (\sin ax)(\cos^m ax)\, dx = -\frac{\cos^{m+1} ax}{(m+1)a}$$

322. $$\int (\sin^m ax)(\cos ax)\, dx = \frac{\sin^{m+1} ax}{(m+1)a}$$

323. $$\int (\cos^m ax)(\sin^n ax)\, dx = \begin{cases} \dfrac{\cos^{m-1} ax \sin^{n+1} ax}{(m+n)a} + \dfrac{m-1}{m+n} \displaystyle\int (\cos^{m-2} ax)(\sin^n ax)\, dx \\ \text{or} \\ -\dfrac{\sin^{n-1} ax \cos^{m+1} ax}{(m+n)a} + \dfrac{n-1}{m+n} \displaystyle\int (\cos^m ax)(\sin^{n-2} ax)\, dx \end{cases}$$

324. $$\int \frac{\cos^m ax}{\sin^n ax}\, dx = \begin{cases} -\dfrac{\cos^{m+1} ax}{(n-1)a \sin^{n-1} ax} - \dfrac{m-n+2}{n-1} \displaystyle\int \frac{\cos^m ax}{\sin^{n-2} ax}\, dx \\ \text{or} \\ \dfrac{\cos^{m-1} ax}{a(m-n) \sin^{n-1} ax} + \dfrac{m-1}{m-n} \displaystyle\int \frac{\cos^{m-2} ax}{\sin^n ax}\, dx \end{cases}$$

INTEGRALS (Continued)

325. $$\int \frac{\sin^m ax}{\cos^n ax} dx = \begin{cases} \dfrac{\sin^{m+1} ax}{a(n-1)\cos^{n-1} ax} - \dfrac{m-n+2}{n-1} \displaystyle\int \frac{\sin^m ax}{\cos^{n-2} ax} dx \\ \text{or} \\ -\dfrac{\sin^{m-1} ax}{a(m-n)\cos^{n-1} ax} + \dfrac{m-1}{m-n} \displaystyle\int \frac{\sin^{m-2} ax}{\cos^n ax} dx \end{cases}$$

326. $$\int \frac{\sin ax}{\cos^2 ax} dx = \frac{1}{a \cos ax} = \frac{\sec ax}{a}$$

327. $$\int \frac{\sin^2 ax}{\cos ax} dx = -\frac{1}{a} \sin ax + \frac{1}{a} \log \tan\left(\frac{\pi}{4} + \frac{ax}{2}\right)$$

328. $$\int \frac{\cos ax}{\sin^2 ax} dx = -\frac{1}{a \sin ax} = -\frac{\csc ax}{a}$$

329. $$\int \frac{dx}{(\sin ax)(\cos ax)} = \frac{1}{a} \log \tan ax$$

330. $$\int \frac{dx}{(\sin ax)(\cos^2 ax)} = \frac{1}{a}\left(\sec ax + \log \tan \frac{ax}{2}\right)$$

331. $$\int \frac{dx}{(\sin ax)(\cos^n ax)} = \frac{1}{a(n-1)\cos^{n-1} ax} + \int \frac{dx}{(\sin ax)(\cos^{n-2} ax)}$$

332. $$\int \frac{dx}{(\sin^2 ax)(\cos ax)} = -\frac{1}{a} \csc ax + \frac{1}{a} \log \tan\left(\frac{\pi}{4} + \frac{ax}{2}\right)$$

333. $$\int \frac{dx}{(\sin^2 ax)(\cos^2 ax)} = -\frac{2}{a} \cot 2ax$$

334. $$\int \frac{dx}{\sin^m ax \cos^n ax} = \begin{cases} -\dfrac{1}{a(m-1)(\sin^{m-1} ax)(\cos^{n-1} ax)} \\ \qquad + \dfrac{m+n-2}{m-1} \displaystyle\int \frac{dx}{(\sin^{m-2} ax)(\cos^n ax)} \\ \text{or} \\ \dfrac{1}{a(n-1)\sin^{m-1} ax \cos^{n-1} ax} \\ \qquad - \dfrac{m+n-2}{n-1} \displaystyle\int \frac{dx}{\sin^m ax \cos^{n-2} ax} \end{cases}$$

335. $$\int \sin(a + bx)\, dx = -\frac{1}{b} \cos(a + bx)$$

336. $$\int \cos(a + bx)\, dx = \frac{1}{b} \sin(a + bx)$$

337. $$\int \frac{dx}{1 \pm \sin ax} = \mp \frac{1}{a} \tan\left(\frac{\pi}{4} \mp \frac{ax}{2}\right)$$

INTEGRALS (Continued)

338. $$\int \frac{dx}{1+\cos ax} = \frac{1}{a}\tan\frac{ax}{2}$$

339. $$\int \frac{dx}{1-\cos ax} = -\frac{1}{a}\cot\frac{ax}{2}$$

*340. $$\int \frac{dx}{a+b\sin x} = \begin{cases} \dfrac{2}{\sqrt{a^2-b^2}}\tan^{-1}\dfrac{a\tan\frac{x}{2}+b}{\sqrt{a^2-b^2}} \\ \text{or} \\ \dfrac{1}{\sqrt{b^2-a^2}}\log\dfrac{a\tan\frac{x}{2}+b-\sqrt{b^2-a^2}}{a\tan\frac{x}{2}+b+\sqrt{b^2-a^2}} \end{cases}$$

*341. $$\int \frac{dx}{a+b\cos x} = \begin{cases} \dfrac{2}{\sqrt{a^2-b^2}}\tan^{-1}\dfrac{\sqrt{a^2-b^2}\tan\frac{x}{2}}{a+b} \\ \text{or} \\ \dfrac{1}{\sqrt{b^2-a^2}}\log\left(\dfrac{\sqrt{b^2-a^2}\tan\frac{x}{2}+a+b}{\sqrt{b^2-a^2}\tan\frac{x}{2}-a-b}\right) \end{cases}$$

*342. $$\int \frac{dx}{a+b\sin x+c\cos x}$$

$$= \begin{cases} \dfrac{1}{\sqrt{b^2+c^2-a^2}}\log\dfrac{b-\sqrt{b^2+c^2-a^2}+(a-c)\tan\frac{x}{2}}{b+\sqrt{b^2+c^2-a^2}+(a-c)\tan\frac{x}{2}}, & \text{if } a^2 < b^2+c^2,\ a \neq c \\ \text{or} \\ \dfrac{2}{\sqrt{a^2-b^2-c^2}}\tan^{-1}\dfrac{b+(a-c)\tan\frac{x}{2}}{\sqrt{a^2-b^2-c^2}}, & \text{if } a^2 > b^2+c^2 \\ \text{or} \\ \dfrac{1}{a}\left[\dfrac{a-(b+c)\cos x-(b-c)\sin x}{a-(b-c)\cos x+(b+c)\sin x}\right], & \text{if } a^2 = b^2+c^2,\ a \neq c. \end{cases}$$

*343. $$\int \frac{\sin^2 x\,dx}{a+b\cos^2 x} = \frac{1}{b}\sqrt{\frac{a+b}{a}}\tan^{-1}\left(\sqrt{\frac{a}{a+b}}\tan x\right) - \frac{x}{b}, \qquad (ab > 0, \text{ or } |a| > |b|)$$

*See note 6—page 431.

INTEGRALS (Continued)

*344. $$\int \frac{dx}{a^2 \cos^2 x + b^2 \sin^2 x} = \frac{1}{ab} \tan^{-1}\left(\frac{b \tan x}{a}\right)$$

*345. $$\int \frac{\cos^2 cx}{a^2 + b^2 \sin^2 cx} dx = \frac{\sqrt{a^2 + b^2}}{ab^2 c} \tan^{-1} \frac{\sqrt{a^2 + b^2} \tan cx}{a} - \frac{x}{b^2}$$

346. $$\int \frac{\sin cx \cos cx}{a \cos^2 cx + b \sin^2 cx} dx = \frac{1}{2c(b - a)} \log (a \cos^2 cx + b \sin^2 cx)$$

347. $$\int \frac{\cos cx}{a \cos cx + b \sin cx} dx = \int \frac{dx}{a + b \tan cx} = \frac{1}{c(a^2 + b^2)}[acx + b \log (a \cos cx + b \sin cx)]$$

348. $$\int \frac{\sin cx}{a \sin cx + b \cos cx} dx = \int \frac{dx}{a + b \cot cx} = \frac{1}{c(a^2 + b^2)}[acx - b \log (a \sin cx + b \cos cx)]$$

*349. $$\int \frac{dx}{a \cos^2 x + 2b \cos x \sin x + c \sin^2 x} = \begin{cases} \dfrac{1}{2\sqrt{b^2 - ac}} \log \dfrac{c \tan x + b - \sqrt{b^2 - ac}}{c \tan x + b + \sqrt{b^2 - ac}}, & (b^2 > ac) \\ \text{or} & \\ \dfrac{1}{\sqrt{ac - b^2}} \tan^{-1} \dfrac{c \tan x + b}{\sqrt{ac - b^2}}, & (b^2 < ac) \\ \text{or} & \\ -\dfrac{1}{c \tan x + b}, & (b^2 = ac) \end{cases}$$

350. $$\int \frac{\sin ax}{1 \pm \sin ax} dx = \pm x + \frac{1}{a} \tan\left(\frac{\pi}{4} \mp \frac{ax}{2}\right)$$

351. $$\int \frac{dx}{(\sin ax)(1 \pm \sin ax)} = \frac{1}{a} \tan\left(\frac{\pi}{4} \mp \frac{ax}{2}\right) + \frac{1}{a} \log \tan \frac{ax}{2}$$

352. $$\int \frac{dx}{(1 + \sin ax)^2} = -\frac{1}{2a} \tan\left(\frac{\pi}{4} - \frac{ax}{2}\right) - \frac{1}{6a} \tan^3\left(\frac{\pi}{4} - \frac{ax}{2}\right)$$

353. $$\int \frac{dx}{(1 - \sin ax)^2} = \frac{1}{2a} \cot\left(\frac{\pi}{4} - \frac{ax}{2}\right) + \frac{1}{6a} \cot^3\left(\frac{\pi}{4} - \frac{ax}{2}\right)$$

354. $$\int \frac{\sin ax}{(1 + \sin ax)^2} dx = -\frac{1}{2a} \tan\left(\frac{\pi}{4} - \frac{ax}{2}\right) + \frac{1}{6a} \tan^3\left(\frac{\pi}{4} - \frac{ax}{2}\right)$$

*See note 6--page 431.

INTEGRALS (Continued)

355. $\int \frac{\sin ax}{(1-\sin ax)^2}\,dx = -\frac{1}{2a}\cot\left(\frac{\pi}{4}-\frac{ax}{2}\right) + \frac{1}{6a}\cot^3\left(\frac{\pi}{4}-\frac{ax}{2}\right)$

356. $\int \frac{\sin x\,dx}{a+b\sin x} = \frac{x}{b} - \frac{a}{b}\int \frac{dx}{a+b\sin x}$

357. $\int \frac{dx}{(\sin x)(a+b\sin x)} = \frac{1}{a}\log\tan\frac{x}{2} - \frac{b}{a}\int \frac{dx}{a+b\sin x}$

358. $\int \frac{dx}{(a+b\sin x)^2} = \frac{b\cos x}{(a^2-b^2)(a+b\sin x)} + \frac{a}{a^2-b^2}\int \frac{dx}{a+b\sin x}$

359. $\int \frac{\sin x\,dx}{(a+b\sin x)^2} = \frac{a\cos x}{(b^2-a^2)(a+b\sin x)} + \frac{b}{b^2-a^2}\int \frac{dx}{a+b\sin x}$

*360. $\int \frac{dx}{a^2+b^2\sin^2 cx} = \frac{1}{ac\sqrt{a^2+b^2}}\tan^{-1}\frac{\sqrt{a^2+b^2}\tan cx}{a}$

*361. $\int \frac{dx}{a^2-b^2\sin^2 cx} = \begin{cases} \frac{1}{ac\sqrt{a^2-b^2}}\tan^{-1}\frac{\sqrt{a^2-b^2}\tan cx}{a}, & (a^2>b^2) \\ \text{or} & \\ \frac{1}{2ac\sqrt{b^2-a^2}}\log\frac{\sqrt{b^2-a^2}\tan cx + a}{\sqrt{b^2-a^2}\tan cx - a}, & (a^2<b^2) \end{cases}$

362. $\int \frac{\cos ax}{1+\cos ax}\,dx = x - \frac{1}{a}\tan\frac{ax}{2}$

363. $\int \frac{\cos ax}{1-\cos ax}\,dx = -x - \frac{1}{a}\cot\frac{ax}{2}$

364. $\int \frac{dx}{(\cos ax)(1+\cos ax)} = \frac{1}{a}\log\tan\left(\frac{\pi}{4}+\frac{ax}{2}\right) - \frac{1}{a}\tan\frac{ax}{2}$

365. $\int \frac{dx}{(\cos ax)(1-\cos ax)} = \frac{1}{a}\log\tan\left(\frac{\pi}{4}+\frac{ax}{2}\right) - \frac{1}{a}\cot\frac{ax}{2}$

366. $\int \frac{dx}{(1+\cos ax)^2} = \frac{1}{2a}\tan\frac{ax}{2} + \frac{1}{6a}\tan^3\frac{ax}{2}$

367. $\int \frac{dx}{(1-\cos ax)^2} = -\frac{1}{2a}\cot\frac{ax}{2} - \frac{1}{6a}\cot^3\frac{ax}{2}$

368. $\int \frac{\cos ax}{(1+\cos ax)^2}\,dx = \frac{1}{2a}\tan\frac{ax}{2} - \frac{1}{6a}\tan^3\frac{ax}{2}$

369. $\int \frac{\cos ax}{(1-\cos ax)^2}\,dx = \frac{1}{2a}\cot\frac{ax}{2} - \frac{1}{6a}\cot^3\frac{ax}{2}$

*See note 6–page 431.

INTEGRALS (Continued)

370. $\int \frac{\cos x\,dx}{a + b\cos x} = \frac{x}{b} - \frac{a}{b}\int \frac{dx}{a + b\cos x}$

371. $\int \frac{dx}{(\cos x)(a + b\cos x)} = \frac{1}{a}\log\tan\left(\frac{x}{2} + \frac{\pi}{4}\right) - \frac{b}{a}\int \frac{dx}{a + b\cos x}$

372. $\int \frac{dx}{(a + b\cos x)^2} = \frac{b\sin x}{(b^2 - a^2)(a + b\cos x)} - \frac{a}{b^2 - a^2}\int \frac{dx}{a + b\cos x}$

373. $\int \frac{\cos x}{(a + b\cos x)^2}\,dx = \frac{a\sin x}{(a^2 - b^2)(a + b\cos x)} - \frac{b}{a^2 - b^2}\int \frac{dx}{a + b\cos x}$

***374.** $\int \frac{dx}{a^2 + b^2 - 2ab\cos cx} = \frac{2}{c(a^2 - b^2)}\tan^{-1}\left(\frac{a + b}{a - b}\tan\frac{cx}{2}\right)$

***375.** $\int \frac{dx}{a^2 + b^2\cos^2 cx} = \frac{1}{ac\sqrt{a^2 + b^2}}\tan^{-1}\frac{a\tan cx}{\sqrt{a^2 + b^2}}$

***376.** $\int \frac{dx}{a^2 - b^2\cos^2 cx} = \begin{cases} \frac{1}{ac\sqrt{a^2 - b^2}}\tan^{-1}\frac{a\tan cx}{\sqrt{a^2 - b^2}}, & (a^2 > b^2) \\ \text{or} & \\ \frac{1}{2ac\sqrt{b^2 - a^2}}\log\frac{a\tan cx - \sqrt{b^2 - a^2}}{a\tan cx + \sqrt{b^2 - a^2}}, & (b^2 > a^2) \end{cases}$

377. $\int \frac{\sin ax}{1 \pm \cos ax}\,dx = \mp\frac{1}{a}\log(1 \pm \cos ax)$

378. $\int \frac{\cos ax}{1 \pm \sin ax}\,dx = \pm\frac{1}{a}\log(1 \pm \sin ax)$

379. $\int \frac{dx}{(\sin ax)(1 \pm \cos ax)} = \pm\frac{1}{2a(1 \pm \cos ax)} + \frac{1}{2a}\log\tan\frac{ax}{2}$

380. $\int \frac{dx}{(\cos ax)(1 \pm \sin ax)} = \mp\frac{1}{2a(1 \pm \sin ax)} + \frac{1}{2a}\log\tan\left(\frac{\pi}{4} + \frac{ax}{2}\right)$

381. $\int \frac{\sin ax}{(\cos ax)(1 \pm \cos ax)}\,dx = \frac{1}{a}\log(\sec ax \pm 1)$

382. $\int \frac{\cos ax}{(\sin ax)(1 \pm \sin ax)}\,dx = -\frac{1}{a}\log(\csc ax \pm 1)$

383. $\int \frac{\sin ax}{(\cos ax)(1 \pm \sin ax)}\,dx = \frac{1}{2a(1 \pm \sin ax)} \pm \frac{1}{2a}\log\tan\left(\frac{\pi}{4} + \frac{ax}{2}\right)$

384. $\int \frac{\cos ax}{(\sin ax)(1 \pm \cos ax)}\,dx = -\frac{1}{2a(1 \pm \cos ax)} \pm \frac{1}{2a}\log\tan\frac{ax}{2}$

*See note 6–page 431.

INTEGRALS (Continued)

385. $$\int \frac{dx}{\sin ax \pm \cos ax} = \frac{1}{a\sqrt{2}} \log \tan\left(\frac{ax}{2} \pm \frac{\pi}{8}\right)$$

386. $$\int \frac{dx}{(\sin ax \pm \cos ax)^2} = \frac{1}{2a} \tan\left(ax \mp \frac{\pi}{4}\right)$$

387. $$\int \frac{dx}{1 + \cos ax \pm \sin ax} = \pm \frac{1}{a} \log\left(1 \pm \tan\frac{ax}{2}\right)$$

388. $$\int \frac{dx}{a^2 \cos^2 cx - b^2 \sin^2 cx} = \frac{1}{2abc} \log \frac{b \tan cx + a}{b \tan cx - a}$$

389. $$\int x(\sin ax)\,dx = \frac{1}{a^2} \sin ax - \frac{x}{a} \cos ax$$

390. $$\int x^2(\sin ax)\,dx = \frac{2x}{a^2} \sin ax - \frac{a^2x^2 - 2}{a^3} \cos ax$$

391. $$\int x^3(\sin ax)\,dx = \frac{3a^2x^2 - 6}{a^4} \sin ax - \frac{a^2x^3 - 6x}{a^3} \cos ax$$

392. $$\int x^m \sin ax\,dx = \begin{cases} -\frac{1}{a}x^m \cos ax + \frac{m}{a}\int x^{m-1} \cos ax\,dx \\ \text{or} \\ \cos ax \sum_{r=0}^{\left[\frac{m}{2}\right]} (-1)^{r+1} \frac{m!}{(m-2r)!} \cdot \frac{x^{m-2r}}{a^{2r+1}} \\ \quad + \sin ax \sum_{r=0}^{\left[\frac{m-1}{2}\right]} (-1)^r \frac{m!}{(m-2r-1)!} \cdot \frac{x^{m-2r-1}}{a^{2r+2}} \end{cases}$$

Note: $[s]$ means greatest integer $\leq s$; $[3\frac{1}{2}] = 3$, $[\frac{1}{2}] = 0$, etc.

393. $$\int x(\cos ax)\,dx = \frac{1}{a^2} \cos ax + \frac{x}{a} \sin ax$$

394. $$\int x^2(\cos ax)\,dx = \frac{2x \cos ax}{a^2} + \frac{a^2x^2 - 2}{a^3} \sin ax$$

395. $$\int x^3(\cos ax)\,dx = \frac{3a^2x^2 - 6}{a^4} \cos ax + \frac{a^2x^3 - 6x}{a^3} \sin ax$$

396. $$\int x^m(\cos ax)\,dx = \begin{cases} \frac{x^m \sin ax}{a} - \frac{m}{a}\int x^{m-1} \sin ax\,dx \\ \text{or} \\ \sin ax \sum_{r=0}^{\left[\frac{m}{2}\right]} (-1)^r \frac{m!}{(m-2r)!} \cdot \frac{x^{m-2r}}{a^{2r+1}} \\ \quad + \cos ax \sum_{r=0}^{\left[\frac{m-1}{2}\right]} (-1)^r \frac{m!}{(m-2r-1)!} \cdot \frac{x^{m-2r-1}}{a^{2r+2}} \end{cases}$$

See note integral 392.

INTEGRALS (Continued)

397. $\int \frac{\sin ax}{x}\,dx = \sum_{n=0}^{\infty} (-1)^n \frac{(ax)^{2n+1}}{(2n+1)(2n+1)!}$

398. $\int \frac{\cos ax}{x}\,dx = \log x + \sum_{n=1}^{\infty} (-1)^n \frac{(ax)^{2n}}{2n(2n)!}$

399. $\int x(\sin^2 ax)\,dx = \frac{x^2}{4} - \frac{x \sin 2ax}{4a} - \frac{\cos 2ax}{8a^2}$

400. $\int x^2(\sin^2 ax)\,dx = \frac{x^3}{6} - \left(\frac{x^2}{4a} - \frac{1}{8a^3}\right) \sin 2ax - \frac{x \cos 2ax}{4a^2}$

401. $\int x(\sin^3 ax)\,dx = \frac{x \cos 3ax}{12a} - \frac{\sin 3ax}{36a^2} - \frac{3x \cos ax}{4a} + \frac{3 \sin ax}{4a^2}$

402. $\int x(\cos^2 ax)\,dx = \frac{x^2}{4} + \frac{x \sin 2ax}{4a} + \frac{\cos 2ax}{8a^2}$

403. $\int x^2(\cos^2 ax)\,dx = \frac{x^3}{6} + \left(\frac{x^2}{4a} - \frac{1}{8a^3}\right) \sin 2ax + \frac{x \cos 2ax}{4a^2}$

404. $\int x(\cos^3 ax)\,dx = \frac{x \sin 3ax}{12a} + \frac{\cos 3ax}{36a^2} + \frac{3x \sin ax}{4a} + \frac{3 \cos ax}{4a^2}$

405. $\int \frac{\sin ax}{x^m}\,dx = -\frac{\sin ax}{(m-1)x^{m-1}} + \frac{a}{m-1} \int \frac{\cos ax}{x^{m-1}}\,dx$

406. $\int \frac{\cos ax}{x^m}\,dx = -\frac{\cos ax}{(m-1)x^{m-1}} - \frac{a}{m-1} \int \frac{\sin ax}{x^{m-1}}\,dx$

407. $\int \frac{x}{1 \pm \sin ax}\,dx = \mp \frac{x \cos ax}{a(1 \pm \sin ax)} + \frac{1}{a^2} \log (1 \pm \sin ax)$

408. $\int \frac{x}{1 + \cos ax}\,dx = \frac{x}{a} \tan \frac{ax}{2} + \frac{2}{a^2} \log \cos \frac{ax}{2}$

409. $\int \frac{x}{1 - \cos ax}\,dx = -\frac{x}{a} \cot \frac{ax}{2} + \frac{2}{a^2} \log \sin \frac{ax}{2}$

410. $\int \frac{x + \sin x}{1 + \cos x}\,dx = x \tan \frac{x}{2}$

411. $\int \frac{x - \sin x}{1 - \cos x}\,dx = -x \cot \frac{x}{2}$

412. $\int \sqrt{1 - \cos ax}\,dx = -\frac{2 \sin ax}{a\sqrt{1 - \cos ax}} = -\frac{2\sqrt{2}}{a} \cos \left(\frac{ax}{2}\right)$

413. $\int \sqrt{1 + \cos ax}\,dx = \frac{2 \sin ax}{a\sqrt{1 + \cos ax}} = \frac{2\sqrt{2}}{a} \sin \left(\frac{ax}{2}\right)$

INTEGRALS (Continued)

414. $\int \sqrt{1+\sin x}\,dx = \pm 2\left(\sin\frac{x}{2} - \cos\frac{x}{2}\right),$

[use + if $(8k-1)\frac{\pi}{2} < x \le (8k+3)\frac{\pi}{2}$, otherwise − ; k an integer]

415. $\int \sqrt{1-\sin x}\,dx = \pm 2\left(\sin\frac{x}{2} + \cos\frac{x}{2}\right),$

[use + if $(8k-3)\frac{\pi}{2} < x \le (8k+1)\frac{\pi}{2}$, otherwise − ; k an integer]

416. $\int \frac{dx}{\sqrt{1-\cos x}} = \pm \sqrt{2}\log\tan\frac{x}{4},$

[use + if $4k\pi < x < (4k+2)\pi$, otherwise − ; k an integer]

417. $\int \frac{dx}{\sqrt{1+\cos x}} = \pm \sqrt{2}\log\tan\left(\frac{x+\pi}{4}\right),$

[use + if $(4k-1)\pi < x < (4k+1)\pi$, otherwise − ; k an integer]

418. $\int \frac{dx}{\sqrt{1-\sin x}} = \pm \sqrt{2}\log\tan\left(\frac{x}{4} - \frac{\pi}{8}\right),$

[use + if $(8k+1)\frac{\pi}{2} < x < (8k+5)\frac{\pi}{2}$, otherwise − ; k an integer]

419. $\int \frac{dx}{\sqrt{1+\sin x}} = \pm \sqrt{2}\log\tan\left(\frac{x}{4} + \frac{\pi}{8}\right),$

[use + if $(8k-1)\frac{\pi}{2} < x < (8k+3)\frac{\pi}{2}$, otherwise − ; k an integer]

420. $\int (\tan^2 ax)\,dx = \frac{1}{a}\tan ax - x$

421. $\int (\tan^3 ax)\,dx = \frac{1}{2a}\tan^2 ax + \frac{1}{a}\log\cos ax$

422. $\int (\tan^4 ax)\,dx = \frac{\tan^3 ax}{3a} - \frac{1}{a}\tan x + x$

423. $\int (\tan^n ax)\,dx = \frac{\tan^{n-1} ax}{a(n-1)} - \int (\tan^{n-2} ax)\,dx$

424. $\int (\cot^2 ax)\,dx = -\frac{1}{a}\cot ax - x$

425. $\int (\cot^3 ax)\,dx = -\frac{1}{2a}\cot^2 ax - \frac{1}{a}\log\sin ax$

426. $\int (\cot^4 ax)\,dx = -\frac{1}{3a}\cot^3 ax + \frac{1}{a}\cot ax + x$

INTEGRALS (Continued)

427. $$\int (\cot^n ax)\,dx = -\frac{\cot^{n-1} ax}{a(n-1)} - \int (\cot^{n-2} ax)\,dx$$

428. $$\int \frac{x}{\sin^2 ax}\,dx = \int x(\csc^2 ax)\,dx = -\frac{x \cot ax}{a} + \frac{1}{a^2} \log \sin ax$$

429. $$\int \frac{x}{\sin^n ax}\,dx = \int x(\csc^n ax)\,dx = -\frac{x \cos ax}{a(n-1)\sin^{n-1} ax} - \frac{1}{a^2(n-1)(n-2)\sin^{n-2} ax} + \frac{(n-2)}{(n-1)} \int \frac{x}{\sin^{n-2} ax}\,dx$$

430. $$\int \frac{x}{\cos^2 ax}\,dx = \int x(\sec^2 ax)\,dx = \frac{1}{a} x \tan ax + \frac{1}{a^2} \log \cos ax$$

431. $$\int \frac{x}{\cos^n ax}\,dx = \int x(\sec^n ax)\,dx = \frac{x \sin ax}{a(n-1)\cos^{n-1} ax} - \frac{1}{a^2(n-1)(n-2)\cos^{n-2} ax} + \frac{n-2}{n-1} \int \frac{x}{\cos^{n-2} ax}\,dx$$

432. $$\int \frac{\sin ax}{\sqrt{1 + b^2 \sin^2 ax}}\,dx = -\frac{1}{ab} \sin^{-1} \frac{b \cos ax}{\sqrt{1 + b^2}}$$

433. $$\int \frac{\sin ax}{\sqrt{1 - b^2 \sin^2 ax}}\,dx = -\frac{1}{ab} \log (b \cos ax + \sqrt{1 - b^2 \sin^2 ax})$$

434. $$\int (\sin ax)\sqrt{1 + b^2 \sin^2 ax}\,dx = -\frac{\cos ax}{2a} \sqrt{1 + b^2 \sin^2 ax} - \frac{1 + b^2}{2ab} \sin^{-1} \frac{b \cos ax}{\sqrt{1 + b^2}}$$

435. $$\int (\sin ax)\sqrt{1 - b^2 \sin^2 ax}\,dx = -\frac{\cos ax}{2a} \sqrt{1 - b^2 \sin^2 ax} - \frac{1 - b^2}{2ab} \log (b \cos ax + \sqrt{1 - b^2 \sin^2 ax})$$

436. $$\int \frac{\cos ax}{\sqrt{1 + b^2 \sin^2 ax}}\,dx = \frac{1}{ab} \log (b \sin ax + \sqrt{1 + b^2 \sin^2 ax})$$

437. $$\int \frac{\cos ax}{\sqrt{1 - b^2 \sin^2 ax}}\,dx = \frac{1}{ab} \sin^{-1} (b \sin ax)$$

438. $$\int (\cos ax)\sqrt{1 + b^2 \sin^2 ax}\,dx = \frac{\sin ax}{2a} \sqrt{1 + b^2 \sin^2 ax} + \frac{1}{2ab} \log (b \sin ax + \sqrt{1 + b^2 \sin^2 ax})$$

INTEGRALS (Continued)

439. $$\int (\cos ax)\sqrt{1 - b^2 \sin^2 ax}\, dx = \frac{\sin ax}{2a}\sqrt{1 - b^2 \sin^2 ax} + \frac{1}{2ab}\sin^{-1}(b \sin ax)$$

440. $$\int \frac{dx}{\sqrt{a + b\tan^2 cx}} = \frac{\pm 1}{c\sqrt{a - b}}\sin^{-1}\left(\sqrt{\frac{a - b}{a}}\sin cx\right), \qquad (a > |b|)$$

[use + if $(2k - 1)\frac{\pi}{2} < x \le (2k + 1)\frac{\pi}{2}$, otherwise − ; k an integer]

FORMS INVOLVING INVERSE TRIGONOMETRIC FUNCTIONS

441. $$\int (\sin^{-1} ax)\, dx = x \sin^{-1} ax + \frac{\sqrt{1 - a^2x^2}}{a}$$

442. $$\int (\cos^{-1} ax)\, dx = x \cos^{-1} ax - \frac{\sqrt{1 - a^2x^2}}{a}$$

443. $$\int (\tan^{-1} ax)\, dx = x \tan^{-1} ax - \frac{1}{2a}\log(1 + a^2x^2)$$

444. $$\int (\cot^{-1} ax)\, dx = x \cot^{-1} ax + \frac{1}{2a}\log(1 + a^2x^2)$$

445. $$\int (\sec^{-1} ax)\, dx = x \sec^{-1} ax - \frac{1}{a}\log(ax + \sqrt{a^2x^2 - 1})$$

446. $$\int (\csc^{-1} ax)\, dx = x \csc^{-1} ax + \frac{1}{a}\log(ax + \sqrt{a^2x^2 - 1})$$

447. $$\int \left(\sin^{-1}\frac{x}{a}\right) dx = x \sin^{-1}\frac{x}{a} + \sqrt{a^2 - x^2}, \qquad (a > 0)$$

448. $$\int \left(\cos^{-1}\frac{x}{a}\right) dx = x \cos^{-1}\frac{x}{a} - \sqrt{a^2 - x^2}, \qquad (a > 0)$$

449. $$\int \left(\tan^{-1}\frac{x}{a}\right) dx = x \tan^{-1}\frac{x}{a} - \frac{a}{2}\log(a^2 + x^2)$$

450. $$\int \left(\cot^{-1}\frac{x}{a}\right) dx = x \cot^{-1}\frac{x}{a} + \frac{a}{2}\log(a^2 + x^2)$$

451. $$\int x[\sin^{-1}(ax)]\, dx = \frac{1}{4a^2}[(2a^2x^2 - 1)\sin^{-1}(ax) + ax\sqrt{1 - a^2x^2}]$$

452. $$\int x[\cos^{-1}(ax)]\, dx = \frac{1}{4a^2}[(2a^2x^2 - 1)\cos^{-1}(ax) - ax\sqrt{1 - a^2x^2}]$$

INTEGRALS (Continued)

453. $\int x^n[\sin^{-1}(ax)]\,dx = \frac{x^{n+1}}{n+1}\sin^{-1}(ax) - \frac{a}{n+1}\int \frac{x^{n+1}\,dx}{\sqrt{1-a^2x^2}}, \qquad (n \neq -1)$

454. $\int x^n[\cos^{-1}(ax)]\,dx = \frac{x^{n+1}}{n+1}\cos^{-1}(ax) + \frac{a}{n+1}\int \frac{x^{n+1}\,dx}{\sqrt{1-a^2x^2}}, \qquad (n \neq -1)$

455. $\int x(\tan^{-1} ax)\,dx = \frac{1+a^2x^2}{2a^2}\tan^{-1} ax - \frac{x}{2a}$

456. $\int x^n(\tan^{-1} ax)\,dx = \frac{x^{n+1}}{n+1}\tan^{-1} ax - \frac{a}{n+1}\int \frac{x^{n+1}}{1+a^2x^2}\,dx$

457. $\int x(\cot^{-1} ax)\,dx = \frac{1+a^2x^2}{2a^2}\cot^{-1} ax + \frac{x}{2a}$

458. $\int x^n(\cot^{-1} ax)\,dx = \frac{x^{n+1}}{n+1}\cot^{-1} ax + \frac{a}{n+1}\int \frac{x^{n+1}}{1+a^2x^2}\,dx$

459. $\int \frac{\sin^{-1}(ax)}{x^2}\,dx = a\log\left(\frac{1-\sqrt{1-a^2x^2}}{x}\right) - \frac{\sin^{-1}(ax)}{x}$

460. $\int \frac{\cos^{-1}(ax)\,dx}{x^2} = -\frac{1}{x}\cos^{-1}(ax) + a\log\frac{1+\sqrt{1-a^2x^2}}{x}$

461. $\int \frac{\tan^{-1}(ax)\,dx}{x^2} = -\frac{1}{x}\tan^{-1}(ax) - \frac{a}{2}\log\frac{1+a^2x^2}{x^2}$

462. $\int \frac{\cot^{-1} ax}{x^2}\,dx = -\frac{1}{x}\cot^{-1} ax - \frac{a}{2}\log\frac{x^2}{a^2x^2+1}$

463. $\int (\sin^{-1} ax)^2\,dx = x(\sin^{-1} ax)^2 - 2x + \frac{2\sqrt{1-a^2x^2}}{a}\sin^{-1} ax$

464. $\int (\cos^{-1} ax)^2\,dx = x(\cos^{-1} ax)^2 - 2x - \frac{2\sqrt{1-a^2x^2}}{a}\cos^{-1} ax$

465.
$$\int (\sin^{-1} ax)^n\,dx = \begin{cases} x(\sin^{-1} ax)^n + \dfrac{n\sqrt{1-a^2x^2}}{a}(\sin^{-1} ax)^{n-1} \\ \qquad -n(n-1)\displaystyle\int (\sin^{-1} ax)^{n-2}\,dx \\ \text{or} \\ \displaystyle\sum_{r=0}^{\left[\frac{n}{2}\right]} (-1)^r \frac{n!}{(n-2r)!}\,x(\sin^{-1} ax)^{n-2r} \\ \qquad + \displaystyle\sum_{r=0}^{\left[\frac{n-1}{2}\right]} (-1)^r \frac{n!\sqrt{1-a^2x^2}}{(n-2r-1)!\,a}(\sin^{-1} ax)^{n-2r-1} \end{cases}$$

Note: $[s]$ means greatest integer $\leq s$. Thus $[3.5]$ means 3; $[5] = 5$, $[\frac{1}{2}] = 0$.

INTEGRALS (Continued)

466. $$\int (\cos^{-1} ax)^n\,dx = \begin{cases} x(\cos^{-1} ax)^n - \dfrac{n\sqrt{1-a^2x^2}}{a}(\cos^{-1} ax)^{n-1} - n(n-1)\displaystyle\int (\cos^{-1} ax)^{n-2}\,dx \\ \text{or} \\ \displaystyle\sum_{r=0}^{[\frac{n}{2}]} (-1)^r \frac{n!}{(n-2r)!} x(\cos^{-1} ax)^{n-2r} - \sum_{r=0}^{[\frac{n-1}{2}]} (-1)^r \frac{n!\sqrt{1-a^2x^2}}{(n-2r-1)!a}(\cos^{-1} ax)^{n-2r-1} \end{cases}$$

467. $$\int \frac{1}{\sqrt{1-a^2x^2}}(\sin^{-1} ax)\,dx = \frac{1}{2a}(\sin^{-1} ax)^2$$

468. $$\int \frac{x^n}{\sqrt{1-a^2x^2}}(\sin^{-1} ax)\,dx = -\frac{x^{n-1}}{na^2}\sqrt{1-a^2x^2}\sin^{-1} ax + \frac{x^n}{n^2a} + \frac{n-1}{na^2}\int \frac{x^{n-2}}{\sqrt{1-a^2x^2}}\sin^{-1} ax\,dx$$

469. $$\int \frac{1}{\sqrt{1-a^2x^2}}(\cos^{-1} ax)\,dx = -\frac{1}{2a}(\cos^{-1} ax)^2$$

470. $$\int \frac{x^n}{\sqrt{1-a^2x^2}}(\cos^{-1} ax)\,dx = -\frac{x^{n-1}}{na^2}\sqrt{1-a^2x^2}\cos^{-1} ax - \frac{x^n}{n^2a} + \frac{n-1}{na^2}\int \frac{x^{n-2}}{\sqrt{1-a^2x^2}}\cos^{-1} ax\,dx$$

471. $$\int \frac{\tan^{-1} ax}{a^2x^2+1}\,dx = \frac{1}{2a}(\tan^{-1} ax)^2$$

472. $$\int \frac{\cot^{-1} ax}{a^2x^2+1}\,dx = -\frac{1}{2a}(\cot^{-1} ax)^2$$

473. $$\int x\sec^{-1} ax\,dx = \frac{x^2}{2}\sec^{-1} ax - \frac{1}{2a^2}\sqrt{a^2x^2-1}$$

474. $$\int x^n\sec^{-1} ax\,dx = \frac{x^{n+1}}{n+1}\sec^{-1} ax - \frac{1}{n+1}\int \frac{x^n\,dx}{\sqrt{a^2x^2-1}}$$

475. $$\int \frac{\sec^{-1} ax}{x^2}\,dx = -\frac{\sec^{-1} ax}{x} + \frac{\sqrt{a^2x^2-1}}{x}$$

476. $$\int x\csc^{-1} ax\,dx = \frac{x^2}{2}\csc^{-1} ax + \frac{1}{2a^2}\sqrt{a^2x^2-1}$$

477. $$\int x^n\csc^{-1} ax\,dx = \frac{x^{n+1}}{n+1}\csc^{-1} ax + \frac{1}{n+1}\int \frac{x^n\,dx}{\sqrt{a^2x^2-1}}$$

INTEGRALS (Continued)

478. $$\int \frac{\csc^{-1} ax}{x^2}\,dx = -\frac{\csc^{-1} ax}{x} - \frac{\sqrt{a^2x^2 - 1}}{x}$$

FORMS INVOLVING TRIGONOMETRIC SUBSTITUTIONS

479. $$\int f(\sin x)\,dx = 2\int f\left(\frac{2z}{1 + z^2}\right)\frac{dz}{1 + z^2}, \qquad \left(z = \tan\frac{x}{2}\right)$$

480. $$\int f(\cos x)\,dx = 2\int f\left(\frac{1 - z^2}{1 + z^2}\right)\frac{dz}{1 + z^2}, \qquad \left(z = \tan\frac{x}{2}\right)$$

***481.** $$\int f(\sin x)\,dx = \int f(u)\frac{du}{\sqrt{1 - u^2}}, \qquad (u = \sin x)$$

***482.** $$\int f(\cos x)\,dx = -\int f(u)\frac{du}{\sqrt{1 - u^2}}, \qquad (u = \cos x)$$

***483.** $$\int f(\sin x, \cos x)\,dx = \int f(u, \sqrt{1 - u^2})\frac{du}{\sqrt{1 - u^2}}, \qquad (u = \sin x)$$

484. $$\int f(\sin x, \cos x)\,dx = 2\int f\left(\frac{2z}{1 + z^2}, \frac{1 - z^2}{1 + z^2}\right)\frac{dz}{1 + z^2}, \qquad \left(z = \tan\frac{x}{2}\right)$$

LOGARITHMIC FORMS

485. $$\int (\log x)\,dx = x\log x - x$$

486. $$\int x(\log x)\,dx = \frac{x^2}{2}\log x - \frac{x^2}{4}$$

487. $$\int x^2(\log x)\,dx = \frac{x^3}{3}\log x - \frac{x^3}{9}$$

488. $$\int x^n(\log ax)\,dx = \frac{x^{n+1}}{n + 1}\log ax - \frac{x^{n+1}}{(n + 1)^2}$$

489. $$\int (\log x)^2\,dx = x(\log x)^2 - 2x\log x + 2x$$

490. $$\int (\log x)^n\,dx = \begin{cases} x(\log x)^n - n\displaystyle\int (\log x)^{n-1}\,dx, & (n \neq -1) \\ \quad \text{or} & \\ (-1)^n n!\,x \displaystyle\sum_{r=0}^{n} \frac{(-\log x)^r}{r!} & \end{cases}$$

*The square roots appearing in these formulas may be plus or minus, depending on the quadrant of x. Care must be used to give them the proper sign.

INTEGRALS (Continued)

491. $$\int \frac{(\log x)^n}{x}\,dx = \frac{1}{n+1}(\log x)^{n+1}$$

492. $$\int \frac{dx}{\log x} = \log(\log x) + \log x + \frac{(\log x)^2}{2\cdot 2!} + \frac{(\log x)^3}{3\cdot 3!} + \cdots$$

493. $$\int \frac{dx}{x \log x} = \log(\log x)$$

494. $$\int \frac{dx}{x(\log x)^n} = -\frac{1}{(n-1)(\log x)^{n-1}}$$

495. $$\int \frac{x^m\,dx}{(\log x)^n} = -\frac{x^{m+1}}{(n-1)(\log x)^{n-1}} + \frac{m+1}{n-1}\int \frac{x^m\,dx}{(\log x)^{n-1}}$$

496. $$\int x^m(\log x)^n\,dx = \begin{cases} \dfrac{x^{m+1}(\log x)^n}{m+1} - \dfrac{n}{m+1}\displaystyle\int x^m(\log x)^{n-1}\,dx \\ \text{or} \\ (-1)^n \dfrac{n!}{m+1} x^{m+1} \displaystyle\sum_{r=0}^{n} \frac{(-\log x)^r}{r!(m+1)^{n-r}} \end{cases}$$

497. $$\int x^p \cos(b\ ln\ x)\,dx = \frac{x^{p+1}}{(p+1)^2 + b^2}\cdot [b \sin(b\ ln\ x) + (p+1)\cos(b\ ln\ x)] + c$$

498. $$\int x^p \sin(b\ ln\ x)\,dx = \frac{x^{p+1}}{(p+1)^2 + b^2}\cdot [(p+1)\sin(b\ ln\ x) - b\cos(b\ ln\ x)] + c$$

499. $$\int [\log(ax+b)]\,dx = \frac{ax+b}{a}\log(ax+b) - x$$

500. $$\int \frac{\log(ax+b)}{x^2}\,dx = \frac{a}{b}\log x - \frac{ax+b}{bx}\log(ax+b)$$

501. $$\int x^m[\log(ax+b)]\,dx = \frac{1}{m+1}\left[x^{m+1} - \left(-\frac{b}{a}\right)^{m+1}\right]\log(ax+b) - \frac{1}{m+1}\left(-\frac{b}{a}\right)^{m+1} \sum_{r=1}^{m+1} \frac{1}{r}\left(-\frac{ax}{b}\right)^r$$

502. $$\int \frac{\log(ax+b)}{x^m}\,dx = -\frac{1}{m-1}\frac{\log(ax+b)}{x^{m-1}} + \frac{1}{m-1}\left(-\frac{a}{b}\right)^{m-1}\log\frac{ax+b}{x} + \frac{1}{m-1}\left(-\frac{a}{b}\right)^{m-1}\sum_{r=1}^{m-2}\frac{1}{r}\left(-\frac{b}{ax}\right)^r, (m > 2)$$

503. $$\int \left[\log\frac{x+a}{x-a}\right]dx = (x+a)\log(x+a) - (x-a)\log(x-a)$$

504. $$\int x^m\left[\log\frac{x+a}{x-a}\right]dx = \frac{x^{m+1} - (-a)^{m+1}}{m+1}\log(x+a) - \frac{x^{m+1} - a^{m+1}}{m+1}\log(x-a) + \frac{2a^{m+1}}{m+1}\sum_{r=1}^{\left[\frac{m+1}{2}\right]} \frac{1}{m-2r+2}\left(\frac{x}{a}\right)^{m-2r+2}$$

See note integral 392.

INTEGRALS (Continued)

505. $\int \frac{1}{x^2}\left[\log \frac{x+a}{x-a}\right] dx = \frac{1}{x}\log\frac{x-a}{x+a} - \frac{1}{a}\log\frac{x^2-a^2}{x^2}$

506. $$\int (\log X)\,dx = \begin{cases} \left(x+\frac{b}{2c}\right)\log X - 2x + \frac{\sqrt{4ac-b^2}}{c}\tan^{-1}\frac{2cx+b}{\sqrt{4ac-b^2}}, & (b^2-4ac<0) \\ \text{or} & \\ \left(x+\frac{b}{2c}\right)\log X - 2x + \frac{\sqrt{b^2-4ac}}{c}\tanh^{-1}\frac{2cx+b}{\sqrt{b^2-4ac}}, & (b^2-4ac>0) \\ \text{where} & \\ X = a+bx+cx^2 & \end{cases}$$

507. $\int x^n(\log X)\,dx = \frac{x^{n+1}}{n+1}\log X - \frac{2c}{n+1}\int\frac{x^{n+2}}{X}dx - \frac{b}{n+1}\int\frac{x^{n+1}}{X}dx$

where $X = a + bx + cx^2$

508. $\int [\log(x^2+a^2)]\,dx = x\log(x^2+a^2) - 2x + 2a\tan^{-1}\frac{x}{a}$

509. $\int [\log(x^2-a^2)]\,dx = x\log(x^2-a^2) - 2x + a\log\frac{x+a}{x-a}$

510. $\int x[\log(x^2\pm a^2)]\,dx = \frac{1}{2}(x^2\pm a^2)\log(x^2\pm a^2) - \frac{1}{2}x^2$

511. $\int [\log(x+\sqrt{x^2\pm a^2})]\,dx = x\log(x+\sqrt{x^2\pm a^2}) - \sqrt{x^2\pm a^2}$

512. $\int x[\log(x+\sqrt{x^2\pm a^2})]\,dx = \left(\frac{x^2}{2}\pm\frac{a^2}{4}\right)\log(x+\sqrt{x^2\pm a^2}) - \frac{x\sqrt{x^2\pm a^2}}{4}$

513. $\int x^m[\log(x+\sqrt{x^2\pm a^2})]\,dx = \frac{x^{m+1}}{m+1}\log(x+\sqrt{x^2\pm a^2}) - \frac{1}{m+1}\int\frac{x^{m+1}}{\sqrt{x^2\pm a^2}}dx$

514. $\int \frac{\log(x+\sqrt{x^2+a^2})}{x^2}dx = -\frac{\log(x+\sqrt{x^2+a^2})}{x} - \frac{1}{a}\log\frac{a+\sqrt{x^2+a^2}}{x}$

515. $\int \frac{\log(x+\sqrt{x^2-a^2})}{x^2}dx = -\frac{\log(x+\sqrt{x^2-a^2})}{x} + \frac{1}{|a|}\sec^{-1}\frac{x}{a}$

INTEGRALS (Continued)

516. $$\int x^n \log(x^2 - a^2)\,dx = \frac{1}{n+1}\left[x^{n+1}\log(x^2-a^2) - a^{n+1}\log(x-a) - (-a)^{n+1}\log(x+a) - 2\sum_{r=0}^{\left[\frac{n}{2}\right]} \frac{a^{2r}x^{n-2r+1}}{n-2r+1}\right]$$

See note integral 392.

EXPONENTIAL FORMS

517. $$\int e^x\,dx = e^x$$

518. $$\int e^{-x}\,dx = -e^{-x}$$

519. $$\int e^{ax}\,dx = \frac{e^{ax}}{a}$$

520. $$\int x\,e^{ax}\,dx = \frac{e^{ax}}{a^2}(ax-1)$$

521. $$\int x^m e^{ax}\,dx = \begin{cases} \dfrac{x^m e^{ax}}{a} - \dfrac{m}{a}\displaystyle\int x^{m-1}e^{ax}\,dx \\ \text{or} \\ e^{ax}\displaystyle\sum_{r=0}^{m}(-1)^r \frac{m!x^{m-r}}{(m-r)!a^{r+1}} \end{cases}$$

522. $$\int \frac{e^{ax}\,dx}{x} = \log x + \frac{ax}{1!} + \frac{a^2x^2}{2\cdot 2!} + \frac{a^3x^3}{3\cdot 3!} + \cdots$$

523. $$\int \frac{e^{ax}}{x^m}\,dx = -\frac{1}{m-1}\frac{e^{ax}}{x^{m-1}} + \frac{a}{m-1}\int \frac{e^{ax}}{x^{m-1}}\,dx$$

524. $$\int e^{ax}\log x\,dx = \frac{e^{ax}\log x}{a} - \frac{1}{a}\int \frac{e^{ax}}{x}\,dx$$

525. $$\int \frac{dx}{1+e^x} = x - \log(1+e^x) = \log\frac{e^x}{1+e^x}$$

526. $$\int \frac{dx}{a+be^{px}} = \frac{x}{a} - \frac{1}{ap}\log(a+be^{px})$$

527. $$\int \frac{dx}{ae^{mx}+be^{-mx}} = \frac{1}{m\sqrt{ab}}\tan^{-1}\left(e^{mx}\sqrt{\frac{a}{b}}\right), \qquad (a>0, b>0)$$

528. $$\int \frac{dx}{ae^{mx}-be^{-mx}} = \begin{cases} \dfrac{1}{2m\sqrt{ab}}\log\dfrac{\sqrt{a}\,e^{mx}-\sqrt{b}}{\sqrt{a}\,e^{mx}+\sqrt{b}} \\ \text{or} \\ \dfrac{-1}{m\sqrt{ab}}\tanh^{-1}\left(\sqrt{\dfrac{a}{b}}\,e^{mx}\right), \qquad (a>0, b>0) \end{cases}$$

INTEGRALS (Continued)

529. $$\int (a^x - a^{-x})\,dx = \frac{a^x + a^{-x}}{\log a}$$

530. $$\int \frac{e^{ax}}{b + ce^{ax}}\,dx = \frac{1}{ac}\log(b + ce^{ax})$$

531. $$\int \frac{x\,e^{ax}}{(1 + ax)^2}\,dx = \frac{e^{ax}}{a^2(1 + ax)}$$

532. $$\int x\,e^{-x^2}\,dx = -\tfrac{1}{2}e^{-x^2}$$

533. $$\int e^{ax}[\sin(bx)]\,dx = \frac{e^{ax}[a\sin(bx) - b\cos(bx)]}{a^2 + b^2}$$

534. $$\int e^{ax}[\sin(bx)][\sin(cx)]\,dx = \frac{e^{ax}[(b - c)\sin(b - c)x + a\cos(b - c)x]}{2[a^2 + (b - c)^2]} - \frac{e^{ax}[(b + c)\sin(b + c)x + a\cos(b + c)x]}{2[a^2 + (b + c)^2]}$$

535. $$\int e^{ax}[\sin(bx)][\cos(cx)]\,dx = \begin{cases} \dfrac{e^{ax}[a\sin(b - c)x - (b - c)\cos(b - c)x]}{2[a^2 + (b - c)^2]} + \dfrac{e^{ax}[a\sin(b + c)x - (b + c)\cos(b + c)x]}{2[a^2 + (b + c)^2]} \\ \text{or} \\ \dfrac{e^{ax}}{\rho}[(a\sin bx - b\cos bx)[\cos(cx - \alpha)] - c(\sin bx)\sin(cx - \alpha)] \\ \text{where} \\ \rho = \sqrt{(a^2 + b^2 - c^2)^2 + 4a^2c^2}, \\ \rho\cos\alpha = a^2 + b^2 - c^2, \qquad \rho\sin\alpha = 2ac \end{cases}$$

536. $$\int e^{ax}[\sin(bx)][\sin(bx + c)]\,dx = \frac{e^{ax}\cos c}{2a} - \frac{e^{ax}[a\cos(2bx + c) + 2b\sin(2bx + c)]}{2(a^2 + 4b^2)}$$

537. $$\int e^{ax}[\sin(bx)][\cos(bx + c)]\,dx = \frac{-e^{ax}\sin c}{2a} + \frac{e^{ax}[a\sin(2bx + c) - 2b\cos(2bx + c)]}{2(a^2 + 4b^2)}$$

538. $$\int e^{ax}[\cos(bx)]\,dx = \frac{e^{ax}}{a^2 + b^2}[a\cos(bx) + b\sin(bx)]$$

INTEGRALS (Continued)

539. $$\int e^{ax}[\cos(bx)][\cos(cx)]\,dx = \frac{e^{ax}[(b-c)\sin(b-c)x + a\cos(b-c)x]}{2[a^2+(b-c)^2]} + \frac{e^{ax}[(b+c)\sin(b+c)x + a\cos(b+c)x]}{2[a^2+(b+c)^2]}$$

540. $$\int e^{ax}[\cos(bx)][\cos(bx+c)]\,dx = \frac{e^{ax}\cos c}{2a} + \frac{e^{ax}[a\cos(2bx+c) + 2b\sin(2bx+c)]}{2(a^2+4b^2)}$$

541. $$\int e^{ax}[\cos(bx)][\sin(bx+c)]\,dx = \frac{e^{ax}\sin c}{2a} + \frac{e^{ax}[a\sin(2bx+c) - 2b\cos(2bx+c)]}{2(a^2+4b^2)}$$

542. $$\int e^{ax}[\sin^n bx]\,dx = \frac{1}{a^2+n^2b^2}\left[(a\sin bx - nb\cos bx)\,e^{ax}\sin^{n-1}bx + n(n-1)b^2\int e^{ax}[\sin^{n-2}bx]\,dx\right]$$

543. $$\int e^{ax}[\cos^n bx]\,dx = \frac{1}{a^2+n^2b^2}\left[(a\cos bx + nb\sin bx)\,e^{ax}\cos^{n-1}bx + n(n-1)b^2\int e^{ax}[\cos^{n-2}bx]\,dx\right]$$

544. $$\int x^m e^x \sin x\,dx = \frac{1}{2}x^m e^x(\sin x - \cos x) - \frac{m}{2}\int x^{m-1}e^x\sin x\,dx + \frac{m}{2}\int x^{m-1}e^x\cos x\,dx$$

545. $$\int x^m e^{ax}[\sin bx]\,dx = \begin{cases} x^m e^{ax}\dfrac{a\sin bx - b\cos bx}{a^2+b^2} - \dfrac{m}{a^2+b^2}\displaystyle\int x^{m-1}e^{ax}(a\sin bx - b\cos bx)\,dx \\ \text{or} \\ e^{ax}\displaystyle\sum_{r=0}^{m}\frac{(-1)^r m!\,x^{m-r}}{\rho^{r+1}(m-r)!}\sin[bx-(r+1)\alpha] \\ \text{where} \\ \rho = \sqrt{a^2+b^2}, \qquad \rho\cos\alpha = a, \qquad \rho\sin\alpha = b \end{cases}$$

546. $$\int x^m e^x \cos x\,dx = \frac{1}{2}x^m e^x(\sin x + \cos x) - \frac{m}{2}\int x^{m-1}e^x\sin x\,dx - \frac{m}{2}\int x^{m-1}e^x\cos x\,dx$$

INTEGRALS (Continued)

547. $$\int x^m e^{ax} \cos bx\, dx = \begin{cases} x^m e^{ax} \dfrac{a \cos bx + b \sin bx}{a^2 + b^2} \\ \qquad - \dfrac{m}{a^2 + b^2} \displaystyle\int x^{m-1} e^{ax}(a \cos bx + b \sin bx)\, dx \\ \text{or} \\ e^{ax} \displaystyle\sum_{r=0}^{m} \dfrac{(-1)^r m!\, x^{m-r}}{\rho^{r+1}(m-r)!} \cos [bx - (r+1)\alpha] \\ \text{where} \\ \rho = \sqrt{a^2 + b^2}, \qquad \rho \cos \alpha = a, \qquad \rho \sin \alpha = b \end{cases}$$

548. $$\int e^{ax}(\cos^m x)(\sin^n x)\, dx = \begin{cases} \dfrac{e^{ax} \cos^{m-1} x \sin^n x[a \cos x + (m+n) \sin x]}{(m+n)^2 + a^2} \\ \qquad - \dfrac{na}{(m+n)^2 + a^2} \displaystyle\int e^{ax}(\cos^{m-1} x)(\sin^{n-1} x)\, dx \\ \qquad + \dfrac{(m-1)(m+n)}{(m+n)^2 + a^2} \displaystyle\int e^{ax}(\cos^{m-2} x)(\sin^n x)\, dx \\ \text{or} \\ \dfrac{e^{ax} \cos^m x \sin^{n-1} x[a \sin x - (m+n) \cos x]}{(m+n)^2 + a^2} \\ \qquad + \dfrac{ma}{(m+n)^2 + a^2} \displaystyle\int e^{ax}(\cos^{m-1} x)(\sin^{n-1} x)\, dx \\ \qquad + \dfrac{(n-1)(m+n)}{(m+n)^2 + a^2} \displaystyle\int e^{ax}(\cos^m x)(\sin^{n-2} x)\, dx \\ \text{or} \\ \dfrac{e^{ax}(\cos^{m-1} x)(\sin^{n-1} x)(a \sin x \cos x + m \sin^2 x - n \cos^2 x)}{(m+n)^2 + a^2} \\ \qquad + \dfrac{m(m-1)}{(m+n)^2 + a^2} \displaystyle\int e^{ax}(\cos^{m-2} x)(\sin^n x)\, dx \\ \qquad + \dfrac{n(n-1)}{(m+n)^2 + a^2} \displaystyle\int e^{ax}(\cos^m x)(\sin^{n-2} x)\, dx \\ \text{or} \\ \dfrac{e^{ax}(\cos^{m-1} x)(\sin^{n-1} x)(a \cos x \sin x + m \sin^2 x - n \cos^2 x)}{(m+n)^2 + a^2} \\ \qquad + \dfrac{m(m-1)}{(m+n)^2 + a^2} \displaystyle\int e^{ax}(\cos^{m-2} x)(\sin^{n-2} x)\, dx \\ \qquad + \dfrac{(n-m)(n+m-1)}{(m+n)^2 + a^2} \displaystyle\int e^{ax}(\cos^m x)(\sin^{n-2} x)\, dx \end{cases}$$

INTEGRALS (Continued)

549. $$\int x\, e^{ax}(\sin bx)\, dx = \frac{x\, e^{ax}}{a^2 + b^2}(a \sin bx - b \cos bx) - \frac{e^{ax}}{(a^2 + b^2)^2}[(a^2 - b^2)\sin bx - 2ab \cos bx]$$

550. $$\int x\, e^{ax}(\cos bx)\, dx = \frac{x\, e^{ax}}{a^2 + b^2}(a \cos bx + b \sin bx) - \frac{e^{ax}}{(a^2 + b^2)^2}[(a^2 - b^2)\cos bx + 2ab \sin bx]$$

551. $$\int \frac{e^{ax}}{\sin^n x} dx = -\frac{e^{ax}[a \sin x + (n-2)\cos x]}{(n-1)(n-2)\sin^{n-1} x} + \frac{a^2 + (n-2)^2}{(n-1)(n-2)} \int \frac{e^{ax}}{\sin^{n-2} x} dx$$

552. $$\int \frac{e^{ax}}{\cos^n x} dx = -\frac{e^{ax}[a \cos x - (n-2)\sin x]}{(n-1)(n-2)\cos^{n-1} x} + \frac{a^2 + (n-2)^2}{(n-1)(n-2)} \int \frac{e^{ax}}{\cos^{n-2} x} dx$$

553. $$\int e^{ax} \tan^n x\, dx = e^{ax} \frac{\tan^{n-1} x}{n-1} - \frac{a}{n-1} \int e^{ax} \tan^{n-1} x\, dx - \int e^{ax} \tan^{n-2} x\, dx$$

HYPERBOLIC FORMS

554. $$\int (\sinh x)\, dx = \cosh x$$

555. $$\int (\cosh x)\, dx = \sinh x$$

556. $$\int (\tanh x)\, dx = \log \cosh x$$

557. $$\int (\coth x)\, dx = \log \sinh x$$

558. $$\int (\operatorname{sech} x)\, dx = \tan^{-1} (\sinh x)$$

559. $$\int \operatorname{csch} x\, dx = \log \tanh \left(\frac{x}{2}\right)$$

560. $$\int x(\sinh x)\, dx = x \cosh x - \sinh x$$

561. $$\int x^n(\sinh x)\, dx = x^n \cosh x - n \int x^{n-1}(\cosh x)\, dx$$

562. $$\int x(\cosh x)\, dx = x \sinh x - \cosh x$$

563. $$\int x^n(\cosh x)\, dx = x^n \sinh x - n \int x^{n-1}(\sinh x)\, dx$$

INTEGRALS (Continued)

564. $\int (\operatorname{sech} x)(\tanh x)\,dx = -\operatorname{sech} x$

565. $\int (\operatorname{csch} x)(\coth x)\,dx = -\operatorname{csch} x$

566. $\int (\sinh^2 x)\,dx = \frac{\sinh 2x}{4} - \frac{x}{2}$

567. $$\int (\sinh^m x)(\cosh^n x)\,dx = \begin{cases} \frac{1}{m+n}(\sinh^{m+1} x)(\cosh^{n-1} x) \\ \qquad + \frac{n-1}{m+n}\int (\sinh^m x)(\cosh^{n-2} x)\,dx \\ \qquad \text{or} \\ \frac{1}{m+n}\sinh^{m-1} x \cosh^{n+1} x \\ \quad - \frac{m-1}{m+n}\int (\sinh^{m-2} x)(\cosh^n x)\,dx, \qquad (m+n \neq 0) \end{cases}$$

568. $$\int \frac{dx}{(\sinh^m x)(\cosh^n x)} = \begin{cases} -\frac{1}{(m-1)(\sinh^{m-1} x)(\cosh^{n-1} x)} \\ \qquad - \frac{m+n-2}{m-1}\int \frac{dx}{(\sinh^{m-2} x)(\cosh^n x)}, \qquad (m \neq 1) \\ \text{or} \\ \frac{1}{(n-1)\sinh^{m-1} x \cosh^{n-1} x} \\ \qquad + \frac{m+n-2}{n-1}\int \frac{dx}{(\sinh^m x)(\cosh^{n-2} x)}, \qquad (n \neq 1) \end{cases}$$

569. $\int (\tanh^2 x)\,dx = x - \tanh x$

570. $\int (\tanh^n x)\,dx = -\frac{\tanh^{n-1} x}{n-1} + \int (\tanh^{n-2} x)\,dx, \qquad (n \neq 1)$

571. $\int (\operatorname{sech}^2 x)\,dx = \tanh x$

572. $\int (\cosh^2 x)\,dx = \frac{\sinh 2x}{4} + \frac{x}{2}$

573. $\int (\coth^2 x)\,dx = x - \coth x$

574. $\int (\coth^n x)\,dx = -\frac{\coth^{n-1} x}{n-1} + \int \coth^{n-2} x\,dx, \qquad (n \neq 1)$

INTEGRALS (Continued)

575. $\int (\operatorname{csch}^2 x)\,dx = -\operatorname{ctnh} x$

576. $\int (\sinh mx)(\sinh nx)\,dx = \frac{\sinh(m+n)x}{2(m+n)} - \frac{\sinh(m-n)x}{2(m-n)}, \qquad (m^2 \neq n^2)$

577. $\int (\cosh mx)(\cosh nx)\,dx = \frac{\sinh(m+n)x}{2(m+n)} + \frac{\sinh(m-n)x}{2(m-n)}, \qquad (m^2 \neq n^2)$

578. $\int (\sinh mx)(\cosh nx)\,dx = \frac{\cosh(m+n)x}{2(m+n)} + \frac{\cosh(m-n)x}{2(m-n)}, \qquad (m^2 \neq n^2)$

579. $\int \left(\sinh^{-1}\frac{x}{a}\right) dx = x\sinh^{-1}\frac{x}{a} - \sqrt{x^2+a^2}, \qquad (a > 0)$

580. $\int x\left(\sinh^{-1}\frac{x}{a}\right) dx = \left(\frac{x^2}{2} + \frac{a^2}{4}\right)\sinh^{-1}\frac{x}{a} - \frac{x}{4}\sqrt{x^2+a^2}, \qquad (a > 0)$

581. $\int x^n(\sinh^{-1} x)\,dx = \frac{x^{n+1}}{n+1}\sinh^{-1} x - \frac{1}{n+1}\int \frac{x^{n+1}}{(1+x^2)^{\frac{1}{2}}}\,dx, \qquad (n \neq -1)$

582. $\int \left(\cosh^{-1}\frac{x}{a}\right) dx = \begin{cases} x\cosh^{-1}\frac{x}{a} - \sqrt{x^2-a^2}, & \left(\cosh^{-1}\frac{x}{a} > 0\right) \\ \text{or} & \\ x\cosh^{-1}\frac{x}{a} + \sqrt{x^2-a^2}, & \left(\cosh^{-1}\frac{x}{a} < 0\right), \end{cases} \qquad (a > 0)$

583. $\int x\left(\cosh^{-1}\frac{x}{a}\right) dx = \frac{2x^2 - a^2}{4}\cosh^{-1}\frac{x}{a} - \frac{x}{4}(x^2-a^2)^{\frac{1}{2}}$

584. $\int x^n(\cosh^{-1} x)\,dx = \frac{x^{n+1}}{n+1}\cosh^{-1} x - \frac{1}{n+1}\int \frac{x^{n+1}}{(x^2-1)^{\frac{1}{2}}}\,dx, \qquad (n \neq -1)$

585. $\int \left(\tanh^{-1}\frac{x}{a}\right) dx = x\tanh^{-1}\frac{x}{a} + \frac{a}{2}\log(a^2 - x^2), \qquad \left(\left|\frac{x}{a}\right| < 1\right)$

586. $\int \left(\coth^{-1}\frac{x}{a}\right) dx = x\coth^{-1}\frac{x}{a} + \frac{a}{2}\log(x^2 - a^2), \qquad \left(\left|\frac{x}{a}\right| > 1\right)$

587. $\int x\left(\tanh^{-1}\frac{x}{a}\right) dx = \frac{x^2 - a^2}{2}\tanh^{-1}\frac{x}{a} + \frac{ax}{2}, \qquad \left(\left|\frac{x}{a}\right| < 1\right)$

588. $\int x^n\left(\tanh^{-1} x\right) dx = \frac{x^{n+1}}{n+1}\tanh^{-1} x - \frac{1}{n+1}\int \frac{x^{n+1}}{1-x^2}\,dx, \qquad (n \neq -1)$

589. $\int x\left(\coth^{-1}\frac{x}{a}\right) dx = \frac{x^2 - a^2}{2}\coth^{-1}\frac{x}{a} + \frac{ax}{2}, \qquad \left(\left|\frac{x}{a}\right| > 1\right)$

590. $\int x^n(\coth^{-1} x)\,dx = \frac{x^{n+1}}{n+1}\coth^{-1} x + \frac{1}{n+1}\int \frac{x^{n+1}}{x^2-1}\,dx, \qquad (n \neq -1)$

INTEGRALS (Continued)

591. $\int (\operatorname{sech}^{-1} x)\, dx = x \operatorname{sech}^{-1} x + \sin^{-1} x$

592. $\int x \operatorname{sech}^{-1} x\, dx = \frac{x^2}{2} \operatorname{sech}^{-1} x - \frac{1}{2}\sqrt{1 - x^2}$

593. $\int x^n \operatorname{sech}^{-1} x\, dx = \frac{x^{n+1}}{n+1} \operatorname{sech}^{-1} x + \frac{1}{n+1} \int \frac{x^n}{(1 - x^2)^{\frac{1}{2}}}\, dx, \qquad (n \neq -1)$

594. $\int \operatorname{csch}^{-1} x\, dx = x \operatorname{csch}^{-1} x + \frac{x}{|x|} \sinh^{-1} x$

595. $\int x \operatorname{csch}^{-1} x\, dx = \frac{x^2}{2} \operatorname{csch}^{-1} x + \frac{1}{2} \frac{x}{|x|}\sqrt{1 + x^2}$

596. $\int x^n \operatorname{csch}^{-1} x\, dx = \frac{x^{n+1}}{n+1} \operatorname{csch}^{-1} x + \frac{1}{n+1} \frac{x}{|x|} \int \frac{x^n}{(x^2 + 1)^{\frac{1}{2}}}\, dx, \qquad (n \neq -1)$

DEFINITE INTEGRALS

597. $\int_0^\infty x^{n-1} e^{-x}\, dx = \int_0^1 \left(\log \frac{1}{x}\right)^{n-1} dx = \frac{1}{n} \prod_{m=1}^{\infty} \frac{\left(1 + \frac{1}{m}\right)^n}{1 + \frac{n}{m}}$

$= \Gamma(n), n \neq 0, -1, -2, -3, \ldots$ (Gamma Function)

598. $\int_0^\infty t^n p^{-t}\, dt = \frac{n!}{(\log p)^{n+1}}, \qquad (n = 0, 1, 2, 3, \ldots \text{ and } p > 0)$

599. $\int_0^\infty t^{n-1} e^{-(a+1)t}\, dt = \frac{\Gamma(n)}{(a+1)^n}, \qquad (n > 0, a > -1)$

600. $\int_0^1 x^m \left(\log \frac{1}{x}\right)^n dx = \frac{\Gamma(n+1)}{(m+1)^{n+1}}, \qquad (m > -1, n > -1)$

601. $\Gamma(n)$ is finite if $n > 0$, $\Gamma(n + 1) = n\Gamma(n)$

602. $\Gamma(n) \cdot \Gamma(1 - n) = \frac{\pi}{\sin n\pi}$

603. $\Gamma(n) = (n - 1)!$ if $n =$ integer > 0

604. $\Gamma(\frac{1}{2}) = 2 \int_0^\infty e^{-t^2}\, dt = \sqrt{\pi} = 1.7724538509 \cdots = (-\frac{1}{2})!$

605. $\Gamma(n + \frac{1}{2}) = \frac{1 \cdot 3 \cdot 5 \ldots (2n - 1)}{2^n}\sqrt{\pi} \qquad n = 1, 2, 3, \ldots$

606. $\Gamma(-n + \frac{1}{2}) = \frac{(-1)^n 2^n \sqrt{\pi}}{1 \cdot 3 \cdot 5 \ldots (2n - 1)} \qquad n = 1, 2, 3, \ldots$

DEFINITE INTEGRALS (Continued)

607. $\int_0^1 x^{m-1}(1-x)^{n-1}\,dx = \int_0^\infty \frac{x^{m-1}}{(1+x)^{m+n}}\,dx = \frac{\Gamma(m)\Gamma(n)}{\Gamma(m+n)} = B(m,n)$

(Beta function)

608. $B(m,n) = B(n,m) = \frac{\Gamma(m)\Gamma(n)}{\Gamma(m+n)}$, where m and n are any positive real numbers.

609. $\int_a^b (x-a)^m(b-x)^n\,dx = (b-a)^{m+n+1}\frac{\Gamma(m+1)\cdot\Gamma(n+1)}{\Gamma(m+n+2)}$,

$(m > -1, n > -1, b > a)$

610. $\int_1^\infty \frac{dx}{x^m} = \frac{1}{m-1}, \qquad [m > 1]$

611. $\int_0^\infty \frac{dx}{(1+x)x^p} = \pi \csc p\pi, \qquad [p < 1]$

612. $\int_0^\infty \frac{dx}{(1-x)x^p} = -\pi \cot p\pi, \qquad [p < 1]$

613. $\int_0^\infty \frac{x^{p-1}\,dx}{1+x} = \frac{\pi}{\sin p\pi}$

$= B(p, 1-p) = \Gamma(p)\Gamma(1-p), \qquad [0 < p < 1]$

614. $\int_0^\infty \frac{x^{m-1}\,dx}{1+x^n} = \frac{\pi}{n \sin \frac{m\pi}{n}}, \qquad [0 < m < n]$

615. $\int_0^\infty \frac{x^a\,dx}{(m+x^b)^c} = \frac{m^{\frac{a+1-bc}{b}}}{b}\left[\frac{\Gamma\left(\frac{a+1}{b}\right)\Gamma\left(c-\frac{a+1}{b}\right)}{\Gamma(c)}\right]$

$\left(a > -1, b > 0, m > 0, c > \frac{a+1}{b}\right)$

616. $\int_0^\infty \frac{dx}{(1+x)\sqrt{x}} = \pi$

617. $\int_0^\infty \frac{a\,dx}{a^2+x^2} = \frac{\pi}{2}$, if $a > 0$; 0, if $a = 0$; $-\frac{\pi}{2}$, if $a < 0$

618. $\int_0^a (a^2-x^2)^{\frac{n}{2}}\,dx = \frac{1}{2}\int_{-a}^a (a^2-x^2)^{\frac{n}{2}}\,dx = \frac{1\cdot 3\cdot 5\ldots n}{2\cdot 4\cdot 6\ldots(n+1)}\cdot\frac{\pi}{2}\cdot a^{n+1}$ (n odd)

619. $\int_0^a x^m(a^2-x^2)^{\frac{n}{2}}\,dx = \begin{cases} \frac{1}{2}a^{m+n+1}B\left(\frac{m+1}{2}, \frac{n+2}{2}\right) \\ \text{or} \\ \frac{1}{2}a^{m+n+1}\frac{\Gamma\left(\frac{m+1}{2}\right)\Gamma\left(\frac{n+2}{2}\right)}{\Gamma\left(\frac{m+n+3}{2}\right)} \end{cases}$

DEFINITE INTEGRALS (Continued)

620. $$\int_0^{\pi/2} (\sin^n x)\,dx = \begin{cases} \displaystyle\int_0^{\pi/2} (\cos^n x)\,dx \\ \text{or} \\ \dfrac{1\cdot 3\cdot 5\cdot 7\ldots(n-1)}{2\cdot 4\cdot 6\cdot 8\ldots(n)}\dfrac{\pi}{2}, & (n \text{ an even integer, } n \neq 0) \\ \text{or} \\ \dfrac{2\cdot 4\cdot 6\cdot 8\ldots(n-1)}{1\cdot 3\cdot 5\cdot 7\ldots(n)}, & (n \text{ an odd integer, } n \neq 1) \\ \text{or} \\ \dfrac{\sqrt{\pi}}{2}\dfrac{\Gamma\left(\frac{n+1}{2}\right)}{\Gamma\left(\frac{n}{2}+1\right)}, & (n > -1) \end{cases}$$

621. $$\int_0^{\infty} \frac{\sin mx\,dx}{x} = \frac{\pi}{2}, \text{ if } m > 0;\ 0, \text{ if } m = 0;\ -\frac{\pi}{2}, \text{ if } m < 0$$

622. $$\int_0^{\infty} \frac{\cos x\,dx}{x} = \infty$$

623. $$\int_0^{\infty} \frac{\tan x\,dx}{x} = \frac{\pi}{2}$$

624. $$\int_0^{\pi} \sin ax \cdot \sin bx\,dx = \int_0^{\pi} \cos ax \cdot \cos bx\,dx = 0, \qquad (a \neq b;\ a, b \text{ integers})$$

625. $$\int_0^{\pi/a} [\sin(ax)][\cos(ax)]\,dx = \int_0^{\pi} [\sin(ax)][\cos(ax)]\,dx = 0$$

626. $$\int_0^{\pi} [\sin(ax)][\cos(bx)]\,dx = \frac{2a}{a^2 - b^2}, \text{ if } a - b \text{ is odd, or 0 if } a - b \text{ is even}$$

627. $$\int_0^{\infty} \frac{\sin x \cos mx\,dx}{x}$$
$$= 0, \text{ if } m < -1 \text{ or } m > 1;\ \frac{\pi}{4}, \text{ if } m = \pm 1;\ \frac{\pi}{2}, \text{ if } m^2 < 1$$

628. $$\int_0^{\infty} \frac{\sin ax \sin bx}{x^2}\,dx = \frac{\pi a}{2}, \qquad (a \leq b)$$

629. $$\int_0^{\pi} \sin^2 mx\,dx = \int_0^{\pi} \cos^2 mx\,dx = \frac{\pi}{2}$$

630. $$\int_0^{\infty} \frac{\sin^2(px)}{x^2}\,dx = \frac{\pi p}{2}$$

DEFINITE INTEGRALS (Continued)

631. $\int_0^\infty \frac{\sin x}{x^p}\,dx = \frac{\pi}{2\Gamma(p)\sin(p\pi/2)}, \qquad 0 < p < 1$

632. $\int_0^\infty \frac{\cos x}{x^p}\,dx = \frac{\pi}{2\Gamma(p)\cos(p\pi/2)}, \qquad 0 < p < 1$

633. $\int_0^\infty \frac{1 - \cos px}{x^2}\,dx = \frac{\pi p}{2}$

634. $\int_0^\infty \frac{\sin px \cos qx}{x}\,dx = \left\{0, \quad q > p > 0; \quad \frac{\pi}{2}, \quad p > q > 0; \quad \frac{\pi}{4}, \quad p = q > 0\right\}$

635. $\int_0^\infty \frac{\cos(mx)}{x^2 + a^2}\,dx = \frac{\pi}{2|a|} e^{-|ma|}$

636. $\int_0^\infty \cos(x^2)\,dx = \int_0^\infty \sin(x^2)\,dx = \frac{1}{2}\sqrt{\frac{\pi}{2}}$

637. $\int_0^\infty \sin ax^n\,dx = \frac{1}{na^{1/n}}\Gamma(1/n)\sin\frac{\pi}{2n}, \qquad n > 1$

638. $\int_0^\infty \cos ax^n\,dx = \frac{1}{na^{1/n}}\Gamma(1/n)\cos\frac{\pi}{2n}, \qquad n > 1$

639. $\int_0^\infty \frac{\sin x}{\sqrt{x}}\,dx = \int_0^\infty \frac{\cos x}{\sqrt{x}}\,dx = \sqrt{\frac{\pi}{2}}$

640. (a) $\int_0^\infty \frac{\sin^3 x}{x}\,dx = \frac{\pi}{4}$ (b) $\int_0^\infty \frac{\sin^3 x}{x^2}\,dx = \frac{3}{4}\log 3$

641. $\int_0^\infty \frac{\sin^3 x}{x^3}\,dx = \frac{3\pi}{8}$

642. $\int_0^\infty \frac{\sin^4 x}{x^4}\,dx = \frac{\pi}{3}$

643. $\int_0^{\pi/2} \frac{dx}{1 + a\cos x} = \frac{\cos^{-1} a}{\sqrt{1 - a^2}}, \qquad (a < 1)$

644. $\int_0^{\pi} \frac{dx}{a + b\cos x} = \frac{\pi}{\sqrt{a^2 - b^2}}, \qquad (a > b \geq 0)$

645. $\int_0^{2\pi} \frac{dx}{1 + a\cos x} = \frac{2\pi}{\sqrt{1 - a^2}}, \qquad (a^2 < 1)$

646. $\int_0^\infty \frac{\cos ax - \cos bx}{x}\,dx = \log\frac{b}{a}$

647. $\int_0^{\pi/2} \frac{dx}{a^2\sin^2 x + b^2\cos^2 x} = \frac{\pi}{2ab}$

DEFINITE INTEGRALS (Continued)

648. $\displaystyle\int_0^{\pi/2} \frac{dx}{(a^2 \sin^2 x + b^2 \cos^2 x)^2} = \frac{\pi(a^2 + b^2)}{4a^3b^3}, \qquad (a, b > 0)$

649. $\displaystyle\int_0^{\pi/2} \sin^{n-1} x \cos^{m-1} x \, dx = \frac{1}{2}\mathrm{B}\left(\frac{n}{2}, \frac{m}{2}\right),$ m and n positive integers

650. $\displaystyle\int_0^{\pi/2} (\sin^{2n+1} \theta) \, d\theta = \frac{2 \cdot 4 \cdot 6 \ldots (2n)}{1 \cdot 3 \cdot 5 \ldots (2n+1)}, \qquad (n = 1, 2, 3 \ldots)$

651. $\displaystyle\int_0^{\pi/2} (\sin^{2n} \theta) \, d\theta = \frac{1 \cdot 3 \cdot 5 \ldots (2n-1)}{2 \cdot 4 \ldots (2n)} \left(\frac{\pi}{2}\right), \qquad (n = 1, 2, 3 \ldots)$

652. $\displaystyle\int_0^{\pi/2} \frac{x}{\sin x} \, dx = 2\left\{\frac{1}{1^2} - \frac{1}{3^2} + \frac{1}{5^2} - \frac{1}{7^2} + \cdots\right\}$

653. $\displaystyle\int_0^{\pi/2} \frac{dx}{1 + \tan^m x} = \frac{\pi}{4}$

654. $\displaystyle\int_0^{\pi/2} \sqrt{\cos \theta} \, d\theta = \frac{(2\pi)^{\frac{3}{2}}}{[\Gamma(\frac{1}{4})]^2}$

655. $\displaystyle\int_0^{\pi/2} (\tan^h \theta) \, d\theta = \frac{\pi}{2 \cos\left(\frac{h\pi}{2}\right)}, \qquad (0 < h < 1)$

656. $\displaystyle\int_0^{\infty} \frac{\tan^{-1}(ax) - \tan^{-1}(bx)}{x} \, dx = \frac{\pi}{2} \log \frac{a}{b}, \qquad (a, b > 0)$

657. The area enclosed by a curve defined through the equation $x^{\frac{b}{c}} + y^{\frac{b}{c}} = a^{\frac{b}{c}}$ where $a > 0$, c a positive odd integer and b a positive even integer is given by

$$\frac{\left[\Gamma\left(\frac{c}{b}\right)\right]^2}{\Gamma\left(\frac{2c}{b}\right)} \left(\frac{2ca^2}{b}\right)$$

658. $I = \displaystyle\iiint_R x^{h-1} y^{m-1} z^{n-1} \, dv$, where R denotes the region of space bounded by the co-ordinate planes and that portion of the surface $\left(\frac{x}{a}\right)^p + \left(\frac{y}{b}\right)^q + \left(\frac{z}{c}\right)^k = 1$, which lies in the first octant and where $h, m, n, p, q, k, a, b, c$, denote positive real numbers is given by

$$\int_0^a x^{h-1} \, dx \int_0^{b\left[1 - \left(\frac{x}{a}\right)^p\right]^{\frac{1}{q}}} y^m \, dy \int_0^{c\left[1 - \left(\frac{x}{a}\right)^p - \left(\frac{y}{b}\right)^q\right]^{\frac{1}{k}}} z^{n-1} \, dz$$

$$= \frac{a^h b^m c^n}{pqk} \frac{\Gamma\left(\frac{h}{p}\right)\Gamma\left(\frac{m}{q}\right)\Gamma\left(\frac{n}{k}\right)}{\Gamma\left(\frac{h}{p} + \frac{m}{q} + \frac{n}{k} + 1\right)}$$

DEFINITE INTEGRALS (Continued)

659. $\int_0^\infty e^{-ax}\,dx = \frac{1}{a}, \qquad (a > 0)$

660. $\int_0^\infty \frac{e^{-ax} - e^{-bx}}{x}\,dx = \log\frac{b}{a}, \qquad (a, b > 0)$

661. $\int_0^\infty x^n e^{-ax}\,dx = \begin{cases} \frac{\Gamma(n+1)}{a^{n+1}}, & (n > -1, a > 0) \\ \text{or} & \\ \frac{n!}{a^{n+1}}, & (a > 0, n \text{ positive integer}) \end{cases}$

662. $\int_0^\infty x^n \exp(-ax^p)\,dx = \frac{\Gamma(k)}{pa^k}, \qquad \left(n > -1, p > 0, a > 0, k = \frac{n+1}{p}\right)$

663. $\int_0^\infty e^{-a^2x^2}\,dx = \frac{1}{2a}\sqrt{\pi} = \frac{1}{2a}\Gamma\left(\frac{1}{2}\right), \qquad (a > 0)$

663a. $\int_0^b e^{-ax^2}\,dx = \frac{1}{2}\sqrt{\frac{\pi}{a}}\ \mathrm{erf}\,(b\sqrt{a})$ Error Function (see page 419)

663b. $\int_b^\infty e^{-ax^2}\,dx = \frac{1}{2}\sqrt{\frac{\pi}{a}}\ \mathrm{erfc}\,(b\sqrt{a})$ Complimentary Error Function (see page 419)

664. $\int_0^\infty x e^{-x^2}\,dx = \frac{1}{2}$

665. $\int_0^\infty x^2 e^{-x^2}\,dx = \frac{\sqrt{\pi}}{4}$

666. $\int_0^\infty x^{2n} e^{-ax^2}\,dx = \frac{1 \cdot 3 \cdot 5 \ldots (2n-1)}{2^{n+1}a^n}\sqrt{\frac{\pi}{a}}$

667. $\int_0^\infty x^{2n+1} e^{-ax^2}\,dx = \frac{n!}{2a^{n+1}}, \qquad (a > 0)$

668. $\int_0^1 x^m e^{-ax}\,dx = \frac{m!}{a^{m+1}}\left[1 - e^{-a}\sum_{r=0}^{m}\frac{a^r}{r!}\right]$

669. $\int_0^\infty e^{\left(-x^2 - \frac{a^2}{x^2}\right)}\,dx = \frac{e^{-2a}\sqrt{\pi}}{2}, \qquad (a \geq 0)$

670. $\int_0^\infty e^{-nx}\sqrt{x}\,dx = \frac{1}{2n}\sqrt{\frac{\pi}{n}}$

DEFINITE INTEGRALS (Continued)

671. $\int_0^\infty \frac{e^{-nx}}{\sqrt{x}} dx = \sqrt{\frac{\pi}{n}}$

672. $\int_0^\infty e^{-ax}(\cos mx)\, dx = \frac{a}{a^2 + m^2}, \qquad (a > 0)$

673. $\int_0^\infty e^{-ax}(\sin mx)\, dx = \frac{m}{a^2 + m^2}, \qquad (a > 0)$

674. $\int_0^\infty x\, e^{-ax}[\sin (bx)]\, dx = \frac{2ab}{(a^2 + b^2)^2}, \qquad (a > 0)$

675. $\int_0^\infty x\, e^{-ax}[\cos (bx)]\, dx = \frac{a^2 - b^2}{(a^2 + b^2)^2}, \qquad (a > 0)$

676. $\int_0^\infty x^n e^{-ax}[\sin (bx)]\, dx = \frac{n![(a + ib)^{n+1} - (a - ib)^{n+1}]}{2i(a^2 + b^2)^{n+1}}, \qquad (i^2 = -1, a > 0)$

677. $\int_0^\infty x^n e^{-ax}[\cos (bx)]\, dx = \frac{n![(a - ib)^{n+1} + (a + ib)^{n+1}]}{2(a^2 + b^2)^{n+1}}, \qquad (i^2 = -1, a > 0)$

678. $\int_0^\infty \frac{e^{-ax} \sin x}{x} dx = \cot^{-1} a, \qquad (a > 0)$

679. $\int_0^\infty e^{-a^2x^2} \cos bx\, dx = \frac{\sqrt{\pi}}{2a} \exp\left(-\frac{b^2}{4a^2}\right), \qquad (ab \neq 0)$

680. $\int_0^\infty e^{-t\cos\phi}\, t^{b-1} \sin (t \sin \phi)\, dt = [\Gamma(b)] \sin (b\phi), \qquad \left(b > 0, -\frac{\pi}{2} < \phi < \frac{\pi}{2}\right)$

681. $\int_0^\infty e^{-t\cos\phi}\, t^{b-1}[\cos (t \sin \phi)]\, dt = [\Gamma(b)] \cos (b\phi), \qquad \left(b > 0, -\frac{\pi}{2} < \phi < \frac{\pi}{2}\right)$

682. $\int_0^\infty t^{b-1} \cos t\, dt = [\Gamma(b)] \cos \left(\frac{b\pi}{2}\right), \qquad (0 < b < 1)$

683. $\int_0^\infty t^{b-1} (\sin t)\, dt = [\Gamma(b)] \sin \left(\frac{b\pi}{2}\right), \qquad (0 < b < 1)$

684. $\int_0^1 (\log x)^n\, dx = (-1)^n \cdot n!$

685. $\int_0^1 \left(\log \frac{1}{x}\right)^{\frac{1}{2}} dx = \frac{\sqrt{\pi}}{2}$

686. $\int_0^1 \left(\log \frac{1}{x}\right)^{-\frac{1}{2}} dx = \sqrt{\pi}$

687. $\int_0^1 \left(\log \frac{1}{x}\right)^n dx = n!$

688. $\int_0^1 x \log (1 - x)\, dx = -\frac{3}{4}$

DEFINITE INTEGRALS (Continued)

689. $\int_0^1 x \log(1+x)\,dx = \frac{1}{4}$

690. $\int_0^1 x^m (\log x)^n\,dx = \frac{(-1)^n n!}{(m+1)^{n+1}}, \qquad m > -1, n = 0, 1, 2, \ldots$

If $n \neq 0, 1, 2, \ldots$ replace $n!$ by $\Gamma(n+1)$.

691. $\int_0^1 \frac{\log x}{1+x}\,dx = -\frac{\pi^2}{12}$

692. $\int_0^1 \frac{\log x}{1-x}\,dx = -\frac{\pi^2}{6}$

693. $\int_0^1 \frac{\log(1+x)}{x}\,dx = \frac{\pi^2}{12}$

694. $\int_0^1 \frac{\log(1-x)}{x}\,dx = -\frac{\pi^2}{6}$

695. $\int_0^1 (\log x)[\log(1+x)]\,dx = 2 - 2\log 2 - \frac{\pi^2}{12}$

696. $\int_0^1 (\log x)[\log(1-x)]\,dx = 2 - \frac{\pi^2}{6}$

697. $\int_0^1 \frac{\log x}{1-x^2}\,dx = -\frac{\pi^2}{8}$

698. $\int_0^1 \log\left(\frac{1+x}{1-x}\right)\frac{dx}{x} = \frac{\pi^2}{4}$

699. $\int_0^1 \frac{\log x\,dx}{\sqrt{1-x^2}} = -\frac{\pi}{2}\log 2$

700. $\int_0^1 x^m\left[\log\left(\frac{1}{x}\right)\right]^n dx = \frac{\Gamma(n+1)}{(m+1)^{n+1}}, \qquad \text{if } m+1>0, n+1>0$

701. $\int_0^1 \frac{(x^p - x^q)\,dx}{\log x} = \log\left(\frac{p+1}{q+1}\right), \qquad (p+1>0, q+1>0)$

702. $\int_0^1 \frac{dx}{\sqrt{\log\left(\frac{1}{x}\right)}} = \sqrt{\pi}$, (same as integral 686)

703. $\int_0^\infty \log\left(\frac{e^x+1}{e^x-1}\right)dx = \frac{\pi^2}{4}$

704. $\int_0^{\pi/2} (\log \sin x)\,dx = \int_0^{\pi/2} \log \cos x\,dx = -\frac{\pi}{2}\log 2$

705. $\int_0^{\pi/2} (\log \sec x)\,dx = \int_0^{\pi/2} \log \csc x\,dx = \frac{\pi}{2}\log 2$

DEFINITE INTEGRALS (Continued)

706. $\int_0^{\pi} x(\log \sin x)\,dx = -\frac{\pi^2}{2}\log 2$

707. $\int_0^{\pi/2} (\sin x)(\log \sin x)\,dx = \log 2 - 1$

708. $\int_0^{\pi/2} (\log \tan x)\,dx = 0$

709. $\int_0^{\pi} \log(a \pm b\cos x)\,dx = \pi \log\left(\frac{a + \sqrt{a^2 - b^2}}{2}\right), \qquad (a \geq b)$

710. $\int_0^{\pi} \log(a^2 - 2ab\cos x + b^2)\,dx = \begin{cases} 2\pi \log a, & a \geq b > 0 \\ 2\pi \log b, & b \geq a > 0 \end{cases}$

711. $\int_0^{\infty} \frac{\sin ax}{\sinh bx}\,dx = \frac{\pi}{2b}\tanh\frac{a\pi}{2b}$

712. $\int_0^{\infty} \frac{\cos ax}{\cosh bx}\,dx = \frac{\pi}{2b}\operatorname{sech}\frac{a\pi}{2b}$

713. $\int_0^{\infty} \frac{dx}{\cosh ax} = \frac{\pi}{2a}$

714. $\int_0^{\infty} \frac{x\,dx}{\sinh ax} = \frac{\pi^2}{4a^2}$

715. $\int_0^{\infty} e^{-ax}(\cosh bx)\,dx = \frac{a}{a^2 - b^2}, \qquad (0 \leq |b| < a)$

716. $\int_0^{\infty} e^{-ax}(\sinh bx)\,dx = \frac{b}{a^2 - b^2}, \qquad (0 \leq |b| < a)$

717. $\int_0^{\infty} \frac{\sinh ax}{e^{bx} + 1}\,dx = \frac{\pi}{2b}\csc\frac{a\pi}{b} - \frac{1}{2a}$

718. $\int_0^{\infty} \frac{\sinh ax}{e^{bx} - 1}\,dx = \frac{1}{2a} - \frac{\pi}{2b}\cot\frac{a\pi}{b}$

719. $\int_0^{\pi/2} \frac{dx}{\sqrt{1 - k^2\sin^2 x}} = \frac{\pi}{2}\left[1 + \left(\frac{1}{2}\right)^2 k^2 + \left(\frac{1\cdot 3}{2\cdot 4}\right)^2 k^4 + \left(\frac{1\cdot 3\cdot 5}{2\cdot 4\cdot 6}\right)^2 k^6 + \cdots\right], \text{ if } k^2 < 1$

719*a*. $\int_0^{\frac{\pi}{2}} \frac{dx}{(1 - k^2 Sin^2 x)^{3/2}} = \frac{\pi}{2}\left[1 + \left(\frac{1}{2}\right)^2 \cdot 3k^2 + \left(\frac{1\cdot 3}{2\cdot 4}\right)^2 \cdot 5k^4 + \left(\frac{1\cdot 3\cdot 5}{2\cdot 4\cdot 6}\right)^2 \cdot 7k^6 + \ldots\right], \text{ if } k^2 < 1$

DEFINITE INTEGRALS (Continued)

720. $\int_0^{\pi/2} \sqrt{1 - k^2 \sin^2 x}\, dx = \frac{\pi}{2}\left[1 - \left(\frac{1}{2}\right)^2 k^2 - \left(\frac{1 \cdot 3}{2 \cdot 4}\right)^2 \frac{k^4}{3} - \left(\frac{1 \cdot 3 \cdot 5}{2 \cdot 4 \cdot 6}\right)^2 \frac{k^6}{5} - \cdots\right]$, if $k^2 < 1$

721. $\int_0^{\infty} e^{-x} \log x\, dx = -\gamma = -0.5772157\ldots$

722. $\int_0^{\infty} e^{-x^2} \log x\, dx = -\frac{\sqrt{\pi}}{4}(\gamma + 2 \log 2)$

723. $\int_0^{\infty} \left(\frac{1}{1 - e^{-x}} - \frac{1}{x}\right) e^{-x}\, dx = \gamma = 0.5772157\ldots$ [Euler's Constant]

724. $\int_0^{\infty} \frac{1}{x}\left(\frac{1}{1 + x} - e^{-x}\right) dx = \gamma = 0.5772157\ldots$

For n even:

725. $\int \cos^n x\, dx = \frac{1}{2^{n-1}} \sum_{k=0}^{\frac{n}{2}-1} \binom{n}{k} \frac{\sin (n - 2k) x}{(n - 2k)} + \frac{1}{2^n}\binom{n}{\frac{n}{2}} x$

726. $\int \sin^n x\, dx = \frac{1}{2^{n-1}} \sum_{k=0}^{\frac{n}{2}-1} \binom{n}{k} \frac{\sin [(n - 2k)(\frac{\pi}{2} - x)]}{2k - n} + \frac{1}{2^n}\binom{n}{\frac{n}{2}} x$

For n odd:

727. $\int \cos^n x\, dx = \frac{1}{2^{n-1}} \sum_{k=0}^{\frac{n-1}{2}} \binom{n}{k} \frac{\sin (n - 2k) x}{(n - 2k)}$

728. $\int \sin^n x\, dx = \frac{1}{2^{n-1}} \sum_{k=0}^{\frac{n-1}{2}} \binom{n}{k} \frac{\sin [n - 2k)(\frac{\pi}{2} - x)]}{2k - n}$

APPENDIX
GLOSSARY OF SYMBOLS AND TERMS

A (mxn)	Matrix with m rows and n columns
α (alpha)	Probability of a Type I error
α_3	Coefficient of skewness
α_4	Coefficient of kurtosis
β (beta)	Probability of a Type II error
1-β	Power of a statistical test
β_o, α	y-intercept in regression model
β_1, β	Slope of linear regression model
β_i	Coeffieient of independent variable x_i in mulitple regression model
β_j	Block effects
b_i, $\hat{\beta}_i$	Least squares estimator of β_i
B (a,b)	Beta function
C_2	Class or interval width; number of defects
χ^2 (chi)	Chi-square distribution statistic
χ_α	Critical value of chi-square distribution
CSCC	Cumulative sum control chart
d_i	Differences for each of n pairs
D_j	j^{th} decile
df	Degrees of freedom
$e = y - \hat{y}$	Error (observed)
E ( )	Expected value
ϵ (epsilon), e_{ij}	Experimental error
f_i	Frequency
F	F-distribution statistic
F′	Substitute F-ratio
F_α	Critical value for F-distribution
f ( )	Probability density function
F ( )	Cumulative distribution function
E, F	Events
E′	Complement of event E
E∪F	Union of events E and F
E∩F	Intersection of events E and F
Γ ( )	Gamma function
G.M.	Geometric mean
H	Test statistic for Kruskal-Wallis nonparametric ANOVA
H_o	Null hypothesis
H_a, H_1	Alternate (or research) hypothesis
H.M.	Harmonic mean
i, j, k	Position number for a particular data point

APPENDIX (continued)
GLOSSARY OF SYMBOLS AND TERMS

I	Identity matrix
$I_x(a,b)$	Incomplete beta function
LCL	Lower control limit (quality control)
M.D.	Mean deviation
MS ( )	Mean square
MSE	Mean square error
M_d	Population median
M_o	Population mode
m'_r	r^{th} sample moment about the origin
m_r	r^{th} sample moment about the mean
$m_x(t)$	Moment generating function (about origin)
$M_x(t)$	Moment generating function (about mean)
μ (mu)	Population mean
μ_d	Mean of differences of *n* pairs
μ'_r	r^{th} population moment about the origin
μ_r	r^{th} population moment about the mean
$\mu'_{(r)}$	r^{th} factorial moment
$\mu_{\bar{x}}$	Mean of the distribution of all possible $\bar{x}$'s
$\mu_{y/x}$	Mean of all y-values at the fixed value of x
n	Sample size (total number of observations in one sample)
N	Population size
$\binom{n}{r}$	Binomial coefficient; number of combinations
p	Probability of an event
P (E/F)	Conditional probability of E given F
P (n,m)	Number of permutations
$P(a<x<b)$	Probability that x has a value between a and b
P_j	j^{th} percentile
q	standardized range
$q = 1 - p$	Probability that an event does not occur
Q_j	j^{th} quartile
r	Linear correlation coefficient for sample data
ρ (rho)	Population correlation coefficient
r_s, ρ_s	Spearman rank correlation coefficient
R	Range of the data
$\bar{R}$	Mean of sample ranges
RMS	Root mean square
s	Sample standard deviation
s^2	Sample variance
σ (lower case sigma)	Population standard deviation

APPENDIX (continued)
GLOSSARY OF SYMBOLS AND TERMS

σ^2	Population variance
$\sigma_{\bar{x}}$	Standard error of the mean (standard deviation of sampling distribution of $\bar{x}$)
SS ( )	Sum of squares
Σ (capital sigma)	Summation notation symbol
t	Student's t-distribution statistic
t_α	Critical value for student's *t*-distribution
τ (tau)	Kendall's rank correlation coefficient
τ_i	Substitute t-ratio; treatment effects
τ_j	Treatment effects
θ	Population proportion; probability of success
$1-\theta$	Probability of failure
u	Number of runs
U	Mann-Whitney U-statistic
UCL	Upper control limit (quality control)
V	Coefficient of variation
w	Sample range
w_i	Weighting factor
W	Standardized sample range
x	Sample measurement
$\bar{x}$	Sample mean
$\tilde{x}$	Sample median
X	Random variable
z	Standard score (z-score)
z_α	Critical value for standard normal distribution statistic
$\lvert\ \rvert$	Absolute value of a number
$=$	Equal to
$\neq$	Not equal to
$<$	Less than
$\leq$	Less than or equal to
$>$	Greater than
$\geq$	Greater than or equal to
$\approx$	Approximately equal to
$\sqrt{}$	Square root symbol

INDEX

(Numbers in parenthesis refer to table numbers)

A

B

C

D

E

F

G

H

I

O

P

Q

R

S

T

U

V

W

Y